Molecular Basis of Pancreas Development and Function

ENDOCRINE UPDATES

Shlomo Melmed, M.D., Series Editor

---

1. E.R. Levin and J.L. Nadler (eds.): Endocrinology of Cardiovascular Function. 1998. ISBN: 0-7923-8217-X
2. J.A. Fagin (ed.): Thyroid Cancer. 1998. ISBN: 0-7923-8326-5
3. J.S. Adams and B.P. Lukert (eds.): Osteoporosis: Genetics, Prevention and Treatment. 1998. ISBN: 0-7923-8366-4.
4. B.-Å. Bengtsson (ed.): Growth Hormone. 1999. ISBN: 0-7923-8478-4
5. C. Wang (ed.): Male Reproductive Function. 1999. ISBN 0-7923-8520-9
6. B. Rapoport and S.M. McLachlan (eds.): Graves' Disease: Pathogenesis and Treatment. 2000. ISBN: 0-7923-7790-7.
7. W. W. de Herder (ed.): Functional and Morphological Imaging of the Endocrine System. 2000. ISBN 0-7923-7923-9
8. H.G. Burger (ed.): Sex Hormone Replacement Therapy. 2001. ISBN 0-7923-7965-9
9. A. Giustina (ed.): Growth Hormone and the Heart. 2001. ISBN 0-7923-7212-3
10. W.L. Lowe, Jr. (ed.): Genetics of Diabetes Mellitus. 2001. ISBN 0-7923-7252-2
11. J.F. Habener and M.A. Hussain (eds.): Molecular Basis of Pancreas Development and Function. 2001. ISBN 0-7923-7271-9

Molecular Basis of Pancreas Development and Function

Editors

Joel F. Habener, M.D.
Laboratory of Molecular Endocrinology
Howard Hughes Medical Institute
Massachusetts General Hospital
Boston, MA

Mehboob A. Hussain, M.D.
Department of Medicine
Clinical and Molecular Endocrinology
New York University Medical Center
New York, NY

Distributors for North, Central and South America:
Kluwer Academic Publishers
101 Philip Drive
Assinippi Park
Norwell, Massachusetts 02061 USA
Telephone (781) 871-6600
Fax (781) 681-9045
E-Mail <kluwer@wkap.com>

Distributors for all other countries:
Kluwer Academic Publishers Group
Distribution Centre
Post Office Box 322
3300 AH Dordrecht, THE NETHERLANDS
Telephone 31 78 6392 392
Fax 31 78 6392 254
E-Mail <services@wkap.nl>

Electronic Services <http://www.wkap.nl>

Library of Congress Cataloging-in-Publication Data

Molecular basis of pancreas development and function / editors, Joel F. Habener, Mehboob A. Hussain.
p. ; cm. -- (Endocrine updates ; 11)
Includes bibliographical references and index.
ISBN 0-7923-7271-9 (hardback : alk. paper)
1. Diabetes--Molecular aspects. 2. Pancreas--Molecular aspects. I. Habener, Joel F. II. Hussain, Mehboob A. III. Series.
[DNLM: 1. Islets of Langerhans--physiology. 2. Endocrine Diseases--physiopathology. WK 800 M718 2001]
RC660 .M5613 2001
616.4'07--dc21

00-051987

Printed on acid-free paper.

Printed in the United States of America

Table of Contents

List of Contributors

Ulf Ahlgren, Ph.D.
University of Umeå, S-90187 Umeå, Sweden
Homeodomain proteins in pancreas development

Gillian M. Beattie, Ph.D.
University of California at San Diego School of Medicine, La Jolla, CA 92037 USA
Gene therapeutic approaches for β-cell replacement

Susan Bonner-Weir, Ph.D.
Joslin Diabetes Center, Boston, MA 02215, USA
Mechanisms of postnatal β-cell mass regulation

Christophe Bonny, Ph.D.
Department of Internal Medicine, CHUV, 1011 Lausanne, Switzerland
Identification, biological functions, and contribution to human diabetes of islet-brain 1

Domenico Bosco, Ph.D.
University of Geneva Medical School, CH-1211 Geneva 4, Switzerland
Communication of islet cells: molecules and functions

Michelle A. Cissell, Ph.D.
Vanderbilt University Medical Center, Nashville, TN 37232, USA
Regulation of pdx-1 gene expression

Christopher A. Crisera, M.D.
New York University Medical Center, New York, N.Y., 10016, USA
Role of mesenchymal-epithelial interactions in pancreas development

Paul Czernichow, M.D.
INSERM U457, Hospital R. Debré, 48 Bd Sérurier, 75019 Paris, France
Soluble factors important for pancreas development

Helena Edlund, Ph.D.
University of Umeå, S-90187 Umeå, Sweden
Homeodomain proteins in pancreas development

Shimon Efrat, Ph.D.
Department of Human Genetics and Molecular Medicine
Sackler School of Medicine, Tel Aviv University,
Ramat Aviv, Tel Aviv 69978, Israel
Development of β-cell lines for transplantation in type 1 diabetes mellitus

Julie C. Evans, B.Sc.
Department of Vascular Medicine and Diabetes Research, School of Postgraduate Medicine and Health Sciences, Barrack Road, Exeter, Devon, UK EX2 5AX
Clinical consequences of genetic defects in β-cell genes

Luis Emilio Flores, Ph.D.
Hagedorn Research Institute, Niels Steensensvej 6, 2820 Gentofte. Denmark
bHLH factors and notch in pancreatic development

Tim M. Frayling, B.Sc., Ph.D.
Department of Vascular Medicine and Diabetes Research, School of Postgraduate Medicine and Health Sciences, Barrack Road, Exeter, Devon, UK EX2 5AX
Clinical consequences of genetic defects in β-cell genes

Kevin Gerrish, M.S.
Vanderbilt University Medical Center, Nashville, TN 37232, USA
Regulation of pdx-1 gene expression

George K. Gittes, M.D.
New York University Medical Center, New York, N.Y., 10016, USA
Role of mesenchymal-epithelial interactions in pancreas development

Catherine Gleason
Pacific Northwest Research Institute and University of Washington,
Seattle, WA 98122 USA
Glucose toxicity of the pancreatic β-cell

Peter Gruss, Ph.D.
Max-Planck Institute of Molecular Biology, 37077 Göttingen, Germany
Pax4 and Pax6 in islet differentiation

Jamie Harmon, Ph.D.
Pacific Northwest Research Institute and University of Washington,
Seattle, WA 98122 USA
Glucose toxicity of the pancreatic β-cell

Andrew T. Hattersley, D.M., F.R.C.P.
Department of Vascular Medicine and Diabetes Research, School of Postgraduate Medicine and Health Sciences, Barrack Road, Exeter, Devon, UK EX2 5AX
Clinical consequences of genetic defects in β-cell genes

Alberto Hayek, M.D.
University of California at San Diego School of Medicine, La Jolla, CA 92037 USA
Gene therapeutic approaches for β-cell replacement

R. Scott Heller, Ph.D.
Hagedorn Research Institute, DK-2820 Gentofte, Denmark
An historical and phylogenetic perspective of islet-cell development
bHLH factors and notch in pancreatic development

George G. Holz, Ph.D.
New York University School of Medicine, New York, NY, USA
Harvard Medical School, Boston, MA, USA
Glucagon-like peptide-1: An insulinotropic hormone with potent growth factor actions at the pancreatic islets of Langerhans

Jan Jensen, Ph.D.,
Hagedorn Research Institute, DK-2820 Gentofte, Denmark
An historical and phylogenetic perspective of islet-cell development
bHLH factors and notch in pancreatic development

Alan S. Kadison, M.D.
New York University Medical Center, New York, N.Y., 10016, USA
Role of mesenchymal-epithelial interactions in pancreas development

C. Ronald Kahn M.D.
Joslin Diabetes Center and Department of Medicine, Harvard Medical School, One Joslin Place, Boston, MA 02215 USA
Genetic models of insulin resistance: alterations in β-cell biology

Willhart Knepel, Ph.D.
University of Göttingen, 37075 Göttingen, Germany
The α-cell and regulation of glucagon gene transcription

Rohit N. Kulkarni M.D. Ph.D.
Joslin Diabetes Center and Department of Medicine, Harvard Medical School, One Joslin Place, Boston, MA 02215 USA
Genetic models of insulin resistance: alterations in β-cell bology

Jack L. Leahy, M.D.
University Of Vermont, Burlington, VT 05405 USA
β-Cell dysfunction and chronic hyperglycaemia

Colin A. Leech, Ph.D.
Howard Hughes Medical Institute, Massachusetts General Hospital
Harvard Medical School, Boston, MA, USA
Glucagon-like peptide-1: An insulinotropic hormone with potent growth factor actions at the pancreatic islets of Langerhans

Fred Levine, M.D.
University of California at San Diego School of Medicine, La Jolla, CA 92037 USA
Gene therapeutic approaches for β-cell replacement

Michael T. Longaker, M.D.
New York University Medical Center, New York, N.Y., 10016, USA
Role of mesenchymal-epithelial interactions in pancreas development

Ole D. Madsen, Ph.D.,
Hagedorn Research Institute, DK-2820 Gentofte, Denmark
An historical and phylogenetic perspective of islet-cell development
bHLH factors and notch in pancreatic development

Mark A. Magnuson, M.D.
Vanderbilt University, Nashville, TN 37232, USA
Use of a cre/loxp strategy in mice to determine the cell-specific roles of glucokinase in mody-2

Thomas S. Maldonado, M.D.
New York University Medical Center, New York, N.Y., 10016, USA
Role of mesenchymal-epithelial interactions in pancreas development

Paolo Meda, M.D.
University of Geneva Medical School, CH-1211 Geneva 4, Switzerland
Communication of islet cells: molecules and functions

Danielle Melloul, Ph. D.
Hadassah University Hospital, Jerusalem, 91120 Israel
Glucose signalling to transcription factors of the insulin gene

Takashi Miki, M.D., Ph.D.
Chiba University, Chiba 260-8670, Japan
The K_{ATP} channel and the sulfonylurea receptor

Helle V. Petersen, Ph.D.
Hagedorn Research Institute, DK-2820 Gentofte, Denmark
An historical and phylogenetic perspective of islet-cell development

Vincent Poitout, D.V.M., Ph.D.
Pacific Northwest Research Institute and University of Washington,
Seattle, WA 98122 USA
Glucose toxicity of the pancreatic β-cell

Catherine Postic, Ph.D.
Vanderbilt University, Nashville, TN 37232, USA
Use of a cre/loxp strategy in mice to determine the cell-specific roles of glucokinase in MODY-2

R. Paul Robertson, M.D.
Pacific Northwest Research Institute and University of Washington,
Seattle, WA 98122 USA
Glucose toxicity of the pancreatic β-cell

Giovanni Sacchi, M.D.
Pacific Northwest Research Institute and University of Washington,
Seattle, WA 98122 USA
Glucose toxicity of the pancreatic β-cell

Susan Samaras, Ph.D.
Vanderbilt University Medical Center, Nashville, TN 37232, USA
Regulation of pdx-1 gene expression

Raphael Scharfmann, Ph.D.
INSERM U457, Hospital R. Debré, 48 Bd Sérurier, 75019 Paris, France
Soluble factors important for pancreas development

Susumu Seino, M.D., D.M.Sci.
Chiba University, Chiba 260-8670, Japan
The K_{ATP} channel and the sulfonylurea receptor

Palle Serup, Ph.D.,
Hagedorn Research Institute, DK-2820 Gentofte, Denmark
An historical and phylogenetic perspective of islet-cell development
bHLH factors and notch in pancreatic development

Roland Stein, Ph.D.
Vanderbilt University Medical Center, Nashville, TN 37232, USA
Regulation of pdx-1 gene expression

Markus Stoffel, M.D., Ph.D.
The Rockefeller University, New York, NY 10021 USA
The role of the hepatocyte nuclear factor network in glucose homeostasis

Yoshito Tananka, M.D.
Pacific Northwest Research Institute and University of Washington, Seattle, WA 98122 USA
Glucose toxicity of the pancreatic β-cell

Bernard Thorens, Ph.D.
University of Lausanne, 1005, Lausanne, Switzerland
Pathophysiology of glut2 in diabetes mellitus

Phuong Oanh T. Tran, Ph.D.
Pacific Northwest Research Institute and University of Washington, Seattle, WA 98122 USA
Glucose toxicity of the pancreatic β-cell

Gérard Waeber, M.D.
Department of Internal Medicine, CHUV, 1011 Lausanne, Switzerland
Identification, biological functions, and contribution to human diabetes of islet-brain 1

Gordon C. Weir, M.D.
Joslin Diabetes Center, Boston, MA 02215, USA
Mechanisms of postnatal β-cell mass regulation

Christopher V.E. Wright, D. Phil.
Vanderbilt University Medical Center, Nashville, TN 37232, USA
Regulation of pdx-1 gene expression

Hideki Yano, M.D., D.M.Sci.
Chiba University, Chiba 260-8670, Japan
The K_{ATP} channel and the sulfonylurea receptor

Xunlei Zhou, Ph.D.
Max-Planck Institute of Molecular Biology, 37077 Göttingen, Germany
Pax4 and Pax6 in islet differentiation

Preface

Diabetes mellitus is rapidly increasing in prevalence throughout both developed and developing countries. The social and economic burden of this disease is estimated to cost 14 billion dollars worldwide. In the USA alone, 15 million individuals are diabetic, nearly half of them unaware of their condition. Complications of diabetes mellitus are the leading causes for blindness, limb amputation and chronic renal failure and kidney transplantation in industrialized countries. Further, diabetes mellitus *per se* and the metabolic derangement associated with diabetes are important risk factors for cardiovascular disease.

Diabetes, as defined by an elevated fasting blood glucose level is presently subdivided in etiologically distinct groups. The most prevalent being type 2 (adult onset) diabetes characterized by insulin resistance and failure of the β-cell to supply insulin in amounts sufficient to meet the body's needs. Type 1 (juvenile) diabetes, most commonly with an onset during childhood and adolescence, is caused by an auto-immune destruction of the pancreatic β-cells. The causations of both type 1 and type 2 diabetes involve a combination of complex genetic traits and environmental influences. A third category are the mature onset diabetes of the young (MODY). This comparatively small group of patients (~10% of diabetes) presents relative early in life (<30 years of age) compared to the more common late onset type 2 diabetes. Because of the clear monogenic inheritance patterns within MODY pedigress, it has been possible to identify distinct genetic loci responsible for islet cell dysfunction and diabetes, mutations in the glucokinase gene and mutations in the transcription factor genes IPF-1, HNF-1α, HNF-1β, HNF-4α, and Beta2/NeuroD.

Concomitant with the identification of genes responsible for diabetes, research on the transcriptional regulation of pancreatic islet genes led to the identification of several transcription factors, which are important not only for the maintenance of the pancreatic β-cell phenotype, but also for development of the pancreas and its endocrine compartment, the islets of Langerhans. Further, the actions of these transcription factors in the islets are altered as a consequence of metabolic derangement that accompanies diabetes (i.e. lipotoxicity, glucotoxicity).

In addition to these advances in understanding the genetic and metabolic causes of islet dysfunctions, the generation of genetic models for the study of insulin resistance (as seen in type 2 diabetes) by ablation of the insulin receptor and downstream signalling molecules have given further insight in the adaptation of pancreatic islet-cell mass in the face of impaired insulin action. This adaptation of islet cell mass involves changes in regeneration and apoptosis of pancreatic endocrine cells. These processes are also accompanied by changes in the transcription factors that are involved in pancreas development and the maintenance of the pancreatic endocrine phenotype.

The purpose of this book is to bring together the many different aspects and the recent discoveries in the understanding of pancreatic endocrine development and its close links to endocrine cell physiology and dysfunction in diabetes. The intention is to combine the knowledge from clinical observations in certain diabetic syndromes with the rapidly growing insights derived from basic molecular biological investigation. At the end of this book, an outlook is provided into a possible future in which the knowledge that is gained from basic studies can be translated into new forms of treatment for diabetes. We hope that this book will serve established investigators, newcomers to the diabetes research community, and clinicians interested in the molecular basis of the syndromes that they encounter.

We gratefully acknowledge the support of this book by Dr. Ralph Stephenson of Pfizer and Drs. Michael Jirousek and Terry Opgenorth of Abbot. We thank Barbara Murphy and Susan Earle of Kluwer Academic Publishers for their help. We thank Richard A.A. Larraga without whose effort this book may never have taken shape, for his heroic, efficient, and indispensable editorial work.

The editors,

Mehboob A. Hussain, M.D.
Department of Medicine
Clinical and Molecular Endocrinology
New York University Medical Center
New York, NY

Joel F. Habener, M.D.
Laboratory of Molecular Endocrinology
Howard Hughes Medical Institute
Massachusetts General Hospital
Boston, MA

June, 2000

1
AN HISTORICAL AND PHYLOGENETIC PERSPECTIVE OF ISLET-CELL DEVELOPMENT

Ole D. Madsen, Ph.D., Palle Serup, Ph.D., Jan Jensen, Ph.D., Helle V. Petersen, Ph.D., and R. Scott Heller, Ph.D.
Hagedorn Research Institute, DK-2820 Gentofte, Denmark

INTRODUCTION

The Discovery of Insulin - a Miraculous Life Saver - only Tamed Diabetes

Before the discovery of insulin the diagnosis of diabetes mellitus was equivalent to being sentenced to death. It was thus a miracle that insulin treatment would rescue the lives of diabetics, and Banting and MacLeod were awarded the Nobel Prize in 1923 for their pioneering work in Toronto (1). As time went by, it became apparent that diabetic patients suffer from late complications such as neuropathy, retinopathy, vascular diseases and kidney failure. Such complications are now ascribed to inappropriate fluctuations in blood glucose levels as revealed in recent clinical trials (DCCT &UKPDS) (2-4). Insulin thus provides a treatment of diabetes - not a cure.

The Danger of Excess Insulin

Insulin controls blood glucose and function through interaction with its receptor to signal glucose uptake in peripheral tissues. Glucose uptake in the brain is independent from insulin. Glucose is also the main energy source for the brain. Insulin is secreted from the pancreatic β-cell (*infra*), but only in response to elevated glucose. Thus, lack of insulin (diabetes) does not immediately affect brain function but the peripheral tissue will 'starve in the sea of plenty' as the increasing blood glucose cannot be utilized. Conversely, excessively high levels of circulating insulin are life-threatening as the periphery will deplete blood glucose levels eventually causing brain failure, coma, and death. Tumours of the pancreatic β-cell (insulinoma) are usually benign but require surgery as they secrete insulin in a glucose-independent way - eventually causing lethal hypoglycaemia. To summarize, only the normal β-cell has a sufficiently proven record of 'knowing' how to release insulin to the circulation to maintain euglycaemia.

The β-Cell and Diabetes

The insulin gene is predominantly active in the pancreatic β-cell of the adult animal. Thus, a unique feature of this cell type is its ability to efficiently transcribe the insulin gene, to mass-produce, to store, and to release insulin appropriately in a glucose-dependent fashion. In type 1 or insulin dependent diabetes (IDDM) a highly selective destruction of the β-cells appears to be the result of an ongoing autoimmune attack (5). The body's only source of insulin becomes depleted as no apparent regeneration seems to occur. In contrast, an immunological memory operates during the lifetime of a type 1 diabetic patient as demonstrated by 'autologous' transplantation of pancreatic tissue between discordant identical twins where the diabetic recipient will accept the pancreas but selectively destroy the β-cells of the fully histocompatible twin (6).

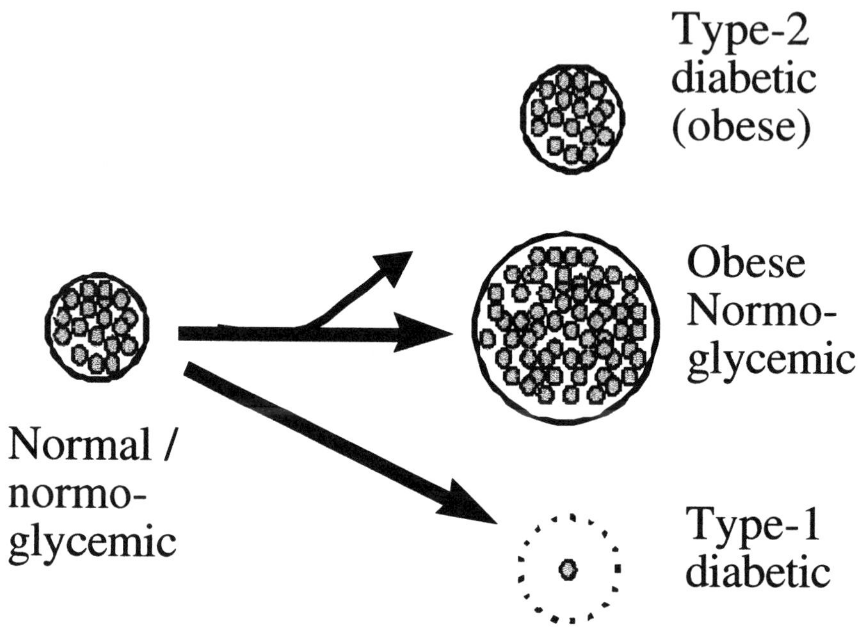

Figure 1. *The β-cell mass adjusts according to needs. β-cell mass increases in obesity. Failure to compensate for increased needs results in Type-2 diabetes. Type-1 diabetes is characterized by a selective and quantitative destruction of β-cells.*

Type 2 or non-insulin dependent diabetes (NIDDM) is characterized by insulin resistance of the periphery. Recently, it has become clearer that the β-cell mass may have a considerable capacity to expand. Obesity and beginning insulin resistance can be counteracted by increasing β-cell mass appropriately to meet the increasing needs for insulin to maintain normoglycaemia (7). The failure of the β-cell mass to compensate for increased needs for insulin may be the hallmark of type 2 diabetes. Thus, a common denominator in the two different types of diabetes is lack of sufficient β-cell mass (Figure 1). Type 2 diabetic patients may become insulin dependent, and such patients may have islet autoimmunity and thus represent a combination of the two types of diabetes (8,9). The dynamics of β-cell mass is discussed *infra*.

The Prospects for Diabetes Treatment

Diabetes (type 2) spreads with an epidemic pace, especially in 3rd world countries, as the western life style becomes adopted (10). It is clear from recent clinical trials that intensive therapy and improved glucose control will reduce, but not eliminate, the risk of diabetes late complications. The negative side of intensified therapy is the concomitant increase in hypoglycaemic episodes. Thus, no current replacement therapy can match the examples of successful whole pancreas or islet transplantation with respect to fully normalizing daily glucose control in diabetic patients (11,12). Such patients are essentially cured of their diabetes but will need continuous immuno-suppression. Only perfect normalization of glucose control can be expected to fully prevent diabetic late complications, and if this is not achieved in future diabetes therapy, the pace by which the costs will increase for the treatment of diabetic late complications may result in a global socio-economic disaster.

On the other hand, there will never be enough human donor pancreata for transplantation, and xenotransplantation of isolated islet material, in addition to requiring great improvements in immuno-suppression, carries an inherent risk of transferring animal viral diseases to humans. Ideally, a strategy based on the possibility to expand human β-cell material retaining fully normal function would be desirable.

Such thoughts have become more realistic as a consequence of great progress in the understanding of how the β-cells form during foetal pancreas development. This aspect will be reviewed in the context of the historical discovery of insulin that is directly linked to the recent breakthroughs in the understanding of pancreas ontogeny. The β-cell will be in focus as revealed by its central position in pancreas phylogeny.

FROM THE DISCOVERY OF INSULIN TO DEVELOPMENTAL BIOLOGY OF THE PANCREAS

From Insulin to the Insulin Gene

After its discovery, insulin attracted much scientific interest and insulin related research became a dominant player in several evolving disciplines of modern natural science (Figure 2). Insulin was soon localized to the islets of Langerhans (13) and was the first protein to be crystallized (14). This was not only a great step forward in the purification of insulin but also a corner stone in the subsequent development of x-ray crystallography to reveal 3-dimensional protein structures. The Nobel Prize was awarded to F. Sanger in 1958 for elucidating the primary structure of insulin (15,16) - and demonstrated for the first time, that a protein has a defined primary structure. The group of the Nobel Laureate X-ray crystallographer, D. Hodgkin with Dr. Blundell and co-workers, elucidated the 3-D structure of insulin (17). R. Yalow received the Nobel Prize in 1977 for establishment of the first radio-immunoassay - and again insulin was the molecule of choice and now accurate measurements of circulating levels of the hormone became possible (see reference (18) for review). Pioneering work of D.F. Steiner on the discovery of proinsulin (19) proved to reveal that polypeptide hormones are commonly produced as larger precursors and are subsequently processed by unique proteases to yield the mature bio-active hormones (see reference (20) for review). Prohormone specific proinsulin antibodies (21) allowed the exact mapping of the intracellular site of proinsulin processing in the β-cell to the trans-Golgi network prior to the formation (or rather maturation) of the typical dense-core insulin secretory granule (22).

The progress in DNA sequencing for which F. Sanger received his second Nobel Prize (shared with W. Gilbert) allowed the determination of the first isolated insulin mRNA (cDNA) by Ullrich (23). In a few years, the sequence of rat and human insulin genes became known (24-26).

Cloning of the insulin genes facilitated the industrial production of recombinant human insulin in microorganisms (27), rather than relying on cumbersome collection and extraction of porcine and bovine pancreata.

The Insulin Promoter, the β-Cell Specific Expression of Insulin, and Pdx1

It remained a puzzle how the insulin-producing cell was able so efficiently to transcribe the insulin gene. Insulin mRNA would constitute as much as 10% of total cellular RNA. The first breakthrough came from the identification of the insulin promoter/enhancer structure, which in *cis* contributed to the tissue specificity of transcriptional control (28-30). Other studies showed that as little as 350-400 bp of the mammalian insulin promoters confer tissue specificity in other species (see reference (31) for review). The hunt for the unique factors, which in *trans* would confer this tissue specificity began.

The identification of such transacting factors revealed members of two major classes of regulatory proteins - namely homeodomain factors (HD) and basic helix-loop-helix (bHLH) factors. It became evident that tissue specificity is likely achieved by a unique combination of abundant and tissue restricted factors (see Figure 2, and chapters by Melloul and Ahlgren & Edlund). The pioneering work of H. Edlund (previously H. Ohlsson) and T. Edlund (32,33) originally identifying IPF-1 (insulin-promoter-factor-1) as a β-cell specific DNA binding complex (34) and the subsequent cloning of the mouse IPF-1 gene revealed a homeodomain protein (35) binding the TAAT-core of the A-elements of the insulin promoter (36). The rat homologue was reported by two groups and revealed it to be less tissue restricted than first anticipated (IDX-1, islet duodenal homeobox-1 (37)) and to possess a transactivation potential also for the somatostatin promoter (STF-1, somatostatin transcription factor-1 (38)). Sequence similarity with XlHbox8 (39) from *Xenopus laevis*, a protein involved in the early cell-autonomous endodermal determination in *Xenopus* embryogenesis (40) indicated that there was more to IPF-1 than just insulin gene regulation. Pancreatic duodenal homeobox (Pdx1) was adopted as the common nomenclature (covering XlHbox8, IPF-1, IDX-1, STF-1, IUF-1(41), or GSF (42)) and has gained widespread acceptance. Pdx1 had proven instrumental in insulin gene regulation (35,43-46). However, the first report on the Pdx1 null mutant mouse lacking the entire pancreas (47) signified a new era for the field of developmental biology of the pancreas. Moreover, a case of pancreatic agenesis in humans was associated with a mutation in the Pdx1 gene (48) and heterozygous relatives would suffer from maturity onset diabetes (MODY, table 1). A similar diabetes is observed in heterozygous (Pdx1+/-) mice (49,50)

Transcription Factors and Pancreas Ontogeny

The Pdx1 knockout first reported by the Edlund laboratory (47,51) and later by Offield et al., (52) proved to be the first in a rapidly growing series of transcription factor null mutants that provided informative pancreatic phenotypes. This has essentially revolutionized the field of pancreatic development and attracted much interest to determine the secrets of the formation of the pancreatic β-cell. Major achievements in the past by the W. Rutter laboratory provided the foundation for the current understanding of pancreas development. In essence, not much happened during the twenty years since the review on the development of the embryonic endocrine pancreas appeared in Handbook of Physiology 1972 by Pictet and Rutter (53). Disputes whether pancreatic endocrine cells were of endodermal (54) or neuroectodermal (55) origin were eventually settled (56). A more recent comprehensive review on pancreas development was produced by Slack in 1995 (57) and several recent reviews on the novel transcription factors and their impact on pancreas development have appeared (58-61).

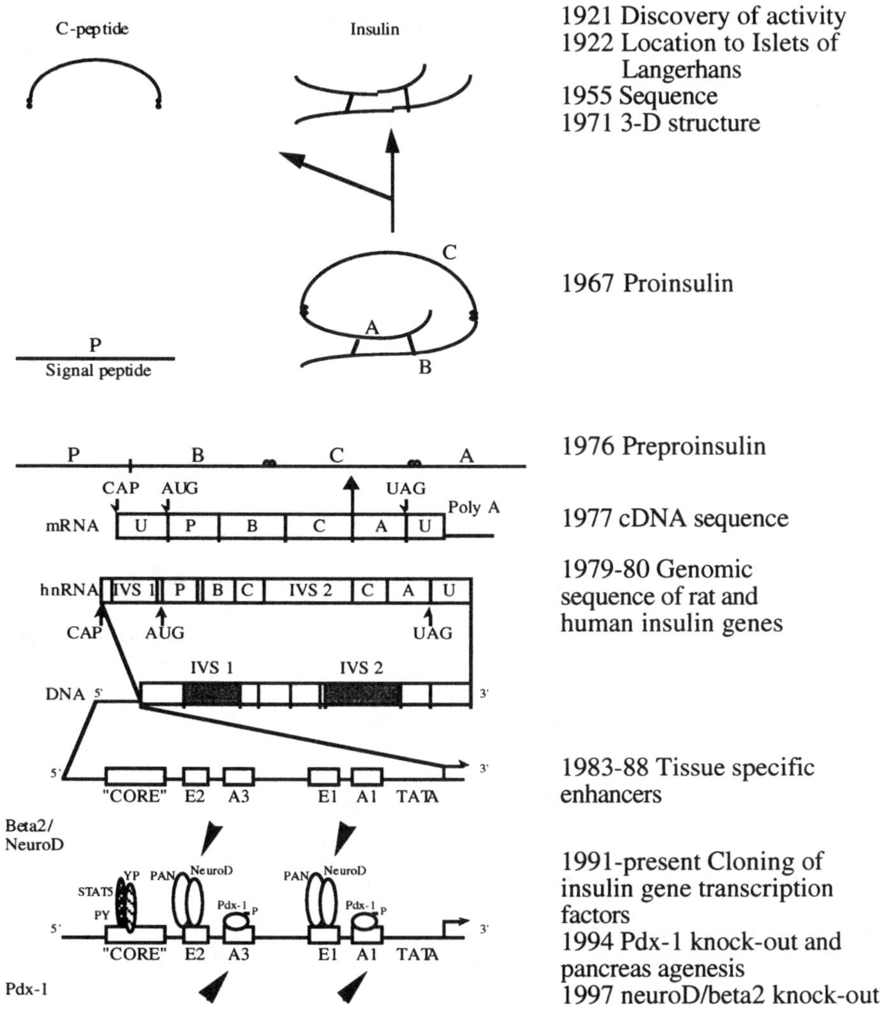

Figure 2. *Selected highlights of the history of insulin. A direct link exists from the discovery of insulin to developmental biology of the pancreas.*

Table 1 lists the various transcription factors, their null-mutant pancreatic phenotypes, as well as the series of recently identified autosomal dominant diabetes genes (MODY) and encoding transcription factors. Much of these data have been thoroughly reviewed in (61) and are not discussed further in great detail (see also chapters by Ahlgren & Edlund, by Zhao & Gruss, and by Stoffel). Exo- versus endocrine fate appears to be controlled by bHLH factors, where lack of p48 leads to failure of exocrine pancreas development (62) while lack of NeuroD (63) drastically reduces endocrine cell number.

Of particular interest is the collection of transcription factors with a β-cell restricted expression in the adult pancreas - including Pdx1, Hlxb9, Pax4, and Nkx6.1 (table 1) and the different mutant phenotypes they produce. In light of the initial reports on the β-cell specific expression pattern of Pdx1 (β-cells constitute approximately 1-2% of the total mass of the adult pancreas) - it was surprising that the Pdx1-/- mouse was apancreatic (47). However, it became apparent that Pdx1 was expressed in a broader region covering the duodenum as well as part of the antral stomach and that it served functions in addition to specifying pancreas, since null-mutants also lacked Brunners glands as well as the antral gastrin producing G-cell (52,64). The pancreas forms as two individual buds on the dorsal and ventral side of the duodenum (53,57). Lack of Pdx1, which normally is expressed at relatively higher levels in all of the epithelial cells in the early buds (Figure 3) (47,65,66), arrested further development of the early forming buds (51,52). The dorsal bud fails to form completely in the Hlxb9 null mutant mice while the ventral pancreas develops but with perturbed islet maturation (67,68). It is thus evident that the initial specifications of the dorsal and the ventral buds are controlled by different mechanisms. The Isl-1 mutant additionally demonstrates that the interaction with the pancreatic mesenchyme differs between the two buds since the absence of dorsal mesenchyme in Isl-1-/- mice results in a secondary failure of dorsal exocrine pancreas formation while ventral exocrine maturation occurs (69). The pax6 mutant lacks α-cells, the Pax4 mutant selectively lacks β- and δ-cells, and the Pax4/Pax6 double mutant has no hormone positive cells (70,71). The Nkx6.1 mutant phenotype has not yet been reported, but the Nkx2.2 mutant has no β-cells but displays a number of hormone-negative cells lacking Nkx6.1. Nkx6.1 is co-expressed with Pdx1 in the early bud-epithelium (66) and this early expression is not affected in the Nkx2.2 mutant (72). β-cell specific deletion of Pdx1 causes loss of β-cell phenotype and diabetes (49) and loss of Nkx6.1 expression. It is thus likely that Nkx6.1 is downstream of Pdx1 and that Nkx2.2 is required for maintaining Nkx6.1 expression in the mature β-cell. It can be concluded that the pancreatic β-cell-specific transcription factors are central in pancreas as well as β-cell ontogeny as they are required at different stages of organ development.

PHYLOGENY OF THE β-CELL AND PANCREAS

The β-Cell - Founder of Pancreatic Evolution?

Thanks to an immense effort by S. Falkmer, who studied the phylogeny of many polypeptide hormones (86,87), we can now focus on his findings regarding the various cell types of the pancreas (88). Proto-chordates have hormone producing cell types known from the mammalian pancreas as scattered cells of the gut epithelium. There is no pancreas in e.g. amphioxus. The first sign of the formation of a distinct organ with pancreatic hormones is in the jawless fish (Agnatha, represented by the hagfishes and lampreys), which are the phylogenetically oldest or earliest still existing vertebrates (chordates). Strikingly, the hagfish has an islet organ composed of 99% β-cells and 1% somatostatin cells. Thus, no α-cells, PP cells nor acinar cells are present in this organ, which is situated as a bud of the common bile duct close to its entry into the duodenum. The islet organ also contain cystic structures of duct-epithelial character. Somatostatin cells are also abundant in the adjacent bile duct epithelium. Dr. Falkmer concludes: "The most remarkable feature of this islet organ is, however, its complete lack of exocrine, acinar, zymogenic pancreatic parenchyma. As a matter of fact, there is no pancreatic gland at all in the hagfish.

Thus, the islets of Langerhans are phylogenetically older than the exocrine pancreatic parenchyma. Thus, it can be concluded that, among the four major islet hormones, it seems as if the insulin cells are the first to appear in a real islet parenchyma, followed by the somatostatin cells, whereas the glucagon and PP cells still lag behind in this respect" (88). As summarized in Figure 4, glucagon and exocrine cells enter the pancreas in the Holocephali group of cartilaginous fish (three existing species include the rabbit-, rat-, and elephant-fish). Later, during evolution, in the Elasmobranchii group of cartilaginous fish such as the shark, the PP cell is present indicating that the 'mammalian-type' of pancreas has existed for more than 350 million years.

The lamprey is different from the hagfish in the sense that it has more than one islet organ situated as buds directly on the primitive gut and not on the bile duct. Otherwise, the organization is the same with all β-cells present in islet parenchyma and none in the gut epithelium (88). It is thus tempting to speculate that the hagfish islet organ represents an equivalent ancestor of the ventral pancreatic bud while the islet organs of the lamprey would represent variants of the dorsal bud. In this respect, it is of interest that inhibition of Hedgehog (hh) signalling in the chicken embryo actually leads to additional pancreas bud formation caudal to the dorsal bud as well as in the distal stomach (89). Sonic Hedgehog (Shh) is expressed throughout the endoderm but remarkably absent in the dorsal and ventral areas of pancreatic bud formation and lack of expression of Shh in the pancreas buds is mandatory for normal pancreatic development (90,91). The suppression of Shh expression in the pancreatic dorsal endoderm is caused by secreted factors from the notochord which in early development is in direct contact with the dorsal endoderm (92).

In the proto-chordate, amphioxus, the insulin cells are scattered in the epithelium of the gut wall (88). In this species insulin and IGF-1 have not diverged. Strikingly, the expression analysis of the amphioxus Pdx1 homologue (AmphiXlox) shows a remarkably confined expression pattern in a stripe of the presumptive gut from the neurula stage through to larvae - as well as in two cells of the neural tube opposite of somite 5 (93). Such data suggest that a region in the amphioxus gut has a specialized function possibly equivalent to the later evolving pancreatic region but prior to the segregation of insulin and IGF-1 as distinct hormones.

β-cells and Brain Evolution?

It is an essential observation that the Agnatha hagfish and lamprey islet organs not only represent the first sign of a pancreas, but also illustrate the fact that all insulin cells are now removed from the gut epithelium into a new organ. This indicates that from Agnatha (e.g. the hagfish) onwards it became important to sense blood glucose rather than gut-glucose. It probably also means that blood glucose has been maintained on defined levels throughout vertebrate evolution (i.e., a period of up to 500 million years).

Table 1. Transcription factors of the pancreas

Transcription factor	Family	Adult pancreatic expression	Null mutant pancreatic phenotype	Mody	Refs.
Pdx1	HD	All β-cells few δ-cells	Lethal early postnatal, diabetes, mice lack pancreas, antral G-cells and Brunners glands, duodenum malformed.	Mody 4	(35,47, 51,52, 64) (73)
ISL-1	LIM/ HD	All islet cells	Lethal, dorsal bud agenesis (mesenchymal faliure), lack of all islet cells.		(69,74)
Nkx 6.1	HD	Only β-cells	?		(75,76)
Nkx2.2	HD	α-, β- and PP-cells; not δ-cells	Lethal early postnatal, diabetes, lack of β-cells, reduced α- and PP cells. Have amylin/Pdx1 positive cells which do not express Nkx6.1.		(72)
Neuro D	bHLH	All islet cells. Part of the IEF-1 transcription complex	Lethal, diabetes Reduced number of islet cells		(63)
E2A (Pan _)	bHLH	Both exo-and endocrine pancreas. Part of the IEF-1 transcription complex	No phenotype		(77)
P48	bHLH	Exocrine acinar cells. Part of the PTF-1 transcription complex	No exocrine pancreas. Islets in spleen.		(62,78)
Pax4	paired/ HD	Only β-cells	Lack of β- and δ-cells; more α-cells		(71)
Pax 6	paired/ HD	All islet cells	No α-cells Other endocrine cell types reduced		(70)
Pax4/6			No islet cells		(70)
Hlxb9	HD	Only β-cells	Dorsal bud agenesis, perturbed ventral endocrine differentiation		(67,68)
HNF4α	SRS	Both exo-and endocrine pancreas.	Non informative. Early lethal	Mody 1	(79,80)
HNF1α	POU/ HD	Both exo-and endocrine pancreas.	Lethal at weaning. Liver failure. Poor β-cell performance, diabetes	Mody 3	(81) (82,84)
HNF1β	POU/ HD			Mody 5	(85)

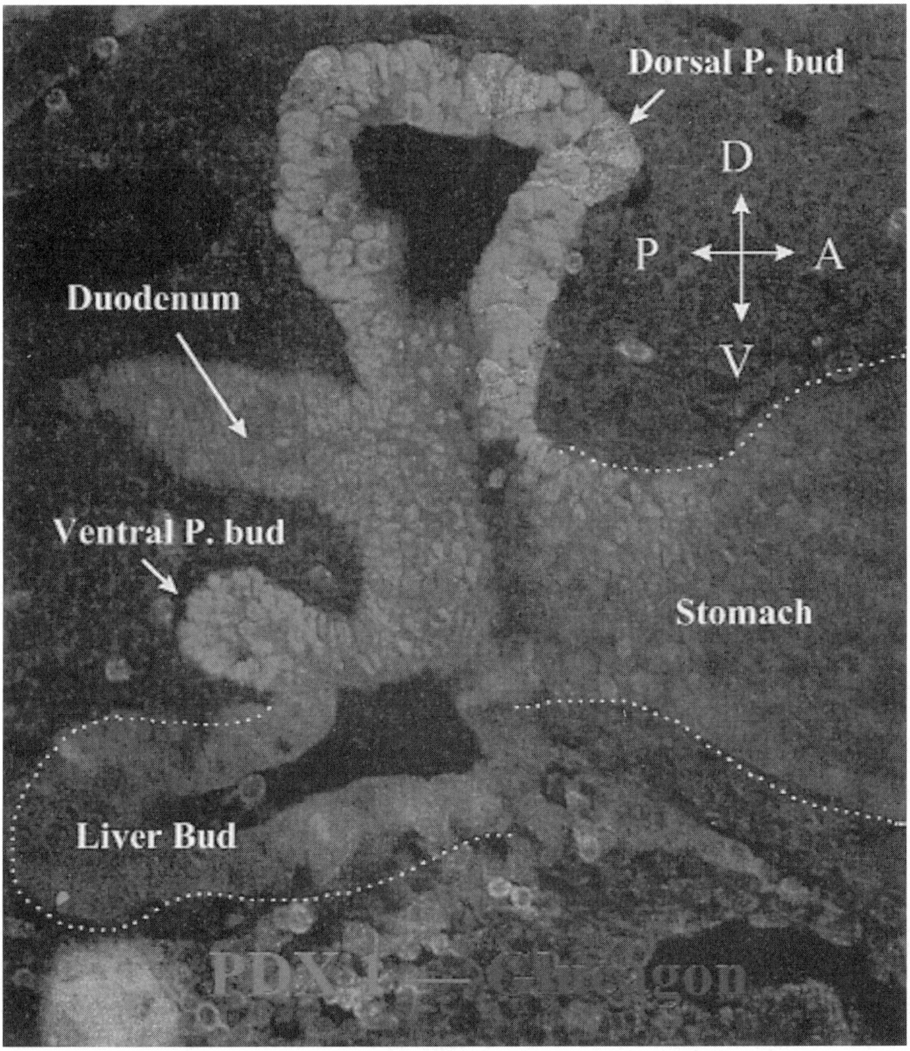

Figure 3. *Embryonic pancreas formation. The ventral and dorsal pancreatic buds are characterized by high level expression of Pdx1 (green) where lower expression is detected in the duodenum and distal stomach. Proglucagon cells appear early in the pancreatic epithelium (red).*

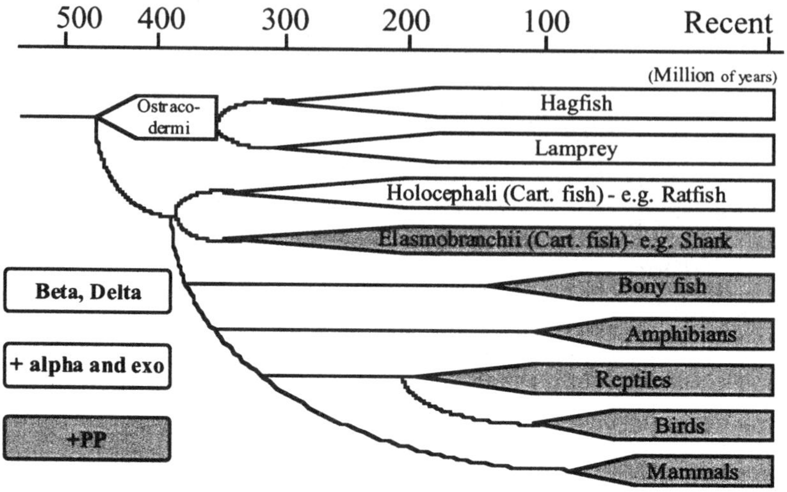

Figure 4. *In hagfish or lampreys the first 'pancreas' is an islet organ of mainly β- and few δ-cells. In the ratfish the α- and exocrine cells have entered the organ - and from sharks an onwards we have the 'mammalian-type' of pancreas (88).*

This circumstance must have been an important prerequisite for the successful evolution of the highly complex vertebrate brain. The greater specialization in glucose sensing of the β-cell (or of the entire islet) – provides a greater safety in ensuring a continuous fuel supply for the evolving brain. At the same time, the individual now became dependent on the performance of the β-cell. Hypoglycaemia, especially, would cause deleterious brain failure and be fatal - and it is reasonable to assume that during evolution the β-cell evolved special features allowing it to take measures against potential hypoglycaemic threats - such as effective mechanisms to reduce the mass of β-cells by the induction of programmed cell death. The existence of such features of the β-cell is exemplified by the post-partum involution of the β-cell mass by apoptosis to adjust to the decreased needs for insulin (94). Similarly, we have reported the down regulation of the endogenous β-cell mass by a subcutaneous insulinoma in the rat, where up to almost 50% of the β-cell mass disappeared by apoptosis while the remainder ceased to produce insulin (95).

Does Ontogeny Recapitulate Phylogeny?

In this context, it is interesting that the very early pancreatic endodermal epithelium actually expresses three β-cell markers of the mature insulin producing cell type, namely Pdx1, Hlxb9 and Nkx6.1. This finding may indicate that the early ontogenic epithelium primarily reflect a β-cell precursor (stem cell) phenotype. This may account for the additional pancreatic cell types that have subsequently been acquired (already residing in the primitive gut-epithelium of the proto-chordates). Interestingly, other β-cell traits, such as Glut2 (96), the NGF-receptor trkA (97) and Pref-1 (98) are also expressed in the epithelium prior to the onset of insulin expression during pancreas development.

Further support of the view that the 'default' pathway of pancreatic differentiation appears to be of the endocrine phenotype, is exemplified by the adopted fate of the epithelium when separated from the surrounding mesenchyme (99,100) (see chapter by Maldonado et al.). Thus, the integration of the exocrine differentiation potential into the pancreatic organ relies on evolution of instructive interactions with the surrounding mesenchyme. This interaction of mesenchyme with pancreatic epithelium was recently characterized to involve mesenchyme derived Fibroblast Growth Factors (FGF-1, -7 and -10) mediating their effect through the FGFR-2 IIIb receptor (101) (see chapter by Scharfmann).

In major contrast to the above concept is the fact that the proglucagon-positive cell type clearly appears much earlier in a fully differentiated form as compared to the β-cell (see also Figure 3). This is, however, not the case in the zebrafish, where the sequence of appearance of hormones is insulin > somatostatin > glucagon, thus strictly following the pattern in phylogeny (102,103). However glucagon-immunoreactivity clearly appears in the extra-pancreatic regions prior to insulin (102) - and such cells would most likely be equivalent to the intestinal L-cell with proglucagon processing to glucagon-like peptide (GLP-1 and GLP-2). Moreover, recent analyses of the early proglucagon positive clusters in rodents reveal that prohormone convertase PC1/3 was expressed (104) which is a characteristic of the intestinal GLP-1 cell (L-cell) rather than of the mature α-cell. PC1/3 is required for generating GLP-1 from the proglucagon precursor (105) and it is thus likely that the early 'glucagon'-clusters found in rodents in fact are GLP-1 producing cell clusters.

CONCLUSIONS AND THE FUTURE PERSPECTIVE

The β-cell has evolved as a specialist in production and delivery of insulin to maintain euglycaemia at all times - and is the ultimate guarantee for the brain that fuel supply will remain constant. This is beyond doubt a very comprehensive task and it is now more evident that β-cell mass can adjust itself according to changes in need (106-109) (Figure 5). Two extreme situations exemplified by threatening hypoglycaemia (caused by a subcutaneous insulinoma in the rat) or by severe insulin resistance (in the double heterozygote knock-out mice IR+/-; IRS-1+/-) - show that β-cells may effectually disappear (95) or increase their mass by up to 30-fold (110), respectively, in attempts to maintain normoglycaemia. IGF-1 receptor signalling and IRS2 appear to be involved in mediating the compensatory growth of β-cells (111,112). Low glucose levels may be fatal to β-cells. A constitutively active apoptotic program seems to exist that requires glucose-induced protein synthesis to be suppressed (113). Additionally, IGF-2 may protect against apoptosis (114).

Diabetes occurs when β-cell mass fails to adjust according to demands (Figure 1). Immune-reactions and cytokines may short-cut circuits normally inhibiting the apoptotic program (115) resulting in IDDM. A regeneration potential resides in the rodent pancreas as shown by partial pancreatectomy (116), by pancreatic duct ligation (117,118), by streptozotocin treatment of newborn rats (119), as well as and by the selective perfusion model where segments of the adult pancreas are exposed to the β-cell toxin, alloxan (120). Especially the latter shows directly that regeneration in the perfused segment occurs from the ducts where neoformation of islets occur while the perfusion-spared segment display β-cell replication in existing islets (120). The expression of ductal markers during islet neogenesis is another strong indication that an islet stem cell potential resides in the ductal epithelium (121). Moreover, Pdx1 is expressed in duct cells at low levels and is upregulated in the regenerating pancreas shortly after partial pancreatectomy (122).

A future goal will be to optimize culture conditions for human foetal pancreas or adult duct-cell preparations to selectively stimulate the growth and differentiation of β-cells (123,124). Important markers can now be used to monitor the success in such attempts including Nkx6.1, Hlxb9 and Pax4. The general low expression of Pdx1 in ductal cells may reflect that all of these would have a stem cell potential. Similarly, extra-insular β-cells are frequently associated with ductules in the adult human pancreas (125) possibly representing continuous neo-formation of β-cells.

Such a controlled expansion is likely an achievable goal within the foreseeable future. It will then be important to investigate to which degree duct cell preparation from a single donor pancreas can be expanded to functional β-cells and it will be equally important that human islet transplantation programs will continue to improve (126). Current progress reports from the International Islet Transplant Registry (ITR) can be found on *http://www.med.uni-giessen.de/itr*. It is likely that a combination of matured islets with ductal cells may further enhance and prolong graft function due to a regenerative potential from the ductal tissue.

Finally, depending on the nature of the critical factors required for β-cell propagation and maturation *in vitro* - a direct application of such factors either systemically or locally to regenerate endogenous pancreas to form β-cells *in vivo* in the diabetic patient could be an additional treatment modality.

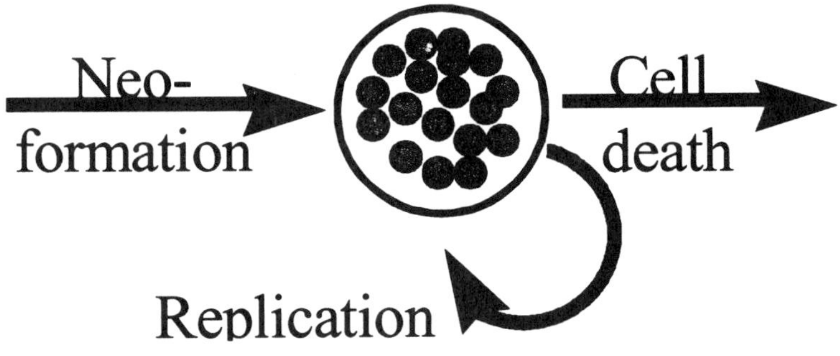

Figure 5. *β-cell mass homeostasis is dependent on neo-formation from ductal precursor cells, replication of existing β-cells and β-cell death (apoptosis).*

ACKNOWLEDGEMENTS

Part of original works on which the present review is based were supported by the Juvenile Diabetes Foundation International, National Institute of Health (grant DK55284) and The Danish National Research Fund. We thank Erna E. Pedersen for skillful technical assistance in immunocytochemistry (Figure 3) and Sture Falkmer and Donald F. Steiner for stimulating discussions.

REFERENCES

1. Banting FG, Best CH. The internal secretion of the pancreas. J Lab Clin Med 1922;7:251-266.
2. The Diabetes Control and Complications Trial Research Group: The effect of intensive treatment of diabetes on the development and progression of long-term complications in insulin-dependent diabetes mellitus. N Engl J Med 1993;329:977-986.
3. UK Prospective Diabetes Study (UKPDS). VIII. Study design, progress and performance. Diabetologia 1991;34:877-90.
4. Colwell JA. Intensive insulin therapy in type II diabetes: rationale and collaborative clinical trial results. Diabetes 1996;45 Suppl 3:S87-90.
5. Lernmark A. Molecular biology of type 1 (insulin-dependent) diabetes mellitus. Diabetologia 1985; 28:195-203.
6. Sutherland DE, Sibley R, Xu XZ, Michael A, Srikanta AM, Taub F, Najarian J, Goetz FC. Twin-to-twin pancreas transplantation: reversal and reenactment of the pathogenesis of type I diabetes. Trans Assoc Amer Physicians 1984;97:80-7.
7. Klöppel G, Löhr M, Habich K, Oberholzer M, Heitz PU. Islet pathology and the pathogenesis of type 1 and type 2 diabetes mellitus revisited. Surv Synth Pathol Res 1985;4:110-25.
8. Tuomi T, Groop LC, Zimmet PZ, Rowley MJ, Knowles W, Mackay IR. Antibodies to glutamic acid decarboxylase reveal latent autoimmune diabetes mellitus in adults with a non-insulin-dependent onset of disease. Diabetes 1993;42:358-362.
9. Turner R, Stratton I, Horton V, Manley S, Zimmet P, Mackay IR, Shattock M, Bottazzo GF, Holman R. UKPDS 25: autoantibodies to islet-cell cytoplasm and glutamic acid decarboxylase for prediction of insulin requirement in type 2 diabetes. UK Prospective Diabetes Study Group [published erratum appears in Lancet 1998 Jan 31;351(9099):376]. Lancet 1997;350:1288-93.
10. Zimmet PZ. Diabetes epidemiology as a tool to trigger diabetes research and care. Diabetologia 1999;42:499-518.
11. Kendall DM, Robertson RP. Pancreas and islet transplantation in humans. Diabetes Metab 1996;22:157-63.
12. Sutherland DE, Gruessner AC, Gruessner RW. Pancreas transplantation: a review. Transplant Proc 1998;30:1940-3.
13. MacLeod JJR. The source of insulin: a study of the effect produced on blood sugar by extracts of the pancreas and principal islets of fishes. J Metab Res 1922;2:149-172.
14. Abel JJ. Crystalline insulin. Proc Natl Acad Sci USA 1926;12:132-136.
15. Ryle AP, Sanger F, Smith LF, Kitai R. The disulfide bonds of insulin. Biochem J 1955;60:541.
16. Sanger F. Chemistry of insulin. Science 1959; 129:1340-1344.
17. Blundell TL, Dodson GG, Hodgkin DC, Mercola D. Insulin: the structure in the crystals and its reflection in chemistry and biology. Adv Protein Chem 1972;26:279-402.
18. Yalow RS. Application of radioimmunologic methods to problems in insulin antigenicity and hormonal assay. In: Luft R, ed. Insulin. Mölndal: A Lindgren&Söner, AB, 1976:149-196.
19. Steiner DF, Oyer PE. The biosynthesis of insulin and a probable precursor of insulin by a human islet cell adenoma. Proc Natl Acad Sci USA 1967;57:473-480.
20. Steiner DF, Rouille Y, Gong Q, Martin S, Carroll R, Chan SJ. The role of prohormone convertases in insulin biosynthesis: evidence for inherited defects in their action in man and experimental animals. Diabetes Metab 1996;22:94-104.
21. Madsen OD, Frank BH, Steiner DF. Human proinsulin-specific antigenic determinants identified by monoclonal antibodies. Diabetes 1984;33:1012-1016.
22. Orci L, Ravazzola M, Amherdt M, Madsen O, Vassalli J-D, Perrelet A. Direct identification of prohormone conversion site in insulin-secreting cells. Cell 1985;42:671-681.
23. Ullrich A, Shine J, Chirgwin J, Pictet R, Tischer E, Rutter WJ, Goodman HM. Rat insulin genes: construction of plasmids containing the coding sequences. Science 1977;196:1313-1319.
24. Cordell B, Bell G, Tischer E, Noto FMD, Ullrich A, Pictet R, Rutter WJ, Goodman HM. Isolation and characterization of a cloned rat insulin gene. Cell 1979;18:533-543.
25. Lomedico P, Rosenthal N, Efstratiadis A, Gilbert W, Kolondner R, Tizard R. The structure and evolution of the two nonallelic rat preproinsulin genes. Cell 1979;18:545-558.
26. Bell GI, Pictet RL, Rutter WJ, Cordell B, Tischer E, Goodman HM. Sequence of the human insulin gene. Nature 1980;284:26-32.
27. Thim L, Hansen MT, Norris K, Hoegh I, Boel E, Forstrom J, Ammerer G, Fiil NP. Secretion and processing of insulin precursors in yeast. Proc Natl Acad Sci USA 1986;83:6766-6770.
28. Walker MD, Edlund T, Boulet AM, Rutter WJ. Cell-specific expression controlled by the 5' flanking regions of the insulin and chymotrypsin genes. Nature 1983;306:557-561.
29. Edlund T, Walker MD, Barr PJ, Rutter WJ. Cell-specific expression of the rat I insulin gene: evidence for role of two distinct 5' flanking elements. Science 1985;230:912-916.
30. Hanahan D. Heritable formation of pancreatic β-cell tumors in transgenic mice expression recombinant insulin/simial virus 40 oncogenes. Nature 1985;315:115-122.

31. Madsen OD, Jensen J, Blume N, Petersen HV, Lund K, Karlsen C, Andersen FG, Jensen PB, Larsson L-I, Serup P. Pancreatic development and maturation of the islet β cell. Studies of pluripotent islet cultures. Eur J Biochem 1996;242:435-445.
32. Ohlsson H, Edlund T. Sequence-specific interactions of nuclear factors with the insulin gene enhancer. Cell 1986;45:35-44.
33. Ohlsson H, Karlsson O, Edlund T. A beta-cell specific protein binds to the two major regulatory sequences of the insulin gene enhancer. Proc Natl Acad Sci USA 1988;85:4228-4231.
34. Ohlsson H, Thor S, Edlund T. Novel insulin promoter- and enhancer-binding proteins that discriminate between pancreatic α- and β-cells. Mol. Endocrinol. 1991;5:897-904.
35. Ohlsson H, Karlsson K, Edlund T. IPF1, a homeodomain-containing transactivator of the insulin gene. EMBO J 1993;12:4251-4259.
36. German M, Ashcroft S, Docherty K, et al. The insulin gene promoter: A simplified nomenclature. Diabetes 1995;44:1002-1004.
37. Miller CP, McGehee RE, Habener JF. IDX-1: a new homeodomain transcription factor expressed in rat pancreatic islets and duodenum that transactivates the somatostatin gene. EMBO J 1994; 13:1145-1156.
38. Leonard J, Peers B, Johnson T, Ferreri K, Lee S, Montminy MR. Characterization of somatostatin transactivating factor-1, a novel homeobox factor that stimulates somatostatin expression in pancreatic islet cells. Mol Endocrinol 1993;7:1275-1283.
39. Wright CVE, Schnegelsberg P, De Robertis EM. XlHbox 8: a novel *Xenopus* homeoprotein restricted to a narrow band of endoderm. Development 1988;104:787-794.
40. Gamer LW, Wright CVE. Autonomous endodermal determination in *Xenopus:* Regulation of expression of the pancreatic gene *XlHbox 8*. Dev Biol 1995;171:240-251.
41. MacFarlane WM, Read ML, Gilligan M, Bujalska I, Docherty K. Glucose modulates the binding activity of the β-cell transcription factor IUF1 in a phosphorylation-dependent manner. Biochem J 1994;303:625-631.
42. Marshak S, Totary H, Cerasi E, Melloul D. Purification of the β-cell glucose-sensitive factor that transactivates the insulin gene differentially in normal and transformed islet cells. Proc Natl Acad Sci USA 1996;93:15057-15062.
43. Petersen HV, Serup P, Leonard J, Michelsen BK, Madsen OD. Transcriptional regulation of the human insulin gene is dependent on the homeodomain protein STF1/IPF1 acting through the CT boxes. Proc Natl Acad Sci USA 1994;91:10465-10469.
44. Peers B, Leonard J, Sharma S, Teitelman G, Montminy MR. Insulin expression in pancreatic islet cells relies in cooperative interactions between the helix-loop-helix factor E47 and the homeobox factor STF-1. Mol Endocrinol 1994;8:1798-1806.
45. Serup P, Petersen HV, Petersen EE, Edlund H, Leonard J, Petersen JS, Larsson L-I, Madsen OD. The homeodomain protein IPF1/STF1 is expressed in a subset of islet cells and promotes rat insulin 1 gene expression dependent on an intact E1 helix-loop-helix factor binding site. Biochem J 1995;310:997-1003.
46. Serup P, Jensen J, Andersen FG, Jørgensen MC, Blume N, Holst JJ, Madsen OD. Induction of insulin and IAPP production in pancreatic islet glucagonoma cells by insulin promoter factor 1. Proc Natl Acad Sci USA 1996;93:9015-9020.
47. Jonsson J, Carlsson L, Edlund T, Edlund H. Insulin-Promoter-Factor 1 is required for pancreas development in mice. Nature 1994;371:606-609.
48. Stoffers DA, Zinkin NT, Stanojevic V, Clarke WL, Habener JF. Pancreatic agenesis attributable to a single nucleotide deletion in the human IPF1 gene coding sequence. Nat Genet 1997;15:106-110.
49. Ahlgren U, Jonsson J, Jonsson L, Simu K, Edlund H. β-cell-specific inactivation of the mouse Ipf1/Pdx1 gene results in loss of the β-cell phenotype and maturity onset diabetes. Genes Dev. 1998;12:1763-1768.
50. Dutta S, Bonner-Weir S, Montminy M, Wright C. Regulatory factor linked to late-onset diabetes? Nature 1998;392.
51. Ahlgren U, Jonsson J, Edlund H. The morphogenesis of the pancreatic mesenchyme is uncoupled from that of the pancreatic epithelium in IPF1/PDX1-deficient mice. Development 1996;122:1409-1416.
52. Offield MF, Jetton TL, Labosky PA, Stein R, Magnuson MA, Hogan BLM, Wright CVE. Pdx-1 is required for pancreatic outgrowth and differentiation of the rostral duodenum. Development 1996;112:983-995.
53. Pictet RL, Rutter WJ. Development of the embryonic endocrine pancreas. In: Steiner DF, Frenkel N, eds. Handbook of Physiology, section 7, vol. 1, American Physiological Society. Washington DC: Williams and Wilkins,1972:25-66.
54. Pictet RL, Rall LB, Phelps P, Rutter WJ. The neural crest and the origin of the insulin-producing and other gastroinstestinal hormone-producing cells. Science 1976;191:191-192.
55. Pearse AGE. Islet cell precursors are neurons. Nature 1982;295:96-97.
56. Percival AC, Slack JMW. Analysis of pancreatic development using a cell lineage label. Exp. Cell Res. 1999; 247:123-132.

57. Slack JMW. Developmental biology of the pancreas. Development 1995;121:1569-1580.
58. Sander M, German MS. The β cell transcription factors and development of the pancreas. J Mol Med 1997;75:327-340.
59. Edlund H. Transcribing Pancreas. Diabetes 1998;47:1817-1823.
60. St-Onge L, Wehr R, Gruss P. Pancreas development and diabetes. Curr Opin Genet Devel 1999;9:295-300.
61. Yamaoka T, Itakura M. Development of pancreatic islets (review). Intl J Mol Med 1999;3:247-261.
62. Krapp A, Knofler M, Ledermann B, Burki K, Berney C, Zoerkler N, Hagenbuchle O, Wellauer P. The bHLH protein PTF1-p48 is essential for the formation of the exocrine and the correct spatial organization of the endocrine pancreas. Genes Dev 1998;12:3752-3763.
63. Naya F, Huang H-P, Qiu Y, Mutoh H, DeMayo F, Leiter A, Tsai M-J. Diabetes, defective pancreatic morphogenesis and abnormal enteroendocrine differentiation in BETA2/NeuroD-deficient mice. Genes Dev 1997;11:2323-2334.
64. Larsson L-I, Madsen OD, Serup P, Jonsson J, Edlund H. Pancreatic-duodenal homeobox 1: Role in gastric endocrine patterning. Mech Dev 1996;60:175-184.
65. Guz Y, Montminy MR, Stein R, Leonard J, Gamer LW, Wright CVE, Teitelman G. Expression of Stf-1, a putative insulin gene transcription factor, in β-cells of pancreas, duodenal epithelium and pancreatic exocrine and endocrine progenitors during ontogeny. Development 1995;121:11-18.
66. Øster A, Jensen J, Serup P, Galante P, Madsen OD, Larsson L-I. Rat endocrine pancreatic development in relation to two homeobox gene products (Pdx-1 and Nkx 6.1). J Histochem Cytochem 1998;46:707-715.
67. Harrison KA, Thaler J, Pfaff SL, Gu H, Kehrl JH. Pancreas dorsal lobe aganesis and abnormal islets of Langerhans in Hlxb9-deficient mice. Nat Genet 1999;23:71-75.
68. Li H, Arber S, Jessell TM, Edlund H. Selective agenesis of the dorsal pancreas in mice lacking homeobox gene Hlxb9. Nat Genet 1999;23:67-70.
69. Ahlgren U, Pfaff SL, Jessel TM, Edlund T, Edlund H. Independent requirement for ISL1 in formation of pancreatic mesenchyme and islet cells. Nature 1997;385:257-260.
70. St-Onge L, Sosa-Pineda B, Chowdhury K, Mansouri A, Gruss P. Pax6 is required for differentiation of glucagon-producing α-cells in mouse pancreas. Nature 1997;397:406-409.
71. Sosa-Pineda B, Chowdhury K, Torres M, Oliver G, Gruss P. The Pax4 gene is essential for differentiation of insulin-producing β cells in the mammalian pancreas. Nature 1997;386:399-402.
72. Sussel L, Kalamaras J, Hartigan-O'Connor DJ, Meneses JJ, Pedersen RA, Rubenstein JLR, German MS. Mice lacking the homeodomain transcription factor Nkx2.2 have diabetes due to arrested differentiation of pancreatic β-cells. Development 1998;125:2213-2221.
73. Stoffers D, Ferrer J, Clarke W, Habener J. Early-onset type-II diabetes mellitus (MODY4) linked to IPF1. Nat Genet 1997;17:138-139.
74. Pfaff SL, Mendelsohn M, Stewart CL, Edlund T, Jessell TM. Requirement for LIM homeobox gene Isl1 in motor neuron generation reveals a motor neoron-dependent step in interneuron differentiation. Cell 1996;84:309-320.
75. Rudnick A, Ling TY, Odagiri H, Rutter WJ, German MS. Pancreatic beta cells express a diverse set of homeobox genes. Proc Natl Acad Sci USA 1994;91:12203-7.
76. Jensen J, Serup P, Karlsen C, Funder TF, Madsen OD. mRNA profiling of rat islet tumors reveals Nkx 6.1 as a β-cell specific homeodomain transcription factor. J Biol Chem 1996;271:18749-18758.
77. Itkin-Ansari P, Bain G, Beattie GM, Mure C, Hayek A, Levine F. E2A gene products are not required for insulin gene expression. Endocrinology 1996;137:3540-3543.
78. Krapp A, Knofler M, Frutiger S, Hughes GJ, Hagenbuchle O, Wellauer P. Thep48 DNA-binding subunit of transcription factor PTF1 is a new exocrine pancreas-specific basic helix-loop-helix protein. EMBO J 1996;15:4317-4329.
79. Chen WS, Manova K, Weinstein DC, Duncan SA, Plump AS, Prezioso VR, Bachvarova RF, Darnell JE. Disruption of the HNF-4 gene, expressed in visceral endoderm, leads to cell death in embryonic ectoderm and impaired gastrulation of mouse embryos. Genes Dev 1994;8:2466-2477.
80. Yamagata K, Furuta H, Oda N, Kaisaki PJ, Menzel S, Cox NJ, Fajans SS, Signorini S, Stoffel N, Bell GI. Mutations in the hepatocyte nuclear factor-4a gene in maturity-onset diabetes of the young (MODY1). Nature 1996;384:458-460.
81. Yamagata K, Oda N, Kaisaki PJ, et al. Mutations in the hepatocyte nuclear factor-1_ gene in maturiti-onset diabetes of the young (MODY3). Nature 1996;384:455-458.
82. Pontoglio M, Barra J, Hadchouel M, Doyen A, Kress C, Bach JP, Babinet C, Yaniv M. Hepatocyte nuclear factor 1 inactivation results in hepatic dysfunction, phenylketonuria, and renal Fanconi syndrome. Cell 1996;84:575-585.

83. Pontoglio M, Sreenan S, Roe M, Pugh W, Ostrega D, doyen A, Pick AJ, Baldwin A, Velho G, Froguel P, Levisetti M, Bonner-Weir S, Bell GI, Yaniv M, Polonsky KS. Defective insulin secretion in hepatocyte nuclear factor 1a-deficient mice. J Clin Invest 1998;101:2215-2222.
84. Lee YH, Sauer B, Gonzales FJ. Laron dwarfism and non-insulin-dependent diabetes mellitus in the hnf-1_ knockout mouse. Mol Cell Biol 1998;18:3059-3068.
85. Horikawa Y, Iwasaki N, Hara M, Furuta H, Hinokio Y, Cockburn BN, Lindner T, Yamagata K, Ogata M, Tomonaga O, Kuroki H, Kasahara T, Iwamoto Y, Bell GI. Mutations in hepatocyte nuclear factor-1b gene (TCF2) associated with MODY. Nat Genet 1997;17:384-385.
86. Falkmer S, El-Salhy M, Titlbach M. Evolution of the neuroendocrine system in vertebrates. A review with particular reference to the phylogeny and postnatal maturation of the islet parenchyma. In: Falkmer S, Håkanson R, Sundler F, eds. Evolution and tumour pathology of the Neuroendocrine System. Amsterdam: Elsevier, 1984:59-87.
87. Falkmer S. Comparative morphology of pancreatic islet in animals. In: Volk BW, Arquilla ER, eds. The Diabetic Pancreas. New York: Plenum Publishing Corporation, 1985:17-52.
88. Falkmer S. Origin of the parenchymal cells of the endocrine pancreas: Some phylogenetic and ontogenetic aspects. In: Mignon M, Jensen RT, eds. Endocrine tumors of the pancreas. Vol. 23. Basel: S Karger, 1995:2-29.
89. Kim SK, Melton DA. Pancreas development is promoted by cyclopamine, a Hedgehog signaling inhibitor. Proc Natl Acad Sci USA 1998;95:13036-13041.
90. Apelqvist Å, Ahlgren U, Edlund H. Sonic hedgehog directs specialised mesoderm differentiation in the intestine and pancreas. Curr Biol 1987;7:801-804.
91. Kim SK, Hebrok M, Melton DA. Notochord to endoderm signaling is required for pancreas development. Development 1997;124:4243-4252.
92. Hebrok M, Kim SK, Melton DA. Notochord repression of endodermal Sonic hedgehog permits pancreas development. Genes Dev 1998;12:1705-1713.
93. Brooke NM, Garcia-Fernández J, Holland PWH. The ParaHox gene cluster is an evolutionary sister of the Hox gene cluster. Nature 1998;392:920-922.
94. Scaglia L, Smith FE, Bonner-Weir S. Apoptosis contributes to the involution of β cell mass in the postpartum rat pancreas. Endocrinology 1995;136:5461-5468.
95. Blume N, Skouv J, Larsson L-I, Holst JJ, Madsen OD. Potent inhibitory effects of transplantable rat glucagonomas and insulinomas on the respective endogenous islet cells are associated with pancreatic apoptosis. J. Clin. Invest 1995;96:2227-2235.
96. Pang K, Mukonoweshuro C, Wong GG. Beta cells arise from glucose transporter type 2 (Glut2)-expressing epithelial cells of the developing rat pancreas. Proc Natl Acad Sci USA 1994;91:9559-9563.
97. Kanaka-Gantenbein C, Tazi A, Czernichow P, Scharfmann R. In vivo presence of the high-affinity NGF receptor TRK-A in the rat pancreas: differential localization during pancreatic development. Endocrinology 1995;136:761-769.
98. Carlsson C, Lindberg DTK, Galante P, Billestrup N, Michelsen B, Larsson LI, Nielsen JH. Growth-hormone and prolactin stimulate the expression of rat preadipocyte factor-1/delta-like protein in pancreatic-islets . Molecular cloning and expression pattern during development and growth of the endocrine pancreas. Endocrinology 1997;138:3940-3948.
99. Gittes GK, Galante PE, Hanahan D, Rutter WJ, Debas HT. Lineage-specific morphogenesis in the developing pancreas: role of mesenchymal factors. Development 1996;122:439-447.
100. Miralles F, Czernichow P, Scharfmann R. Follistatin regulates the relative proportions of endocrine versus exocrine tissue during pancreatic development. Development 1998;125:1017-1024.
101. Miralles F, Czernichow P, Ozaki K, Itoh N, Scharfmann R. Signaling through fibroblast growth factor receptor 2b plays a key role in the development of the exocrine pancreas. Proc Natl Acad Sci USA 1999;96:6267-6272.
102. Argenton F, Zecchin E, Bortolussi M. Early appearance of pancreatic hormone-expressing cells in the zebrafish embryo. Mech Dev 1999;87:217-221.
103. Milewski WM, Duguay SJ, Chan SJ, Steiner DF. Conservation of PDX-1 structure, function and expression in zebrafish. Endocrinology 1998;139:1440-1449.
104. Lee YC, Damholt AB, Billestrup N, Kisbye T, Galante P, Michelsen B, Kofod H, Nielsen JH. Developmental expression of proprotein convertase 1/3 in the rat. Mol Cell Endocrinol 1999;In press.
105. Rouille Y, Kantengwa S, Irminger JC, Halban PA. Role of the prohormone convertase PC3 in the procession of proglucagon to glucagon-like peptide 1. J Biol Chem 1997;272:32810-32816.
106. Hellerstrom C. The life story of the pancreatic β cell. Diabetologia 1984;26:393-400.
107. Bonner-Weir S. Regulation of pancreatic beta-cell mass in vivo. Rec Prog Horm Res 1994;49:91-104.
108. Vinik A, Pittenger G, Rafaeloff R, Rosenberg L, Duguid W. Determinants of pancreatic islet cell mass: a balance between neogenesis and senescence/apoptosis. Diabetes Rev. 1996;4:235-236.
109. Finegood DT, Scaglia L, Bonner-weir S. Dynamics of the β cell mass in the growing rat pancreas. Diabetes 1995;44:249-256.

110. Brüning JC, Winnay J, Bonner-Weir S, Taylor SI, Accili D, Kahn CR. Development of a novel polygenic model of NIDDM in mice heterozygous for IR and IRS-1 null alleles. Cell 1997;88:561-572.
111. Withers D, Gutierrez J, Towery H, Burks D, Ren J, Previs S, Zhang Y, Bernal D, Pons S, Shulman G, Bonner-Weir S, White M. Disruption of IRS-2 causes type 2 diabetes in mice. Nature 1998;391:900-904.
112. Withers DJ, Burks DJ, Towery HH, Altamuro SL, Flint CL, White MF. Irs-2 coordinates Ifg-1 receptor-mediated b-cell development and peripheral insulin signalling. Nat Genet 1999;23:32-40.
113. Hoorens A, Van de Casteele M, Klöppel G, Pipeleers D. Glucose promotes survival of rat pancreatic beta cells by activating synthesis of proteins which suppress a constitutive apoptotic program. J Clin Invest 1996;98:1568-74.
114. Petrik J, Arany E, Mcdonald TJ, Hill DJ. Apoptosis in the pancreatic islet cells of the neonatal rat is associated with a reduced expression of insulin-like growth factor II that may act as a survival factor. Endocrinology 1998;139:2994-3004.
115. Mandrup-Poulsen T. The role of interleukin-1 in the pathogenesis of IDDM. Diabetologia 1996;39:1005-1029.
116. Bonner-Weir S, Baxter LA, Schuppin GT, Smith FE. A second pathway for regeneration of adult exocrine and endocrine pancreas - a possible recapitulation of embryonic development. Diabetes 1993;42:1715-1720.
117. Wang RN, Klöppel G, Bouwens L. Duct-cell to islet-cell differentiation and islet growth in the pancreas of duct-ligated adult rats. Diabetologia 1995;38:1404-1411.
118. Rafaeloff R, Pittenger GL, Barlow SW, Qin XF, Yan B, Rosenberg L, Duguid WP, Vinik AI. Cloning and sequencing of the pancreatic islet neogenesis associated protein (INGAP) gene and its expression in islet neogenesis in hamsters. J Clin Invest 1997;99:2100-2109.
119. Wang RN, Bouwens L, Klöppel G. Beta-cell proliferation in normal and streptozotocin-treated newborn rats: site, dynamics and capacity. Diabetologia 1994;37:1088-1096.
120. Waguri M, Yamamoto K, Miyagawa JI, Tochino Y, Yamamori K, Kajimoto Y, Nakajima H, Watada H, Yoshiuchi I, Itoh N, Imagawa A. Demonstration of two different processes of beta-cell regeneration in a new diabetic mouse model induced by selective perfusion of alloxan. Diabetes 1997;46.
121. Bouwens L, Wang R-N, Blay ED, Pipeleers DG, Klöppel G. Cytokeratins as markers of ductal cell differentiation and islet neogenesis in the neonatal rat pancreas. Diabetes 1994;43:1279-1283.
122. Sharma A, Zangen DH, Reitz P, Taneja M, Lissauer ME, Miller CP, Weir GC, Habener JF, Bonner-Weir S. The homeodomain protein IDX-1 increases after an early burst of proliferation during pancreatic regeneration. Diabetes 1999;48:507-513.
123. Kerr-Conte J, Pattou F, Lecomte-Houcke M, Xia Y, Boilly B, Proye C, Lefebvre J. Ductal cyst formation in collagen-embedded adult human islet preparations. A means to the reproduction of nesidioblastosis in vitro. Diabetes 1996;45:1108-1114.
124. Beattie GM, Cirulli V, Lopez AD, Hayek A. Ex vivo expansion of human pancreatic endocrine cells. J. Clin. Endocrinol. Metab. 1997;82:1852-1856.
125. Bouwens L, Pipeleers DG. Extra-insular beta cells associated with ductules are frequent in adult human pancreas. Diabetologia 1998;41:629-633.
126. Roep BO, Stobbe I, Duinkerken G, vanRood JJ, Lernmark Å, Keymeulen B, Pipeleers D, Claas FHJ, deVries RRP. Auto-and alloimmune reactivity to human islet allografts transplanted into type 1 diabetic patients. Diabetes 1999;48:484-490.

2
GLUCOSE SIGNALLING TO TRANSCRIPTION FACTORS OF THE INSULIN GENE

Danielle Melloul, Ph.D.
Hadassah University Hospital, Jerusalem, 91120 Israel

In the adult, insulin is expressed exclusively in the pancreatic β-cells. This hormone is essential to the control of mammalian glucose homeostasis and it is influenced by nutrients and hormonal factors. Although considerable progress has been made in understanding the molecular mechanisms that confer tissue-specificity and metabolic responsiveness on insulin gene expression, we are only beginning to comprehend the complexities involved. In β-cells, glucose is the primary physiological regulator of insulin secretion and biosynthesis. This chapter will focus on the transcriptional control of the insulin gene by glucose, and on the transcription factors mediating this effect.

TRANSCRIPTIONAL REGULATION OF INSULIN GENE EXPRESSION

β-cell-restricted expression of the insulin gene relies on the interaction of 5'-flanking sequence motifs in the promoter region with a number of ubiquitous and islet-specific transcription factors. These interactions determine the temporal expression of the gene and its inducibility by physiological stimuli (for reviews, see references 1-3). Most of the studies on the regulation of insulin gene expression were conducted with rat insulin I and II and the human genes. They share a number of conserved cis- elements in their 5'-flanking region (4,5) and are probably regulated by similar transacting factors. Among such elements, the E and A boxes appear to be the major determinants of β-cell specific insulin gene expression (6). The E boxes (El and E2), with the consensus CANNTG, bind transcription factors of the helix-loop-helix family (bHLH) (7-15). Indeed, transfection studies in insulin-producing cells show that motifs El and E2 are important for the tissue-specific expression of insulin. The El box binds IEF1 that is composed of bHLH proteins such as E12 and/or E47. These interact with the cell-type-restricted bHLH protein NeuroD/BETA2 that is expressed in pancreatic and neuroendocrine cells and is an important regulator of pancreatic development (16) and of insulin gene expression (13). Interestingly, disruption of the E2A gene has no effect on the β-cell phenotype (14), indicating a redundancy between members of the bHLH gene family. In contrast to rat insulin I, the human insulin 5'-flanking region does not contain the second consensus E2 box, but the corresponding sequence binds the HLH protein USF (17).

Additional prominent regulatory elements containing AT rich sequences, the A boxes (A1-A5) (6), bind factors that belong to the homeodomain-containing protein family. The most conserved A1 and A3 boxes in the insulin promoter bind the Pancreatic Duodenal Homeobox-1 (pdx-1) transcription factor, the mammalian homolog of the *Xenopus laevis* XlHbox8 (18), and previously described as ipf-1 (19), STF-1 (20), IDX-1 (21), GSF (22,23), and IUF-1 (24). The name pdx-1 will be used throughout this chapter to designate this protein. Pdx-1 is a transactivator of islet-specific glucose transporter 2 (25), glucokinase (26), and particularly of the insulin gene (19,23,27). Gene disruption experiments in mice show that pdx-1 is needed for pancreas formation (28). Moreover, the pattern of its expression and its ability to stimulate insulin gene transcription strongly suggest that pdx-1 functions both in early commitment of the primitive gut to a pancreatic fate and in the maturation of the pancreatic β-cells (29-36).

The picture emerging from studies on the transcriptional control of insulin gene expression is that some of the identified cis-acting regulatory sequences are common to several genes, and that utilization of these elements apparently varies among the individual genes. In the rat insulin I gene, the A3 and A4 boxes bind several homeodomain-containing proteins such as isl-1 (37), cdx-3 and lmx-1 (38), HNF1-α (39) and Oct (unpublished results). Factors binding to the A3-A4 boxes of the rat insulin I gene function synergistically with E2A-encoded proteins in transfected foetal islets, as well as in β-cell lines (32,38,40). Indeed, lmx (38) or pdx-1 (and more specifically the N-terminal and the homeodomain regions) (41) act synergistically with a member of the bHLH family of transcription factors, the E47 protein, to activate rat insulin I gene expression. Thus, tissue-specific expression appears to depend on a combination of transcription factors, only some of which are restricted to the β-cell.

GLUCOSE-REGULATED EXPRESSION OF THE INSULIN GENE

Because of its central role in metabolic control, tight regulation of insulin production and release is critical. Inducible transcription may well depend upon the very same sequences in the promoter/enhancer regions that control the cell-type specificity of the insulin gene. In pancreatic β-cells, glucose is the major regulator of insulin biosynthesis and secretion. The stimulatory effect of high glucose levels on insulin synthesis has been extensively investigated. Recent studies have shown that glucose can both positively (short- and medium-term exposure) and negatively (chronic exposure) regulate insulin gene expression. Experiments with rat and human islets, as well as β-cell lines, indicated that glucose regulates insulin gene expression by both stimulating transcription and inhibiting proinsulin mRNA degradation. Early effects of glucose are increased translation of pre-existing proinsulin mRNA. Delayed effects are the stimulation of new proinsulin mRNA production (42-50). However, more sensitive methods for detecting insulin transcript levels reveal that transcription is initiated within minutes of glucose stimulation, thereby suggesting that also short term glucose signalling leads to the elevation of cytoplasmic insulin mRNA levels (51,52).

The glucose-responsiveness of the insulin gene is mediated by cis-acting elements within the 5' flanking region relative to the transcription start site (22,23,27,48,49,53-55). It appears that in β-cells, several elements within the insulin promoter combine to provide the full glucose response of the intact promoter and that more than one transcription factor is regulated by glucose. Most likely, glucose controls the metabolic response elements by regulating the protein factors that bind to them. Of the elements contributing to the activation of insulin gene transcription by glucose, the most extensively studied are shown in Figure 1:

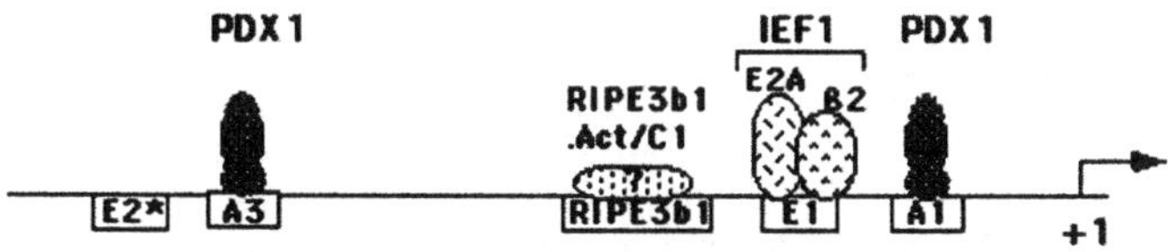

Figure 1. *Potential mediators of the glucose effect on human insulin gene expression: cis-acting regulatory elements of the gene (depicted as boxes, according to the nomenclature of German et al. (6)) and their binding proteins. The * relates to the human insulin sequence (CACCGG), which differs slightly from the E consensus sequence (CANNTG).*

pdx-1 and RIPE3b1-Act (or C1) binding to the respective A3 and RIPE3b1 elements were potentiated in glucose-stimulated cells. However little (54) or no increase (55, and unpublished data) in the E1 binding complex (IEF1) was observed. More recently, an additional glucose-responsive element in the human insulin gene (-292/-243) was reported in primary cultured islet cells, the shorter sequence -292/-263 binding a glucose-responsive complex (56).

The Glucose-Responsive Trans-Acting Factor RIPE3b1

To identify the cis-acting control elements within the rat insulin II gene that are responsible for regulating glucose-stimulated expression in the β-cell, the effect of glucose concentration was analysed on a series of transfected 5'-flanking deletion mutant constructs. It was shown that glucose-induced transcription of the rat insulin II gene is mediated by sequences located between -126 and -91 bp relative to the transcription start site. This region contains two cis-acting elements that are essential in directing β-cell-specific expression of the rat insulin II gene, the insulin control element (ICE; -100 to -91 bp) and RIPE3b1 (-115 to -107 bp). Mutations in RIPE3b1 and ICE elements within the rat insulin II promoter reduce glucose-inducible expression to a similar extent, thereby supporting their role in the glucose-responsive transcription of the rat insulin II gene and as independent mediators of this response (57). RIPE3b1 binding activity was selectively induced by high glucose concentrations. In contrast, binding to other insulin cis-acting element sequences, like ICE and RIPE3a2 (-108 to -99 bp), was unaffected (55). The RIPE3b1-activator has not been isolated, and our knowledge of the signalling pathway leading to the glucose-induced binding activity is limited. The RIPE3b1 -activator can also be regulated in β-cells by several physiological effectors such as mannose and pyruvate, implying the generation of a common signal(s) during glucose metabolism that mediates both insulin transcription and secretion (57). In the human insulin gene, a C2 element (adjacent to the E2-like motif) was shown to bind a factor, D0, which exhibits similar properties to RIPE3b1. Its binding was abolished by both the oxidizing agent diamide and the alkylating agent N-ethylmaleimide, suggesting that expression of the insulin gene may be regulated by a redox-dependent pathway involving the RIPE3b1 -activator or a RIPE3b1-like factor (58).

The Glucose-Responsive Transcription Factor pdx-1

The role of the pdx-1 protein in glucose-regulated expression of the insulin gene has been more extensively studied than the above described transcription factors.

German et al. (48) first showed that the Far-Flat (FF) minienhancer element of the rat insulin I gene (around -200 to -250) mediated the glucose-stimulated transcription of a reporter gene in transfected fetal rat islets. Using normal adult rat and human islets we have further mapped the glucose-sensitive element to sequences -193 to -227 that contain the highly conserved A3 motif (22) (see Figure 1).

The glucose effect on the pdx-1 DNA binding domain
Several years ago, we first identified an islet-specific nuclear protein whose DNA binding to the A3 sequence of the human insulin gene was modulated by extracellular glucose levels within a relatively short period of time (Figure 2A). We originally named this protein GSF, for Glucose Sensitive Factor. A point mutation in the sequence -206 to -227 of the human A3 element abolished the binding of pdx-1 to its recognition site (Figure 2B). Islets transfected with the wild type human insulin promoter exhibited substantially increased activity when incubated in high versus low glucose concentrations. In sharp contrast, the single mutation in the pdx-1 binding site, within the context of the insulin promoter, completely abolished the stimulatory effect of high glucose concentrations (Figure 2C). These results demonstrate that the A3 motif is crucial to glucose sensing in the human insulin gene (23). Similar findings by Petersen et al. (27) support the suggested physiological role of pdx-1 as one of the important factors in the glucose-regulated expression of the insulin gene. The protein corresponding to GSF was purified, and its amino acid sequence matched that of the previously described ipf-1/pdx-1 protein (23), providing direct evidence of its involvement in glucose-responsiveness. The human cDNA coding for pdx-1 has been isolated and its DNA sequence has been determined. Sequence comparison between the human and rodent pdx-1 showed a high degree of conservation (23). Thus, in addition to its essential roles in the development and differentiation of pancreatic islets and in β-cell-specific gene expression, pdx-1 mediates the glucose effect on insulin gene transcription in differentiated β-cells.

The glucose effect on the pdx-1 activation domain
Is transcriptional activation of the insulin promoter by glucose primarily the result of a gain in its DNA binding activity or does it also affect the transcriptional activation domain of pdx-1? In an attempt to resolve this issue, we mapped the human pdx-1 (hpdx-1) domains implicated in the transcriptional activation, using a trans-activation assay based on the Gal4 system. We constructed chimeric proteins containing the heterologous DNA binding portion of Gal4 protein (59) fused to portions of hpdx-1. Hybrid molecules containing the full length hpdx-1 protein (aa 1-283: Gal4-full length: G1), the N-terminal (aa 1-120: Gal4-N-term: G2) or the C-terminal (aa 190-283: Gal4-C-term: G6) domains, were co-transfected into Hela and βTC6 cells with a plasmid containing in tandem multiple binding sites for Gal4 upstream of the reporter CAT gene. Whereas the activation domain was contained within the N-terminal region of the hpdx-1, the full length protein or the C-terminal part had low or no transcriptional activity in transiently transfected cells. These results concur with reports from several groups which have shown that the transactivation domain of the rodent pdx-1 resides in the N-terminus of the molecule (41,60).

To determine whether these sequences are involved in mediating the glucose effect on transcriptional activation, the different constructs were transiently transfected into adult islets and incubated in low and high glucose concentrations. The CAT activities obtained from such transfections showed that the full-length protein had a mild transactivation effect (less than two-fold) and thus the glucose-stimulated transcriptional activity resided within the first 120 amino acids. The C-terminus of the molecule remained silent at both glucose concentrations. Sequence comparison of amino acids 1-120 of the N-terminal domain between human pdx-1 (23), mouse ipf-1 (19), rat STF-1/IDX-1 (20,21) and the frog XlHbox8 homolog (18), reveals a very high degree of conservation. The identical amino acids in the different pdx-1 homologues are labeled A, B, C, D boxes in Figure 3. A series of N-termini were tested in normal adult rat islets incubated in medium containing 2 or 20 mM glucose.

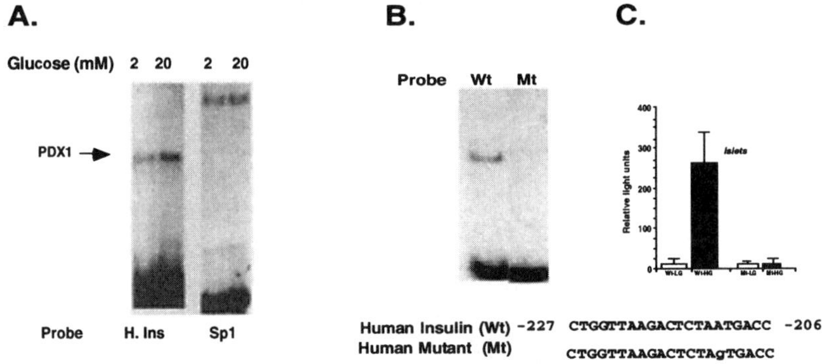

Figure 2. *A) Isolated rat islets were incubated in 2mM and 20 mM glucose for 20 min. Extracted nuclear proteins were incubated with the labeled human insulin sequence (H. Ins.) or with the control SP1 binding site. The complexes were separated using the electrophoretic mobility shift assay (EMSA). B) A single mutation abolishes GSF binding to its recognition site. Islet nuclear extracts were tested for PDX1 binding, using the labeled wild type (Wt) and the mutant form (Mt) of the human insulin sequence. Protein-DNA complexes were resolved by EMSA. C) Glucose inducibility of the insulin gene. Normal adult rat islets were transfected with plasmids containing the luciferase reporter gene controlled by the human insulin wild type promoter extending from +1 to -364 (WT), or by the same promoter, into which a single point mutation in the pdx-1 binding site had been introduced (Mt). The islets were then incubated in low (WT-LG or Mt-LG) or high glucose concentrations (WT-HG or Mt-HG) and luciferase activity was measured. Reprinted in part, from reference 23.*

Significant CAT activity was only detected in islets cultivated at the high glucose concentration (20 mM) and maximal glucose-stimulated transcriptional activity (six-fold) was obtained in islets transfected with the wild type (aa 1-120 in G2) or the A box-deleted form (aa 20-120 in G4) of the N-terminal domain (Figure 3). However, removal of the last 23 amino acids (aa 1-97 in G3) or of the B box (aa 50-120 in G5) completely abolished the glucose effect on transcription. To prove that the high glucose effect on transactivation is specific to the N-terminal region of the hpdx-1 portion of the chimeric protein, the Gal4-VP16 chimeric transcription factor was used as control (90). Furthermore, Petersen et al. (61) showed that the N-terminal domain (aa 1-149) of the rat pdx-1 was also regulated by the metabolizable mannose but not by 2-deoxy-glucose that is not metabolized in cells.

The low transcriptional activity exhibited by the wild type Gal4-hpdx-1 fusion protein may be due to one or more mechanisms. Activation and repression domains in pdx-1 could function by engaging different components of the basal transcriptional complex. Alternatively, these regions might interact with different surfaces of the same transcriptional component or compete directly with each other for a common binding site within the transcriptional machinery. Another possibility of a direct interaction between the N-terminal and the C-terminal sequences of pdx-1 is that, under certain conditions, e.g. following exposure of the islets to high glucose concentrations, could be relieved. A mechanism converting this protein from an inactive state to a state of positive or negative activity would conceivably turn on its diverse functions in a regulated manner, following a stimulus such as glucose. Summing up the evidence accumulated so far, glucose not only increases the pdx-1 DNA binding activity but also stimulates its transactivation potency.

Long-term effects of glucose on insulin gene expression and transcription factors

Several recent studies have shown that chronic elevation of the blood glucose concentration in man and in experimental animals reduces insulin secretion as well as β-cell insulin content. This has led to the concept of "glucose toxicity" (see chapters on glucotoxicity). As described in the first part of this chapter, short-term regulation of the insulin gene appears to be modulated by several transcription factors: pdx-1, the RIPE3b1-activator (or C1) and possibly IEF1. Robertson and co-workers (62-65) have demonstrated reduced binding of both pdx-1 and RIPE3b1-Act following chronic exposure of the insulinoma cell line HIT-T15 to high glucose concentrations, while in βTC6 cells, another insulinoma line, the binding of only RIPE3b1-Act (65) was affected. Thus, the role of insulin transcription factors in overall insulin gene expression remains controversial, one reason being the variability associated with the specific β-cell line investigated. It was, therefore, important to assess the effect of chronic exposure to high glucose concentrations in normal adult human islets. Indeed, several β-cell functions were impaired when cultured human islets were chronically exposed to high glucose concentrations. Thus, within a few days, glucose-induced insulin release was markedly reduced and islet insulin content diminished. This was accompanied by a major reduction in insulin mRNA and in the transcriptional activity of the human insulin promoter. Restoration of glucose concentrations to normal partially reversed these deleterious effects (91). We tested whether the observed loss in human insulin promoter activity was because of changes in the binding of the above mentioned transcription factors. We found a marked reduction in pdx-1 binding to the human insulin A3 element in islets chronically exposed to high glucose concentrations for four and nine days, which fell to 60% and 45%, respectively, of the binding intensity obtained at normal glucose concentrations (Figure 4A). The specific binding activity of RIPE3b1-Act in these cells was also reduced, albeit to a much lesser extent, at days 4 and 9, dropping to 73% and 83%, respectively, of the control. In contrast, IEF1 binding to the rat insulin promoter I E1 element was unaffected (Figure 4A). The described decline in pdx-1 binding appears to correlate largely with the reduction in pdx-1 mRNA, as measured by RT-PCR (Figure 4B). In addition, the reverse experiment showed, to a certain degree, the recovery of both insulin and pdx-1 mRNA levels.

Thus, the reduction in insulin gene expression and the subsequent decline in proinsulin biosynthesis, combined with β-cell hypersecretion caused by elevated glucose concentrations, i.e. a prolonged imbalance between insulin synthesis and secretion is responsible for the diminished hormone stores.

More recently, it was shown that the transcription factor c/EBP β is upregulated in the β-cell lines HIT-15 and INS-1 (66), in the Zucker fatty (fa/fa) rat, as well as in 90% pancreatectomized rats, where it was associated with the manifestation of hyperglycaemia during the development of diabetes (67). c/EBP beta inhibits insulin promoter activity in β-cell lines by directly interacting with one of the second activation domains of the bHLH protein E47.

Further studies with islets are necessary to elucidate the molecular mechanisms accountable for the deleterious effects of high glucose concentrations on insulin gene transcription and on the activity and/or expression of the transcription factors responsible for these phenomena. It has been suggested that glycation and reactive oxygen species, which are generated *in vivo* under chronic hyperglycaemia, may serve as mediators of such effects (68).

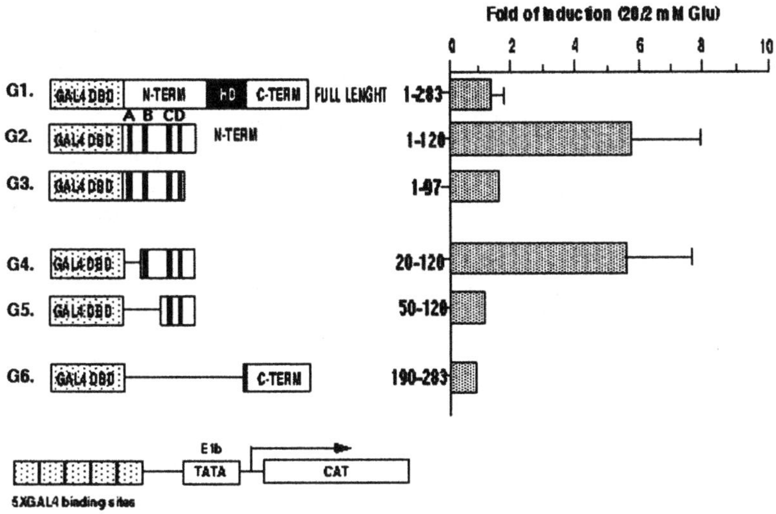

Figure 3. *The N-terminal domain of hpdx-1 confers glucose-mediated transactivation in rat islets. Various sequences of hpdx-1 were fused to the Gal4 DNA binding domain (Gal4-DBD). The structure of the full-length hpdx-1 is schematically represented in plasmid G1. HD in the black box represents the homeodomain, which is flanked by the N- and the C-terminal domains. For constructs G2-G6, numbers indicate the fused hpdx-1amino acids sequences. The conserved A-D boxes in the N-terminal domain are represented by bars. The chimeric plasmids were cotransfected into cultured rat islets with the CAT reporter plasmid, controlled by 5 copies of the Gal4 binding site and the internal control plasmid CMV-β-galactosidase. Results representing the mean ± S.D. of three to six independent experiments are depicted as fold activation of the normalized CAT activity of islets incubated in 20 versus 2 mM glucose. Reprinted in part, from reference 90.*

STIMULUS-TRANSCRIPTION COUPLING IN THE β-CELL

The β-cell is equipped to respond to increases in blood glucose levels by accelerating the rate of hexose metabolism, as well as stimulating insulin release and production. The important elements involved in glucose sensing are the non-rate-limiting glucose transporter, Glut2 (69)› and the high Km hexokinase, the β-cell-specific glucokinase (70). The regulation of proinsulin biosynthesis in pancreatic β-cells is vital for maintaining optimal insulin stores for glucose-induced insulin release.

The signalling pathway/s implicated in the induction of insulin gene transcription by glucose is unclear. Detailed studies on glucose-induced insulin secretion in β-cells show that it is initiated by closure of the ATP-regulated potassium channels. This results in depolarization of the membrane, with subsequent opening of the voltage-dependent calcium channels, causing a rise in cytosolic calcium.

Several lines of evidence indicate that glucose metabolism is essential to β-cell specific induced-gene expression. Ferrer et al (71) showed that the metabolizable sugars mannose and glyceraldehyde enhanced proinsulin and GLUT2 transporter mRNA levels. This was in contrast to the lack of stimulation by the nonmetabolizable analogue 2-deoxy-D-glucose, pointing to a common signalling mechanism(s) in glucose regulation of proinsulin and GLUT2 gene expression. Gasa et al. (72) also reported that expression of the islet amyloid polypeptide (IAPP) gene is regulated by signals deriving from glucose metabolism. The findings that insulin gene expression is inhibited by calcium channel blockers (48,51) and activated following β-cell membrane depolarization (73), suggest that the observed stimulatory effect is mediated by calcium, although this concept has been contested (44,53). It is, however, conceivable that at least one component involved in the transmission of the glucose stimulus for β-cell-specific gene expression activates a calcium-dependent pathway/s.

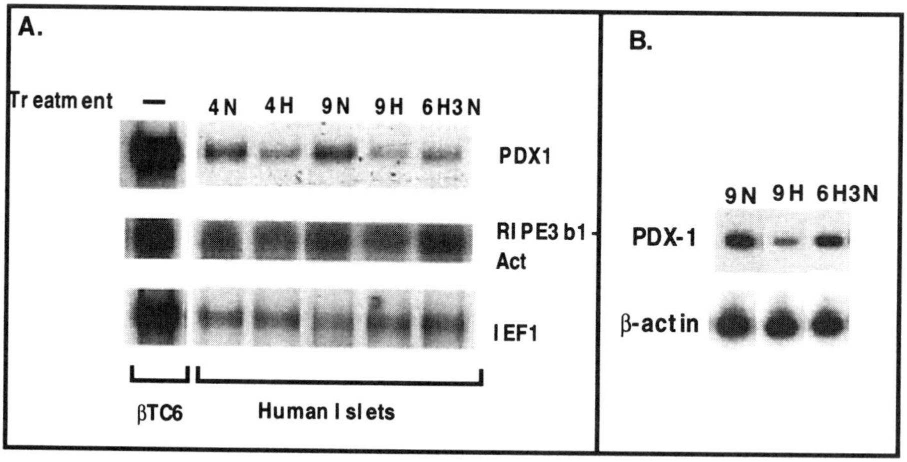

Figure 4. *Effect of chronic exposure to high glucose on binding activities of human islet nuclear proteins to insulin-promoter regulatory elements.* ***A)*** *Nuclear proteins were extracted from human islets treated for 4 and 9 days in 5.5 mM (4N, 9N) or 33 mM glucose (4H, 9H) or, in the reverse experiment, maintained for 6 days in high glucose then switched to normal glucose concentrations for 3 days (6H3N). The extracts were incubated with labeled sequences of human A3, rat II RIPE3b1 or rat I IEF1/E1 insulin gene elements. βTC6 cell extracts were used as a β-cell specific control.* ***B)*** *Quantitative PCR of pdx-1 mRNAs from cultured human islets incubated for 9 days at different glucose concentrations. RNA isolated from human islets treated as described in A) was reverse transcribed. The corresponding cDNAs were amplified by PCR, using oligonucleotides complementary to sequences in the human β-actin and pdx-1 genes. The intensity of the radiolabeled β-actin band was used to normalize mRNA levels. Reprinted in part, from ref. 91.*

Two general mechanisms have evolved for the rapid and accurate transmission of signals from cell-surface receptors to the nucleus. Both are associated with protein phosphorylation. One mechanism depends on the regulated translocation of activated protein kinases from the cytoplasm to the nucleus, where they phosphorylate target transcription factors. In the second, transcription factors are maintained in a latent state in the cytoplasm and are translocated into the nucleus upon activation. Most commonly, regulation is achieved by reversible phosphorylation. The rapid changes in the binding of pdx-1 to the human probe shown in Figure 1A may imply a post-translational modification, rather than *de novo* protein synthesis. Indeed, no difference in binding properties was observed when cycloheximide was added to medium containing low or high glucose concentrations (data not shown). The possibility that the post-translational event relates to the degree of glycosylation of the protein was tested in islets following variations in extracellular glucose levels. The results ruled out this prospect, in spite of the presence of a potential glycosylation site, according to the deduced sequence of pdx-1 in the homeobox domain (not shown).

β-cell glucose metabolism activates a variety of signalling pathways, several of which presumably regulate insulin gene transcription. Because cAMP can augment insulin mRNA levels (43,48) it has been proposed that the cAMP pathway contributes directly to glucose-stimulated insulin transcription. We tested whether incubation of the β-cells in the presence of forskolin, which raises the level of intracellular cAMP, would mimic the increased pdx-1 binding activity observed following incubation of islets in high glucose concentrations. The finding that no additional effect on pdx-1 binding was obtained in islet cells treated with low or high glucose concentrations in the presence of forskolin indicates that elevated cAMP does not contribute to the glucose effect (data not shown, 24). It is more likely that cAMP induces insulin gene expression through the stimulated interaction of transcription factor CREB with its recognition site (74,76).

Protein phosphorylation is a major mechanism for controlling gene expression in response to extracellular stimuli. It is considered that different extracellular stimuli elicit distinct transcriptional responses by activating specific protein kinases that uniquely phosphorylate sequence-specific transcription factors (77,78).

In the β-cell, glucose and ligands acting at the cell surface regulate insulin release by modulating the concentrations of intracellular second messengers. These mediators mainly modulate the activities of regulated protein kinases that, in turn, phosphorylate substrates on serine/threonine residues. Signalling pathways involving activation of kinases such as protein kinase A (PKA), protein kinase C (PKC), members of the calcium calmodulin- dependent kinases (CaMK) and of the mitogen activated protein kinases (MAPK), have been described in the pancreatic β-cell (79). However, the mechanism(s) by which glucose metabolism modulates their activity, leading to modification of the phosphorylation state of insulin transcription factors and, consequently, the rate of insulin gene transcription, remains obscure.

Macfarlane et al. (24) reported that in human islets, or in the mouse β-cell line MIN6, the effect of high glucose concentrations on pdx-1 binding to DNA is dependent on glucose metabolism, as it was inhibited by mannoheptulose. Most importantly, the glucose effect was mimicked by serine/threonine phosphatase inhibitors. This indicates that induction of the DNA binding activity relates to changes in the phosphorylation state of the protein. The glucose-stimulated binding of pdx-1 to DNA and the pdx-1-dependent gene transcription were both prevented by a specific inhibitor of stress-activated p38 MAPK (p38 kinase) (80). The same group (81) showed, by Western blotting and an electrophoretic mobility shift assay, that in human islets of Langerhans incubated in low glucose concentrations pdx-1 is present as an inactive 31-kDa protein localized exclusively in the cytoplasm. Transfer of the islets to high glucose concentrations resulted in rapid conversion of PDX1 to an active 46-kDa form that was found predominantly in the nucleus. Overexpression of p38 kinase mimicked the glucose effect on pdx-1 and also stimulated pdx-1-dependent transcription of the human insulin gene promoter. However, using antibodies raised against the N-terminal domain of the human pdx-1 and *Xenopus laevis* XlHbox8 proteins we could not detect a 31 KDa form of pdx-1 in islets incubated in low glucose concentrations. It is not clear whether this discrepancy is due to the different antibodies used in identifying the protein. Furthermore, Rafiq et al. (82) monitored glucose-induced changes in the subcellular localization of transfected pdx-1 labelled with a c-myc epitope tag, using laser-scanning confocal microscopy. In the majority of cells maintained at a low extracellular glucose concentration, pdx-1.c-myc immunoreactivity was confined to the nuclear periphery. Incubation of cells at stimulatory glucose concentrations caused a rapid redistribution of the chimera to the nucleoplasm, in parallel with the stimulation of the transcriptional activity of an insulin promoter construct. Apparently, the glucose signalling pathways that modulate the phosphorylation of pdx-1 (24,61,80,81) trigger its movement from the cytoplasm or the nuclear periphery to the nucleoplasm, thereby enhancing the trans-activational capacity of this factor in β-cells.

Mitogen-activated protein kinases play a major role in the regulation of transcription factor activity in response to extracellular stimuli (77,78). MAPKs have been implicated in phosphorylation and activation of a wide array of transcription factors in mammals and yeast (77,83). For example, whereas the c-Jun transcription factor is specifically phosphorylated by a distinct MAPK or a subgroup of closely related MAPKs (78), the single ternary complex transcription factor (TCF)/Elk-1 is phosphorylated by several MAPKs that respond to different stimuli (84,85).

The role played by MAPKs in the regulation of insulin secretion from rat islets of Langerhans has been investigated by examining the glucose effect on islet MAPK activity and measuring the secreted insulin. Persaud et al. (86) reported that in isolated islets high glucose concentration had a small (less than two-fold) stimulatory effect on MAPK activity. In contrast, in the rat insulinoma cell line INS-1, Frodin et al. (88) found that glucose metabolism led to the activation of ERK1, a member of the MAPK family, and that although its increased activity correlated with stimulated insulin-secretion, ERKs were also activated by agents that did not promote secretion. Furthermore, Khoo and Cobb (89) showed that in these cells ERK1 and ERK2 are activated up to 15-fold by glucose. Although ERK activation was dependent on glucose metabolism, insulin secretion was normal even when ERKs activity was blocked. The variable degree of MAPK activation by glucose stresses once again the differences between normal and transformed islet cells. However, the conclusion that emerges from these studies is that ERK activation is neither sufficient nor crucial for inducing secretion (86-89). In addition, in INS-1 cells glucose elicited a marked translocation of ERKs to the nucleus, suggesting their possible role in glucose-dependent nuclear events in β-cells. Interestingly, the p38 kinase, which was shown to be activated by glucose in MIN6 insulinoma cells (80), was only slightly responsive (1.5-fold) (89).

It may be some time before the complexity of glucose signalling to insulin transcription factors is fully resolved. A series of potential activated protein kinases in β-cells may respond to extracellular signals such as Ca-dependent protein kinases and/or members of the MAP kinase family. The identification of specific phosphorylated sites modified by variations in extracellular glucose concentrations is of crucial importance in determining the specific kinases involved in such regulation.

ACKNOWLEDGEMENTS

The author is indebted to Prof. E. Cerasi for his longstanding collaboration and invaluable aid and wishes to express her gratitude to S. Marshak, E. Ben Shushan, G. Leibovitch, R. Oron, as well as to all the members of the Department of Endocrinology and Metabolism, for their contributions. This work was supported by grants from the Juvenile Diabetes Foundation and the Israel Academy of Sciences.

REFERENCES

1. Stein R. Regulation of insulin gene transcription. Trends Endocrinol & Metab 1993;4:96-101.
2. Dumonteil E, Philippe J. Insulin gene: organization, expression and regulation. Diabetes Metab1996;22:164-73.
3. Docherty K, Clark AR. Nutrient regulation of insulin gene expression. Faseb J 1994;8:20-7.
4. Steiner DF, Chan SJ, Welsh JM, Kwok SC. Structure and evolution of the insulin gene. Annu Rev Genet 1985;19:463-84.
5. Sander M, German MS. The beta cell transcription factors and development of the pancreas. J Mol Med 1997;75:327-40.
6. German M, Ashcroft S, Docherty K, et al. The insulin gene promoter. A simplified nomenclature. Diabetes 1995; 44:1002-4.
7. Murre C, McCaw PS, Baltimore D. A new DNA binding and dimerization motif in immunoglobulin enhancer binding, daughterless, MyoD, and myc proteins. Cell 1989; 56:777-83.
8. Walker MD, Park CW, Rosen A, Aronheim A. A cDNA from a mouse pancreatic beta cell encoding a putative transcription factor of the insulin gene. Nucleic Acids Res 1990;18:1159-66.
9. Shibasaki Y, Sakura H, Takaku F, Kasuga M. Insulin enhancer binding protein has helix-loop-helix structure. Biochem Biophys Res Commun 1990;170:314-21.
10. Cordle SR, Henderson E, Masuoka H, Weil PA, Stein R. Pancreatic beta-cell-type-specific transcription of the insulin gene is mediated by basic helix-loop-helix DNA-binding proteins. Mol Cell Biol 1991;11:1734-8.
11. German MS, Blanar MA, Nelson C, Moss LG, Rutter WJ. Two related helix-loop-helix proteins participate in separate cell-specific complexes that bind the insulin enhancer. Mol Endocrinol 1991;5:292-9.
12. Peyton M, Moss LG, Tsai MJ. Two distinct class A helix-loop-helix transcription factors, E2A and BETA1, form separate DNA binding complexes on the insulin gene E box. J Biol Chem 1994;269:25936-41.
13. Naya FJ, Stellrecht CM, Tsai MJ. Tissue-specific regulation of the insulin gene by a novel basic helix-loop-helix transcription factor. Genes Dev 1995;9:1009-19.
14. Itkin-Ansari P, Bain G, Beattie G M, Murre C, Hayek A, Levine F. E2A gene products are not required for insulin gene expression. Endocrinology 1996;8:3540-3.
15. Sharma A, Henderson E, Gamer L, Zhuang Y, Stein R. Analysis of the role of E2A-encoded proteins in insulin gene transcription. Mol Endocrinol 1997;11:1608-17.
16. Naya FJ, Huang HP, Qiu Y, et al. Diabetes, defective pancreatic morphogenesis, and abnormal enteroendocrine differentiation in BETA2/neuroD-deficient mice. Genes Dev 1997;11:2323-34.

17. Read ML, Clark AR, Docherty K. The helix-loop-helix transcription factor USF (upstream stimulating factor) binds to a regulatory sequence of the human insulin gene enhancer. Biochem J 1993;295:233-7.
18. Wright CV, Schnegelsberg P, De Robertis EM. XlHbox 8: a novel Xenopus homeo protein restricted to a narrow band of endoderm. Development 1989;105:787-94.
19. Ohlsson H, Karlsson K, Edlund T. IPF1, a homeodomain-containing transactivator of the insulin gene. Embo J 1993;12:4251-9.
20. Leonard J, Peers B, Johnson T, Ferreri K, Lee S, Montminy MR. Characterization of somatostatin transactivating factor-1, a novel homeobox factor that stimulates somatostatin expression in pancreatic islet cells. Mol Endocrinol 1993;7:1275-83.
21. Miller CP, McGehee RE, Jr., Habener JF. IDX-1: a new homeodomain transcription factor expressed in rat pancreatic islets and duodenum that transactivates the somatostatin gene. Embo J 1994;13:1145-56.
22. Melloul D, Ben-Neriah Y, Cerasi E. Glucose modulates the binding of an islet-specific factor to a conserved sequence within the rat I and the human insulin promoters. Proc Natl Acad Sci USA 1993;90:3865-9.
23. Marshak S, Totary H, Cerasi E, Melloul D. Purification of the beta-cell glucose-sensitive factor that transactivates the insulin gene differentially in normal and transformed islet cells. Proc Natl Acad Sci USA 1996;93:15057-62.
24. MacFarlane WM, Read ML, Gilligan M, Bujalska I, Docherty K. Glucose modulates the binding activity of the beta-cell transcription factor IUF1 in a phosphorylation-dependent manner. Biochem J 1994;303:625-31.
25. Waeber G, Thompson N, Nicod P, Bonny C. Transcriptional activation of the GLUT2 gene by the IPF-1/STF-1/IDX-1 homeobox factor. Mol Endocrinol 1996;10:1327-34.
26. Watada H, Kajimoto Y, Umayahara Y, et al. The human glucokinase gene beta-cell-type promoter: an essential role of insulin promoter factor 1/PDX-1 in its activation in HIT-T15 cells. Diabetes 1996;45:1478-88.
27. Petersen HV, Serup P, Leonard J, Michelsen BK, Madsen OD. Transcriptional regulation of the human insulin gene is dependent on the homeodomain protein STF1/IPF1 acting through the CT boxes. Proc Natl Acad Sci USA 1994;91:10465-9.
28. Jonsson J, Carlsson L, Edlund T, Edlund H. Insulin-promoter-factor 1 is required for pancreas development in mice. Nature 1994;371:606-9.
29. Slack JM. Developmental biology of the pancreas. Development 1995;121:1569-80.
30. Jonsson J, Ahlgren U, Edlund T, Edlund H. IPF1, a homeodomain protein with a dual function in pancreas development. Int J Dev Biol 1995;39:789-98.
31. Guz Y, Montminy MR, Stein R, et al. Expression of murine STF-1, a putative insulin gene transcription factor, in beta cells of pancreas, duodenal epithelium and pancreatic exocrine and endocrine progenitors during ontogeny. Development 1995;121:11-8.
32. Serup P, Petersen HV, Pedersen EE, et al. The homeodomain protein IPF-1/STF-1 is expressed in a subset of islet cells and promotes rat insulin 1 gene expression dependent on an intact E1 helix-loop-helix factor binding site. Biochem J 1995;310:997-1003.
33. Ahlgren U, Jonsson J, Edlund H. The morphogenesis of the pancreatic mesenchyme is uncoupled from that of the pancreatic epithelium in IPF1/PDX1-deficient mice. Development 1996;122:1409-16.
34. Offield MF, Jetton TL, Labosky PA, et al. PDX-1 is required for pancreatic outgrowth and differentiation of the rostral duodenum. Development 1996;122:983-95.
35. Madsen OD, Jensen J, Blume N, et al. Pancreatic development and maturation of the islet B cell. Studies of pluripotent islet cultures. Eur J Biochem 1996;242:435-45.
36. Ahlgren U, Jonsson J, Jonsson L, Simu K, Edlund H. Beta-cell-specific inactivation of the mouse Ipf1/Pdx1 gene results in loss of the beta-cell phenotype and maturity onset diabetes. Genes Dev 1998;12:1763-8.
37. Karlsson O, Thor S, Norberg T, Ohlsson H, Edlund T. Insulin gene enhancer binding protein Isl-1 is a member of a novel class of proteins containing both a homeo- and a Cys-His domain. Nature 1990;344:879-82.
38. German MS, Wang J, Chadwick RB, Rutter WJ. Synergistic activation of the insulin gene by a LIM-homeo domain protein and a basic helix-loop-helix protein: building a functional insulin minienhancer complex. Genes Dev 1992;6:2165-76.

39. Emens LA, Landers DW, Moss LG. Hepatocyte nuclear factor 1 alpha is expressed in a hamster insulinoma line and transactivates the rat insulin I gene. Proc Natl Acad Sci U S A 1992;89:7300-4.
40. Peers B, Leonard J, Sharma S, Teitelman G, Montminy MR. Insulin expression in pancreatic islet cells relies on cooperative interactions between the helix loop helix factor E47 and the homeobox factor STF-1. Mol Endocrinol 1994;8:1798-806.
41. Peshavaria M, Henderson E, Sharma A, Wright CV, Stein R. Functional characterization of the transactivation properties of the PDX-1 homeodomain protein. Mol Cell Biol 1997;17:3987-96.
42. Brunstedt J, Chan SJ. Direct effect of glucose on the preproinsulin mRNA level in isolated pancreatic islets. Biochem Biophys Res Commun 1982;106:1383-1389.
43. Nielsen DA, Welsh M, Casadaban MJ, Steiner DF. Control of insulin gene expression in pancreatic beta-cells and in an insulin-producing cell line, RIN-5F cells. I. Effects of glucose and cyclic AMP on the transcription of insulin mRNA. J Biol Chem 1985;260:13585-9.
44. Welsh M, Nielsen DA, MacKrell AJ, Steiner DF. Control of insulin gene expression in pancreatic beta-cells and in an insulin-producing cell line, RIN-5F cells. II. Regulation of insulin mRNA stability. J Biol Chem 1985;260:13590-4.
45. Hammonds P, Schofield PN, Ashcroft SJ, Sutton R, Gray DW. Regulation and specificity of glucose-stimulated insulin gene expression in human islets of Langerhans. FEBS Lett 1987;223:131-7.
46. Hammonds P, Schofield PN, Ashcroft SJ. Glucose regulates preproinsulin messenger RNA levels in a clonal cell line of simian virus 40-transformed β cells. FEBS Lett 1987;213:149-54.
47. Nagamatsu S, Grodsky GM. Glucose-regulated proinsulin processing in isolated islets from rat pancreas. Diabetes 1988;37:1426-31.
48. German MS, Moss LG, Rutter WJ. Regulation of insulin gene expression by glucose and calcium in transfected primary islet cultures. J Biol Chem 1990;265:22063-6.
49. Redmon JB, Towle HC, Robertson RP. Regulation of human insulin gene transcription by glucose, epinephrine, and somatostatin. Diabetes 1994;43:546-51.
50. Wang J, Shen L, Najafi H, et al. Regulation of insulin preRNA splicing by glucose. Proc Natl Acad Sci USA 1997;94:4360-5.
51. Efrat S, Surana M, Fleischer N. Glucose induces insulin gene transcription in a murine pancreatic beta- cell line. J Biol Chem 1991;266:11141-3.
52. Leibiger B, Moede T, Schwarz T, et al. Short-term regulation of insulin gene transcription by glucose. Proc Natl Acad Sci USA 1998;95:9307-12.
53. Goodison S, Kenna S, Ashcroft SJ. Control of insulin gene expression by glucose. Biochem J 1992;285:563-8.
54. German MS, Wang J. The insulin gene contains multiple transcriptional elements that respond to glucose. Mol Cell Biol 1994;14:4067-75.
55. Sharma A, Stein R. Glucose-induced transcription of the insulin gene is mediated by factors required for beta-cell-type-specific expression. Mol Cell Biol 1994;14:871-9.
56. Sander M, Griffen SC, Huang J, German MS. A novel glucose-responsive element in the human insulin gene functions uniquely in primary cultured islets. Proc Natl Acad Sci USA 1998;95:11572-7.
57. Sharma A, Fusco-DeMane D, Henderson E, Efrat S, Stein R. The role of the insulin control element and RIPE3b1 -activator in glucose-stimulated transcription of the insulin gene. Mol Endocrinol 1995;9:1468-76.
58. Read ML, Masson MR, Docherty K. A RIPE3b1-like factor binds to a novel site in the human insulin promoter in a redox-dependent manner. FEBS Lett 1997;418:68-72.
59. Sadowski I, Ptashne M. A vector for expressing GAL4(1-147) fusions in mammalian cells. NucleicAcids Res 1989;17:7539.
60. Lu M, Miller C, Habener JF. Functional regions of the homeodomain protein IDX-1 required for transactivation of the rat somatostatin gene. Endocrinology 1996;137:2959-67.
61. Petersen HV, Peshavaria M, Pedersen AA, et al. Glucose stimulates the activation domain potential of the PDX-1 homeodomain transcription factor. FEBS Lett 1998;431:362-6.
62. Olson LK, Sharma A, Peshavaria M, et al. Reduction of insulin gene transcription in HIT-T15 beta cells chronically exposed to a supraphysiologic glucose concentration is associated with loss of STF-1 transcription factor expression [published erratum appears in Proc Natl Acad Sci USA 1995 Nov 21;92(24):11322]. Proc Natl Acad Sci USA 1995;92:9127-31.

63. Sharma A, Olson LK, Robertson RP, Stein R. The reduction of insulin gene transcription in HIT-T15 beta cells chronically exposed to high glucose concentration is associated with the loss of RIPE3b1 and STF-1 transcription factor expression. Mol Endocrinol 1995;9:1127-34.
64. Moran A, Zhang HJ, Olson LK, Harmon JS, Poitout V, Robertson RP. Differentiation of glucose toxicity from beta cell exhaustion during the evolution of defective insulin gene expression in the pancreatic islet cell line, HIT-T15. J Clin Invest 1997;99:534-9.
65. Poitout V, Olson LK, Robertson RP. Chronic exposure of betaTC-6 cells to supraphysiologic concentrations of glucose decreases binding of the RIPE3b1 insulin gene transcription activator. J Clin Invest 1996;97:1041-6.
66. Lu M, Seufert J, Habener JF. Pancreatic beta-cell-specific repression of insulin gene transcription by CCAAT/enhancer-binding protein beta. Inhibitory interactions with basic helix-loop-helix transcription factor E47. J Biol Chem 1997;272:28349-59.
67. Seufert J, Weir GC, Habener JF. Differential expression of the insulin gene transcriptional repressor CCAAT/enhancer-binding protein beta and transactivator islet duodenum homeobox-1 in rat pancreatic beta cells during the development of diabetes mellitus. J Clin Invest 1998;101:2528-39.
68. Matsuoka T, Kajimoto Y, Watada H, et al. Glycation-dependent, reactive oxygen species-mediated suppression of the insulin gene promoter activity in HIT cells. J Clin Invest 1997;99:144-50.
69. Thorens B, Sarkar HK, Kaback HR, Lodish HF. Cloning and functional expression in bacteria of a novel glucose transporter present in liver, intestine, kidney, and beta-pancreatic islet cells. Cell 1988;55:281-90.
70. Matschinsky FM. Glucokinase as glucose sensor and metabolic signal generator in pancreatic beta-cells and hepatocytes. Diabetes 1990;39:647-52.
71. Ferrer J, Gomis R, Fernandez Alvarez J, Casamitjana R, Vilardell E. Signals derived from glucose metabolism are required for glucose regulation of pancreatic islet GLUT2 mRNA and protein. Diabetes 1993;42:1273-80.
72. Gasa R, Gomis R, Casamitjana R, Novials A. Signals related to glucose metabolism regulate islet amyloid polypeptide (IAPP) gene expression in human pancreatic islets. Regul Pept 1997;68:99-104.
73. Leibiger IB, Leibiger B, Moede T, Berggren PO. Exocytosis of insulin promotes insulin gene transcription via the insulin receptor/PI-3 kinase/p70 s6 kinase and CaM kinase pathways. Mol Cell 1998;1:933-8.
74. Philippe J, Missotten M. Functional characterization of a cAMP-responsive element of the rat insulin I gene. J Biol Chem 1990;265:1465-9.
75. Oetjen E, Diedrich T, Eggers A, Eckert B, Knepel W. Distinct properties of the cAMP-responsive element of the rat insulin I gene. J Biol Chem 1994;269:27036-44.
76. Eggers A, Siemann G, Blume R, Knepel W. Gene-specific transcriptional activity of the insulin cAMP-responsive element is conferred by NF-Y in combination with cAMP response element-binding protein. J Biol Chem 1998;273:18499-508.
77. Hill CS, Treisman R. Transcriptional regulation by extracellular signals: mechanisms and specificity. Cell 1995;80:199-211.
78. Karin M, Hunter T. Transcriptional control by protein phosphorylation: signal transmission from the cell surface to the nucleus. Curr Biol 1995;5:747-57.
79. Jones PM, Persaud SJ. Protein kinases, protein phosphorylation, and the regulation of insulin secretion from pancreatic beta-cells. Endocr Rev 1998;19:429-61.
80. Macfarlane WM, Smith SB, James RF, et al. The p38/reactivating kinase mitogen-activated protein kinase cascade mediates the activation of the transcription factor insulin upstream factor 1 and insulin gene transcription by high glucose in pancreatic beta-cells. J Biol Chem 1997;272:20936-44.
81. Macfarlane WM, McKinnon CM, Felton-Edkins ZA, Cragg H, James RF, Docherty K. Glucose stimulates translocation of the homeodomain transcription factor PDX1 from the cytoplasm to the nucleus in pancreatic beta-cells. J Biol Chem 1999;274:1011-6.
82. Rafiq I, Kennedy HJ, Rutter GA. Glucose-dependent translocation of insulin promoter factor-1 (IPF-1) between the nuclear periphery and the nucleoplasm of single MIN6 beta-cells. J Biol Chem 1998;273:23241-7.
83. Herskowitz I. MAP kinase pathways in yeast: for mating and more. Cell 1995;80:187-97.
84. Cavigelli M, Dolfi F, Claret FX, Karin M. Induction of c-fos expression through JNK-mediated TCF/Elk-1 phosphorylation. Embo J 1995;14:5957-64.

85. Whitmarsh AJ, Shore P, Sharrocks AD, Davis RJ. Integration of MAP kinase signal transduction pathways at the serum response element. Science 1995;269:403-7.
86. Persaud SJ, Wheeler-Jones CP, Jones PM. The mitogen-activated protein kinase pathway in rat islets of Langerhans: studies on the regulation of insulin secretion. Biochem J 1996;313:119-24.
87. Burns CJ, Howell SL, Jones PM, Persaud SJ. Glucose-stimulated insulin secretion from rat islets of Langerhans is independent of mitogen-activated protein kinase activation. Biochem Biophys Res Commun 1997;239:447-50.
88. Frodin M, Sekine N, Roche E, et al. Glucose, other secretagogues, and nerve growth factor stimulate mitogen-activated protein kinase in the insulin-secreting beta-cell line, INS-1. J Biol Chem 1995;270:7882-9.
89. Khoo S, Cobb MH. Activation of mitogen-activating protein kinase by glucose is not required for insulin secretion. Proc Natl Acad Sci USA 1997;94:5599-604.
90. Ben Shushan E, Cerasi E, Melloul D. Regulation of the insulin gene by glucose: Stimulation of transactivation potency of the human PDX-1 N-terminal domain. DNA Cell Biol 1999;18:471-79.
91. Marshak S, Leibowitz G, Bertuzzi F, Socci C, Kaiser N, Gross J, Cerasi E, Melloul D. Impaired β-Cell functions induced by chronic exposure of cultured human pancreatic islets to high glucose. Diabetes 1999;48(6).

3
β-CELL DYSFUNCTION AND CHRONIC HYPERGLYCAEMIA

Jack L. Leahy, M.D.
University of Vermont, Burlington, VT 05405 USA

INTRODUCTION

Type 2 diabetes mellitus is a complex illness with both genetic and environmental pathogenic elements. Disturbed insulin secretion (*β-cell dysfunction*) and tissue insulin insensitivity *(insulin resistance)* are jointly found, and there is controversy as to which comes first, and how they interact to lead to diabetes mellitus. Studies in high risk populations for type 2 diabetes have delineated the natural history of type 2 diabetes mellitus (Figure 1): yet undefined genetic mutation(s) combine with metabolic and lifestyle factors to cause the diabetes phenotype. Insulin resistance and β-cell dysfunction are shown at the bottom of Figure 1: they are present to some degree before glucose intolerance is detectable. The environmental factors aggravate insulin resistance (obesity, inactivity, aging, and pregnancy) or the β-cell dysfunction (electrolyte abnormalities, several drugs, and malnutrition). However, the insulin resistance typically worsens little during the early stages of the disease, when glucose intolerance progresses to overt fasting hyperglycaemia. Instead, the factor determining whether diabetes occurs is β-cell function. As long as β-cells compensate for the insulin resistance through increased insulin secretion, glycaemia can be controlled. Frank diabetes is seen when the β-cell compensation is lost – i.e. *β-cell failure* (1-3).

An important observation made in the late 1970s was that a period of intensive glycaemic control improves insulin secretion in persons with type 2 diabetes (4,5). An active research field has evolved to investigate how the diabetes metabolic milieu negatively affects the β-cell - the term *glucose toxicity* was coined in reference to that concept (6,7). More recently, detrimental effects of elevated levels of free fatty acids on β-cell function have been studied - so-called *lipotoxicity* (8,9). Other potential explanations for the β-cell failure in diabetes are that islet amyloid deposits which are found in type 2 diabetes may lower the functional β-cell mass (10), and speculation that altered β-cell growth factors and/or apoptosis-induced β-cell death may cause the β-cell mass to decline (11). However, the latter two entail a loss of β-cells, which would not acutely reverse with intensive glycaemic control. To summarize, the basis for the β-cell failure in type 2 diabetes is presumed to be multifactorial.

Our laboratory investigates diabetic rodents to better understand the reversible component of β-cell failure. Rats share many features with human type 2 diabetes mellitus in terms of abnormal β-cell function, and make it possible to perform biochemical and molecular studies of isolated islets which is impossible in humans.

We summarize here a working model for the β-cell dysfunction, based on a concept of β-cell "overwork" or "exhaustion" (12).

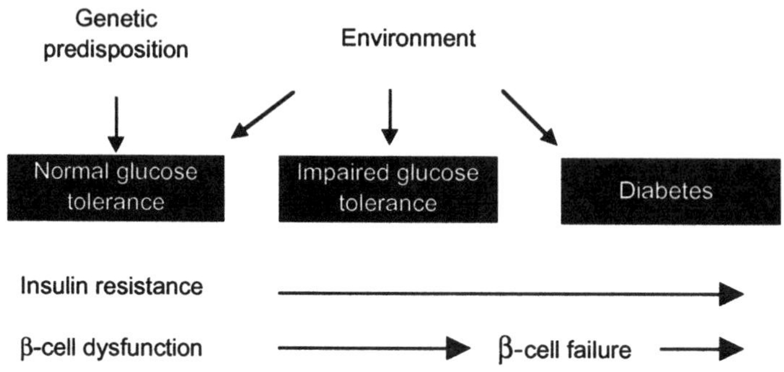

Figure 1. *Schematic for the pathogenesis of type 2 diabetes.*

90% PANCREATECTOMY RAT MODEL

This chapter focuses on studies that we have performed in 90% pancreatectomy (Px) rats. Pancreatectomy is performed by abrading pancreatic tissue off the blood vessels using cotton applicators (13). The surgery is well tolerated - the rats grow normally on standard chow diets - and results in mild sustained hyperglycaemia of 1-2 mM above normal within a week of the surgery. A source of confusion has been that some groups report much higher levels of glycaemia in 90% Px rats, presumably because of removal of more than 90% of pancreatic tissue. In these latter situations, marked hyperglycaemia or other associated metabolic changes may alter β-cell function in ways other than with the mild hyperglycaemia we see. Our studies have been performed to investigate the β-cell failure that occurs during the transition from glucose intolerance to fasting hyperglycaemia; thus, it is crucial to use animals which present with a mild degree of hyperglycaemia.

Natural History of Insulin Secretion in the 90% Pancreatectomy Rat Model

Our initial studies mapped out the natural history of β-cell function in 90% Px rats in order to identify when β-cell failure occurs. Insulin secretion was studied using the *in situ* perfused pancreas (a standard organ perfusion system) at weekly intervals after the surgery. Figure 2 shows mean insulin levels in response to perfusion of 16.7 mM glucose or 16.7 mM glucose + 10 mM arginine. The latter combination mimics the nutrient-induced insulin secretion as occurs with meals - so-called *glucose potentiation* (data from references 14 and 15).

One-week post surgery, insulin responses after administration of both perfusates are normal when adjusted for the reduced β-cell mass (≈20% of normal). Two weeks post surgery, the insulin responses are still relatively intact. By three weeks, the insulin response to 16.7 mM glucose falls by 80% as compared to the one-week post-pancreatectomy value, and glucose-potentiated insulin secretion is also reduced, (although the percentage of decline is somewhat less). The cause is not a loss of β-cells since β-cell mass is increasing during this time period (13).

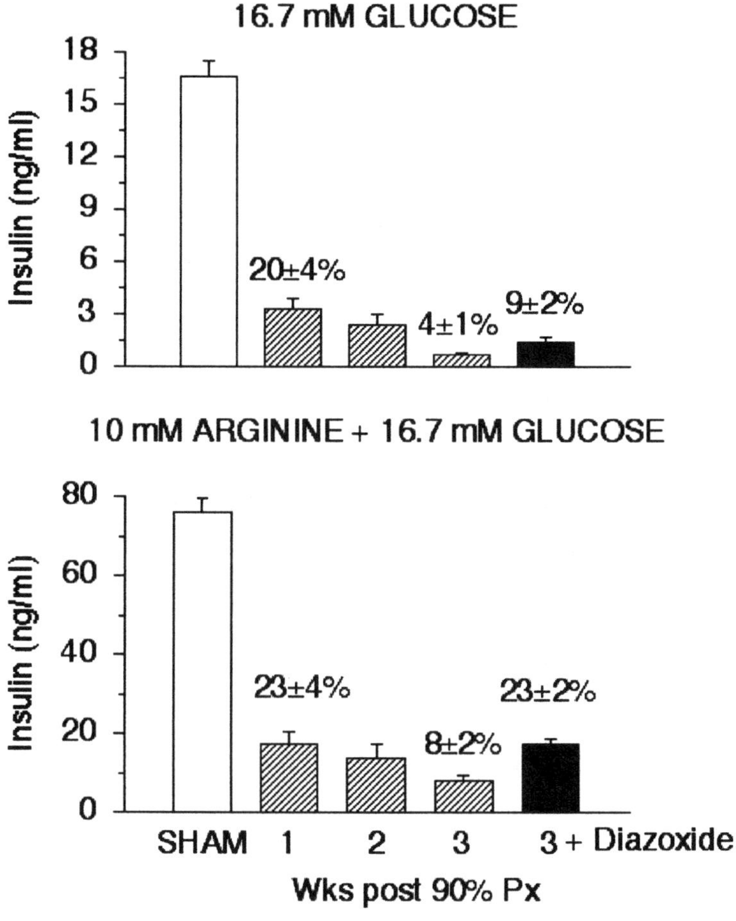

Figure 2. *Natural history of insulin secretion following a 90% pancreatectomy (Px) in rats. Insulin secretion to 16.7 mM glucose and 16.7 mM glucose + 10 mM arginine was assessed with the in situ perfused pancreas at weekly intervals after a 90% Px. Mean insulin responses are shown by the height of the bars; the percentage values above the Px bars are the fractional output (%) versus the 1-week shams (open bars). At three weeks post surgery, both insulin responses of the Px rats fell, showing the onset of β-cell failure. A 5 day treatment period with diazoxide partially blocked the fall in glucose-induced insulin secretion, and normalized that to glucose + arginine (solid bars). Data reprinted with permission from references 14 and 15.*

β-cell Hypersensitivity to Glucose

We initially interpreted the findings in Figure 2 that β-cell function was "normal" until the third week after 90% pancreatectomy. That conclusion proved incorrect when, at one week, we perfused pancreata at glucose concentrations different from 16.7 mM, and found left-shifted curves for both glucose-induced insulin secretion and for glucose potentiation (Figure 3). This observation is crucial in the concept of the "overworked β-cell." Initially it was unclear how the small degree of hyperglycaemia of the Px rats (1-2 mM above normal) could overwork a β-cell. The answer is depicted in Figure 3. At their usual level of glycaemia (9-10 mM), β-cells from the Px rats function close to 100% of secretory capacity as compared to the 10% of control rats at their physiological glycaemia level (7-8 mM). Subsequent studies detailed below show that this β-cell hypersensitivity for glucose plays a dual role in the natural history of this disease. Initially, the resulting insulin hypersecretion counters the insulin resistance or lowered β-cell mass to prevent hyperglycaemia. However, in those who progress to diabetes, β-cell glucose sensitivity further increases to a degree that can not be maintained, ultimately leading to β-cell failure.

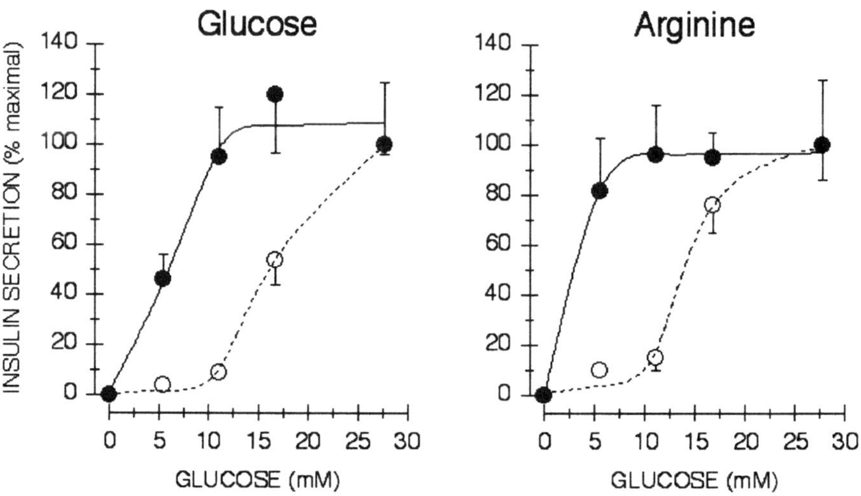

Figure 3. *β-cell glucose hypersensitivity in 90% pancreatectomy (Px) rats. Sham-operated (EKE) and 90% Px rats (JKJ) that were 1 week post surgery underwent in situ pancreas perfusion for 15 minutes using 5.5, 11.1, 16.7 or 27.7 mM glucose followed by an additional 15 minutes of the same glucose concentration + 10 mM arginine. Each point represents the mean effluent insulin concentration from a unique group of rats (n=3-4). Mean insulin responses at each glucose concentration were calculated, and expressed as % of the results at 27.7 mM glucose (% maximal). Note the marked left shift of the curves in the 90% Px rats so that at their usual plasma glucose level (10.6 mM glucose 90% Px rats and 8.1 mM glucose shams in this study), Px β-cells functioned near 100% of secretory capacity versus the normal 10%. Reprinted with permission from reference 14.*

Reversal Studies

Diazoxide, which is an inhibitor of insulin secretion, prevents β-cell dysfunction in rats made hyperglycaemic by 48-hour glucose infusion (16). This observation raises the possibility that β-cell exhaustion or overwork rather than hyperglycaemia *per se* is the basis for glucose toxicity. Ninety-percent Px rats treated with diazoxide orally for five days have clearly improved insulin secretion. In particular, the glucose-potentiated insulin response to arginine is restored to normal (Figure 2) (15). These results support a β-cell exhaustion effect in 90% Px rats. However, a concern is whether some unique effect of diazoxide is operative. We tested this possibility by lowering insulin secretion in 90% Px rats by an alternative approach than diazoxide treatment – a 40-hour fast. In this situation a three-fold increase of glucose-potentiated insulin secretion and a three-fold increase in pancreatic insulin content was found (17). The concept was further tested by causing a hyperstimulated insulin secretion in nondiabetic rats using a high dose infusion of the insulin secretagogue tolbutamide (glucose was also infused to preserve normoglycaemia): insulin content fell by 50% and there was a parallel reduction of insulin secretory responses (18). The results suggest that (nonsustainable) hyperstimulation of insulin secretion, i.e. β-cell overwork, plays a major role in the hyperglycaemia-associated β-cell dysfunction in 90% Px rats. Further, these studies show a linear correlation between the percent change in the pancreatic insulin content (up or down) and insulin secretory responses. We thus proposed that a failure to preserve the insulin content at a required level is the basis for the β-cell dysfunction. Grill and colleagues (19) and Ling et al. (20) have come to similar conclusions based on studies of islets cultured with high glucose. Our data thus imply a link between the amount of insulin that is stored and how much insulin is secreted in response to a particular stimulus, in particular glucose-potentiated secretion. Extrapolations of this idea are that anything that alters the ability of β-cells to store insulin normally will impair insulin secretory responses, and in turn, a reduction of insulin secretion in those situations could paradoxically improve insulin secretory function - so-called *β-cell rest*. As described above, our studies have shown this effect with diazoxide and fasting in 90% Px rats. Importantly, diazoxide, fasting, and somatostatin have also been reported to paradoxically increase insulin secretion in type 2 diabetes (21-23), establishing the relevance of our studies to humans.

Model for β-cell overwork

The model that we have developed from these observations (Figure 4) is a cascade of functional changes in β-cells that are initiated when the need for insulin secretion is increased, as might occur in states of insulin resistance or reduced β-cell mass. The first event is that β-cell glucose sensitivity increases so that insulin output is augmented, thus maintaining the level of glycaemia. In contrast, if even mild hyperglycaemia develops, the cascade on the right of Figure 4 progresses and culminates in reduced insulin secretion. The mechanism for β-cell failure is multifactorial, but our results suggest reduced cellular stores of insulin to be an important pathogenic element. The model also shows a raised proinsulin to insulin ratio resulting from the overworked β-cell cascade.

WHAT IS THE BIOCHEMICAL BASIS FOR GLUCOSE HYPERSENSITIVITY PRECEDING β-CELL FAILURE?

We investigated this question in three normoglycaemic rodent models of β-cell adaptation, insulin resistant spontaneously hypertensive rats (24), rats made hyperinsulinemic by a glucose infusion (25), and following a 60% Px in rats (26). All of these models are characterized by a heightened β-cell glucose sensing so that insulin secretion is enhanced at normal and elevated levels of glycaemia - in contrast, basal insulin secretion, which is loosely defined as insulin secretion below 5mM glucose, is unaffected. The biochemical basis for this adaptation proves to be an increased activity of glucokinase, the important regulatory enzyme for β-cell glucose sensing. Immunoblot analysis shows little to no change in its cellular content, suggesting an increased catalytic activity of GK as the basis for the increased glucose sensing and the increase in insulin secretion in the models documented above. Several investigators have supported the idea of variable catalytic activity for β-cell glucokinase. A recent study provides evidence for a yet undefined regulatory protein interacting with GK (27).

Additional mechanisms are known that alter β-cell glucose sensing and induce a compensatory adaptation of insulin secretion. Best studied is pregnancy during which β-cell glucokinase and hexokinase levels increase to counter the insulin resistance, presumably secondary to the effects of prolactin and placental hormones (28,29). An additional model studied is that of compensatory hyperinsulinemia found in models of insulin resistance with marked hypertriglyceridemia. The glucose-sensing pattern for insulin secretion is different from the three models already described, in that basal insulin secretion is markedly increased (30). Elevated levels of fatty acid metabolites in β-cells are thought to cause altered glucose sensing, and we have studied islets cultured with fatty acid to investigate the mechanism. Basal glucose consumption and insulin secretion are increased (30-32). In this model phosphofructokinase (PFK) activity is increased because of 1) increased PFK gene expression and production; and 2) decreased synthesis/content of citrate, which is a potent inhibitor of PFK activity (33,34). These changes lead to a decreased cellular G6P concentration because of its increased metabolism. G6P is a potent inhibitor of hexokinase. Thus, in this model of hypertriglyceridemia, increased hexokinase activity appears to be the basis for increased glucose sensing in β-cells and enhances basal insulin secretion (35).

Referring to Figure 4, these results show a repertoire of mechanisms in the β-cell that lead to compensatory changes in their glucose sensing and function to maintain euglycemia in situations of chronically altered insulin demands (i.e. insulin resistance). The ability to alter β-cell sensitivity to glucose is central to the adaptive response of β-cells. To maintain equilibrium in the "new" adapted state, insulin stores (i.e. insulin production) need to be maintained at a high level. Diabetes develops when this compensatory mechanism fails.

WHAT CAUSES THE INSULIN CONTENT TO BECOME SUBNORMAL IN DIABETES?

An important question at this point is what are the mechanisms that cause the insulin content of β-cells to decrease? We suggest a dual mechanism: increased β-cell hexokinase activity, and the inability of β-cells to upregulate proinsulin synthesis to keep up with the insulin secretion. These results suggest a regulatory change other than glucokinase.

Increased β-cell Hexokinase Activity

As previously described, our studies in nondiabetic models reveal no change in basal insulin secretion (24-26). Glucokinase activity is upregulated which leads to a compensatory increase in glucose stimulated insulin secretion (glucokinase has a K_m of 10-12 mM glucose). At normal levels of glycaemia, insulin secretion is increased less than twice of normal in these models. In contrast, in diabetic 90% Px rats, basal insulin secretion is increased and the shape of the curve in Figure 3 is different from normal. Because of the changed shape, insulin secretion, despite only modestly increased glucose levels is increased five- to ten-fold in Px rats as compared to controls.

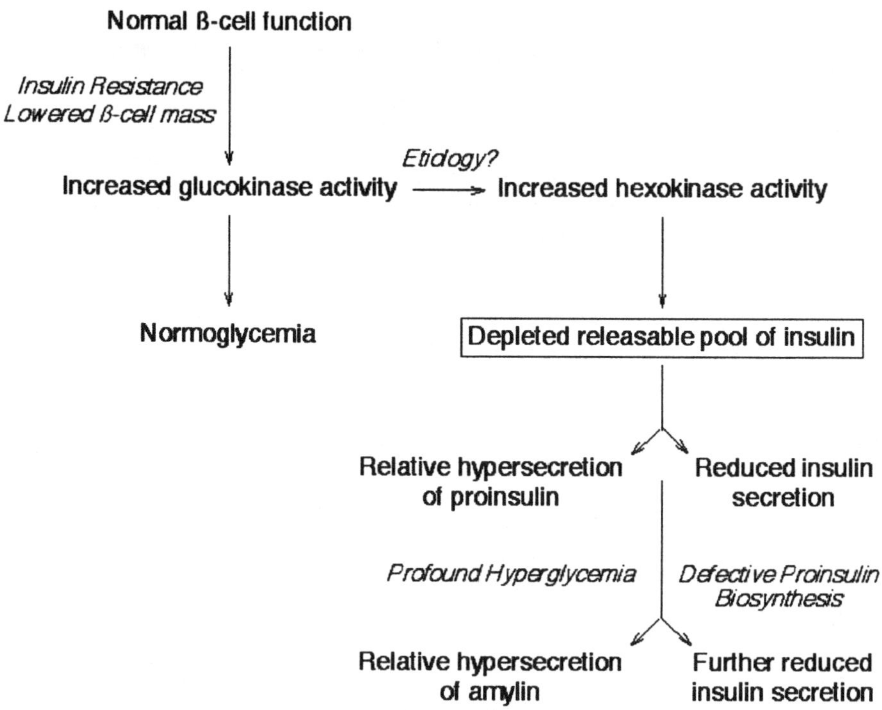

Figure 4. *Proposed schema for the overworked β-cell hypothesis based on our own data and that of others from animal models, and studies conducted in man.*

We investigated the molecular basis for the left-shifted curve in isolated islets of 90% Px rats. Increased hexokinase V_{max} is the dominant change in islet glucose utilization (36). In contrast, in nondiabetic models (including 60% Px rats) the dominant finding is enhanced glucokinase activity. This suggests that hyperglycaemia or an associated metabolic defect causes hexokinase activity and subsequently basal insulin secretion to increase. Additional support for this idea is increased islet hexokinase V_{max} and basal insulin secretion rates in rats made hyperglycaemic by 48 hours of glucose infusion, but not in normoglycaemic/hyperinsulinemic rats (25). Most definitive is the study by Cockburn in diabetes prone ZDF rats before and after onset of diabetes in which the prediabetic period is characterized by increased islet glucokinase activity as opposed to a marked increase in hexokinase activity and basal insulin secretion when hyperglycaemia is established (37). Thus, hyperglycaemia is typically accompanied by enhanced β-cell hexokinase activity that results in a very high level of insulin output. Whether hyperglycaemia precedes the increased hexokinase activity or *vice versa* is not known. Neither is there information on the control and biochemistry of the increased hexokinase activity in islets. This marked increase in insulin output sets the stage for its exceeding the capacity for proinsulin synthesis as detailed next.

Mismatch between Proinsulin Synthesis and Insulin Secretion
Many investigators in this field would state that impaired proinsulin synthesis leads to the subnormal insulin content in 90% Px rats. This stems from the observation that when β-cells are chronically exposed to high glucose levels, proinsulin gene expression is impaired because of altered transcriptional regulation *in vitro* (38,39) as well as *in vivo* (40). Another possibility for reduced insulin stores in 90% Px rats is that β-cells normally secrete 10%-20% of their maximal capacity and can increase secretion rates by five- to ten-fold (Figure 3). In contrast, proinsulin synthesis which is also glucose regulated, can be maximally upregulated only two- to three-fold from baseline levels (41,42). A situation in which both proinsulin synthesis and insulin secretion are fully upregulated would lead to a mismatch between production and secretion leading to a reduction in insulin stores. Our results in 90% Px rats are consistent with this idea. Proinsulin synthesis increases three-fold over the controls (17). In contrast, insulin secretion increases 5-10-fold. Similar conclusions have been drawn from experiments with isolated islets cultured at high glucose levels (20).

WHAT IS THE LINK BETWEEN A LOWERED INSULIN CONTENT AND SUBNORMAL INSULIN SECRETION?

How then does a 20%-40% reduction of islet insulin content (as found in most diabetes models) manifest itself in altered insulin secretory response? One possibility is that a portion of stored insulin is contained in a releasable pool, and that a reduction of insulin in this particular pool causes the subnormal insulin responses to glucose stimulation. The other possibility would be that the insulin content of individual granules is reduced. Conceptually, the first possibility is defective granule mobilization and the second is defective granule content.

Diabetic rats (43-45) and humans (46,47) have an increased serum amylin to insulin ratio. The mildly diabetic 90% Px rats have normal stored and secreted ratios of amylin to insulin. In contrast, both ratios are doubled in much more hyperglycaemic 95% Px rats (43). Our interpretation of this result is that the lowered insulin responses (especially postprandial) that characterize the transition from glucose intolerance to overt hyperglycaemia are seen because the releasable pool of insulin is depleted, i.e. the granule composition of insulin is relatively normal in early stages of glucose intolerance. In contrast, as glycaemia rises (of which the threshold level has not been determined), the toxic effect of hyperglycaemia on proinsulin synthesis as described above leads to insulin depletion of granules and, as a consequence, further deterioration of insulin secretion, now manifest as a raised secreted amylin to insulin ratio.

RAISED RATIO OF PROINSULIN TO INSULIN

Type 2 diabetics have a raised serum ratio of proinsulin and its conversion intermediates relative to insulin (48). The presumed cause is a relative hypersecretion of these peptides. Hyperglycaemia rather than increased insulin demand is linked to the pathogenesis of this finding. States of increased insulin secretion without hyperglycaemia - such as obesity - have a normal to subnormal proinsulin to insulin ratio (49). Two hypotheses have been proposed to explain how hyperglycaemia causes a hypersecretion of proinsulin-like peptides. The first postulates a shortened transit time from granule packaging to release, such that peptide processing is incomplete at the time of release of granule content into the circulation. The second postulates a defective proinsulin processing machinery.

We measured the proinsulin to insulin ratio in pancreas extracts and portal vein samples (obtained during pancreas perfusion) from 90% Px rats. The ratio of proinsulin-like peptides relative to insulin is increased in the pancreas and portal vein samples of these diabetic rats (50). This suggests that the storage, and subsequent secretion, of material enriched in proinsulin-like peptides is the primary defect. Studies of diabetic sand rats (51) and type 2 diabetics (52) have made the same conclusion.

In normal rats, 48-hour glucose infusions allow variable levels of glycaemia to be attained based on the concentration of glucose in the infusate. In this model (53), the pancreatic proinsulin to insulin ratio increases in rats rendered hyperglycaemic as compared to normoglycaemic littermates. The increase is caused by a fall in the insulin content, not an increase in the proinsulin content as might be expected with defective proinsulin processing. The data are consistent with the hypothesis of a hyperstimulated insulin secretion causing release of granules before peptide processing is complete. Further supporting this hypothesis: diazoxide treatment prevents the fall in insulin content and the proinsulin to insulin ratio remains normal. *In vitro*, pancreatic extracts of diabetic rats can completely process proinsulin to insulin. This further suggests that *in vivo* the decreased transit time of insulin granules is responsible for incomplete proinsulin processing (53-55).

CONCLUSIONS

The studies described herein have focused on the β-cell dysfunction that predisposes to the transition from normoglycaemia to overt frank diabetes. Our results have led to the model shown in Figure 4, which is based on a concept of β-cell overwork or exhaustion.

Following the onset of insulin resistance or insufficient β-cell mass, glucose sensing by the β-cell is altered such that insulin secretion is enhanced while glucose levels remain relatively unchanged. The mechanism behind this is increased glucokinase activity. Increased proinsulin synthesis compensates for increased demand, and normoglycaemia is maintained indefinitely at this new equilibrium (left hand side of Figure 4).

In contrast, genetic predisposition to type 2 diabetes does not allow sustained β-cell compensatory response. An important event is the onset of increased β-cell hexokinase activity (for unknown reasons). In this situation, insulin secretion surpasses production, and the pool of releasable insulin granules falls below what is needed for normal β-cell secretory function. A second effect is the granules that are released are enriched in proinsulin-like peptides. As hyperglycaemia worsens, proinsulin gene expression is disturbed at the transcriptional level. The secretory granules in β-cells are now relatively devoid of insulin that exacerbates the insulin secretory deficiency, and is manifest as a rise in the secreted ratio of amylin to insulin. What role this might play in the islet amyloid deposits that are found in type 2 diabetes is unknown (10). One would predict from this model that when insulin resistance is present, drugs that improve insulin sensitivity should have a beneficial effect because of the reduced insulin secretion which has been observed in diabetic rodents (56). Prevention of the vicious cycle of β-cell exhaustion at a very early stage may thus be the adequate treatment strategy for patients prone to develop type 2 diabetes mellitus.

REFERENCES

1. Leahy JL. Natural history of β-cell dysfunction in NIDDM. Diabetes Care 1990;13:992-1010.
2. Saad MF, Knowler WC, Pettitt DJ, Nelson RG, Charles MA, Bennett PH. A two-step model for development of non-insulin dependent diabetes. Am J Med 1991;90:229-35.
3. Beck-Neilsen H, Groop LC. Metabolic and genetic characterization of prediabetic state. Sequence of events leading to non-insulin dependent diabetes mellitus. J Clin Invest 1994;94:1714-21.
4. Turner RC, Holman RR. Beta-cell function during insulin or chlorpropamide treatment of maturity-onset diabetes mellitus. Diabetes 1978;27(Suppl 1):241-6.
5. Kosaka K, Kuzuya T, Akanuma Y, Hagura R. Increase in insulin response after treatment of overt maturity-onset diabetes is independent of the mode of treatment. Diabetologia 1980;18:23-8.
6. Rossetti L, Giaccari A, DeFronzo RA. Glucose toxicity. Diabetes Care 1990;13:610-30.
7. Yki-Järvinen H. Glucose toxicity. Endocr Rev 1992;13:415-31.
8. Unger RH. Lipotoxicity in the pathogenesis of obesity-dependent NIDDM. Genetic and clinical implications. Diabetes 1995;44:863-70.
9. Prentki M, Corkey BE. Are the β-cell signalling molecules malonyl CoA and cytosolic long-chain acyl-CoA implicated in multiple tissue defects of obesity and NIDDM? Diabetes 1996;45:273-83.
10. Kahn SE, Andrikopoulos S, Verchere CB. Islet amyloid: a long recognized but underappreciated pathological feature of type 2 diabetes. Diabetes 1999;48:241-53.
11. Pick A, Clark J, Kubstrup C, Levisetti M, Pugh W, Bonner-Weir S, Polonsky KS. Role of apoptosis in failure of beta-cell mass compensation for insulin resistance and beta-cell defects in the male Zucker diabetic fatty rat. Diabetes 1998;47:358-64.
12. Leahy JL. β-cell dysfunction with chronic hyperglycaemia: the "overworked β-cell" hypothesis. Diabetes Revs 1996;4:298-319.
13. Bonner-Weir S, Trent DF, Weir GC. Partial pancreatectomy in the rat and subsequent defect in glucose-induced insulin release. J Clin Invest 1983;71:1544-53.
14. Leahy JL, Bumbalo LM, Chen C. Beta-cell hypersensitivity for glucose precedes loss of glucose-induced insulin secretion in 90% pancreatectomized rats. Diabetologia 1993;36:1238-44.
15. Leahy JL, Bumbalo LM, Chen C. Diazoxide causes recovery of β–cell glucose responsiveness in 90% pancreatectomized diabetic rats. Diabetes 1994;43:173-9.
16. Sako Y, Grill VE. Coupling of β-cell desensitization by hyperglycaemia to excessive stimulation and circulating insulin in glucose-infused rats. Diabetes 1990;39:1580-3.
17. Hosokawa YA, Hosokawa H, Chen C, Leahy JL. Mechanism of impaired glucose-potentiated insulin secretion in diabetic 90% pancreatectomy rats: Study using GLP-1 (7-37). J Clin Invest 1996;97:180-6.
18. Hosokawa YA, Leahy JL. Parallel reduction of pancreas insulin content and insulin secretion in 48-h tolbutamide-infused normoglycaemic rats. Diabetes 1997;46:808-13.
19. Björklund A, Grill V. β-cell insensitivity *in vitro*: reversal by diazoxide entails more than one event in stimulus-secretion coupling. Endocrinology 1993;132:1319-28.
20. Ling Z, Kiekins R, Mahler T, Schuit FC, Pipeleers-Marichal M, Sener A, Klöppel G, Malaisse WJ, Pipeleers DG. Effects of chronically elevated glucose levels on the functional properties of rat pancreatic β-cells. Diabetes 1996;45:1774-82.
21. Greenwood RH, Mahler RF, Hales CN. Improvement in insulin secretion in diabetes after diazoxide. Lancet 1976;1:444-7.
22. Féry F, Balasse EO. Glucose metabolism during the starved-to-fed transition in obese patients with NIDDM. Diabetes 1994;43:1418-25.
23. Laedtke T, Schmitz O, Porksen N, Veldhuis J, Butler P. Mechanism of impaired pulsatile insulin secretion in NIDDM? Diabetes 1996;45(Suppl. 2):40A.
24. Chen C, Hosokawa H, Bumbalo LM, Leahy JL. Mechanism of compensatory hyperinsulinemia in normoglycaemic insulin resistant SHR rats: augmented enzymatic activity of glucokinase in β-cells. J Clin Invest 1994;94:399-404.
25. Chen C, Bumbalo LM, Hosokawa H, Leahy JL. Increased catalytic activity of glucokinase in isolated islets from hyperinsulinemic rats. Diabetes 1994;43:684-9.
26. Leahy JL, Liu YQ, Sun X-J, Nevin PW. β-cell adaptation in normoglycaemic 60% pancreatectomy rats: increased islet glucokinase activcity and IRS-2 content. Diabetes 1999;48(Suppl. 1):A236.
27. Tiedge M, Steffeck H, Elsner M, Lenzen S. Metabolic regulation, activity state, and intracellular binding of glucokinase in insulin secreting cells. Diabetes 1999;48:514-23.
28. Parsons JA, Brelje TC, Sorenson RL. Adaption of islets of Langerhans to pregnancy: increased islet cell proliferation and insulin secretion correlates with the onset of placental lactogen secretion. Endocrinology 1992;130:1459-66.

29. Sorenson RL, Brelje TC. Adaptation of islets of Langerhans to pregnancy: beta-cell growth, enhanced insulin secretion and the role of lactogenic hormones. Horm Metab Res 1997;29:301-7.
30. Milburn JL Jr, Hirose H, Lee YH, Nagasawa Y, Ogawa A, Ohneda M, BeltrandelRio H, Newgard CB, Johnson JH, Unger RH. Pancreatic β-cells in obesity. Evidence for induction of functional, morphologic, and metabolic abnormalities by increased long chain fatty acids. J Biol Chem 1995;270:1295-9.
31. Hosokawa H, Corkey BE, Leahy JL. Beta-cell hypersensitivity to glucose following 24-h exposure of rat islets to fatty acids. Diabetologia 1997;40:392-7.
32. Zhou YP, Grill VE. Long-term exposure of rat pancreatic islets to fatty acids inhibits glucose-induced insulin secretion and biosynthesis through a glucose fatty acid cycle. J Clin Invest 1994;93:870-6.
33. Liu YQ, Tornheim K, Leahy JL. Shared biochemical properties of glucotoxicity and lipotoxicity in islets to lower citrate synthase activity and increase phosphofructokinase activity. Diabetes 1998;47:1889-93.
34. Liu YQ, Tornheim K, Leahy JL. Fatty acid-induced beta cell hypersensitivity to glucose. Increased phosphofructokinase activity and lowered glucose-6-phosphate content. J Clin Invest 1998;101:1870-5.
35. Giroix M-H, Sener A, Pipeleers DG, Malaisse WJ. Hexose metabolism in pancreatic islets. Inhibition of hexokinase. Biochem J 1984;223:447-53.
36. Hosokawa H, Hosokawa YA, Leahy JL. Upregulated hexokinase activity in isolated islets from diabetic 90% pancreatectomized rats. Diabetes 1995;44:1328-33.
37. Cockburn BN, Ostrega DM, Sturis J, Kubstrup K, Polonsky KS, Bell GI. Changes in pancreatic islet glucokinase and hexokinase activities with increasing age, obesity, and the onset of diabetes. Diabetes 1997;46:1434-9.
38. Olson LK, Sharma A, Peshavaria M, Wright CV, Towle HC, Robertson RP, Stein R. Reduction of insulin gene transcription in HIT-T15 beta cells chronically exposed to a supraphysiologic glucose concentration is associated with loss of STF-1 transcription factor expression. Proc Natl Acad Sci USA 1995;92:9127-31.
39. Robertson RP, Olson LK, Zhang H-J. Differentiating glucose toxicity from glucose desensitization: a message from the insulin gene. Diabetes 1994;43:1085-9.
40. Zangen DH, Bonner-Weir S, Lee CH, Latimer JB, Miller CP, Habener JF, Weir GC. Reduced insulin, GLUT2, and IDX-1 in β-cells after partial pancreatectomy. Diabetes 1996;46:258-64.
41. Ashcroft SJH. Glucoreceptor mechanism and the control of insulin release and biosynthesis. Diabetologia 1980;18:5-15.
42. Schuit FC, Kickens R, Pipeleers DG. Measuring the balance between insulin synthesis and insulin release. Biochem Biophys Res Comm 1991;178:1182-7.
43. Leahy JL, Fineman MS. Impaired phasic insulin and amylin secretion in diabetic rats. Am J Physiol 1998;38:E457-62.
44. Gedulin B, Cooper GJ, Young AA. Amylin secretion from the perfused pancreas: dissociation from insulin and abnormal elevation in insulin-resistant diabetic rats. Biochem Biophys Res Commun 1991;180:782-9.
45. Inoue K, Hisatomi A, Umeda F, Nawata H. Relative hypersecretion of amylin to insulin from rat pancreas after neonatal STZ treatment. Diabetes 1992;41:723-7.
46. Butler PC, Chou J, Carter WB, Wang YN, Bu BH, Chang D, Chang JK, Rizza R. Effects of meal ingestion on plasma amylin concentration in NIDDM and nondiabetic humans. Diabetes 1990;39:752-6.
47. Kautzky-Willer A, Thomaseth K, Ludvik B, Nowotny P, Rabensteiner D, Waldhäusl W, Pacini G, Prager R. Elevated islet amyloid pancreatic polypeptide and proinsulin in lean gestational diabetes. Diabetes 1997;46:607-14.
48. Rhodes CJ, Alarcón C. What beta-cell defect could lead to hyperproinsulinemia in NIDDM? Some clues from recent advances made in understanding the proinsulin-processing mechanism. Diabetes 1994;43:511-7.
49. Koivisto VA, Yki-Järvinen H, Hartling SV, Pelkonen R. The effect of exogenous hyperinsulinemia on proinsulin secretion in normal man, obese subjects, and patients with insulinoma. J Clin Endocrinol Metab 1986;63:1117-20.
50. Leahy JL, Halban PA, Weir GC. Relative hypersecretion of proinsulin in a rat model of non-insulin-dependent diabetes mellitus. Diabetes 1991;40:985-9.
51. Gadot M, Leibowitz G, Shafrir E, Cerasi E, Gross DJ, Kaiser N. Hyperproinsulinemia and insulin deficiency in the diabetic *Psammomys obesus*. Endocrinology 1994;135:610-6.
52. Kahn SE, Halban PA. Release of incompletely processed proinsulin is the cause of the disproportionate proinsulinemia of NIDDM. Diabetes 1997;46:1725-32.
53. Leahy JL. Increased proinsulin/insulin ratio in pancreas extracts of hyperglycaemic rats. Diabetes 1993;42:22-7.
54. Gadot M, Ariav Y, Cerasi E, Kaiser N, Gross DJ. Hyperproinsulinemia in the diabetic *Psammomys obesus* is a result of increased secretory demand on the β-cell. Endocrinology 1995;136:4218-23.

55. Alarcón C, Leahy JL, Schuppin GT, Rhodes CJ. Increased secretory demand rather than a defect in the proinsulin conversion mechanism causes hyperproinsulinemia in a glucose-infusion rat model of non insulin dependent diabetes mellitus. J Clin Invest 1995;95:1032-9.
56. Sreenan S, Sturis J, Pugh W, Burant CF, Polonsky KS. Prevention of hyperglycaemia in the Zucker diabetic fatty rat by treatment with metformin or troglitazone. Am J Physiol 1996;34:E742-7.

4

GLUCOSE TOXICITY OF THE PANCREATIC β-CELL

R. Paul Robertson, M.D., Jamie Harmon, Ph.D., Yoshito Tananka, M.D., Giovanni Sacchi, M.D., Phuong Oanh T. Tran, Ph.D., Catherine Gleason, Vincent Poitout, D.V.M., Ph.D.

Pacific Northwest Research Institute and University of Washington, Seattle, WA 98122 USA

INTRODUCTION

For purposes of this chapter, glucose toxicity is defined as pathophysiologic and largely irreversible damage to the pancreatic islet β-cell caused by chronic exposure to supraphysiologic glucose concentrations. This leads to profound disturbances in insulin synthesis, which in turn leads to decreased insulin content and secretion. Using various experimental models, many authors have described negative effects of glucose on β-cell function and termed these effects variously as glucose toxicity, β-cell exhaustion, or glucose desensitization (1-50). While the distinction between β-cell exhaustion and glucose toxicity is not always clear, we favor the concept that the two lie in a pathophysiologic continuum. β-cell exhaustion is the earlier form and likely to be reversible, whereas glucose toxicity is the later form and less reversible. In marked contrast, we view "glucose desensitization" as a temporary, physiological state of β-cell refractoriness induced by repeated or prolonged exposure to high glucose concentrations, which is reversed in a time-dependent manner after restoration of normal glucose concentrations. This term implies an intrinsic and reversible alteration in stimulus-secretion coupling rather than damage to the β-cell.

Glucose is the primary regulator of insulin exocytosis from the β-cell and also a major regulator of insulin gene transcription and proinsulin processing (51-58). This chapter focuses on the hypothesis that glucose toxicity of the β-cell is the paradoxical inhibition of insulin gene expression by glucose. The majority of experiments used to formulate the concept of glucose toxicity have been performed with transformed islet cell lines as research tools. The use of cell lines rather than isolated islets has been necessary because it is practically impossible to maintain pancreatic islets in primary culture for much longer than six weeks. In contrast, islet cell lines can be maintained in culture for more than one year. Additionally, some newer information about glucose toxicity from long-term *in vivo* experiments using diabetic rodent models is forthcoming and will be discussed.

HIT-T15 CELLS AS A MODEL OF GLUCOSE TOXICITY

Santerre et al. (59) introduced HIT-T15 cells, the first glucose-responsive β-cell line. This line was derived from simian virus 40 transformation of Syrian hamster pancreatic islets. It raised immediate interest because it had the important feature of regulated insulin secretion. In these cells, glucose stimulates insulin release in a concentration-dependent manner and insulin secretion responds to physiologic inhibition of insulin secretion by epinephrine, somatostatin, and prostaglandin E_2. Although other glucose-responsive cell lines were subsequently derived, and although some of these cell lines provide greater magnitudes of insulin secretion, the HIT-T15 cell line remains the most responsive in terms of fold-increments above basal secretion when challenged with glucose (34). However, this cell line has two disadvantages. First, it has a left-shifted glucose concentration-insulin response curve as compared to isolated pancreatic islets (34,60). Second, early in its history investigators noted a disappointing loss of glucose-induced insulin secretion after the cells had been split and passaged over 80 times.

We observed that HIT-T15 cells chronically cultured to passages 80 and above not only lost glucose-induced insulin secretion, but also had decreased insulin content and insulin mRNA (Figures 1-3).

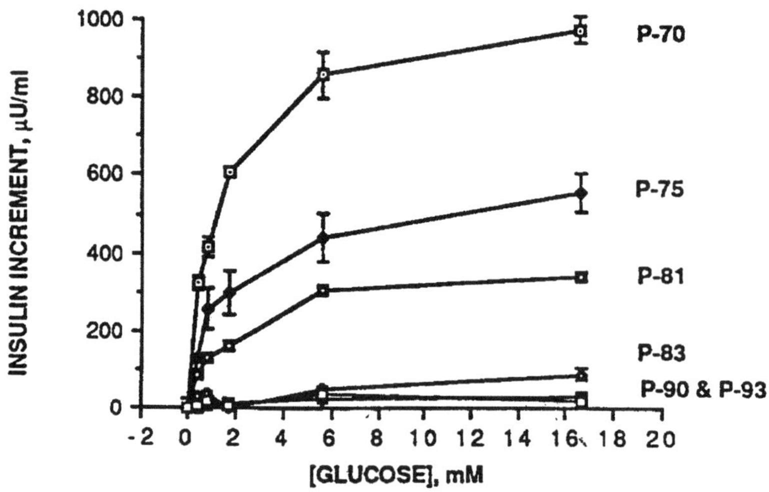

Figure 1. *Passage-dependent loss of glucose-induced insulin secretion from HIT cells serially grown from passage 70 through passage 93. Reprinted with permission from reference (34).*

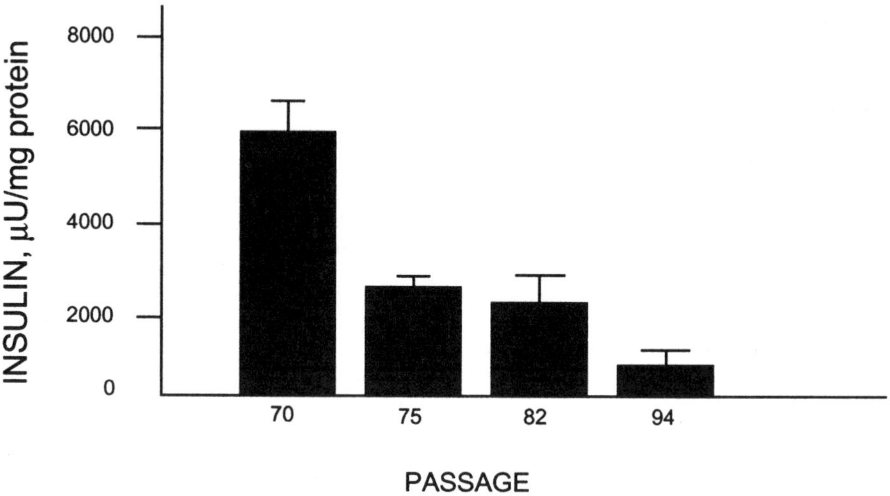

Figure 2. *Passage-dependent decrements in insulin content of HIT cells grown serially from passage 70 through passage 94. Reprinted with permission from reference (34).*

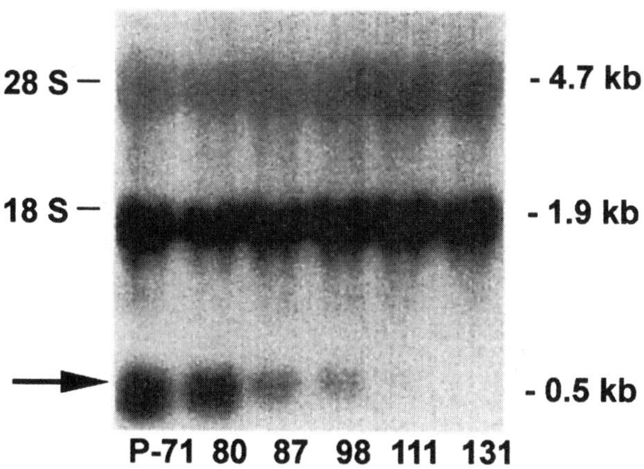

Figure 3. *Passage-dependent decrements in insulin mRNA levels in HIT cells cultured serially from passage 71 through 131. Arrow designates insulin mRNA. Reprinted with permission from reference (36).*

At this time, we were using the same culture media used by all other investigators studying the HIT-T15 cell line, namely, RPMI-1640. It occurred to us that this media contained 11.1 mM glucose and that this concentration exceeded the maximal stimulatory glucose concentration for insulin secretion by the cells by a factor of at least 5. This prompted us to compare the behaviour of the cells when they were cultured in media containing a more physiologic glucose concentration from passages in the low 70s through passages into the low 100s. We observed that late passages of HIT-T15 cells cultured serially in RPMI-1640 media containing 0.8 mM glucose retained glucose-induced insulin secretion and had higher insulin content and levels of insulin mRNA than cells cultured in RPMI-1640 containing 11.1 mM glucose. Thus, we suggested that the supraphysiologic glucose concentration in RPMI-1640, which was routinely used to culture HIT-T15 cells, had caused glucose toxicity and that this toxicity might be explained by molecular mechanisms involving insulin gene expression and subsequent insulin synthesis (36). Although chronic culture of the cells for up to 6-7 months was accompanied by a slight increase in cell population doubling times, the changes we observed in insulin mRNA and insulin content could not be ascribed to this variable because cell population doubling times were not significantly different for a given passage whether the media contained 0.8 or 11.1 mM glucose (Figure 4).

To elucidate the mechanism for paradoxically glucose-induced decreased insulin gene expression, we performed experiments to determine whether this phenomenon was associated with decreases in insulin gene promoter activity and altered transcription factor binding to the insulin promoter. HIT-T15 cells that were transiently transfected with a Chloramphenicol Acetyl Transferase (CAT) reporter gene controlled by the 5'-regulatory domain of the human insulin gene (INSCAT). Early passages of cells cultured in supraphysiologic glucose concentrations readily expressed INSCAT, whereas late passages expressed only 29% of the CAT activity.

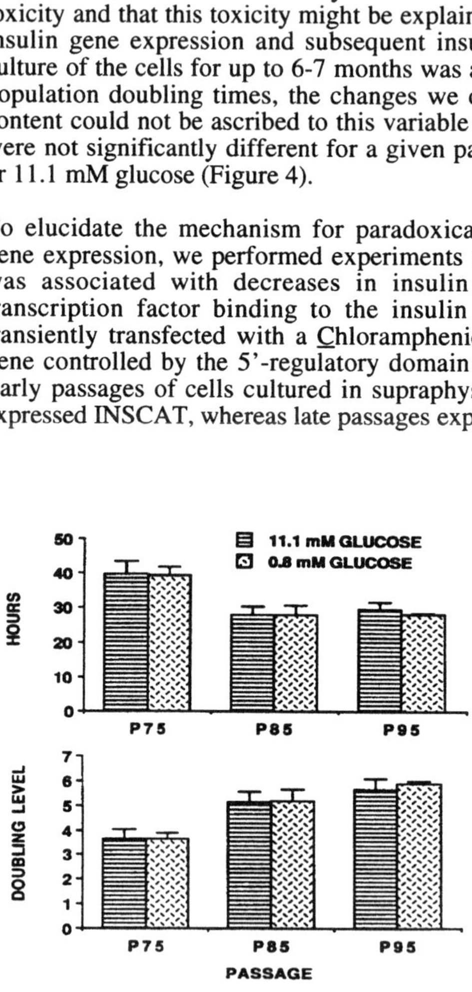

Figure 4. *Comparison of HIT cell population doubling times and cumulative doubling levels in passages 75, 85, and 95. Cells were serially cultured either in 11.1 mM or 0.8 mM glucose. Reprinted with permission from reference (36).*

However, late passages of cells cultured in 0.8 mM glucose, rather than 11.1 mM glucose, retained the ability to express CAT activity to a level of 70-100% of the activity observed in earlier passages (Figure 5). By electrophoretic mobility shift assays, we observed that late passages of cells cultured in 11.1 mM glucose lost the ability to form a nuclear protein-DNA complex with specific motifs of the human insulin promoter (Figure 6) (37).

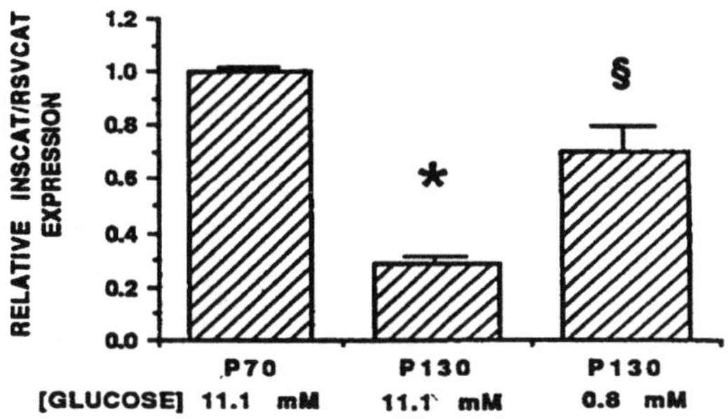

Figure 5. *Preservation of CAT activity in late passages of HIT cells grown in 0.8 mM glucose rather than 11.1 mM glucose. Reprinted with permission from reference (37).*

Although we gave the name Glucose-Sensitive Transcription Factor (GSTF) for this putative DNA binding factor, it soon became apparent that it was identical to IUF-1 (61). Later, PDX-1 became clear that GSTF/IUF-1 is identical to the transcription factors STF-1, pdx-1, and IDX-1 (62). For purposes of simplicity, we will use the term STF-1 in this chapter to refer to this transcription factor.

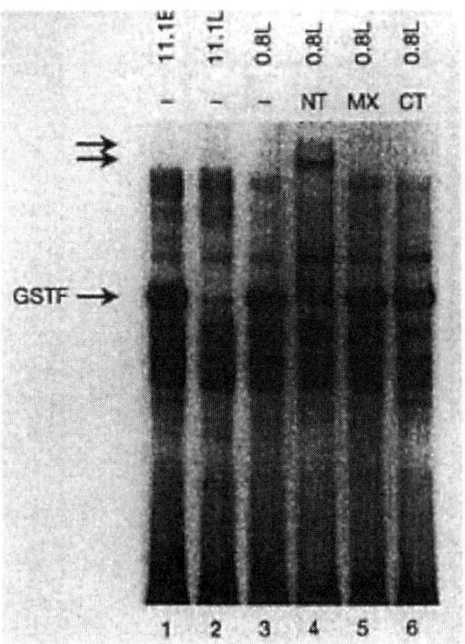

Figure 6. *Supershift of the GSTF complex with an affinity-purified anti-N-terminal XIHbox 8 antibody. Equal concentrations (5 μg) of HIT [11.1E], HIT [0.8L], and HIT [11.1L] protein extract were analyzed for GSTF binding (lanes 1-6) using a human insulin (-230/-201) probe. The effect of the affinity-purified Mox-1 and N- and C-terminal XIGbox 8 antibody (4 μl) on GSTF complex formation was analyzed. The GSTF complex is labelled and the supershifted complexes are indicated with arrows. Lane 1 HIT [11.1E} alone; lane 2 HIT [11.1L] alone; lane 3, HIT [0.8L] alone; lane 4, HIT [0.8L] plus N-terminal XIHbox 8 antibody; lane 5, HIT [0.8L] plus Mox-1 antibody; lane 6, HIT [0.8L] plus C-terminal XIHbox 8 antibody. Reprinted with permission from reference (38).*

When the motif in the insulin promoter that is bound by STF-1 is mutated, INSCAT activity is markedly decreased in early and late passages of HIT-T15 cells, thereby demonstrating the importance of this regulator for insulin transcription (Figure 7) (37). Western analysis reveals that STF-1 protein is reduced in HIT-T15 cells that are chronically cultured in supraphysiologic, but not physiologic, glucose concentrations (Figure 8) (38). We concluded that the molecular mechanism by which chronic exposure of pancreatic islet β-cells to high glucose concentrations can paradoxically decrease insulin gene expression, i.e., glucose toxicity, involves alteration of the ability of STF-1 to bind to the insulin gene promoter.

STF-1 mRNA was also markedly reduced in cells chronically cultured in supraphysiologic glucose concentration (38). This decrease in STF-1 mRNA could not be accounted for by changes in the rate of STF-1 gene transcription as assessed by nuclear run-on analysis. Interestingly, an apparent accumulation of 6.4 kb RNA detected by northern analysis suggested that this larger species might be STF-1 precursor RNA. We hypothesized that the glucotoxic effects might have as a site of action post-transcriptional processing of STF-1 RNA, that might prevent the normal accumulation of the 2.3 and 1.9 kb STF-1 mRNAs.

In work by Sharma et al. (39) we also observed the disappearance of binding by another transcription factor: RIPE-3b1-activator after prolonged culture in high glucose. As with STF-1, binding of RIPE-3b1-activator was reduced in parallel with the decreases in insulin gene expression in HIT-T15 cells chronically cultured in media containing 11.1 mM glucose. In contrast, the insulin control element (ICE) activator, another important transcription factor of the insulin gene did not show any change in DNA-biding in the same experiments. These observations were consistent with the conclusion that glucotoxic effects on insulin gene expression involved not only interference with STF-1, but also interference with RIPE-3b1-activator availability to the insulin promoter.

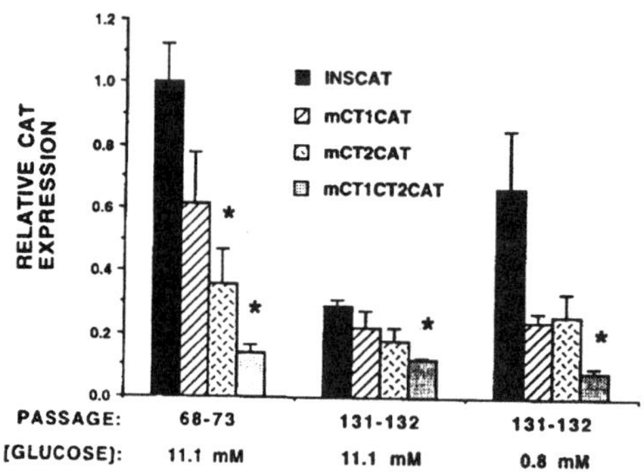

Figure 7. Functional analysis of the CT motifs contained within the human insulin gene promoter. Early and late passages of HIT cells serially passaged in 11.1 mM and 0.8 mM glucose were transiently transfected with INSCAT with the CT1 (mCT1CAT), CT2 (mCT2CAT), or both the CT1 and CT2 (mCT1CT2CAT) motifs mutated. Reprinted with permission from reference (37).

In cells chronically cultured at supraphysiologic glucose concentrations. RIPE-3b1 binding activity decreases below 25% of control by passage 81. STF-1 binding remains at normal levels up to passage 100 and does not decrease to 25% of control until passage 106 (Figure 9). These findings suggest that the loss of RIPE-3b1-activator binding may play an early, dominant role in glucotoxic events (40).

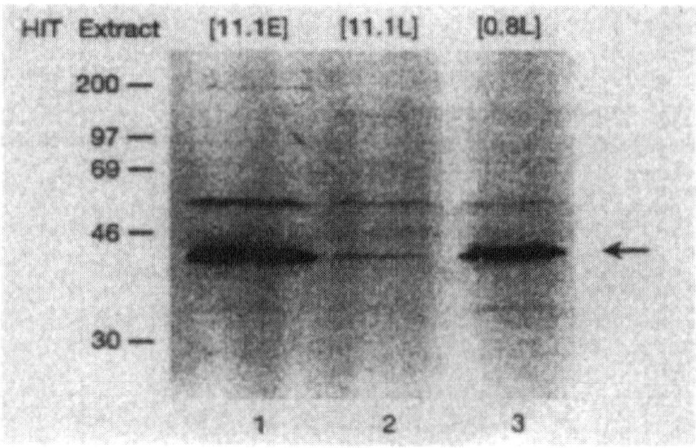

Figure 8. *Expression of STF-1 in HIT-T15 cells chronically cultured in 11.1 mM glucose. Each lane contains 30 μg of HIT[11.1E], HIT[0.8L], or GIT[11.1L] nuclear extract protein. The blot was probed with the affinity-purified N-terminal XIHbox 8 antibody. The position of the STF-1 protein is indicated by the arrow and the migration of various molecular mass (kDa) markers is shown. Densitometric scanning of the blot demonstrated that STF-1 immunoreactivity in HIT[11.1L] cells was <1% of that observed in HIT[11.1E] and HIT[0.8L] cells. Reprinted with permission from reference (38).*

Reconstitution of late passage glucotoxic cells with STF-1 cDNA partially (approximately 40% of control levels) restores insulin promoter activity (40). This raised the question whether the remaining 60% might be attributable to loss of RIPE-3b1-activator binding. Unfortunately, similar studies of RIPE-3b1-activator reconstitution cannot yet be performed because the RIPE-3b1-activator gene has not yet been cloned. Control studies were performed in another glucotoxic cell line, late passages of βTC-6 cells chronically cultured in media containing a supraphysiologic glucose concentration. They are deficient in RIPE-3b1-activator but not STF-1 and STF-1 transfection has no effect on insulin promoter activity in either late or early passage cells. When HIT-T15 cells are cultured in 11.1 mM glucose from passage 75-99 and then switched to 0.8 mM glucose at passage 100 and carried to passage 146, the glucotoxic effects are barely reversible. Insulin gene expression returns to approximately 20% of control after switching to a media containing the lower glucose concentration (Figure 11). Inhibition of insulin secretion with somatostatin had no effect on insulin gene expression in cells cultured in 11.1 mM glucose (Figures 12 and 13) (41). Thus, the glucotoxic effects are not simply because of temporary exhaustion of insulin synthesis, content or secretion.

Glucose toxicity in β-cell lines may also be related to other transcription factors. The transcription factor C/EBPβ is expressed in pancreatic β-cells, is up-regulated by supraphysiological glucose levels and inhibits insulin promoter activity in β-cell lines. HIT-T15 cells transiently co-transfected with C/EBPβ expression plasmid and the reporter-gene construct -410INS-LUC have less reporter activity than observed in the absence of the C/EBPβ plasmid. Nonetheless, mutation of the C/EBPβ binding site does not affect the inhibition of the mutated rat insulin 1 gene promoter by C/EBPβ. Hence, this transcription factor inhibits the rat insulin 1 gene promoter through interaction with *cis*-elements other than C/EBPβ box or their corresponding transcription factors (45).

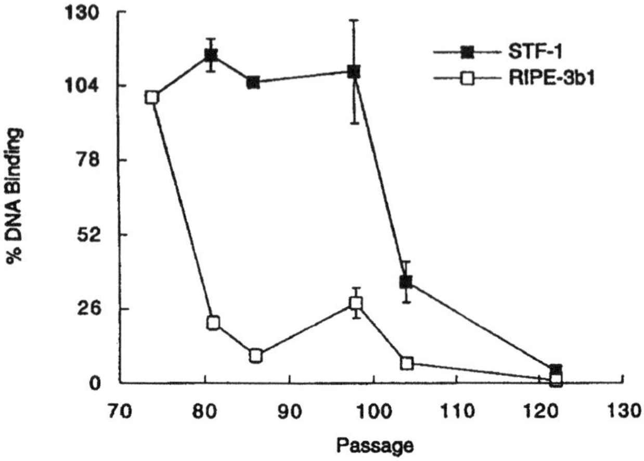

Figure 9. *Relative protein binding of the insulin promoter. Nuclear extracts from various passages of HIT-T15 cells were analyzed by EMSA and quantitated by densitometry, using a Phosphor Imager. Passage-dependent decreases are schematically represented, with percent binding normalized to the protein binding in p74. Data are presented as means ± SE for three to five independent experiments. Some error bars lie within the symbol boundaries. Reprinted with permission from reference (40).*

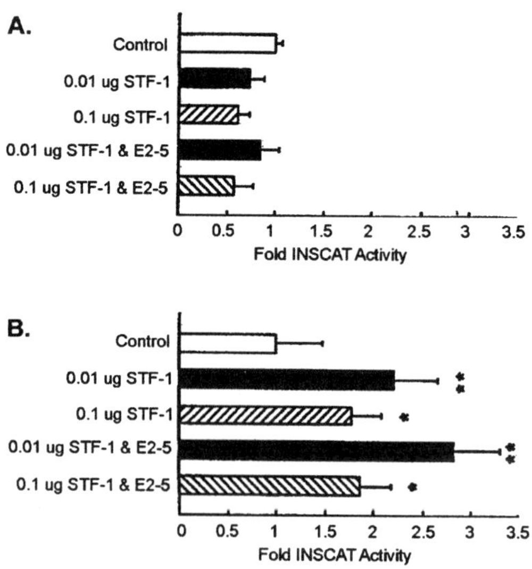

Figure 10. *Reconstitution of HIT-T15 cells with STF-1 and E2-5 expression vectors. HIT-T15 cells were transiently transfected with INSCAT (control), co-transfected with INSCAT plus 0.01 μg STF-1, 0.01 μg each of STF-1 and E2-5, or 0.1 μg each of STF-1 and E2-5 into early (p71-74) passage (A), or late (p118-122) passage (B) cells. Data are presented as means ± SE for four independent experiments with duplicate observations. *P < 0.05; **p < 0.01. Reprinted with permission from reference (40).*

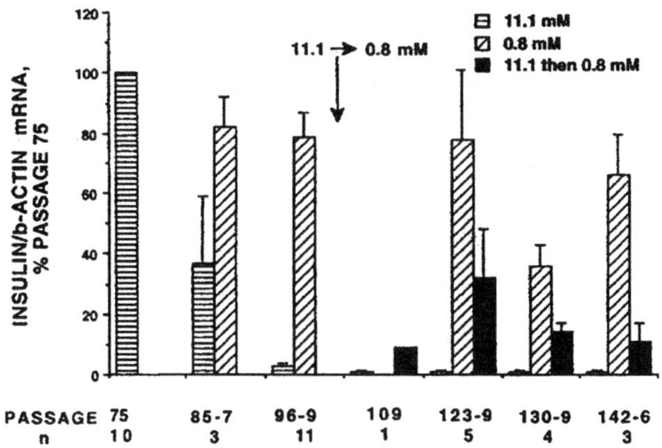

Figure 11. *Illustration of disappearance of insulin mRNA in cells cultured in 11.1 mM glucose, preservation of insulin mRNA in cells cultured in 0.8 mM glucose, and partial restoration of insulin mRNA in cells cultured in 11.1 mM glucose from passage 75 to 100 and then switched to 0.8 mM glucose from passage 100 to 146. Reprinted with permission from reference (41).*

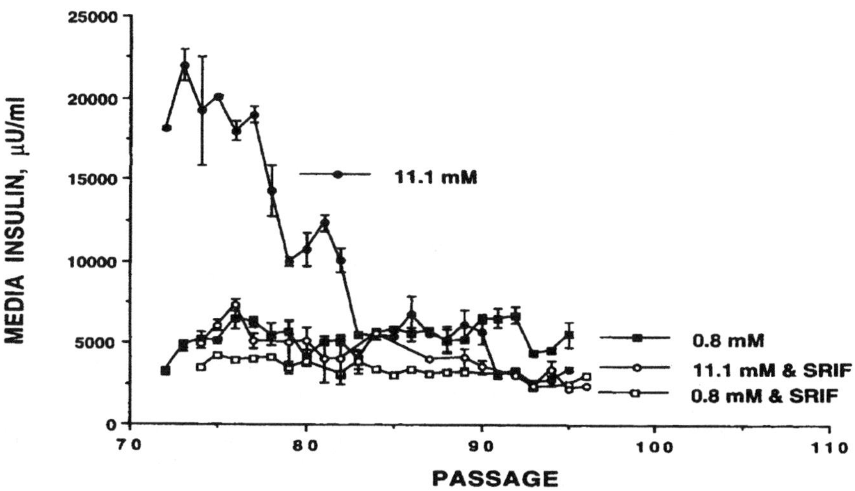

Figure 12. *Media insulin levels in HIT cells from passage 74 to 100 grown in RPMI-1640 medium containing 10% FCS under four conditions: 0.8 mM glucose; 0.8 mM glucose plus 10-6 M SRIF. Each week, aliquots of cells growing under the experimental media conditions were transferred to 12-well plates and continued in their respective experimental media. After 48 h, media insulin concentration was determined and was normalized for protein content. Reprinted with permission from reference (41).*

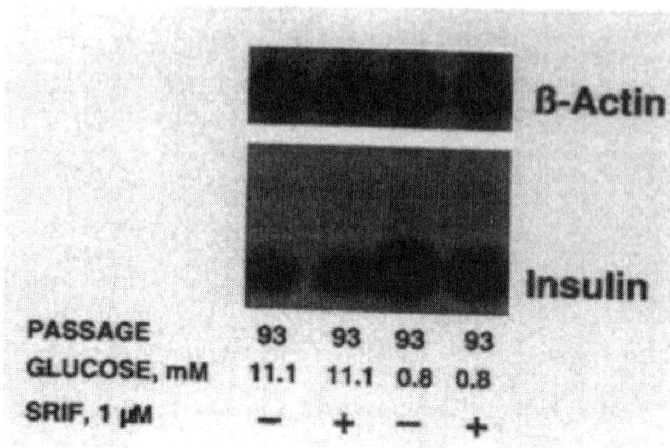

Figure 13. Analysis of mRNA levels in late passage HIT cells (passage 93) grown under the four experimental conditions described in Figure 5. Cells were subcultured in absence of SRIF for 48 hrs prior to analysis. Reprinted with permission from reference (41).

Interestingly, reversible glucose-induced decreases in insulin gene expression are found after short-term exposure to high glucose concentrations in INS-1 cells, a cell line that has the ability to secrete insulin response at physiological glucose concentrations. Binding activity of STF-1 and RIPE-3b1-activator to the insulin promoter diminishes after only 48-hour exposure to elevated glucose concentrations (44). Although these observations do not fall into our definition of glucose toxicity, i.e., largely irreversible decreases in insulin gene expression after long-term exposure to high glucose concentrations, they suggest that similar molecular mechanisms may be implicated in temporary down-regulation of insulin gene expression over a short time frame in INS-1 cells. This phenomenon is not observed in HIT-T15 cells after 48 hours of exposure to media containing supraphysiologic glucose concentrations.

βTC-6 Cells as a Model of Glucose Toxicity

The βTC-6 cell line was derived from transgenic mice harbouring the large T antigen of simian virus 40 driven by the rat insulin II promoter and secretes insulin in response to glucose (65). βTC-6 cells were chronically cultured from passage 35 to 76 in 0.8 or 11.1 mM glucose. At the higher glucose concentration progressive decreases in glucose-induced insulin secretion, insulin content, and insulin mRNA levels were detected (Figures 14-16) (42).

Decrease in insulin mRNA in βTC-6 cells is not due to decreased stability of insulin mRNA (42). Activity of the reporter plasmid INSCAT is decreased to 50% when cells are cultured in 11.1 mM glucose whereas no loss of activity is observed in cells cultured in 0.8 mM glucose (Figure 17).

RIPE-3b1-activator binding also diminishes in late passages cultured under supraphysiologic glucose concentrations, whereas STF-1 binding remained unchanged (Figure 18). Whether or not the βTC-6 cell line eventually loses STF-1 binding is unclear because we have not carried these cultures beyond passage 84. We conclude that decreased binding of RIPE-3b1-activator alone might be responsible for the decrease in insulin promoter activity and insulin gene expression in βTC-6 cells cultured chronically in high glucose concentrations. These data reinforce our concept that RIPE-3b1-activator is adversely affected early in the course of developing glucose toxicity in β-cell lines and that its loss plays a major role in the loss of insulin gene expression, content, and secretion (Figure 19).

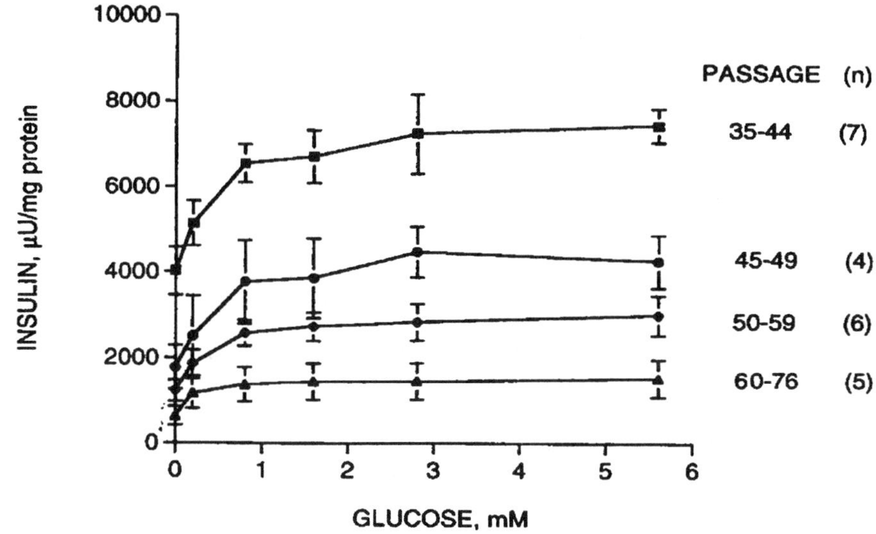

Figure 14. *Glucose-induced insulin secretion in βTC-6 cells serially passaged in RPMI-1640 containing 11.1 mM glucose from passage 35 to 76. βTC-6 cells at various passages were incubated for 2 h in the presence of increasing glucose concentrations. Each curve represents the mean±SE for n experiments performed in duplicate. Both basal and maximally stimulated insulin release gradually decreased as passage number increased (ANOVA; P<0.0001).*

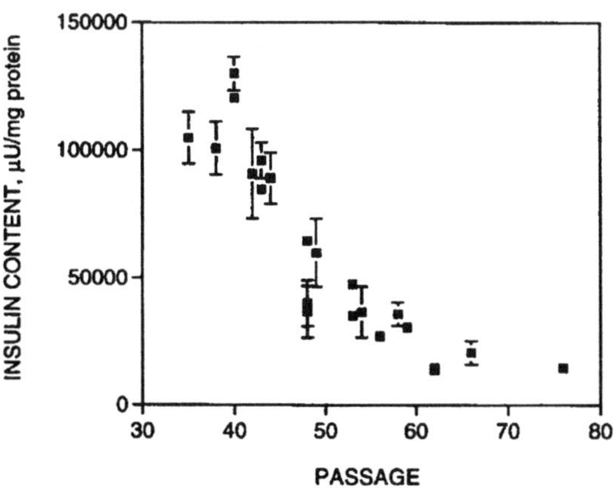

Figure 15. *Intracellular insulin in βTC-6 cells serially passaged in RPMI-1640 containing 11.1 mM glucose from passage 35 to 76. Intracellular insulin was measured after acidified ethanol extraction. Each datum represents the mean±SD for an individual experiment performed in duplicate. Intracellular insulin decreased as passage number increased (ANOVA;P<0.0001). Reprinted with permission from reference (42).*

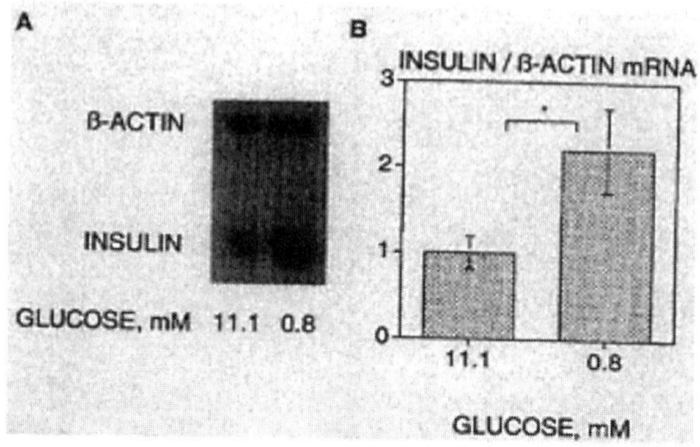

Figure 16. *Northern analysis of insulin mRNA in βTC-6 cells cultured in either 11.1 or 0.8 mM glucose for 20-27 sk.* ***A)*** *Representative experiment performed at passage 57.* ***B)*** *Densitometric analysis of insulin mRNA from 5 experiments performed at passage 55-62. Data are expressed as mean±SE relative density of insulin mRNA/β-actin mRNA. Cells chronically cultured in 0.8 mM glucose had more insulin mRNA than cells chronically cultured in 11.1 mM glucose. *P<0.05. Reprinted with permission from reference (42).*

In control experiments, we have used an α-cell line, the αTC-1/9 cell, which is a clonal cell derived from islet cell tumours obtained from transgenic mice in which the large T antigen SV-40 was expressed in islet cells under control of the proglucagon gene promoter (64). These cells were cultured for 30 passages in media containing various glucose concentrations. Population doubling times as well as levels of glucagon mRNA, glucagon content, and glucagon secretion were assessed. We found no differences in population doubling times when comparing the earlier passages (P43) and the later passages (P64). In marked contrast to our studies of insulin gene expression in β-cell lines, glucagon gene expression, content, and secretion remain preserved in αTC-1/9 cells despite chronic passaging in media containing glucose concentrations ranging from physiologic to supraphysiologic (3.0, 5.5, 11.1, and 16.7 mM) (65). In both static incubations and perifusion studies, glucagon secretion is not diminished in cells cultured under high glucose concentrations (Figure 20). Similarly, neither glucagon content nor glucagon gene expression as detected by northern analysis are reduced (Figure 21). We conclude that the glucotoxic effects observed in HIT-T15 cells and βTC-6 cells are specific to β-cell lines and not a generalized effect that applies to this α-cell line. Isolated rat islets cultured for up to 6 weeks in supraphysiological (16.7 mM) glucose concentrations have insulin mRNA amounts that are half of those found in controls (5.6 mM) (66). GLUT2 protein and mRNA levels are not affected in the same experiment (66).

Zucker Diabetic Fatty (ZDF) Rats as Models of Glucose Toxicity

To establish physiological relevance, the *in vitro* experiments we have described assessing molecular mechanisms of glucose toxicity must be replicated *in vivo*. To this end, we have recently carried out studies using Zucker diabetic fatty (ZDF) rats. The ZDF animals are homozygous for deficiency of the leptin receptor, and develop obesity and hyperglycaemia with decreased insulin gene expression after 6-7 weeks of age (67-71). The lean counterpart of the ZDF animal is the Zucker lean control (ZLC) which does not have deficiency in leptin receptors and does not develop hyperglycaemia. Previous experiments by Seufert et al. (46) established that development of hyperglycaemia in this animal model is associated with the loss of insulin gene expression and IDX-1 (STF-1) protein by western analysis. Interestingly, the transcription factor C/EBPβ, a repressor of insulin promoter activity, was found to be up-regulated in association with hyperglycaemia in the ZDF animal. Similar observations were made in a 90% pancreatized rat model of diabetes studied by the same authors (46).

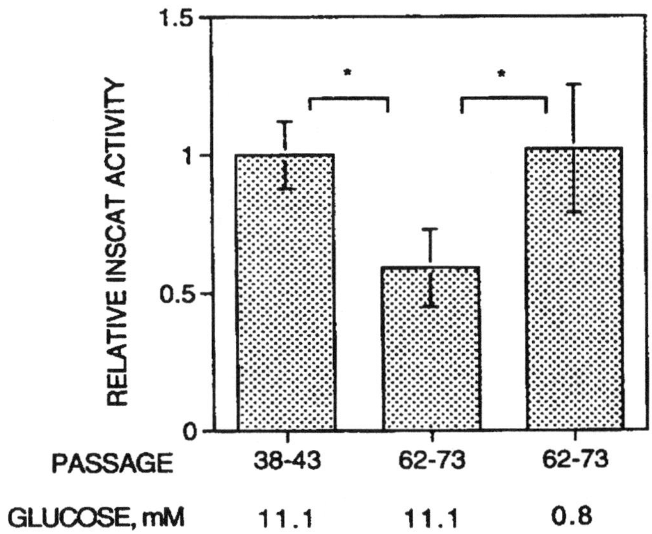

Figure 17. *Early passages (38-43) of βTC-6 cells or late passages (62-73) of βTC-6 cells cultured in either 11.1 or 0.8 mM glucose were transiently transfected with INSCAT. The relative expressions of INSCAT to RSVCAT are normalized to expression observed in early passage βTC-6 cells. Late passages of cells chronically cultured in 11.1 mM glucose had decreased INSCAT activity as compared to early passage cells. In contrast, INSCAT activity was preserved in late passage cells chronically cultured in 0.8 mM glucose. Data represent the mean±SE for five independent experiments with duplicate observations* (n = *5). *P<0.01. Reprinted with permission from reference (42).*

In attempts to link a cause and effect relationship between the development of hyperglycaemia and the subsequent loss of STF-1 and insulin gene expression in this animal model, we designed experiments in which hyperglycaemia was prevented by the drug troglitazone. Four groups of animals were examined. ZLC and ZDF animals were either treated or not treated with troglitazone given orally from 6 weeks of age. By 16 weeks of age we observed that the ZDF animals developed hyperglycaemia and marked decreases in STF-1 mRNA, STF-1 binding to the insulin promoter, insulin mRNA levels and glucose-induced insulin secretion. Troglitazone prevented the development of hyperglycaemia in the ZDF animals and this prevention was associated with preserved STF-1 mRNA, STF-1 binding, insulin mRNA, and glucose-stimulated insulin secretion (72). We interpreted these findings to be consistent with the hypothesis that progressive hyperglycaemia in this animal model causes secondary effects on insulin gene expression that are associated with a decrease in STF-1 gene expression. We do not rule out that the beneficial effects of troglitazone might be partially explained by the avoidance of another pathophysiologic state, lipotoxicity (73-75), since this drug has also been reported to decrease circulating triglycerides and free fatty acids. To differentiate glucose toxic effects from lipotoxic effects will require experimentation with drugs that lower glucose levels but not blood lipid or intraislet triglyceride levels, as well as experiments with lipid-lowering agents that do not affect glucose levels.

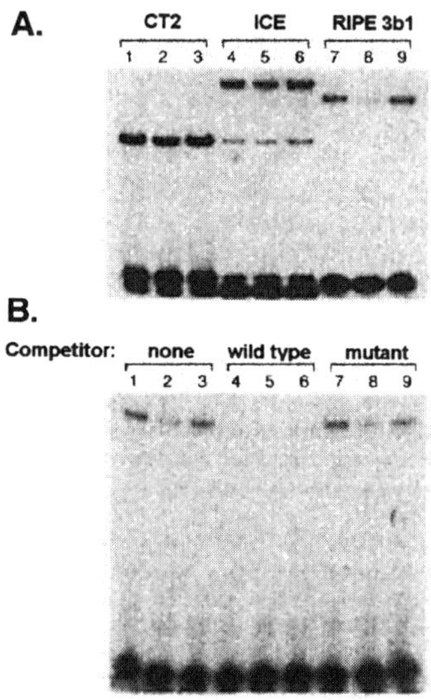

Figure 18. *EMSA analysis of nuclear extracts from early passage of βTC-6 cells and late passage of βTC-6 cells chronically cultured in 0.8 or 11.1 mM glucose. A) EMSA using P-labeled sequences to the CT2 (lanes 1-3), ICE/E1 (lanes 4-6), and RIPE3b1 (lanes 7-9) binding sites. Lanes 1, 4, and 7: nuclear extract from βTC-6 cells passage 71 chronically cultured in 0.8 mM glucose. Using oligodeoxynucleotides to the RIPE3b1 sequence, a major DNA/protein complex was present in early passage cells and late passage cells cultured in 0.8 mM glucose (lanes 7 and 9), but was reduced in late passage cells cultured in 11.1 mM glucose (lane 8). B) EMSA using P-labeled sequence to the RIPE3b1. Lanes 1, 4, and 7: nuclear extract from βTC-6 cells passage 71 chronically cultured in 0.8 mM glucose. Competitor added: lanes 4-6: 200-fold excess of unlabeled wild type sequence; lanes 7-9: 200-foldexcess of unlabeled mutant sequence. Similar results were obtained for two independent experiments for each condition. Reprint with permission from reference (42).*

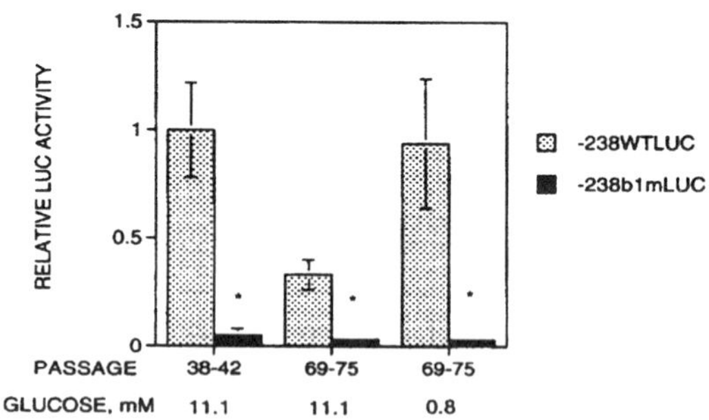

Figure 19. *Functional analysis of the RIPE3b1 binding site. Early passages of βTC-6 cells or late passages of βTC-6 cells cultured in 0.8 or 11.1 mM glucose were transiently transfected with either the wild type vector –238WTLUC or the mutant vector –238b1mLUC. The relative –238LUC/RSVLUC expressions were normalized to the expression observed in early passage cells. Mutation of the RIPE3b1 binding site almost abolished the insulin promoter expression in all three conditions. Data represent the mean±SE for four independent experiments with duplicate observations (n = 4). *P<0.05 vs. wild type vector. Reprinted with permission from reference (42).*

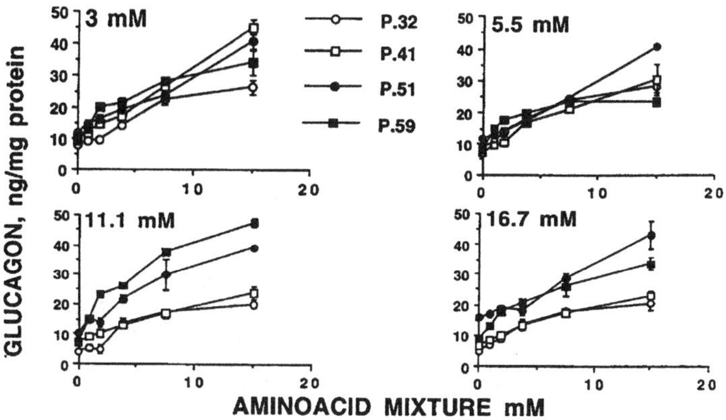

Figure 20. *Glucagon responses during static incubations of αTC-1/9 cells that had been chronically cultured in RPMI 1640 media containing 3.0, 5.5, 11.1, or 16.7 mM glucose. The passages examined were 32, 41, 51, and 59. Stimulation was provided by increasing concentrations of a mixture of amino acids. Glucagon secretion was not decreased in the older cells that had been cultured in high glucose concentrations. Reprinted with permission from reference (65).*

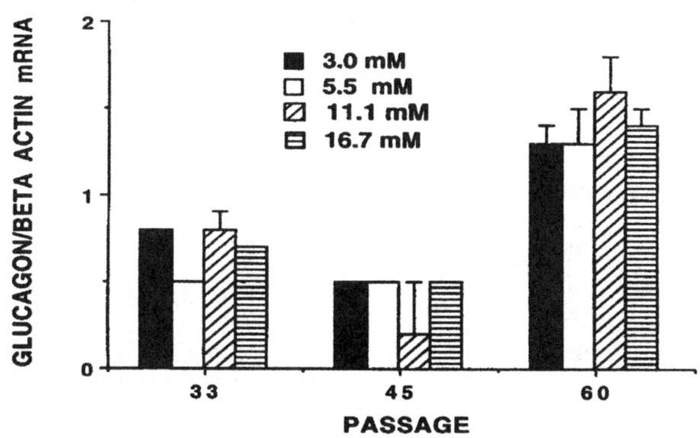

Figure 21. *Glucagon/β actin mRNA levels in αTC-1/9 cells chronically cultured from passage 33 through 60 in media containing 4 different glucose concentrations. Reprinted with permission from reference (65).*

In other recent experiments, we evaluated the hypothesis that one mechanism of glucose toxicity might be chronic oxidative stress. The rationale for performing these experiments is that hyperglycaemia is known to be associated with clinical oxidative stress in diabetic patients and that auto-oxidation of glucose is known to generate reactive oxygen species (76-80). In these experiments, either n-acetyl-cysteine (NAC), a potent antioxidant (81,82), or placebo was injected in ZDF animals. ZLC control animals were treated likewise. Treatment was begun at 6 weeks of age and carried through 12 weeks of age. Serum measures of chronic oxidative stress were higher in the ZDF rats that developed hyperglycaemia compared to the ZLC rats and to ZDF rats treated with NAC. Hyperglycaemia, decreased glucose tolerance, decreased insulin secretion, decreased STF-1 binding to the insulin promoter, and decreased insulin gene expression were found in the ZDF animals treated with placebo. In contrast, the ZDF animals treated with NAC failed to develop hyperglycaemia and had preserved STF-1 binding, insulin gene expression and nearly normal insulin secretion and glucose tolerance (83). We observed similar findings in parallel studies using aminoguanidine, a drug that is both an antioxidant and an inhibitor of glycosylation (84-87). In this context, it is interesting to note that troglitazone is also an antioxidant (88).

SPECULATION: IMPACT OF GLUCOSE TOXICITY ON THE PATHOGENESIS OF TYPE 2 DIABETES MELLITUS

This chapter has focused on potential molecular mechanisms of glucose toxicity. What role might glucose toxicity play in the pathogenesis of type 2 diabetes mellitus? This form of diabetes, which has variably been termed adult-onset diabetes or noninsulin-dependent diabetes, usually begins in the 5th decade of life and is silent in its onset. Eventually, the patient becomes aware of the disease because of significantly elevated glucose concentrations, which are associated with loss of glucose in the urine, increased urinary volume, and weight loss. It is speculated that the time elapsed between onset of the disease and its full symptomatic expression may be as long as 5 to 10 years. In this context, we view the cause of type 2 diabetes mellitus to be a combination of defective insulin secretion and peripheral insulin resistance. As this combination leads to the development of frank hyperglycaemia, it seems likely that continued exposure to elevated circulating glucose concentrations over the years before the disease is detected might secondarily cause glucose toxic effects on the islet β-cell. Moreover, once detected, if the disease is not optimally treated to return the patient to normal glucose levels, he may experience continued exposure to the toxic effects of supraphysiologic concentrations of glucose. In this context, glucotoxicity might lead to an ever-downward spiralling negative effect on the insulin synthetic machinery of the β-cell, leading in turn to more extreme hyperglycaemia.

If our findings using β-cell lines and ZDF rats have relevance to this disease, it can be predicted that there is an initial element of reversible glucose desensitization, followed later by β-cell exhaustion of the islet, in the early years after the establishment of hyperglycaemia. With time, however, a non-reversible component of hyperglycaemia emerges that is glucose toxicity-related. If true, this circumstance is reminiscent of the experiments previously cited by Moran et al. (41) in which approximately only 20% of the loss in insulin gene expression and insulin secretion in glucotoxic HIT-T15 cells could be reversed by switching the culture media from a high glucose concentration to a low concentration. This emphasizes the need for meticulous regulation of glycaemia in type 2 diabetic patients, as has already been demonstrated by Ohkubo et al. (89) in non-islet studies of secondary complications of this disease.

REFERENCES

1. Rossetti L, Giaccari A, DeFronzo RA. Glucose Toxicity. Diabetes Care 1990;13:610-630.
2. Yki-Jarvinen H. Glucose Toxicity. Endocr Rev 1992;13:415-431.
3. Leahy JL. Impaired beta-cell function with chronic hyperglycemia: "overworked beta-cell" hypothesis. Diabetes Rev 1996;4:298-319.
4. Flatt PR, Abdel-Wahab YHA, Boyd AC, Barnett CR, F.P.M. OH. Pancreatic beta-cell dysfunction and glucose toxicity in non-insulin-dependent diabetes. Proc Nutr Soc 1997;56:243-262.
5. Robertson RP. Type II diabetes, glucose "non-sense," and islet desensitization. Diabetes 1989;38:1501-1505.

6. Robertson RP, Olson LK, Zhang H-J. Differentiating glucose toxicity from glucose desensitization: a new message from the insulin gene. Diabetes 1994;43:1085-1089.
7. Robertson RP, Olson LK, Redmon JB, Zhang H-J, Towle HC. Glucose toxicity and the insulin gene. In: Draznin G, LeRoith D, eds. Molecular Biology of Diabetes, Part I: Humana Press Inc., 1994:195-212.
8. Grodsky GM, Curry DL, Bennett LL, Rodrigo JJ. Factors influencing different rates of insulin release in vitro. Acta Diabetologia Latina 1968;5:140-161.
9. Grodsky GM. A new phase of insulin secretion. How will it contribute to our understanding of beta-cell function? Diabetes 1989;38:673-678.
10. Grodsky GM, Bolaffi JL. Desensitization of the insulin-secreting beta cell. J Cell Biochem 1992;48:3-11.
11. Giroix M-H, Serradas P, Portha B. The desensitization of normal beta-cells to glucose *in vitro* is transient and not related to high glucose levels. Endocrinology 1989;125:1999-2007.
12. Thibault C, Laury M-C, Bailbe D, Ktorza A, Portha B. Effect of prolonged *in vivo* glucose infusion on insulin secretion in rats with previous glucose intolerance. Endocrinology 1992;130:2521-2527.
13. Efendic S, Lins PE, Cerasi E. Potentiation and inhibition of insulin release in man following priming with glucose and with arginine-effect of somatostatin. Acta Endocrinologia 1979;90:259-271.
14. Glaser B, Leibovich G, Nesher R, Hartling S, Binder C, Cerasi E. Improved beta-cell function after intensive insulin treatment in severe non-insulin-dependent diabetes. Acta Endocrinologia 1988;118:365-373.
15. Kaiser N, Corcos AP, Sarel I, Cerasi E. Monolayer culture of adult rat pancreatic islets on extracellular matrix: modulation of B-cell function by chronic exposure to high glucose. Endocrinology 1991;129:2067-2076.
16. Gross DJ, Leibowitz G, Cerasi E, Kaiser N. Increased susceptibility of islets from diabetes-prone *psammomys obesus* to the deleterious effects of chronic glucose exposure. Endocrinology 1996;137:5610-5615.
17. Liu YQ, Tornheim K, Leahy JL. Shared biochemical properties of glucotoxicity and lipotoxicity in islets decrease citrate synthase activity and increase phosphofructokinase activity. Diabetes 1998;47:1889-1893.
18. Leahy JL, Bonner-Weir S, Weir GC. Minimal chronic hyperglycemia is a critical determinant of impaired insulin secretion after an incomplete pancreatectomy. J Clin Invest 1988;81:1407-1414.
19. Leahy JL, Bumbalo LM, Chen C. Beta-cell hypersensitivity for glucose precedes loss of glucose-induced insulin secretion in 90% pancreatectomized rats. Diabetologia 1993;36:1238-1244.
20. Xia M, Hokin LE, Laychock SG. Rat pancreatic islets cultured at hyperglycemic glucose concentrations have altered phosphoinositide turnover, inositol phosphate production and ATP levels. Endocrine 1994;2:741-747.
21. Boden G, Ruiz J, Kim C-J, Chen X. Effects of prolonged glucose infusion on insulin secretion, clearance, and action in normal subjects. Am J Physiol 1996:E251-E258.
22. Purrello F, Rabuazzo AM, Anello M, Patane G. Effects of prolonged glucose stimulation on pancreatic beta cells: from increased sensitivity to desensitization. Acta Diabetol 1996;33:253-256.
23. Kosaka K, Kuzuya T, Akanuma Y, Hagura R. Increase in insulin response after treatment of overt maturity-onset diabetes is independent of the mode of treatment. Diabetologia 1980;18:23-28.
24. Rossetti L, Shulman GI, Zawalich W, DeFronzo RA. Effect of chronic hyperglycemia on in vivo insulin secretion in partially pancreatectomized rats. J Clin Invest 1987;80:1037-1044.
25. Ling Z, Kiekens R, Mahler T, et al. Effects of chronically elevated glucose levels on the functional properties of rat pancreatic β-cells. Diabetes 1996;45:1774-1782.
26. Sako Y, Grill VE. Coupling of β-cell desensitization by hyperglycemia to excessive stimulation and circulating insulin in glucose-infused rats. Diabetes 1990;39:1580-1583.
27. Urata Y, Yamamoto H, Goto S, et al. Long exposure to high glucose concentration impairs the responsive expression of y-glutamylcysteine synthetase by interleukin-1b and tumor necrosis factor-a in mouse endothelial cells. J Biol Chem 1996;271:15146-15152.
28. Pehuet-Figoni M, Ballot E, Bach J-F, Chatenoud L. Aberrant function and long-term survival of mouse β-cells exposed in vitro to high glucose concentrations. Cell Transplant 1994;3:445-451.
29. Davalli AM, Ricordi C, Socci C, et al. Abnormal sensitivity to glucose of human islets cultured in high glucose medium: partial reversibility after an additional culture in a normal glucose medium. J Clin Endocrinol Metab 1991;72:202-208.
30. Bedoya FJ, Jeanrenaud B. Insulin secretory response to secretagogues by perifused islets from chronically glucose-infused rats. Diabetes 1991;40:15-19.
31. Eizirik DL, Strandell E, Sandler S. Prolonged exposure of pancreatic islets isolated from "pre-diabetic" non-obese diabetic mice to a high glucose concentration does not impair beta-cell function. Diabetologia 1991;34:6-11.
32. Svensson C, Sandler S, Hellerstrom C. Lack of long-term b-cell glucotoxicity *in vitro* in pancreatic islets isolated from two mouse strains (C57BL/6J; C5BL/KsJ) with different sensitivities of the b-cells to hyperglycaemia *in vivo*. J Endocrinol 1992;136:289-296.

33. Ling Z, Pipeleers DG. Prolonged exposure of human β-cells to elevated glucose levels results in sustained cellular activation leading to a loss of glucose regulation. J Clin Invest 1996;98:2805-2812.
34. Zhang HJ, Walseth TF, Robertson RP. Insulin secretion and cAMP metabolism in HIT cells. Reciprocal and serial passage-dependent relationships. Diabetes 1989;38:44-8.
35. Kilpatrick ED, Robertson RP. Differentiation between glucose-induced desensitization of insulin secretion and b-cell exhaustion in the HIT-T15 cell line. Diabetes 1998;47:606-611.
36. Robertson RP, Zhang H-J, Pyzdrowski KL, Walseth TF. Preservation of insulin mRNA levels and insulin secretion in HIT cells by avoidance of chronic exposure to high glucose concentrations. J Clin Invest 1992;90:320-325.
37. Olson LK, Redmon JB, Towle HC, Robertson RP. Chronic exposure of HIT cells to high glucose concentrations paradoxically decreases insulin gene transcription and alters binding of insulin gene regulatory protein. J Clin Invest 1993;92:514-519.
38. Olson LK, Sharma A, Peshavaria M, et al. Reduction of insulin gene transcription in HIT-T15 β-cells chronically exposed to a supraphysiologic glucose concentration is associated with loss of STF-1 transcription factor expression. Proc Natl Acad Sci USA 1995;92:9127-9131.
39. Sharma A, Olson LK, Robertson RP, Stein R. The reduction of insulin gene transcription in HIT-T15 β-cells chronically exposed to high glucose concentration is associated with the loss of RIPE3b1 and STF-1 transcription factor expression. Mol Endocrinol 1995; 9:1127-1134.
40. Harmon JS, Tanaka Y, Olson LK, Robertson RP. Reconstitution of glucotoxic HIT-T15 cells with somatostatin transcription factor-1 partially restores insulin promoter activity. Diabetes 1998;47:900-904.
41. Moran A, Zhang HJ, Olson LK, Harmon JS, Poitout V, Robertson RP. Differentiation of glucose toxicity from beta cell exhaustion during the evolution of defective insulin gene expression in the pancreatic islet cell line, HIT-T15. J Clin Invest 1997;99:534-9.
42. Poitout V, Olson LK, Robertson RP. Chronic exposure of betaTC-6 cells to supraphysiologic concentrations of glucose decreases binding of the RIPE3b1 insulin gene transcription activator. J Clin Invest 1996;97:1041-6.
43. Eizirik DL, Korbutt GS, Hellerstrom C. Prolonged exposure of human pancreatic islets to high glucose concentrations in vitro impairs the beta-cell function. J Clin Invest 1992;90:1263-8.
44. Olson LK, Qian J, Poitout V. Glucose rapidly and reversibly decreases INS-1 cell insulin gene transcription via decrements in STF-1 and C1 activator transcription factor activity. Mol Endocrinol 1998;12:207-19.
45. Lu M, Seufert J, Habener JF. Pancreatic beta-cell-specific repression of insulin gene transcription by CCAAT/enhancer-binding protein beta. Inhibitory interactions with basic helix-loop-helix transcription factor E47. J Biol Chem 1997;272:28349-59.
46. Seufert J, Weir GC, Habener JF. Differential expression of the insulin gene transcriptional repressor CCAAT/enhancer-binding protein beta and transactivator islet duodenum homeobox-1 in rat pancreatic beta cells during the development of diabetes mellitus. J Clin Invest 1998;01:2528-39.
47. Schmeltz R, Wendorff HJ, Field JB. Effect of control of blood glucose on plasma insulin responses to various stimuli in secondary failures to oral hypoglycemic agents and in newly diagnosed, maturity onset, ketosis-resistant diabetics. J Clin Endocrinol Metab 1978;46:519-27.
48. Garvey WT, Olefsky JM, Griffin J, Hamman RF, Kolterman OG. The effect of insulin treatment on insulin secretion and insulin action in type II diabetes mellitus. Diabetes 1985;34:222-34.
49. Vague P, Moulin JP. The defective glucose sensitivity of the β–cell in non insulin dependent diabetes. Improvement after twenty hours of normoglycaemia. Metabolism 1982;31:139-42.
50. Flax H, Matthews DR, Levy JC, Coppack SW, Turner RC. No glucotoxicity after 53 hours of 6.0 mmol/l hyperglycaemia in normal man. Diabetologia 1991;34:570-5.
51. Giddings SJ, Chirgwin J, Permutt MA. Effects of glucose on proinsulin messenger RNA in rats in vivo. Diabetes 1982;31:624-9.
52. Welsh M, Nielsen DA, MacKrell AJ, Steiner DF. Control of insulin gene expression in pancreatic beta-cells and in an insulin-producing cell line, RIN-5F cells. II. Regulation of insulin mRNA stability. J Biol Chem 1985;260:13590-4.
53. Koranyi L, James DE, Kraegen EW, Permutt MA. Feedback inhibition of insulin gene expression by insulin. J Clin Invest 1992;89:432-6.
54. Philippe J, Pacheco I, Meda P. Insulin gene transcription is decreased rapidly by lowering glucose concentrations in rat islet cells. Diabetes 1994;43:523-8.
55. Petersen HV, Peshavaria M, Pedersen AA, et al. Glucose stimulates the activation domain potential of the PDX-1 homeodomain transcription factor. FEBS Letters 1998;431:362-6.
56. Leibiger B, Moede T, Schwarz T, et al. Short-term regulation of insulin gene transcription by glucose. Proc Natl Acad Sci USA 1998;95:9307-12.
57. Macfarlane WM, McKinnon CM, Felton-Edkins ZA, Cragg H, James RFL, Docherty K. Glucose stimulates translocation of the homeodomain transcription factor PDX1 from the cytoplasm to the nucleus in pancreatic beta-cells [In Process Citation]. J Biol Chem 1999;274:1011-6.
58. Zhang HJ, Petersen B, Robertson RP. Variable regulation by insulin of insulin gene expression in HIT-T15 cells. Diabetologia 1994;37:559-66.

59. Santerre RF, Cook RA, Crisel RM, et al. Insulin synthesis in a clonal cell line of simian virus 40-transformed hamster pancreatic beta cells. Proc Natl Acad Sci USA 1981;78:4339-43.
60. Robertson RP, Tsai P, Little SA, Zhang HJ, Walseth TF. Receptor-mediated adenylate cyclase-coupled mechanism for PGE2 inhibition of insulin secretion in HIT cells. Diabetes 1987;36:1047-53.
61. Boam DS, Clark AR, Docherty K. Positive and negative regulation of the human insulin gene by multiple trans-acting factors. J Biol Chem 1990;265:8285-96.
62. German M, Ashcroft S, Docherty K, et al. The insulin gene promoter. A simplified nomenclature [letter]. Diabetes 1995;44:1002-4.
63. Efrat S, Linde S, Kofod H, et al. Beta-cell lines derived from transgenic mice expressing a hybrid insulin gene-oncogene. Proc Natl Acad Sci USA 1988;85:9037-41.
64. Powers AC, Efrat S, Mojsov S, Spector D, Habener JF, Hanahan D. Proglucagon processing similar to normal islets in pancreatic alpha- like cell line derived from transgenic mouse tumor. Diabetes 1990;39:406-14.
65. Sacchi G, Zhang H-J, Robertson RP. Glucsoe toxicity and alpha cell function. Diabetologia 1996;42:A13.
66. Briaud I, Rouault C, Reach G, Poitout V. Long-term exposure of isolated rat islets to supraphysiologic glucose concentrations decreases insulin mRNA levels. Metabolism 1999;48:319-323.
67. Tokuyama Y, Sturis J, DePaoli AM, et al. Evolution of beta-cell dysfunction in the male Zucker diabetic fatty rat. Diabetes 1995;44:1447-57.
68. Sreenan S, Sturis J, Pugh W, Burant CF, Polonsky KS. Prevention of hyperglycemia in the Zucker diabetic fatty rat by treatment with metformin or troglitazone. Am J Physiol 1996;271:E742-7.
69. Ohtani KI, Shimizu H, Sato N, Mori M. Troglitazone (CS-045) inhibits beta-cell proliferation rate following stimulation of insulin secretion in HIT-T 15 cells. Endocrinology 1998;139:172-8.
70. Pick A, Clark J, Kubstrup C, et al. Role of apoptosis in failure of beta-cell mass compensation for insulin resistance and beta-cell defects in the male Zucker diabetic fatty rat. Diabetes 1998;47:358-64.
71. Wang MY, Koyama K, Shimabukuro M, Mangelsdorf D, Newgard CB, Unger RH. Overexpression of leptin receptors in pancreatic islets of Zucker diabetic fatty rats restores GLUT-2, glucokinase, and glucose- stimulated insulin secretion. Proc Natl Acad Sci USA 1998;95:11921-6.
72. Harmon JD, Oseid EA, Gleason CE, Tanaka Y, Hunter-Berger KK, Robertson RP. Prevention of hyperglycemia and glucotoxic effects on insulin gene expression by troglitazone in ZDF rats. J Invest Med 1999;47:29A.
73. Zhou YT, Shimabukuro M, Lee Y, et al. Enhanced de novo lipogenesis in the leptin-unresponsive pancreatic islets of prediabetic Zucker diabetic fatty rats: role in the pathogenesis of lipotoxic diabetes. Diabetes 1998;47:1904-8.
74. Gremlich S, Bonny C, Waeber G, Thorens B. Fatty acids decrease IDX-1 expression in rat pancreatic islets and reduce GLUT2, glucokinase, insulin, and somatostatin levels. J Biol Chem 1997;272:30261-9.
75. Shimabukuro M, Zhou YT, Lee Y, Unger RH. Troglitazone lowers islet fat and restores beta cell function of Zucker diabetic fatty rats. J Biol Chem 1998;273:3547-50.
76. Wolff SP, Dean RT. Glucose autoxidation and protein modification. The potential role of 'autoxidative glycosylation' in diabetes. Biochem J 1987;245:243-250.
77. Yoshida K, Hirokawa J, Tagami S, Kawakami Y, Urata Y, Kondo T. Weakened cellular scavenging activity against oxidative stress in diabetes mellitus: regulation of glutathione synthesis and efflux. Diabetologia 1995;38:201-10.
78. Matsuoka T-a, Kajimoto Y, Watada H, et al. Glycation-dependent, reactive oxygen species-mediated suppression of the insulin gene promoter activity in HIT cells. J Clin Invest 1997;99:144-150.
79. Traverso N, Menini S, Cosso L, et al. Immunological evidence for increased oxidative stress in diabetic rats. Diabetologia 1998;41:265-70.
80. Sano T, Umeda F, Hashimoto T, Nawata H, Utsumi H. Oxidative stress measurement by in vivo electron spin resonance spectroscopy in rats with streptozotocin-induced diabetes. Diabetologia 1998;41:1355-60.
81. Cotgreave IA. N-acetylcysteine: pharmacological considerations and experimental and clinical applications. Adv Pharmacol 1997;38:205-27.
82. Pieper GM, Siebeneich W. Oral administration of the antioxidant, N-acetylcysteine, abrogates diabetes-induced endothelial dysfunction. J Cardiovasc Pharmacol 1998;32:101-5.
83. Tanaka Y, Gleason CE, Oseid EA, et al. Prevention of glucose toxicity in HIT-T15 cells and ZDF rats by an antioxidant, N-acetyl-l-cysteine. Proc Natl Acad Sci USA 1999;96:10857-62.
84. Giardino I, Fard AK, Hatchell DL, Brownlee M. Aminoguanidine inhibits reactive oxygen species formation, lipid peroxidation, and oxidant-induced apoptosis. Diabetes 1998;47:1114-20.
85. Tajiri Y, Moller C, Grill V. Long-term effects of aminoguanidine on insulin release and biosynthesis: evidence that the formation of advanced glycosylation end products inhibits β-cell function. Endocrinology 1997;138:273-80.

86. Purrello F, Vetri M, Gatta C, Gullo D, Vigneri R. Effects of high glucose on insulin secretion by isolated rat islets and purified beta-cells and possible role of glycosylation. Diabetes 1989;38:1417-22.
87. Bucala R, Model P, Cerami A. Modification of DNA by reducing sugars: a possible mechanism for nucleic acid aging and age-related dysfunction in gene expression. Proc Natl Acad Sci USA 1984;81:105-9.
88. Fujiwara T, Ohsawa T, Takahashi S, et al. Troglitazone, a new antidiabetic agent possessing radical scavenging ability, improved decreased skin blood flow in diabetic rats. Life Sci 1998;63:2039-47.
89. Ohkubo Y, Kishikawa H, Araki E, et al. Intensive insulin therapy prevents the progression of diabetic microvascular complications in Japanese patients with non-insulin- dependent diabetes mellitus: a randomized prospective 6-year study. Diabetes Res Clin Pract 1995;28:103-17.

5

THE α-CELL AND REGULATION OF GLUCAGON GENE TRANSCRIPTION

Willhart Knepel, Ph.D.
University of Göttingen, 37075 Göttingen, Germany

INTRODUCTION

The glucagon gene in mammals is a single copy gene that is expressed in a highly tissue-restricted fashion (1). Best known is its expression in α-cells of the pancreatic islets, but it is also expressed in intestinal L-cells, a few neurones in the brain and, at very low levels, the thymus (1-4). Using all six exons of the glucagon gene, a single common transcript and proglucagon prohormone is generated in the pancreas, intestine, and brain (1-3). However, tissue-specific post-translational processing results in the formation of peptides that have distinctly different bioactivities (1). The intestinal L-cells process proglucagon predominantly to glucagon-like peptide 1 (GLP-1), GLP-2, and oxyntomodulin that play important roles in the regulation of insulin secretion, intestinal epithelial proliferation, and intestinal glucose absorption, respectively (2,5). GLP-1 formed in the brain modulates the action of leptin and the central control of feeding (2). In contrast, in pancreatic islets, cleavage of proglucagon results predominantly in the formation of glucagon and, to a lesser extent, GLP-1 (1).

Glucagon is a peptide hormone of 29 amino acids and a biologic antagonist of insulin. After secretion into the portal circulation, glucagon acts on the liver to enhance hepatic fuel production through glycogenolysis, gluconeogenesis, and ketogenesis (6-8). By stimulating glucose output from the liver, glucagon secures an adequate glucose supply for the body's organs including exercising muscles and the brain, for which glucose is normally the sole source of energy. Glucagon thus plays an important role in the body's defence against hypoglycaemia. Since, in the resting state, about 75 percent of basal hepatic glucose production is glucagon-mediated, glucagon may well be essential for life, which could account for the absence of cases of isolated glucagon deficiency. Inactivating mutations of the glucagon gene seem to be incompatible with survival. Abnormal regulation of glucagon gene expression and relative hyperglucagonemia contribute to impaired glucose tolerance in diabetes mellitus (6-8).

THE MOLECULAR MECHANISM OF PANCREATIC ISLET α-CELL-SPECIFIC ACTIVATION OF GLUCAGON GENE TRANSCRIPTION

Because of the fact that every cell of an organism possesses in its nucleus all genes, it is obvious that highly efficient mechanisms exist which ensure the specific activation of a given gene in a particular cell type. The terminally differentiated pancreatic islets are composed of phenotypically distinct hormone-producing cells, the more prominent of which are the cells that produce glucagon (α), insulin (β), and somatostatin (δ). Pancreatic islet cell-specific gene expression is controlled at the transcriptional level. Experiments using transgenic mice (9,10), cell-free *in vitro* transcription systems (11) and gene transfer into cultured tumour cell lines (12,13) suggest that pancreatic α-cell-specific activation of the glucagon gene is conferred by the 5'-flanking region of the glucagon gene. A fragment of the glucagon gene extending about 1,300 base pairs (bp) upstream of the cap site directs transcription to pancreatic α-cells and the brain, but not to the intestine, of transgenic mice (9,10) suggesting that different tissue-specific enhancer elements mediate activation of glucagon gene transcription in the pancreas and intestine. A reporter fusion gene containing 350 bp of the 5'-flanking region of the glucagon gene is sufficient for cell-specific activation of transcription in glucagon-producing pancreatic islet tumour cell lines (12,13) as well as in nuclear protein extracts from these cell lines (11). Although these cells were originally derived from pancreatic endocrine cells and have retained many characteristics of fully differentiated normal pancreatic islet cell types, it has to be kept in mind that results derived from transformed cell lines may not represent the actual *in vivo* situation and that such findings need to be confirmed for adult animals. It is thus not known whether 350 bp of the 5'-flanking region of the glucagon gene are sufficient to activate glucagon gene transcription specifically in pancreatic α-cells *in vivo*.

Gene transcription depends on the one hand on the so-called general transcription machinery that, under suitable conditions, assembles as a multiprotein complex including TATA box-binding protein and RNA polymerase II around the start site of transcription of the gene. However, efficiency, cell-specificity, and regulation of gene transcription is conferred by proteins, called transcription factors that bind in a sequence-specific manner to DNA and, upon DNA binding, interact with the general transcription machinery to stimulate or to inhibit gene transcription. The transcriptional activity of the glucagon gene 5'-flanking region is thus conferred by interacting transcription factors. Experiments using transient transfections of various glucagon reporter fusion genes into islet and non-islet cell lines as well as *in vitro* protein-DNA binding assays (*in vitro* DNase I footprinting) identified three regions within 350 bp of the 5'-flanking region that interact with nuclear proteins and function as major transcriptional control elements (13). The so-called G2 (from about -170 to -200) and G3 (from about -235 to -270) elements appear to display islet-specific enhancer-like properties inasmuch as they enhance expression in some phenotypically distinct pancreatic islet cell lines but not in several non-islet cell lines; the promoter element G1 (from about -50 to -100) has low transcriptional activity of its own but is required to mediate transcriptional activation by G2 and G3 (13). Although the presence of G1 does not prevent transactivation of the glucagon or thymidine kinase promoter by homologous or viral enhancer elements in non-islet cell lines or islet cell lines with β- or δ-cell phenotypes (13,14), studies in which glucagon promoter fragments were fused to homologous or heterologous enhancer elements provide some evidence that the proximal glucagon promoter including the G1 element may play a role in restricting glucagon gene transcription to cell lines with α-cell phenotype (13,15).

Underscoring the importance of the G1, G2, and G3 control elements for glucagon gene transcription is the fact that the 5'-flanking sequences of the rat and human glucagon gene have been highly conserved during evolution, with 95 and 97% homology for G1 and G2, respectively (13). Notably, the first 125 bp 5' of the cap site of the rat gene has 91% homology with the human gene sequences. The more distal sequences are less well conserved since rat G3 has only 75% homology with human G3, a percentage which is similar to the overall homology of the first 300 bp (13).

After the initial description of the G1, G2, and G3 control elements, many interacting protein complexes were detected in *in vitro* DNase I footprinting or electrophoretic mobility shift assays with nuclear extracts from islet or non-islet cell lines, suggesting that a great number of islet-specific or more widely expressed transcription factors bind and regulate the glucagon gene. Several of these proteins have now been identified at the molecular level (Figure 1).

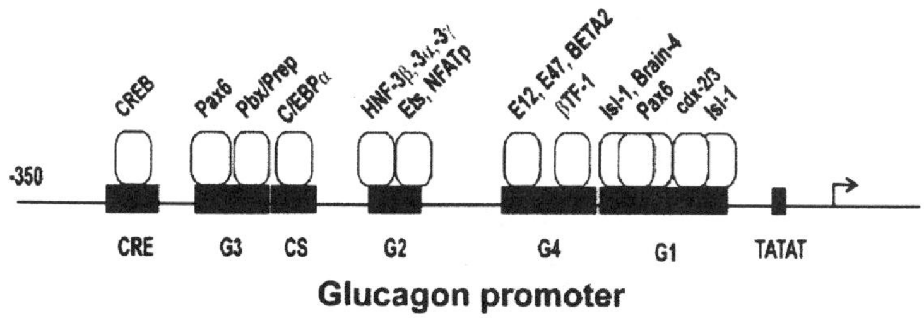

Figure 1. *Control elements within the 5'-flanking region of the rat glucagon gene and transcription factors that are known to bind these elements. The arrow indicates the start site of transcription. CRE, cAMP response element; CS, C/EBP binding site.*

TRANSCRIPTION FACTORS OF THE G1 ELEMENT

The G1 element contains AT-rich motifs (15) characteristic of core elements that bind homeodomain-containing transcription factors. These observations suggest that the islet cell-specific expression of the glucagon gene may be mediated by one or more homeobox-containing proteins expressed in pancreatic α-cells. Several homeodomain proteins of distinct classes have indeed been shown to be able to bind to the G1 element and to be present in G1-binding nuclear protein complexes from glucagon-expressing pancreatic islet cell lines, including the LIM domain homeobox protein Isl-1 (16), the *caudal*-related homeodomain protein cdx-2/3 (17,18), and the pit-oct-unc (POU) homeobox transcription factor brain-4 (19) (Figure 1). Isl-1 plays an important role in islet development (20) and is expressed in all classes of islet cells in the adult (20). The observation that Isl-1 is detected as part of a high molecular weight complex in nuclear extracts from the glucagon-producing pancreatic islet cell line InR1-G9 by electrophoretic mobility shift assays (16) suggests that protein-protein interactions may be important for the formation of a transcriptionally active Isl-1 complex on the glucagon gene promoter which, however, remains to be shown. In contrast to Isl-1, overexpression of cdx-2/3 activates the glucagon promoter in BHK fibroblasts (17) or InR1-G9 cells (18), whereas a mutation of the major cdx-2/3 binding site within G1 decreases glucagon reporter gene activity in InR1-G9 cells (15). These data indicate that cdx-2/3 positively regulates transcriptional activity of the glucagon gene in α-cell lines. However, brain-4 showed in BHK fibroblasts a four- to fivefold stronger glucagon reporter gene-activating capability compared to that of cdx-2 (19). By immunofluorescence staining, abundant brain-4 immunoreactivity in adult rat pancreas localizes to nuclei of glucagon-producing cells located in the mantle of the rat islet, whereas cdx-2 immunoreactivity is detected at various intensities in a few scattered cells throughout adult rat islets but does not show a clear localization to the glucagon-producing cells in the islet periphery; cdx-2 is, however, found in abundance in gut epithelial cells (19). It may thus be possible, according to this relative tissue distribution, that brain-4 is the predominant regulator of the glucagon gene in pancreatic islet α-cells (and in the brain), whereas cdx-2/3 is the predominant tissue-specific factor binding to the G1 element in proglucagon-expressing cells of the intestine. However, the function of brain-4 for activation of the glucagon gene in normal pancreatic α-cells remains to be confirmed *in vivo.*

In addition to Isl-1, cdx-2/3, and brain-4, the G1 element interacts also with the transcription factor Pax6 (Figure 1) (see further below), which contains both, a homeodomain and a paired domain. Furthermore, there is evidence for the binding of additional, not yet identified proteins to the G1 element (15). Since some of the binding sites of these factors within G1 seem to overlap intensively, it is likely that some of the G1-binding transcription factors may interact, a first example being the recently described transcriptionally co-operative complex of Pax6 with cdx-2/3 on the G1 element (21,22). Cdx-2/3 preferentially binds to the 3' AT-rich site within G1, which partially overlaps, with the Pax6 site (21,22). Based on a proposed model of protein-DNA contacts (21) Pax6 and cdx-2/3 contact the major groove of the DNA at the same nucleotides but the geometry of the paired domain and the homeodomain would place the DNA binding domains adjacent to each other. Brain-4 preferentially binds to the 5' AT-rich site within G1 (19), which is contained completely within the Pax6 site (21). This may not necessarily prohibit simultaneous binding of Pax6 and brain-4 since the somatostatin upstream element (UE) gives an example of Pax6 binding simultaneously with another homeodomain protein. In the case of the somatostatin UE, Pax6 and Pdx1 bind to completely overlapping binding sites and together contribute to the β/δ-cell specificity of this enhancer element (21,23). It will be interesting to see how Pax6 and brain-4 interact on the G1 element, which may be important for pancreatic α-cell-specific expression of the glucagon gene.

Just upstream of the G1 element the glucagon promoter contains a region (G4) that, similar to control elements in the insulin gene, contains adjacent binding sites for Pdx1 and the basic region helix-loop-helix proteins E2A (E12/E47/E2/5) and Beta2 (NeuroD) (Figure 1). The binding of Pdx1 to the glucagon promoter was detected with a nuclear protein complex from a rat pancreatic insulinoma cell line (RIN 1046-38) that was initially called βTF-1 (24) and was later molecularly identified as the homeobox protein Pdx1 (also called IDX-1, STF-1, IPF-1) (25). Although Pdx1 activates the insulin and somatostatin promoter and is important for pancreas formation (26), the lack of Pdx1 expression in the majority of glucagon-producing α-cells (26) excludes a role for Pdx1 in glucagon gene transcription in mature islets. Beta2 is expressed in all endocrine cells of the pancreas (27). However, the binding affinity of Beta2/E47 heterodimers to the site in the glucagon promoter is much lower when compared with sites in the insulin promoter (28) and the overexpression of Beta2 in non-islet cells does not activate a glucagon reporter gene although it does activate the insulin gene (Figure 2) (U. Leinemann and W. Knepel, unpublished observation). Thus, a role for Beta2 in the regulation of glucagon gene transcription remains to be shown.

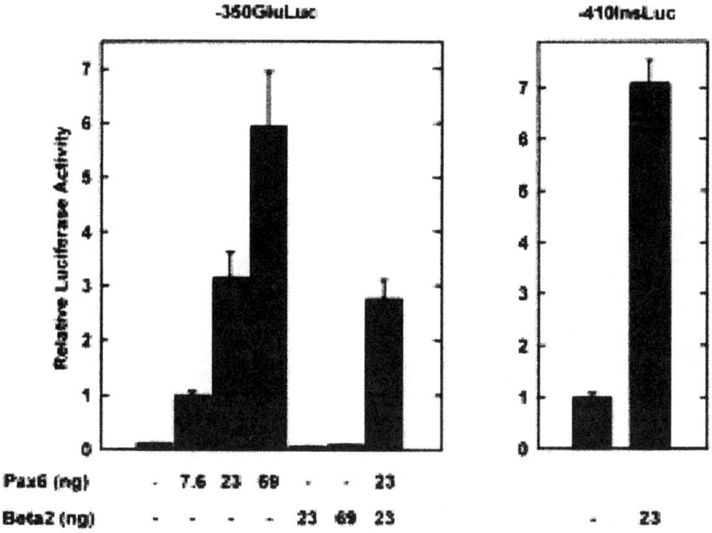

Figure 2. *Overexpression of Pax6, but not Beta2, activates glucagon gene transcription in a non-islet cell line. Reporter genes containing 350 bp of the 5'-flanking region of the rat glucagon gene (-350GluLuc) or 410 bp of the 5'-flanking region of the rat insulin I gene (-410InsLuc) were transiently transfected into JEG cells together with the indicated amounts of expression vectors encoding Pax6 (pBAT14.mPAX6) or Beta2 (pCDM8.BETA2). Activation by Beta2 of -410InsLuc served as a positive control. Values are mean ± S.E. of six experiments.*

TRANSCRIPTION FACTORS OF THE G2 ELEMENT

Hepatocyte nuclear factor (HNF) proteins were initially believed to be expressed only in the liver. They have been classified into several groups according to the structure of their DNA-binding domains. The HNF-3 proteins (HNF-3α, -3β, -3γ) are members of the HNF-3/*forkhead* transcription factor family that share a so-called winged-helix DNA-binding domain (29). HNF-3α, -3β, and -3γ are expressed early during development and are transcriptional activators that co-ordinately regulate the expression of a number of liver-specific genes (29). All three proteins are also expressed in pancreatic islets and phenotypically distinct pancreatic islet cell lines (30-34). A sequence within G2 shares extensive homology with reported HNF-3 binding sites (Figure 3). From -181 to -192, ten of the twelve bases match the HNF-3 consensus-binding site (35), suggesting that HNF-3 proteins may be involved in glucagon gene transcription. Consistent with this view, a nuclear protein complex binding to this sequence and contained in nuclear extracts from two glucagon-producing pancreatic islet cell lines (InR1-G9, αTC2) was identified as HNF-3β (30,33). HNF-3β was initially postulated to negatively regulate G2 transcriptional activity, since HNF-3β repressed the activity of glucagon promoter constructs in transfected InR1-G9 cells (30). Whether this observation might be attributable to nonphysiological overexpression of HNF-3β leading to squelching of promoter activity or to an imbalance of HNF-3β levels relative to those of other transcription factors is not clear. In contrast, deletion of the HNF-3β-binding site leads to a major loss of G2 transcriptional activity (33), implying that HNF-3 proteins clearly activate glucagon gene transcription through the G2 enhancer. This is directly supported by findings in cotransfection assays showing that HNF-3β as well as HNF-3α and HNF-3γ transactivate glucagon reporter constructs in non-islet HepG2 (33) or BHK cells (34). However, transactivation by HNF-3β in pancreatic α-cell lines requires protein binding to a site closely associated with the HNF-3β site within G2 (33). The protein binding to this site has not yet been molecularly identified. The fact that its binding to G2 depends on a sequence motif, GGAA (Figure 3) (33), which is known as an essential purine-rich core of binding sites for Ets proteins (36,37) as well as cross-competition binding experiments (33) suggest that this protein may be related to the Ets family of transcription factors. All these data provide strong evidence for the positive action of HNF-3 proteins on glucagon gene transcription; functionally interacting with a factor possibly related to Ets family proteins (Figure 1).

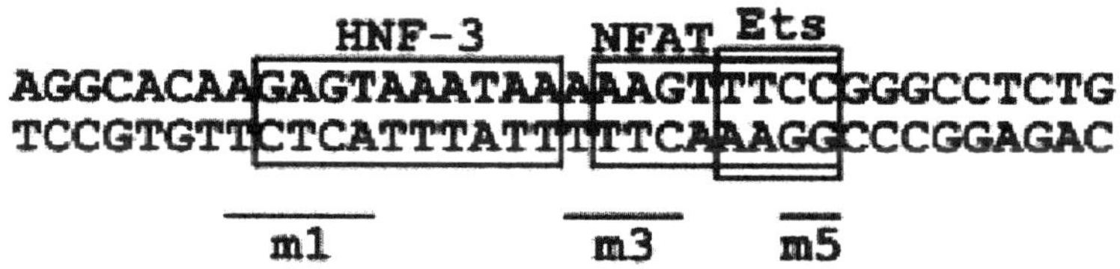

Figure 3. *The G2 wild-type sequence. The boxed sequence motifs show the homology to the HNF-3 consensus binding site as well as the GGAA motif, an essential purine-rich core of binding sites for members of the Ets family of transcription factors. Also boxed is a sequence, 5'-GGAAACTT-3', which shares extensive homology with a sequence in the murine IL-2 gene that binds transcription factors of the NFAT family. The bases mutated in mutants 1, 3, and 5 (33) are indicated.*

Mice with a targeted deletion in the HNF-3β gene die around embryonic day 10 to 11 (38,39) precluding assessment of glucagon gene expression in the endocrine pancreas in the absence of HNF-3β. Mice homozygous for a null mutation in the HNF-3α gene (HNF-3α$^{-/-}$) survive embryonic development but die of severe hypoglycaemia within fourteen days after birth (34). These HNF-3α$^{-/-}$ mice can store glycogen in the liver and express normally HNF-3 target genes involved in hepatic gluconeogenesis. However, plasma glucagon levels are markedly reduced, as is the cellular content of steady-state glucagon mRNA levels in pancreatic islet α-cells (34). These results thus identify HNF-3α as an essential positive activator of the glucagon gene *in vivo*. At the same time they also strengthen the view that glucagon is essential for survival. Although an indirect effect of HNF-3α on glucagon gene expression cannot be excluded, the available data suggests strongly that HNF-3α directly activates glucagon gene transcription in the endocrine pancreas *in vivo*. HNF-3α is thus the first and only transcription factor whose role in glucagon gene transcription has so far been demonstrated *in vivo*.

Noteworthy, the sequence of the HNF-3 binding site within G2 of the human glucagon gene differs from the sequence in the rat glucagon gene in two positions in a way that does not match the HNF-3 consensus-binding motif (eight out of twelve bases in human G2 match the HNF-3 consensus) (13,35). The consequence, if any, of this alteration for HNF-3 binding and function is not yet known.

TRANSCRIPTION FACTORS OF THE G3 ELEMENT AND THE ROLE OF PAX6

The glucagon G3 enhancer element comprises two domains, A and B, that bind distinct cellular proteins (40). The domain A contains a sequence motif which is present also in the upstream element (UE) of the rat somatostatin gene and the enhancer 1 (E1) element of the rat insulin I gene (Figure 4) (14) and which is therefore called pancreatic islet cell-specific enhancer sequence, PISCES (Figure 4). These elements, however, display different pancreatic islet cell-type-specific activities (14). Multiple copies of the PISCES motif are sufficient to selectively stimulate transcriptional activity of a luciferase reporter gene in various phenotypically distinct pancreatic islet cell lines without affecting expression in several non-islet cell lines (42). Because mutation studies have demonstrated that the PISCES element is important for the activity of each of the three hormone gene promoters (14,40,42), the PISCES motif and its binding factor appear to be a key component of the transcription complexes co-ordinately directing insulin, glucagon, and somatostatin gene transcription in distinct islet cell types.

PISCES
Pancreatic islet cell-specific enhancer sequences

		Match to PISCES Consensus
Glucagon-G3 (-263/-252)	TTTCACGCCTGA	12/12
Glucagon-G1 (-73/-84)	TTTCTCATCTGT	9/12
Insulin-E1 (-309/-320)	TTTTCCACCTCA	11/12
Somatostatin-UE (-81/-92)	TTTTACGCACCA	10/12
PISCES Consensus	TTTYACRCCTSA	
Pax6 consensus	A--TTCACGCMTSA-TKM-Y	11/12

Figure 4. *Comparison between the PISCES motif and the Pax6 paired domain consensus binding site. PISCES, pancreatic islet cell-specific enhancer sequences. The PISCES consensus motif is determined by alignment of the two rat glucagon gene control elements G3 and G1, the enhancer-1 element of the rat insulin I gene (Insulin-E1), and the upstream element (UE) of the rat somatostatin gene. The numbers given in parentheses designate the number of bp from the transcriptional start sites of the respective genes. The Pax6 paired domain consensus binding site was taken from Epstein et al. (41). W, A or T; K, G or T; M, A or C; Y, T or C; R, A or G; S, G or C.*

The PISCES motif found in the rat insulin I E1 element is, however, at that position not conserved in the human insulin gene (43). The PISCES motifs of the rat glucagon G3, somatostatin UE, and insulin I E1 elements cross-compete for the binding of a nuclear protein that is found in all islet cell types (42) and that has been identified as the transcription factor Pax6 (44). Pax6 contains two DNA-binding domains, a paired domain and a homeodomain (45,46), and the PISCES motif shows high homology to part of the consensus recognition site of the Pax6 paired domain (Figure 4) (41,47,48). The Pax6 paired domain recognition site is unusually long (20 bp) because in contrast to most other Pax proteins the Pax6 paired domain contacts DNA not only through its N-terminal subdomain but also through its C-terminal subdomain (47,48). The bp 16 to 20 at the 3' end of the Pax6 paired domain recognition sequence make major groove contacts with the recognition helix of the C-terminal subdomain (48) and are not included in the PISCES motif (Figure 4). Thus, the way in which Pax6 interacts with the PISCES motifs in the various enhancer elements could be different with possibly significant functional consequences.

Pancreatic islets express the Pax6 gene as at least two isoforms, only one of which binds the PISCES motif (49). An alternatively spliced exon (exon 5a) results in the insertion of a 14-amino acid peptide in the N-terminal subdomain of the Pax6 paired domain and in unique DNA-binding properties (47). The Pax6 paired domain binds very well the PISCES motif, whereas the extended paired domain (Pax6-5a) does not (Figure 5) (49). The glucagon gene contains a PISCES motif not only in G3 but also in G1 (Figure 4) and each PISCES motif appears to be important for glucagon promoter activity, since the mutation of the PISCES motif within G3 and also within G1 lead to a marked reduction in glucagon promoter activity (Figure 6) (R. Grzeskowiak and W. Knepel, unpublished observation). Furthermore, Pax6 is a powerful activator of the glucagon promoter in a non-islet cell line (Figure 2) and a GAL4-Pax6 fusion protein restores transcriptional activity of a glucagon promoter construct in which the PISCES motifs have been mutated into binding sites of the yeast transcription factor GAL4 (Figure 6). All these data strongly suggest that Pax6, acting through the PISCES motif, is a major transcriptional activator of the glucagon gene in islet cell lines.

However, when a PISCES-luciferase reporter gene, that exhibits strong transcriptional activity in pancreatic islet cell lines (42), was used to generate transgenic mice, the PISCES motif directed gene expression in the adult eye, cerebellum, and discrete brain areas, consistent with the tissue distribution of Pax6, whereas no reporter gene expression was found in pancreatic islets (Figure 7) (49). The lack of PISCES-mediated transcription in adult islets of transgenic mice indicates that the Pax6 protein(s) expressed in adult pancreatic islets function differently from the ones in the eye, cerebellum, and islet cell lines. It is possible that islet hormone gene transcription in normal islets *in vivo* is maintained independently of Pax6. Alternatively, Pax6 by itself may not be sufficient for transcriptional activation in normal islets and may depend on the interaction with additional proteins. On the somatostatin UE, Pax6 has been shown to bind simultaneously with Pdx1 to completely overlapping sites and to thereby confer transcriptional activity in an islet cell line (23) whereas a complex consisting of Pdx1 and a Pbx/Prep1 heterodimer, reported previously (50), appears to be dispensable (23). There is also evidence for Pax6 complex formation on the glucagon G1 element (*supra*). Within the glucagon G3 element, cellular proteins bind to domain B closely associated with the Pax6 binding site (40). Although the binding of these proteins is competed for by some typical binding sites of winged-helix proteins (51), more recent data show that binding sites of certain homeodomain proteins are more powerful competitors for protein binding to domain B of G3 (S. Herzig and W. Knepel, manuscript in preparation). Furthermore, right next to G3 is a C/EBPα binding site that can mediate transactivation of the glucagon gene by C/EBPα (52). Whether and how these proteins interact with Pax6 is unknown. Although Pax6 is required for islet formation and the differentiation of glucagon-producing α-cells in mouse pancreas (53), the role of Pax6 in glucagon gene transcription *in vivo* remains to be established.

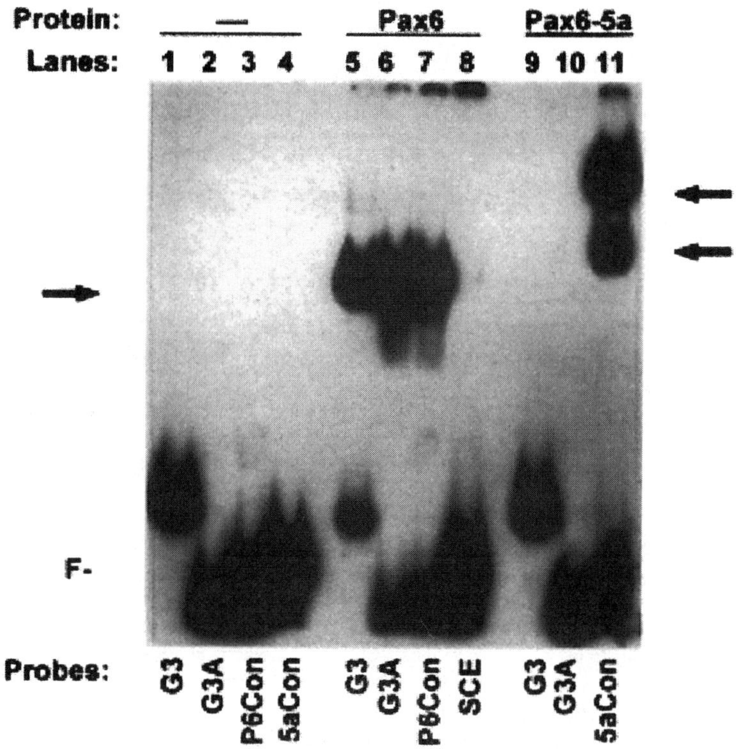

Figure 5. *The paired domain of Pax6, but not the splice variant Pax6-5a, binds the PISCES motif as revealed by electrophoretic mobility shift assay. The bacterially expressed Pax6 or Pax6-5a paired domains were incubated with the probes indicated. G3 and G3A (domain A of G3) contain the PISCES motif. P6Con and 5aCon contain high affinity consensus binding sites for the Pax6 and Pax6-5a paired domains, respectively, and served as positive controls. SCE contains the cAMP response element of the rat somatostatin gene and served as negative control. F, free probe. Specific complexes formed by Pax6 and Pax6-5a are indicated by arrows on the left and right, respectively. Pax6-5a has been shown to form several complexes when incubated with labelled 5aCon (47). Reproduced with permission from Beimesche et al. (49).*

A UNIQUE COMBINATION OF TRANSCRIPTION FACTORS

It is obvious that none of the transcription factors so far known to bind and regulate the glucagon gene is specific for pancreatic α-cells or exhibits a pattern of expression that is the same as that of the glucagon gene. These factors are expressed also in other pancreatic endocrine cells or in other tissues like the intestine (cdx-2/3), the liver (HNF-3 proteins), and the brain (brain-4, Isl-1, Beta2, Pax6). The finding that pancreatic islets share some transcription factors with the brain suggests a molecular explanation for the fact that pancreatic endocrine cells possess some characteristics of neurones. Although HNF-3 proteins and possibly brain-4 and Pax6 appear to be of major importance for glucagon gene transcription, at this time it has to be concluded that pancreatic islet α-cell-specific activation of the glucagon gene is conferred by a unique combinatorial and spatial arrangement of multiple transcription factors that synergistically activate the glucagon gene.

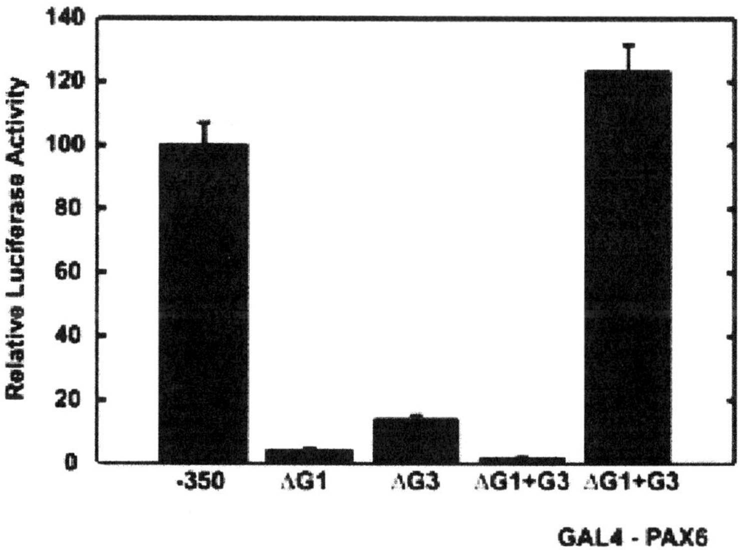

Figure 6. *The PISCES sequence both within G3 and G1 confers basal transcriptional activity to the glucagon promoter which, when lost by mutation, can be restored by Pax6. The PISCES motif within G3, G1, or both was mutated in a way to convert it into a DNA-binding site of the yeast transcription factor GAL4. Reporter fusion genes containing 350 bp of the 5'-flanking region of the rat glucagon gene with wild-type sequence (-350) or with internal mutations of the PISCES motif in G1 (ΔG1), G3 (ΔG3) or G1 and G3 (ΔG1+G3) were transiently transfected into the glucagon-producing pancreatic islet cell line InR1-G9. When indicated, an expression vector encoding Pax6 fused to the DNA-binding domain of GAL4 (GAL4-PAX6) was cotransfected. Values are means ± S.E. of six experiments.*

SIGNALLING PATHWAYS TO THE GLUCAGON GENE AND TARGETED TRANSCRIPTION FACTORS

To satisfy the fuel needs of the tissues of an organism; hepatic glucose and ketone production must be adjusted to the ever-varying supply and demand. Glucagon plays an important role in such metabolic adjustments. Thus, a great number of neural hormonal and metabolic messengers act on pancreatic islet cells and regulate the synthesis and secretion of pancreatic islet hormones. They act through distinct intracellular second messenger pathways including cAMP, calcium, and diacylglycerol. During exercise, glucose utilization by the muscles increases markedly and hypoglycaemia would supervene if there were not a stimulation of glucagon secretion mediated through the sympathetic nervous system. The transmitter of the sympathetic nervous system, noradrenaline, hereby acts on β-adrenergic cell-surface receptors leading to an increase in cAMP levels (6,7). In a subpopulation of α-cells, cAMP levels may be raised also by GLP-1 and glucagon itself (54,55). Glucagon-producing islet cells show spontaneous electrical activity (56) that is controlled by secretagogues in a way leading to an increase in cytosolic calcium concentration. Whereas L-arginine increases spike frequency (56), noradrenaline through cAMP increases the influx of calcium associated with each action potential (57). Activation of the parasympathetic nervous system stimulates glucagon secretion through acetylcholine acting on M3 muscarinic acetylcholine receptors that activate phospholipase C, generating inositol 1,4,5-trisphosphate and diacylglycerol, an activator of protein kinase C isoforms (58,59). The response of glucagon during a meal varies. The stimulation of glucagon secretion by amino acids like L-arginine and activation of the parasympathetic nervous system is suppressed under conditions of excess glucose. Thus, during a carbohydrate-rich meal hyperglycaemia and insulin inhibit glucagon secretion (6-8). Lack of inhibition by insulin contributes to the relative hyperglucagonemia in diabetes mellitus (6-8). Whereas the tight control of hormone secretion is critical for minute-to-minute metabolic adjustments, regulation of hormone synthesis is important in order to maintain the long-term responsiveness. Consistent with this view, cAMP, calcium, diacylglycerol, and insulin have been shown to regulate glucagon gene transcription. A summary of the signalling pathways to the glucagon gene and the transcription factors involved is shown in Figure 8.

THE CYCLIC AMP SIGNALLING PATHWAY

By transient transfections of both wild-type and mutant glucagon-reporter fusion genes into pancreatic islet cell lines it was shown that cAMP stimulates glucagon gene transcription through a cAMP response element (CRE) with the core octamer sequence TGACGTCA (from -291 to -298) (60) (Figure 8). The binding of cAMP to the regulatory subunits of protein kinase A releases the catalytic subunits which migrate into the nucleus and phosphorylate the transcription factor CREB bound to the glucagon CRE (60-63). CREB is a member of the basic region leucine zipper family of proteins (64). The leucine zipper is a dimerization domain and appears to form a continuous α-helix with the basic region, so that the basic region leucine zipper dimer is oriented almost perpendicular to the DNA axis. Numerous contacts to DNA bases and phosphate oxygens are made by basic region residues (65). CREB is a ubiquitously expressed protein and is now known to confer cAMP responsiveness to a great number of genes that carry a CREB binding site related to the consensus motif TGACGTCA (64).

Cyclic AMP stimulates the transactivating potential of CREB (66). The phosphorylation of CREB at serine-119 (in CREB-327) by protein kinase A allows CREB to bind and thereby recruit the coactivator CREB-binding protein (CBP) or the highly related protein p300 through their KIX domain (67-74). CBP/p300 then stimulate transcription by promoting chromatin remodelling, providing a molecular platform for additional cofactors, and contacting components of the general transcription machinery. These multiple functions are served by distinct regions of CBP. The middle region of CBP exhibits histone acetyltransferase activity that is required for CREB function (75), possibly because the acetylation of specific lysine residues located within the highly basic amino-terminal domains of the core histones may relax chromatin structure (76). Chromatin remodelling may also be favoured by recruiting RNA helicase A that binds to the Cys/His-rich region 3 (C/H3) of CBP and may locally unwind promoter DNA (77). Microinjection studies in Rat-1 fibroblasts revealed that CREB-mediated transcription requires the assembly of p/CAF and p/CIP on CBP as additional co-activators (75). The C/H3 region of CBP interacts *in vitro* with the basal transcription factor TFIIB (68), and the C- and N-termini of CBP bind TATA box-binding protein (78,79). Through its C/H3 region and RNA helicase A, CBP can associate with functional RNA polymerase II complexes (77), further supporting a role for CBP in the interaction between CREB and the basal transcription apparatus. These studies thus suggest that, in response to cAMP, CREB positions a specific CBP - p/CAF - p/CIP-coactivator complex that mediates transcriptional activation. However, it is unclear whether all CRE-containing genes exhibit the same requirements for the components of the CREB coactivator complex. The 12S adenovirus E1A protein can bind to the C/H3 region of CBP disrupting protein-protein interactions and inhibit CREB/CBP-dependent transcription (71,80,81). Recent studies show that whereas the 12S E1A protein inhibits cAMP-induced activation of a GAL4-CREB fusion protein in pancreatic islet cell lines, it enhances the cAMP-induced stimulation of the glucagon promoter (M. Chilla, E. Oetjen, R. Blume, and W. Knepel, submitted for publication). These results suggest that the CBP/p300-coactivator complex is differentially used by CREB anchored to the glucagon promoter. This differential use of CBP may reflect the assembly of a promoter-specific CBP-coactivator complex that allows the promoter-specific integration of the cAMP-induced signalling pathway and other signalling systems leading to a glucagon gene transcriptional response that secures appropriate blood glucose levels.

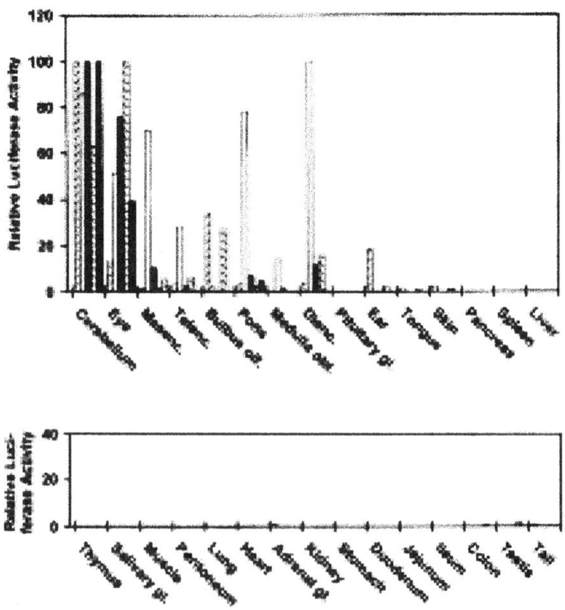

Figure 7. *PISCES-reporter transgene expression in adult transgenic mice. Four copies of the PISCES motif (domain A of G3) were placed in front of the minimal herpes simplex virus thymidine kinase promoter (from -81 to +52) and linked to the luciferase reporter gene (4xG3AT81Luc). Luciferase reporter enzyme activity was measured in the indicated tissues from five independent transgenic lines carrying the 4xG3AT81Luc transgene. For each independent transgenic line, luciferase activity measured in the tissue with highest activity is set as 100 and luciferase activity measured in the other tissues is expressed relative to that. Mesenc., mesencephalon; Telenc., telencephalon; Bulbus olf., bulbus olfactorius; Medulla obl., medulla oblongata; Dienc., diencephalon; gl., gland. Reproduced with permission from Beimesche et al. (49).*

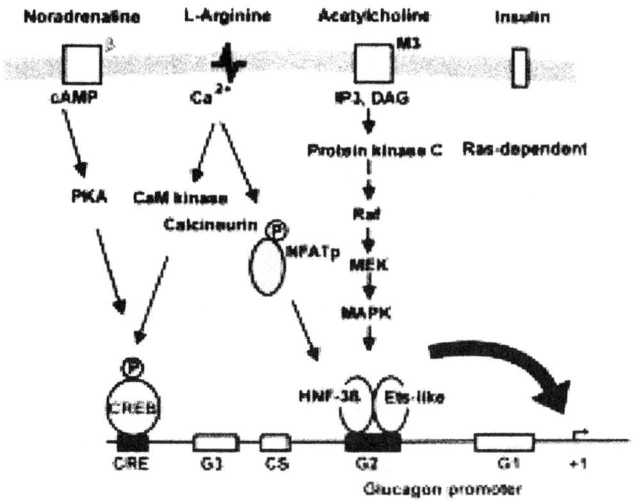

Figure 8. *Signalling pathways to the glucagon gene. CRE, cAMP response element; CS, C/EBP binding site; PKA, protein kinase A; CaM kinase, calcium/calmodulin-dependent protein kinase; MAPK, mitogen-activated protein kinase; MEK, MAPK/extracellular signal-regulated kinase kinase; IP3, inositol 1,4,5-trisphosphate; DAG, diacylglycerol; β, β-adrenergic receptor; M3, M3 muscarinic acetylcholine receptor.*

STIMULATION OF GLUCAGON GENE TRANSCRIPTION BY MEMBRANE DEPOLARIZATION AND CALCIUM INFLUX

Like neurones, endocrine cells of the pancreatic islets are electrically excitable. Using pancreatic islet cell lines, it has been shown that membrane depolarization stimulates glucagon gene transcription through the influx of calcium via voltage-dependent, L-type calcium channels, and an increase in the cytosolic free calcium concentration (82). Mapping studies demonstrated that at least two elements confer calcium responsiveness to the glucagon gene, one being the glucagon CRE (82,83). The same serine residue of CREB (serine-119 in CREB-327) that is phosphorylated by protein kinase A and that is important for transcriptional activation of CREB, is phosphorylated both *in vitro* and *in vivo* also by several other kinases including calcium/calmodulin-dependent (CaM) protein kinases (84). As has been demonstrated before in neuronal PC12 pheochromocytoma cells (84), CREB was shown, by using GAL4-CREB fusion proteins, to function as a depolarization-regulated transcription factor in pancreatic islet cells (82). Membrane depolarization and cAMP have synergistic effects on glucagon CRE-mediated transcription (82), the mechanism of which is unclear but may be due to the fact that CaM kinase activity may not only phosphorylate CREB and thereby induce the recruitment of CBP but also increase CBP transcriptional activity as has been shown recently in the mouse pituitary cell line AtT20 (85). Thus, the calcium signal may be transmitted via CaM kinases and CREB to the glucagon CRE (Figure 8).

Membrane depolarization relies also on calcineurin phosphatase activity for activation of CREB/CRE-mediated glucagon gene transcription in pancreatic islet cells (Figure 8). This is indicated by the observation that the immunosuppressive drugs cyclosporin A and FK506 (Tacrolimus) block calcineurin activity in islet cells and at the same concentrations also inhibit depolarization-induced CREB/CRE-mediated transcription (83,86,87). Calcineurin is a calcium/calmodulin-dependent protein phosphatase. Cyclosporin A and FK506 do not interfere with the calcium-induced phosphorylation of CREB at serine 119 (87). This suggests the existence of an additional, calcineurin-sensitive phosphorylation that directly or indirectly interferes with the transcriptional competence of serine 119-phosphorylated CREB. Although this calcineurin substrate is still unknown, recent experiments suggest that calcineurin phosphatase activity may be required for calcium-induced CBP activity in islet cells (E. Oetjen and W. Knepel, unpublished observation).

Interestingly, cyclosporin A and FK506 inhibit CREB/CRE-directed transcription not only in pancreatic islet cells but also in several other cell lines including Jurkat T-cells (88). When taken together with recent evidence for an essential role of CREB in T-cell activation and proliferation (89,90), inhibition of CREB/CRE-mediated transcription by cyclosporin A and FK506 may be a molecular mechanism of the immunosuppressive effect of these clinically important drugs (88,91).

The G2 element of the glucagon promoter has been identified as a second calcium response element of the glucagon gene (92). Some of the transcription factors involved appear to be different from those that confer basal activity to this element. By electrophoretic mobility shift assays, membrane depolarization was found to induce the binding of a nuclear complex with NFATp-like immunoreactivity to the G2 element (Figure 9) (92). NFATp was originally characterized as the pre-existing cytoplasmic component of a transcription factor in T-cell hybridomas implicated in the induction of several cytokine genes during the immune response (93). NFATp has been molecularly cloned (93) and is now known to be a member of a family of transcription factors that contain at least four members and share a 300-amino acid DNA-binding domain distantly related to the Rel homology region (93). In resting T-cells, NFATp resides in the cytoplasm and is fully phosphorylated; following stimulation, it rapidly becomes dephosphorylated by calcineurin activated by an increase in cytosolic calcium concentration, and NFATp then translocates to the nucleus (93,94). The G2 element contains a typical NFAT-binding site, 5'-GGAAACTT-3' (Figure 3).

The expression of NFATp in pancreatic islet αTC2 cells was confirmed by RT-PCR of NFATp mRNA as well as by Western blotting (92). Inhibition of calcineurin phosphatase activity by FK506 blocked both the depolarization-caused induction of nuclear NFATp binding and G2-mediated transcription. The latter was also prevented by mutating the binding sites for NFATp or HNF-3β within G2 (92). Taken together, these data suggest that the molecular mechanism by which glucagon gene transcription is induced by membrane depolarization and calcium influx in pancreatic islet cells through the G2 element may be consistent with a model in which calcium activates calcineurin phosphatase activity which then, probably by direct dephosphorylation, induces the translocation of NFATp from the cytosol to the nucleus where it co-operates with HNF-3β at the G2 element to stimulate transcription (Figure 10).

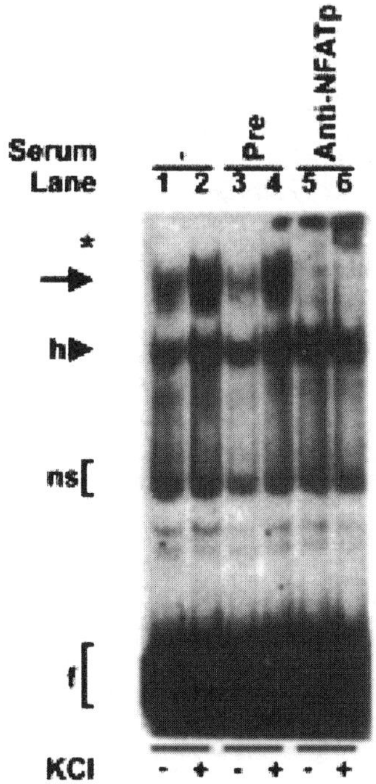

Figure 9. *Membrane depolarization induces nuclear protein binding to the G2 element, which is recognized by an antiserum specifically directed against NFATp. Electrophoretic mobility shift assay. Labelled G2 was incubated with nuclear extracts prepared from glucagon-producing pancreatic islet αTC2 cells that had been stimulated for 60 minutes with high potassium-induced membrane depolarization (KCl, 45 mM) or had been left unstimulated. Pre-immune serum (Pre) or anti-NFATp antiserum (Anti-NFATp) was added to the binding reaction as indicated on top of the lanes. The arrow indicates the depolarization-induced protein binding. h, bands representing the binding of HNF-3β; ns, non-specific bands; f, free probe. Reproduced with permission from Fürstenau et al. (92).*

Transcription factors of the NFAT family are known to co-operate with AP-1 proteins in T-cells for calcium-dependent activation of cytokine genes (93). In the IL-2 enhancer, NFAT and AP-1 together form a highly stable co-operative complex, wherein the so-called insert region of NFATc lies closest to the spacer region of cFos/cJun, allowing a single arginine residue in the c-Jun spacer (Arg-285) to make an especially important contact (95,96). The studies on the glucagon gene (92) show a novel pairing of NFATp with the cell-specific transcription factor HNF-3β in islet cells to form a novel calcium response element in the glucagon gene.

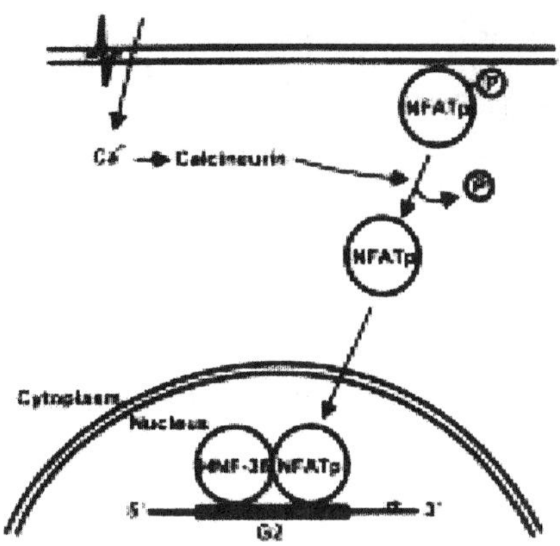

Figure 10. *Novel pairing of NFATp with the cell-specific transcription factor HNF-3β in islet cells to form a novel calcium response element in the glucagon gene. Recent results suggest a model in which membrane depolarization and calcium influx activate calcineurin phosphatase activity that then, probably by direct dephosphorylation, induces the translocation of NFATp from the cytosol to the nucleus where it co-operates with HNF-3β to stimulate transcription. Reproduced with permission from Fürstenau et al. (92).*

The N-terminal transactivation domain of NFATp has been shown to recruit the co-activators p300/CBP (97). The NFATp-CBP interaction may involve the C/H3 region of CBP that is distinct from the CBP CREB-binding domain, KIX (97). Thus, co-operative recruitment of a common coactivator by CREB, binding to the CRE, and NFATp, binding together with HNF-3β to G2, is a potential explanation for the observation (92) that depolarization responsiveness is conferred to the glucagon promoter by a synergistic interaction between G2 and the CRE (Figure 11).

STIMULATION OF GLUCAGON GENE TRANSCRIPTION BY PROTEIN KINASE C AND RAS

Early studies show that activation of protein kinase C with 12-*O*-tetradecanoylphorbol-13-acetate (TPA) increases steady-state glucagon mRNA levels and stimulates the formation of nascent glucagon RNA transcripts in nuclei from the RIN 1056-A islet cell line that simultaneously expresses multiple islet hormones, including glucagon (98), suggesting that glucagon gene transcription is regulated via a protein kinase C-activated pathway. This conclusion was confirmed recently by transient transfections of glucagon-reporter fusion genes into a more differentiated pancreatic islet cell line with α-cell phenotype, αTC2 (33). A protein kinase C response element was mapped to the G2 element (33). Like TPA, overexpression of oncogenic Ras (V-12 Ras) stimulated G2-mediated transcription whereas overexpression of a dominant negative Ras mutant (N-17 Ras) blocked the effect of TPA (33). Thus, the G2 element confers basal activity, calcium responsiveness, and protein kinase C/Ras responsiveness (Figure 8). A mutational analysis showed that the mutations in mutant 3 (Figure 3), which interfere with NFAT binding (92), abolished the transcriptional activation of G2 by membrane depolarization, whereas basal activity and protein kinase C responsiveness were not inhibited (33,92). In contrast, the mutations in mutant 1 and mutant 5 (Figure 3), which interfere, respectively, with HNF-3β and Ets-like protein/NFAT binding (33), decreased basal activity, depolarization responsiveness, as well as protein kinase C responsiveness (33,92). These data suggest that protein kinase C responsiveness, like basal activity, is conferred to the glucagon G2 element by HNF-3β functionally interacting with a protein that binds to a closely associate site with sequence similarity to binding sites of Ets family proteins (Figure 8).

These studies on the glucagon gene in pancreatic islet cells expand the functions of HNF-3β and possibly other HNF-3 proteins to include a role in calcium- and protein kinase C /Ras-regulated gene transcription. HNF-3β was first defined as a transcription factor involved in developmental and cell-specific gene transcription (*supra*). Subsequently, it has been suggested that HNF-3β synergizes with the glucocorticoid receptor in the liver to confer glucocorticoid responsiveness to the tyrosine aminotransferase gene (99). The results obtained in studies on the glucagon gene suggest that HNF-3β potentiates transcriptional activation by the calcium-regulated transcription factor NFATp (*supra*) and synergizes with an Ets-like transcription factor to confer Ras and protein kinase C responsiveness. Thus, HNF-3β is able to co-operate with several regulated transcription factors and in this way seems to function as a mediator of environmental signals in tissues in which it is expressed. Diverse protein kinase C response elements, including AP-1 and NF-κB sites, have already been described (100,101). The glucagon protein kinase C response element differs from these elements not only by DNA sequence and interacting proteins but also by the lack of a major effect of TPA on protein binding. The glucagon protein kinase C response element may have, however, some limited similarity to an element in the *c-fos* promoter. TPA activates *c-fos* via the serum response element, which interacts with a serum response factor dimer and a ternary complex factor, of which more than one may exist, belonging to a subgroup of the Ets-domain family that includes Elk-1, SAP-1, and SAP-2 (36). Thus, the tissue-specific transcription factor HNF-3β, interacting with possibly an Ets-related protein at the glucagon G2 element, represents a novel protein kinase C response unit.

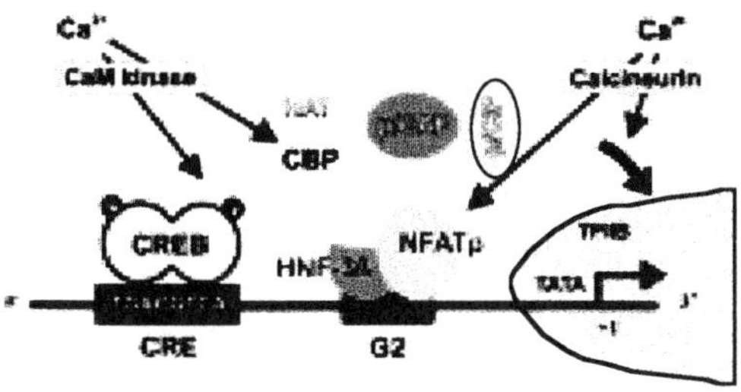

Figure 11. *Model for co-operative recruitment of a common coactivator, CBP, by CREB, binding to the CRE, and NFATp, binding together with HNF-3β to G2 in response to membrane depolarization and calcium influx. The model assumes that an increase in the cytosolic free calcium concentration activates CaM kinases that on the one hand phosphorylate CREB at serine-119, which allows CREB to bind CBP, and on the other hand increase the transcriptional activity of CBP. Calcium also activates calcineurin phosphatase activity that on the one hand is required for the calcium-induced transcriptional activity of CBP and on the other hand induces the nuclear translocation of NFATp. CRE, cAMP response element; TF, transcription factor; CBP, CREB-binding protein; HAT, histone acetyltransferase; p/CAF, p300/CBP-associated factor; p/CIP, p300/CBP-interacting protein; CaM kinase, calcium/calmodulin-dependent protein kinase.*

Protein kinase C can induce nuclear responses indirectly by activating protein kinase cascades leading to the nucleus (102-105). Although protein kinase C has multiple effector systems, protein kinase C controls the mitogen-activated protein kinases (MAPKs) by acting on Raf, probably through direct phosphorylation and activation of Raf (102,103,106,107). Thus, protein kinase C could stimulate Raf kinase, which leads through the MAPK/extracellular signal-regulated kinase kinase (MEK)-MAPK cascade to the activation of the glucagon protein kinase C response element in a Ras-dependent manner. Recent experiments support this view (Figure 8) (U. Fürstenau, L. Klinge, C. Dellas, and W. Knepel, unpublished observation). Members of the Ets family of transcription factors contain putative MAPK phosphorylation sites and have been shown to be phosphorylated by MAPKs *in vitro* (36) and to mediate the TPA/MAPK activation of the c-fos serum response element (107,108). Therefore, the suggested Ets-related protein, rather than HNF-3β, may be the target of the protein kinase C signalling pathway within the glucagon G2 element (Figure 8).

REGULATION OF GLUCAGON GENE TRANSCRIPTION BY GLUCOSE AND INSULIN

Hypoglycaemia and hyperglycaemia have been shown to increase and decrease, respectively, glucagon gene expression *in vivo* (109,110). However, the relative role of plasma glucose levels *per se*, plasma insulin levels or a combination of both in this regulation is still unclear (111,112). Insulin has been shown to inhibit glucagon gene transcription in the glucagon-producing pancreatic islet cell line InR1-G9 (113). However, the mechanism involved remains unclear. The insulin receptor is a tyrosine kinase and has been shown to signal through phosphatidylinositide 3-kinase, 3-phosphoinositide-dependent protein kinases, protein kinase B, and glycogen synthase kinase-3 to stimulate glycogen synthesis (114-116). Related signalling pathways may mediate other metabolic effects of insulin (114-116). An insulin responsive element in the 5'-flanking region of the rat glucagon gene, the G3 element, has been proposed (117). In another study, this element was, however, dispensable for inhibition by insulin of glucagon gene transcription (J. Amin, E. Oetjen, R. Grzeskowiak, and W. Knepel, unpublished observation).

INTEGRATION OF MULTIPLE SIGNALLING PATHWAYS

It became apparent in recent years that multiple positively acting (cAMP, calcium, protein kinase C, Ras) and negatively acting (glucose, insulin) signalling pathways converge on the glucagon gene 5'-flanking region. The involvement of HNF-3β as an essential component of a calcium- and protein-kinase C/Ras-responsive element gives an example how signalling pathways are tied directly to cell-specific control of gene transcription. The ability of protein kinase C and membrane depolarization to potentiate cAMP-induced glucagon gene transcription in a synergistic fashion (33,82) may be physiologically important. By virtue of this synergism, these distinct stimuli may participate in a cross talk between intracellular signalling systems that in α-cells integrates multiple stimuli to an appropriate transcriptional response of the glucagon gene.

REFERENCES

1. Habener JF, Drucker DJ, Mojsov S, Knepel W, Philippe J. Biosynthesis of glucagon. In: Samols E, ed. The endocrine pancreas. New York: Raven Press, 1991:53-71.
2. Drucker DJ. Glucagon-like peptides. Diabetes 1998;47:159-69.
3. Drucker DJ, Asa S. Glucagon gene expression in vertebrate brain. J Biol Chem 1988; 263:13475-8.
4. Throsby M, Homo-Delarche F, Chevenne D, Goya R, Dardenne M, Pleau JM. Pancreatic hormone expression in the murine thymus: localization in dendritic cells and macrophages. Endocrinology 1998;139:2399-406.
5. Stümpel F, Scholtka B, Hunger A, Jungermann K. Enteric glucagon 37 rather than pancreatic glucagon 29 stimulates glucose absorption in rat intestine. Gastroenterology 1998;115:1-10.
6. Unger RH, Orci L. Glucagon and the A cell (first part). New Engl J Med 1981;304:1518-24.
7. Unger RH, Orci L. Glucagon and the A cell (second part). New Engl J Med 1981;304:1575-80.
8. Lefebvre PJ. Glucagon and its family revisited. Diabetes Care 1995;18:715-30.
9. Efrat S, Teitelman G, Anwar M, Ruggiero D, Hanahan D. Glucagon gene regulatory region directs oncoprotein expression to neurones and pancreatic α cells. Neuron 1988;1:605-13.
10. Lee YC, Asa SL, Drucker DJ. Glucagon gene 5'-flanking sequences direct expression of simian virus 40 lage T antigen to the intestine, producing carcinoma of the large bowel in transgenic mice. J Biol Chem 1992;267:10705-8.
11. Knepel W. Transcriptional control of pancreatic islet hormones gene expression. Exp Clin Endocrinol 1993;101:39-45.

12. Drucker DJ, Philippe F, Jepeal L, Habener JF. Glucagon gene 5'-flanking sequences promote islet cell-specific gene transcription. J Biol Chem 1987;262:15659-65.
13. Philippe J, Drucker DJ, Knepel W, Jepeal L, Misulovin Z, Habener JF. Alpha-cell-specific expression of the glucagon gene is conferred to the glucagon promoter element by the interactions of DNA-binding proteins. Mol Cell Biol 1988;8:4877-88.
14. Knepel W, Vallejo M, Chafitz JA, Habener JF. The pancreatic islet-specific glucagon G3 transcription factors recognize control elements in the rat somatostatin and insulin-I genes. Mol Endocrinol 1991;5:1457-66.
15. Morel C, Cordier-Bussat M, Philippe J. The upstream promoter element of the glucagon gene, G1, confers pancreatic alpha cell-specific expression. J Biol Chem 1995;270:3046-55.
16. Wang M, Drucker DJ. The LIM domain homeobox gene *isl-1* is a positive regulator of islet-specific proglucagon gene transcription. J Biol Chem 1995;270:12646-52.
17. Jin T, Drucker DJ. Activation of proglucagon gene transcription through a novel promoter element by the caudal-related homeodomain protein cdx-2/3. Mol Cell Biol 1996;16:19-28.
18. Jin T, Trinh DKY, Wang F, Drucker DJ. The caudal homeobox protein cdx-2/3 activates endogenous proglucagon gene expression in InR1-G9 islet cells. Mol Endocrinol 1997;11:203-9.
19. Hussain MA, Lee J, Miller CP, Habener JF. POU domain transcription factor brain 4 confers pancreatic α-cell-specific expression of the proglucagon gene through interaction with a novel proximal promoter G1 element. Mol Cell Biol 1997;17:7186-94.
20. Ahlgren U, Pfaff SL, Jessell TM, Edlund T, Edlund H. Independent requirement for ISL1 in formation of pancreatic mesenchyme and islet cells. Nature 1997;385:257-60.
21. Andersen FG, Heller RS, Petersen HV, Jensen J, Madsen OD, Serup P. Pax6 and Cdx2/3 form a functional complex on the rat glucagon gene promoter G1-element. FEBS Lett 1999;445:306-10.
22. Ritz-Laser B, Estreicher A, Klages N, Saule S, Philippe J. Pax-6 and Cdx-2/3 interact to activate glucagon gene expression on the G_1 control element. J Biol Chem 1999;274:4124-32.
23. Andersen FG, Jensen J, Heller RS, Petersen HV, Lasson LI, Madsen OD, Serup P. Pax6 and Pdx1 form a functional complex on the rat somatostatin gene upstream enhancer. FEBS Lett 1999;445:315-20.
24. Kruse F, Rose SD, Swift GH, Hammer RE, MacDonald RJ. An endocrine-specific element is an integral component of an exocrine-specific pancreatic enhancer. Genes Dev 1993;7:774-86.
25. Swift GH, Liu Y, Rose SD, Bischof LJ, Steelman S, Buchberg AM, Wright CVE, MacDonald RJ. An endocrine-exocrine switch in the activity of the pancreatic homeodomain protein PDX1 through formation of a trimeric complex with PBX1b and MRG1 (MEIS2). Mol Cell Biol 1998;18:5109-20.
26. Habener JF, Stoffers DA. A newly discovered role of transcription factors involved in pancreas development and the pathogenesis of diabetes mellitus. Proc Assoc Am Physicians 1998;110:12-21.
27. Naya FJ, Huang HP, Qiu Y, Mutoh H, DeMayo FJ, Leiter AB, Tsai MJ. Diabetes, defective pancreatic morphogenesis, and abnormal enteroendocrine differentiation in BETA2/NeuroD-deficient mice. Genes Dev 1997;11:2323-34.
28. Dumonteil E, Laser B, Constant I, Philippe J. Differential regulation of the glucagon and insulin I gene promoters by the basic helix-loop-helix transcription factors E47 and BETA2. J Biol Chem 1998;273:19945-54.
29. Lai E, Clark KL, Burley SK, Darnell JE. Hepatocyte nuclear factor 3/fork head or "winged helix" proteins: A family of transcription factors of diverse biologic function. Proc. Natl Acad Sci USA 1993;90:10421-3.
30. Philippe J, Morel C, Prezioso VR. Glucagon gene expression is negatively regulated by hepatocyte nuclear factor 3ß. Mol Cell Biol 1994;14:3514-23.
31. Cockell M, Stolarczyk D, Frutiger S, Hughes GJ, Hagenbüchle O, Wellauer PK. Binding sites for hepatocyte nuclear factor 3ß or 3_ and pancreas transcription factor 1 are required for efficient expression of the gene encoding pancreatic _ -amylase. Mol Cell Biol 1995;15:1933-41.
32. Vaisse C, Kim J, Espinosa R, Le Beau MM, Stoffel M. Pancreatic islet expression studies and polymorphic DNA markers in the genes encoding hepatocyte nuclear factor-3α, -3β, -3γ, -4γ, and -6. Diabetes 1997;46:1364-7.
33. Fürstenau U, Schwaninger M, Blume R, Kennerknecht I, Knepel W. Characterization of novel protein kinase C response element in the glucagon gene. Mol Cell Biol 1997;17:1805-16.
34. Kaestner KH, Katz J, Liu Y, Drucker DJ, Schütz G. Inactivation of the winged helix transcription factor HNF3α affects glucose homeostasis and islet glucagon gene expression in vivo. Genes Dev 1999;13:495-504.
35. Overdier DG, Porcella A, Costa RH. The DNA-binding specificity of the hepatocyte nuclear factor 3/forkhead domain is influenced by amino acid residues adjacent to the recognition helix. Mol Cell Biol 1994;14:2755-66.
36. Janknecht R, Nordheim A. Gene regulation by Ets proteins. Biochim Biophys Acta 1993;1155:346-56.
37. Wasylyk B, Hahn SL, Giovane A. The Ets family of transcription factors. Eur J Biochem 1993;211:7-18.

38. Ang SL, Rossant J. HNF-3ß is essential for node and notochord formation in mouse development. Cell 1994;78:561-74.
39. Weinstein DC, Ruiz i Altaba A, Chen WS, Hoodless P, Prezioso VR, Jessell TM, Darnell JE Jr. The winged-helix transcription factor HNF-3ß is required for notochord development in the mouse embryo. Cell 1994;78:575-88.
40. Knepel W, Jepeal L, Habener JF. A pancreatic islet cell-specific enhancer-like element in the glucagon gene contains two domains binding distinct cellular proteins. J Biol Chem 1990;265:8725-35.
41. Epstein J, Cai J, Glaser T, Jepeal L, Maas R. Identification of a Pax paired domain recognition sequence and evidence for DNA-dependent conformational changes. J Biol Chem 1994;269:8355-61.
42. Wrege A, Diedrich T, Hochhuth C, Knepel W. Transcriptional activity of domain A of the rat glucagon G3 element conferred by an islet-specific nuclear protein that also binds to similar pancreatic islet cell-specific enhancer sequences (PISCES). Gene Expr 1995;4:205-16.
43. Yildiz N, Diedrich T, Knepel W. Nuclear protein binding and functional activity of a variant insulin gene found in non-insulin-dependent diabetes mellitus. Exp Clin Endocrinol Diabetes 1996;104:218-27.
44. Sander M, Neubüser A, Kalamaras J, Ee HC, Martin GR, German MS. Genetic analysis reveals that Pax6 is required for normal transcription of pancreatic hormone genes and islet development. Genes Dev 1997;11:1662-73.
45. Walther C, Gruss P. *Pax-6*, a murine paired box gene, is expressed in the developing CNS. Development 1991;113:1435-49.
46. Mansouri A, Hallonet M, Gruss P. *Pax* genes and their roles in cell differentiation and development. Curr Opin Cell Biol 1996;8:851-7.
47. Epstein JA, Glaser T, Cai J, Jepeal L, Walton DS, Maas RL. Two independent and interactive DNA-binding subdomains of the Pax6 paired domain are regulated by alternative splicing. Genes Dev 1994;8:2022-34.
48. Xu W, Rould MA, Jun S, Desplan C, Pabo CO. Crystal structure of a paired domain-DNA complex at 2.5 Å resolution reveals structural basis for Pax developmental mutations. Cell 1995;80:639-50.
49. Beimesche S, Neubauer A, Herzig S, Grzeskowiak R, Diedrich T, Cierny I, Scholz D, Alejel T, Knepel W. Tissue-specific transcriptional activity of a pancreatic islet cell-specific enhancer sequence/Pax6-binding site determined in normal adult tisues in vivo using transgenic mice. Mol Endocrinol 1999;13:718-28.
50. Goudet G, Delhalle S, Biemar F, Martial JA, Peers B. Functional and cooperative interactions between the homeodomain PDX1, Pbx, and Prep1 factors on the somatostatin promoter. J Biol Chem 1999;274:4067-73.
51. Diedrich T, Fürstenau U, Knepel W. Glucagon gene G3 enhancer: evidence that activity depends on combination of an islet-specific factor and a winged helix protein. Biol Chem 1997;378:89-98.
52. Hochhuth C, Neubauer A, Knepel W. Transactivation of the rat glucagon gene promoter by the CCAAT/enhancer-binding protein. Endocrine 1994;2:833-9.
53. St-Onge L, Sosa-Pineda B, Chowdhury K, Mansouri A, Gruss P. *Pax6* is required for differentiation of glucagon-producing α-cells in mouse pancreas. Nature 1997; 387:406-9.
54. Kiefer TJ, Heller RS, Unson CG, Weir GC, Habener JF. Distribution of glucagon receptors on hormone-specific endocrine cells of rat pancreatic islets. Endocrinology 1996;137:5119-25.
55. Heller RS, Kieffer TJ, Habener JF. Insulinotropic glucagon-like peptide I receptor expression in glucagon-producing α-cells of the rat endocrine pancreas. Diabetes 1997;46:785-91.
56. Rorsman P, Hellman B. Voltage-activated currents in guinea pig pancreatic $_{-2}$ cells. J Gen Physiol 1988;91:223-42.
57. Rorsman P. Two types of Ca^{2+} currents with different sensitivities to organic Ca^{2+} channel antagonists in guinea pig pancreatic α_2 cells. J Gen Physiol 1988;91:243-54.
58. Van der Zee EA, Buwalda B, Strubbe JH, Strosberg AD, Luiten PGM. Immunocytochemical localization of muscarinic acetylcholine receptors in the rat endocrine pancreas. Cell Tissue Res 1992;269:99-106.
59. Verspohl EJ, Tacke R, Mutschler E, Lambrecht G. Muscarinic receptor subtypes in rat pancreatic islets: binding and functional studies. Eur J Pharmacol 1990;178:303-11.
60. Knepel W, Chafitz J, Habener JF. Transcriptional activation of the rat glucagon gene by the cyclic AMP-responsive element in pancreatic islet cells. Mol Cell Biol 1990;10:6799-6804.
61. Oetjen E, Diedrich T, Eggers A, Eckert B, Knepel W. Distinct properties of the cAMP-responsive element of the rat insulin I gene. J Biol Chem 1994;269:27036-44.
62. Drucker DJ, Campos R, Reynolds R, Stobie K, Brubaker PL. The rat glucagon gene is regulated by a protein kinase A-dependent pathway in pancreatic islet cells. Endocrinology 1991;128:394-400.
63. Miller CP, Lin JC, Habener JF. Transcription of the rat glucagon gene by the cyclic AMP response element-binding protein CREB is modulated by adjacent CREB-associated proteins. Mol Cell Biol 1993;13:7080-90.

64. Meyer TE, Habener JF. Cyclic adenosine 3', 5'-monophosphate response element binding protein (CREB) and related transcription-activating deoxyribonucleic acid-binding proteins. Endocr Rev 1993;14:269-90.
65. Ellenberger TE, Brandl CJ, Struhl K, Harrison SC. The GCN4 basic region leucine zipper binds DNA as a dimer of uninterrupted α helices: crystal structure of the protein-DNA complex. Cell 1992;71:1223-37.
66. Gonzalez G, Montminy MR. Cyclic AMP stimulates somatostatin gene transcription by phosphorylation of CREB at serine 133. Cell 1989;59:675-80.
67. Chrivia JC, Kwok RPS, Lamp N, Hagiwara M, Montminy MR, Goodmann RH. Phosphorylated CREB binds specifically to the nuclear protein CBP. Nature 1993;365:855-9.
68. Kwok RPS, Lundblad JR, Chrivia JC, Richards JP, Bächinger HP, Brennan RG, Roberts SGE, Green MR, Goodman RH. Nuclear protein CBP is a coactivator for the transcription factor CREB. Nature 1994;370:223-6.
69. Arias J, Alberts AS, Brindle P, Claret FX, Smeal T, Karin M, Feramisco J, Montminy M. Activation of cAMP and mitogen responsive genes relies on a common nuclear factor. Nature 1994;370:226-8.
70. Parker D, Ferreri K, Nakajima T, LaMorte VJ, Evans R, Koerber SC, Hoeger C, Montminy MR. Phosphorylation of CREB at Ser-133 induces complex formation with CREB-binding protein via a direct mechanism. Mol Cell Biol 1996;16:694-703.
71. Lundblad JR, Kwok RPS, Laurance ME, Harter ML, Goodman RH. Adenoviral E1A-associated protein p300 as a functional homologue of the transcriptional co-activator CBP. Nature 1995;374:85-8.
72. Eckner R. p300 and CBP as transcriptional regulators and targets of oncogenic events. Biol Chem 1996;377:685-8.
73. Parker D, Jhala US, Radhakrishnan I, Yaffe MB, Reyes C, Shulman AI, Cantley LC, Wright PE, Montminy M. Analysis of an activator:coactivator complex reveals an essential role for secondary structure in transcriptional activation. Mol Cell 1998;2:353-9.
74. Hua QX, Jia WH, Bullock BP, Habener JF, Weiss MA. Transcriptional activator-coactivator recognition: nascent folding of a kinase-inducible transactivation domain predicts its structure on coactivator binding. Biochemistry 1998;37:5858-66.
75. Korzus E, Torchia J, Rose DW, Xu L, Kurokawa R, McInerney EM, Mullen TM, Glass CK, Rosenfeld MG. Transcription factor-specific requirements for coactivators and their acetyltransferase functions. Science 1998;279:703-7.
76. Mymryk JS, Smith MM. Influence of the adenovirus 5 E1A oncogene on chromatin remodelling. Biochem Cell Biol 1997;75:95-102.
77. Nakajima T, Uchida C, Anderson SF, Lee CG, Hurwitz J, Parvin JD, Montminy M. RNA helicase A mediates association of CBP with RNA polymerase II. Cell 1997;90:1107-12.
78. Yuan W, Condorelli G, Caruso M, Felsani A, Giordano A. Human p300 protein is a coactivator for the transcription factor MyoD. J Biol Chem 1996;271:9009-13.
79. Dallas PB, Yaciuk P, Moran E. Characterization of monoclonal antibodies raised against p300: both p300 and CBP are present in intracellular TBP complexes. J Virol 1997;71:1726-31.
80. Flint J, Shenk T. Viral transactivating proteins. Annu Rev Genet 1997;31:177-212.
81. Arany Z, Newsome D, Oldread E, Livingston DM, Eckner R. A family of transcriptional adaptor proteins targeted by the E1A oncoprotein. Nature 1995;374:81-4.
82. Schwaninger M, Lux G, Blume R, Oetjen E, Hidaka H, Knepel W. Membrane depolarization and calcium influx induce glucagon gene transcription in pancreatic islet cells through the cyclic AMP-responsive element. J Biol Chem 1993;268:5168-77.
83. Schwaninger M, Blume R, Oetjen E, Lux G, Knepel W. Inhibition of cAMP-responsive element-mediated gene transcription by cyclosporin A and FK506 after membrane depolarization. J Biol Chem 1993;268:23111-5.
84. Ghosh A, Greenberg ME. Calcium signalling in neurones: molecular mechanisms and cellular consequences. Science 1995;268:239-47.
85. Chawla S, Hardingham GE, Quinn DR, Bading H. CBP: a signal regulated transcriptional coactivator controlled by nuclear calcium and CaM kinase IV. Science 1998;281:1505-9.
86. Schwaninger M, Blume R, Oetjen E, Knepel W. The immunosuppressive drugs cyclosporin A and FK506 inhibit calcineurin phosphatase activity and gene transcription mediated through the cAMP-responsive element in a nonimmune cell line. Naunyn-Schmiedeberg's Arch Pharmacol 1993;348:541-5.
87. Schwaninger M, Blume R, Krüger M, Lux G, Oetjen E, Knepel W. Involvement of the Ca^{2+}-dependent phosphatase calcineurin in gene transcription that is stimulated by cAMP trough cAMP response elements. J Biol Chem 1995;270:8860-6.
88. Krüger M, Schwaninger M, Blume R, Oetjen E, Knepel W. Inhibition of CREB- and cAMP response element-mediated gene transcription by the immunosuppressive drugs cyclosporin A and FK506 in T cells. Naunyn-Schmiedeberg's Arch Pharmacol 1997; 356:433-40.

89. Barton K, Muthusamy N, Chanyangam M, Fischer C, Clendenin C, Leiden JM. Defective thymocyte proliferation and IL-2 production in transgenic mice expressing a dominant-negative form of CREB. Nature 1996;379:81-5.
90. Rudolph D, Tafuri A, Gass P, Hämmerling GJ, Arnold B, Schütz G. Impaired foetal T cells development and perinatal lethality in mice lacking the cAMP response element binding protein. Proc Natl Acad Sci USA 1998;95:4481-6.
91. Siemann G, Blume R, Grapentin D, Oetjen E, Schwaninger M, Knepel W. Inhibition of CREB/CRE-mediated transcription by the immunosuppressive drugs cyclosporin A and FK506 depends on the promoter context. Mol Pharmacol 1999;1094-1100.
92. Fürstenau U, Schwaninger M, Blume R, Jendrusch EM, Knepel W. Characterization of a novel calcium response element in the glucagon gene. J Biol Chem 1999;274:5851-60.
93. Rao A, Luo C, Hogan PG. Transcription factors of the NFAT family: regulation and function. Annu Rev Immunol 1997;15:707-47.
94. Crabtree GR. Generic signals and specific outcomes: signalling through Ca^{2+}, calcineurin, and NF-AT. Cell 1999;96:611-4.
95. Wolfe SA, Zhou P, Dötsch V, Chen L, You A, Ho SN, Crabtree GR, Wagner G, Verdine GL. Unusual rel-like architecture in the DNA-binding domain of the transcription factor NFATc. Nature 1997;385:172-6.
96. Peterson BR, Sun LJ, Verdine GL. A critical arginine residue mediates cooperativity in the contact interface between transcription factors NFAT and AP-1. Proc Natl Acad Sci USA 1996;93:13671-6.
97. Garcia-Rodriguez C, Rao A. Nuclear factor of activated T cells (NFAT)-dependent transactivation regulated by the coactivators p300/CREB-binding protein (CBP). J Exp Med 1998;187:2031-6.
98. Philippe J, Drucker DJ, Habener JF. Glucagon gene transcription in an islet cell line is regulated via a protein kinase C-activated pathway. J Biol Chem 1987;262:1823-8.
99. Nitsch D, Boshart M, Schütz G. Activation of the tyrosine aminotransferase gene is dependent on synergy betweeen liver-specific and hormone-responsive elements. Proc Natl Acad Sci USA 1993;90:5479-83.
100. Boyle WJ, Smeal T, Defize LHK, Angel P, Woodgett JR, Karin M, Hunter T. Activation of protein kinase C decreases phosphorylation of c-Jun at sites that negatively regulate its DNA-binding activity. Cell 1991;64:573-84.
101. Thanos D, Maniatis T. NF-_B: A lesson in family values. Cell 1995;80:529-32.
102. Burgering BMT, Bos JL. Regulation of Ras-mediated signalling: more than one way to skin a cat. Trends Biochem Sci 1995;20:18-22.
103. Cano E, Mahadevan LC. Parallel signal processing among mammalian MAPKs. Trends Biochem Sci 1995;20:117-22.
104. Nishizuka Y. Intracellular signalling by hydrolysis of phospholipids and activation of protein kinase C. Science 1992;258:607-14.
105. Olson EN, Burgess R, Staudinger J. Protein kinase C as a transducer of nuclear signals. Cell Growth Diff 1993;4:699-705.
106. Kolch W, Heidecker G, Kochs G, Hummel R, Vahidi H, Mischak H, Finkenzeller G, Marmé D, Rapp UR. Protein kinase C_ activates RAF-1 by direct phosphorylation. Nature 1993;364:249-52.
107. Whitmarsh AJ, Shore P, Sharrocks AD, Davis RJ. Integration of MAP kinase signal transduction pathways at the serum response element. Science 1995;269:403-7.
108. Hill CS, Wynne J, Treisman R. The Rho family GTPases RhoA, Rac1, and CDC42Hs regulate transcriptional activation by SRF. Cell 1995;81:1159-70.
109. Chen L, Komiya I, Inman L, McCorkle K, Alam T, Unger RH. Molecular and cellular responses of islets during perturbations of glucose homeostasis determined by in situ hybriditation histochemistry. Proc Natl Acad Sci USA 1989;86:1367-71.
110. Chen L, Komiya I, Inman L, O'Neil J, Appel M, Alam T, Unger RH. Effects of hypoglycaemia and prolonged fasting on insulin and glucagon gene expression. J Clin Invest 1989;84:711-14.
111. Shi ZQ, Rastogi KS, Lekas M, Efendic S, Drucker DJ, Vranic M. Glucagon response to hypoglycaemia is improved by insulin-independent restoration of normoglycaemia in diabetic rats. Endocrinology 1996;137:3193-9.
112. Dumonteil E, Magnan C, Ritz-Laser B, Meda P, Dussoix P, Gilbert M, Ktorza A, Philippe J. Insulin, but not glucose lowering corrects the hyperglucagonemia and increased proglucagon messenger ribonucleic acid levels observed in insulinopenic diabetes. Endocrinology 1998;139:4540-6.
113. Philippe J. Glucagon gene transcription is negatively regulated by insulin in a hamster islet cell line. J Clin Invest 1989;84:672-7.
114. Cohen P, Alessi DR, Cross DAE. PDK1, one of the missing links in insulin signal transduction? FEBS Lett 1997;410:3-10.
115. Alessi DR, Cohen P. Mechanism of activation and function of protein kinase B. Curr Opin Genet Dev 1998;8:55-62.
116. Shepherd PR, Whithers DJ, Siddle K. Phosphoinositide 3-kinase: the key switch mechanism in insulin signalling. J Biochem 1998;333:471-90.

117. Philippe J. Insulin regulation of the glucagon gene is mediated by an insulin-responsive DNA element. Proc Natl Acad Sci USA 1991;88:7224-7.

6

THE K_{ATP} CHANNEL AND THE SULFONYLUREA RECEPTOR

Susumu Seino, M.D., D.M.Sci., Takashi Miki, M.D., Ph.D., and Hideki Yano, M.D., D.M.Sci.
Chiba University, Chiba 260-8670, Japan

INTRODUCTION

ATP-sensitive K^+ channels (K_{ATP} channels) were first described in cardiac myocytes (1) and were subsequently found in many other tissues including pancreatic β-cells (2-5), skeletal muscle (6), smooth muscle (7), brain (8), pituitary (9), and kidney (10) and in mitochondria (11). K_{ATP} channels were originally characterized by inhibition when the ATP concentration at the cytoplasmic surface was increased (12). It is now known that regulation of K_{ATP} channel activity is complex, involving factors including nucleotide diphosphates such as ADP, Mg^{2+}, and phosphatidylinositol bisphosphate (13-18). K_{ATP} channels play important roles in endocrine cells, muscles, and neurones, by coupling metabolic state to membrane potential (12,19,20). In pancreatic β-cells, K_{ATP} channels regulate glucose-induced insulin secretion. Inhibition of the K_{ATP} channels by glucose depolarizes the β-cell membrane, leading to opening of the voltage-dependent calcium channels (VDCCs), and allowing calcium influx. The rise in intracellular calcium concentration ($[Ca^{2+}]_i$) in the β-cell triggers exocytosis of the insulin granules. While the K^+ channel opener diazoxide inhibits insulin secretion by activating the K_{ATP} channels, sulfonylureas such as glibenclamide, which is widely used in the treatment of type 2 diabetes mellitus, stimulate insulin release by inhibiting the K_{ATP} channels (21,22) (Figure 1). The cloning of members of the inwardly rectifying K^+ channel subfamily Kir6.0 and the sulfonylurea receptors has clarified the structure of K_{ATP} channels and revealed a new paradigm of channel/receptor assembly. Molecular biological and molecular genetic studies of K_{ATP} channels have also provided insight into the pathophysiological roles of the K_{ATP} channels in pancreatic β-cells.

STRUCTURE AND FUNCTION OF THE PANCREATIC β-CELL K_{ATP} CHANNEL

The Inwardly Rectifying K^+ Channel Subfamily Member Kir6.2

cDNA encoding Kir6.1, a member of the Kir family (Kir6.0 subfamily) with two transmembrane segments was cloned from a cDNA library constructed from rat islet mRNA (23). Although Kir6.1 is expressed widely in tissues including pancreatic islets, heart, skeletal muscle, and brain, it is not expressed in any of the insulin-secreting cell lines examined. Kir6.1 and SUR2B reconstitute ATP-insensitive, smooth muscle (24-27). The Kir6.1 is also suggested to be present in the mitochondria as well as in plasma membrane (28).

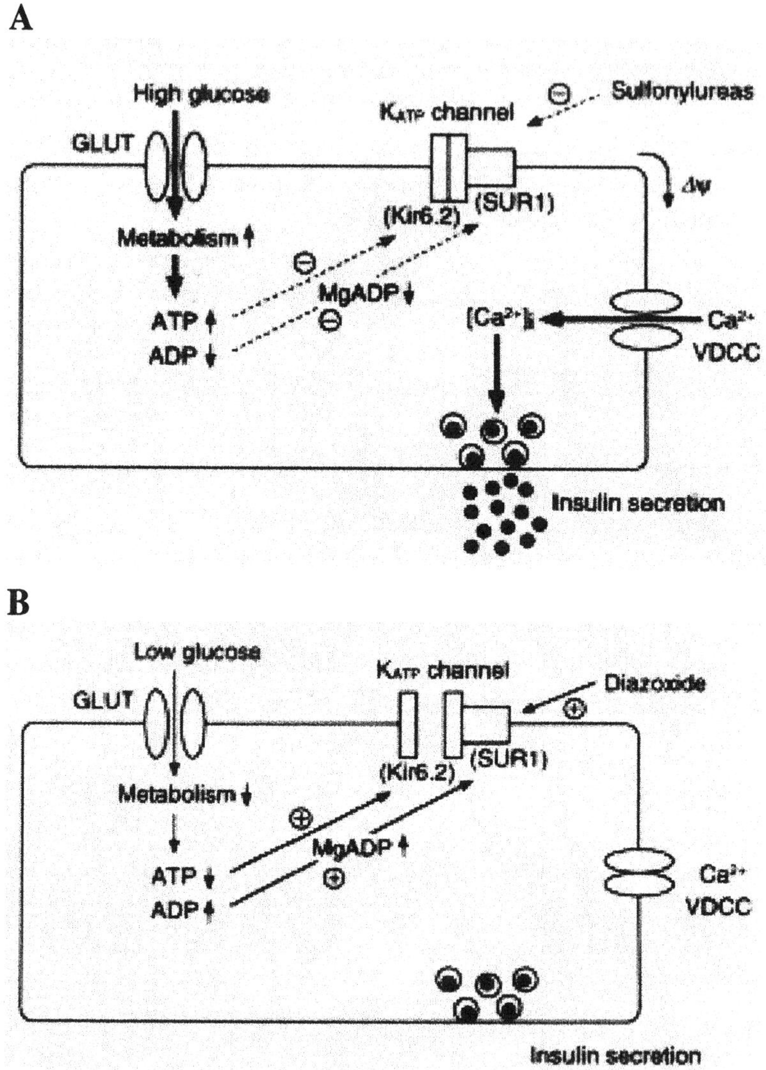

Figure 1. *Major pathway of insulin secretion via the K_{ATP} channels. A) Inhibition of the pancreatic β-cell K_{ATP} channel. An increase in glucose metabolism results in an increase in the ATP concentration and a decrease in the ADP concentration. An increase in ATP/ADP ratio inhibits the K_{ATP} channel. Sulfonylureas also inhibit the channel through SUR1, depolarizing the β-cell membrane, opening the voltage-dependent calcium channel (VDCC), and stimulating exocytosis of the insulin granules.* ***B)*** *Activation of the pancreatic β-cell K_{ATP} channel. A decrease in glucose metabolism results in decreased ATP concentration and increased ADP concentration. A decrease in ATP/ADP ratio activates the K_{ATP} channel. The K^+ channel opener, diazoxide, also activate the channel through SUR1.*

Human Kir6.1, is a nucleotide diphosphate-activated and glibenclamide-sensitive K^+ channel resembling the nucleotide diphosphate-dependent (K_{NDP}) K^+ channels in vascular vessels, and the gene, *KCNJ8*, was mapped to chromosome 12p11.23 using fluorescence in situ hybridization (29); the gene contains 3 exons spanning about 10 kb. Using Kir6.1 cDNA as a probe, Kir6.2, an isoform of Kir6.1, was subsequently cloned. Mouse Kir6.2 is a protein of 390 amino acids that shares 71% amino acid identity (82% similarity) with rat Kir6.1. Human and rat Kir6.2 also were cloned. Although the Gly-Tyr-Gly motif in the H5 region, which is thought to be critical for K^+ ion selectivity, is highly conserved in inwardly rectifying K^+ channels, the amino acid sequence of this motif in both Kir6.1 and Kir6.2 is Gly-Phe-Gly, suggesting that this motif may be unique in the Kir6.0 subfamily (Figure 2). Two potential protein kinase A-dependent phosphorylation sites (Thr-224 and Ser-372) in Kir6.2 are conserved in all species in which Kir6.2 has been identified. Kir6.2 mRNA is expressed at high levels in pancreatic islets, the glucose-responsive insulin-secreting cell lines MIN6 (mouse) and HIT-T15 (hamster), and the glucagon-secreting cell line αTC-6, and at lower levels in heart, skeletal muscle, brain, and the rat insulinoma cell line RINm5F (30). It is also expressed at very low levels in the pituitary and the pituitary-derived cell line AtT-20. *In situ* hybridization and immunohistochemistry reveal that Kir6.2 is present in the insulin-secreting β-cells, glucagon-secreting α–cells, and somatostatin-secreting δ–cells in pancreatic islets (31). The Kir6.2 gene has no intron in the protein-coding region. Human Kir6.2 gene, *KCNJ11*, was mapped to 11p15.1 by fluorescence in situ hybridization (33). The sequence obtained from the one lambda clone at the 3' end of the SUR1 gene matched a part of the gene encoding Kir6.2; a sense primer near the 3' end of the SUR1 gene and an antisense primer near the 5' end of the Kir6.2 gene amplified an approximately 4.5-kb fragment (30,32). Thus, the two genes are clustered at 11p15.1, with the Kir6.2 gene immediately to the 3' side of the SUR1 gene. Recently, Evans et al. (34) reported an 86-kb fragment of human genomic DNA from chromosome 11p14.3 that contains the entire sequence of human Kir6.2 and the 3' end of SUR1.

The Sulfonylurea Receptor

The sulfonylurea receptor (now called SUR1) that shows high affinity for glibenclamide was cloned from HIT and RINm5F cDNA libraries (32). Hamster SUR1 and rat SUR1 have been reported to be a 1581 and a 1582 amino acid protein, respectively. The difference in size might be an alternative splice site at the 5'-boundary of exon 17 (35). SUR1 has multiple putative transmembrane segments and two Nucleotide Binding Folds (or Domains) (NBFs or NBDs) (32) in the cytoplasmic side. As with Cystic Fibrosis Transmembrane conductance Regulator (CFTR), P-glycoprotein (P-gp), and Multi-drug Resistance associated Protein (MRP), SUR1 is a member of the ABC superfamily (36). Each NBF contains the Walker A and B motifs and the SGGQ ABC signature (37), which are thought to be important in nucleotide regulation of the functional activities of ABC proteins (36). Although SUR1 was originally proposed to have 13 transmembrane segments, it has recently been proposed to represent a 17 transmembrane segment model, based on sequence alignments of SUR1 and members of the MRP gene subfamily (38) (Figure 3). In this model, in addition to two Transmembrane Domains (TMD1 and TMD2), each of which consists of six transmembrane segments, SUR1 has another transmembrane domain (TMD0) consisting of five transmembrane segments in the N-terminal region. However, the precise membrane topology needs to be established. There are two potential N-linked glycosylation sites in hamster (Asn-10, Asn-1050), rat (Asn-10, Asn-1049 according to Aguilar-Bryan et al. (32)), and human (Asn-10, Asn-1049) SUR1: one in the extracellular N-terminus and one in the extracellular region between the 12th and 13th (38) transmembrane segment. There are three potential protein kinase A-dependent phosphorylation sites in rat SUR1 (Thr-278, Ser-1448, Ser-1500), four in hamster (Thr278, Ser-950, Ser-1447, Ser-1501), and four in human (Thr-949, Ser-1446, Ser-1500, and Ser-1571).

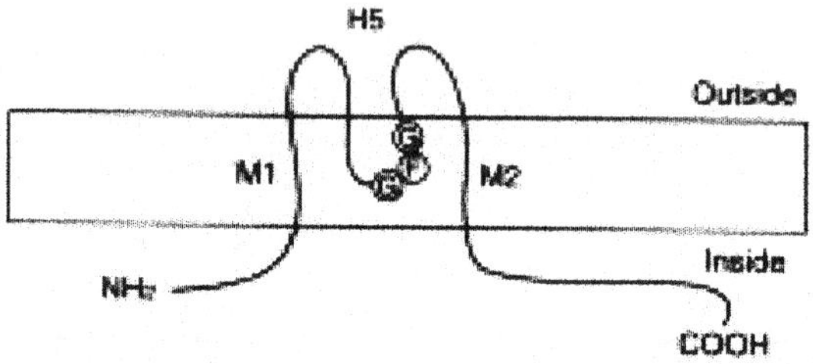

Figure 2. *Putative membrane topology of Kir6.2. M1 and M2 represent transmembrane domains. The K^+ ion-permeable domain, H5, also is shown. The motif GFG is thought to be critical for K^+ ion selectivity.*

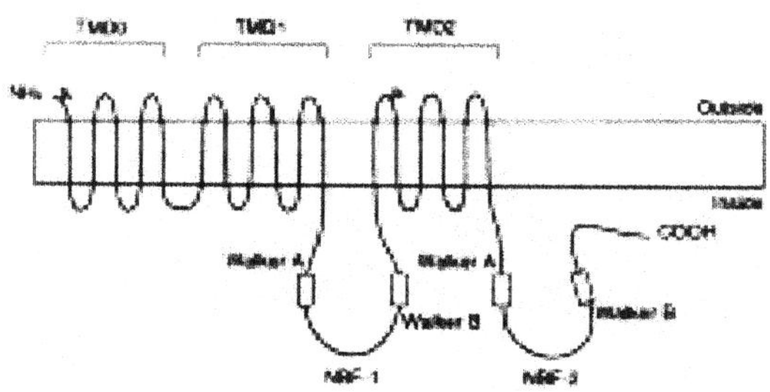

Figure 3. *Putative membrane topology of SUR1. A 17 transmembrane segment model based on Tusnady et al. (38) is shown. SUR1 is thought to have three transmembrane domains, TMD0, TMD1, and TMD2, which consist of five, six, and six transmembrane segments, respectively.*

Expression of recombinant rodent SUR1 in COSm6 cells exhibits high affinity for ^{125}I iodoglibenclamide binding (K_D ~10 nM) (32). SUR1 is expressed at high levels in pancreatic islets, HIT and MIN6 cells, and at moderate to low levels in RINm5F and αTC-6 cells. *In situ* hybridization histochemistry shows that SUR1 is expressed in not only β-cells but also α, δ, and PP-cells (39). cDNA encoding an isoform of SUR1, SUR2 (now called SUR2A) was subsequently cloned (40). Rat SUR2 is a protein of 1545 amino acids sharing 68% amino acid identity with hamster SUR1 and also similar membrane topology. There are three potential N-linked glycosylation sites in rat SUR2: one in the extracellular N-terminus (Asn-9) and two in the extracellular region between the 6th and 7th (Asn-330 and Asn-331) transmembrane segments (according to Tusnady et al. (38)). There are two potential protein kinase A-dependent phosphorylation sites: one (T-632) in the 11th and 12th, and the other (S-1464) in the intracellular C-terminal region in rat SUR2A. The affinity of SUR2A for sulfonylureas is ~500 times lower than that of SUR1 when they are expressed in COS1 cells (40). SUR2A cannot be photolabelled with ^{125}I-iodoglibenclamide under the same conditions that photolabel SUR1, indicating that SUR2A is a low affinity receptor (40). Several variants of SUR2 have been identified. One variant, SUR2B, differs from SUR2A by 42 amino acids in the C-terminus, but is similar in the C-terminus to SUR1 (41). While SUR2A is expressed predominantly in heart and skeletal muscle (40), SUR2B is expressed ubiquitously (41). In addition to these main transcripts, other alternative spliced mRNAs also have been identified (SUR2AΔ14: a deletion of exon 14 (42), SUR2AΔ17 and Δ17,18: a deletion of exon 17 or exon 17 plus 18(43)). Recently, SUR2AΔ17 has been shown to be predominant in skeletal muscle, gut, and bladder and may affect the ATP sensitivity of the K_{ATP} channel, altering the burst pattern (44). However, it is not clear whether exon skipped mRNAs other than Δ17 are functional or physiologically important. The human SUR1 gene, spanning 39 exons over 100 kb of DNA, was localized on the short arm of chromosome 11, at 11p15.1 (33). The human SUR2 gene, spanning 38 exons over 100 kb (42), localizes on the short arm of chromosome 12 at 12p11.12. To date, no disease has been reported to be associated with the SUR2 gene.

Reconstitution of Pancreatic β-cell K_{ATP} Channels
Coexpression of Kir6.2 and SUR1 in COS-1 cells reconstitutes weakly inwardly rectifying channel K^+ currents with unitary conductance of ~76 pS in the presence of 140 mM K^+ on both sides of the membrane. The reconstituted K^+ channel (Kir6.2/SUR1 channel) currents are inhibited by ATP with half-maximal inhibition (K_i) at ~10 μM in the presence of Mg^{2+}. The reconstituted currents are also inhibited by adenyl-5'-yl imidodiphosphate (AMP-PNP), a non-hydrolysable ATP analog. Glibenclamide blocks the reconstituted K^+ channel currents, while diazoxide stimulates them. Metabolic poisoning with oligomycin and 2-deoxy-glucose remarkably stimulates $^{86}Rb^+$ efflux through Kir6.2/SUR1 channels reconstituted in COSm6 cells (30), and it is inhibited by glibenclamide and stimulated by diazoxide (45). Thus, the properties of K^+ channel currents reconstituted from Kir6.2 and SUR1 are similar to those of the K_{ATP} channel currents in native pancreatic β-cells, indicating that Kir6.2 and SUR1 couple to form the functional pancreatic β-cell type K_{ATP} channel. Differing combinations of the Kir6.2 or Kir6.1 and the SUR1 or SUR2 variants comprise K_{ATP} channels with distinct nucleotide and pharmacological sensitivities: Kir6.2 and SUR2A constitute cardiac type and, probably, skeletal muscle type K_{ATP} channels (40); Kir6.2 and SUR2B make up the smooth muscle type channel (41). Kir6.1 and SUR2B reconstitute the vascular smooth muscle type channel (24).

The Pancreatic β-cell K_{ATP} Channel: Kir6.2/SUR1 is a hetero-octamer
Reconstitution of K_{ATP} channel currents by coexpression of Kir6.2 and SUR1 suggests strongly that they are physically associated. When Kir6.2 and SUR1 are coexpressed in COSm6 cells, both subunits are photolabelled with ^{125}I-azidoglibenclamide (46). Physical association of Kir6.2 and SUR1 is further confirmed by co-purification of the complex glycosylated SUR1 and Kir6.2 species (47). Using the specific antibody to Kir6.2, Kir6.2 and SUR1 proteins coimmunoprecipitate from a mixture of Kir6.2 and SUR1 *in vitro*-translated proteins and from COS-7 cells transfected with both Kir6.2 and SUR1. The largest highly glycosylated SUR1/Kir6.2 complex is estimated to be ~950 kD, suggesting hetero-octameric structure of the four SUR1 subunits (~170 kD) and four Kir6.2 subunits (~45 kD). The stoichiometry of the SUR1/Kir6.2 channel is confirmed by constructing fusion proteins of SUR1 and Kir6.2 subunits. The properties of channels reconstituted from SUR1-Kir6.2 (1:1) fusion protein including unitary conductance, ATP-sensitivity, and glibenclamide-sensitivity are similar to those of the K_{ATP} channels reconstituted from monomeric SUR1 subunits and monomeric Kir6.2 subunits (46-48), suggesting a 1:1 stoichiometry to be sufficient for functional expression of the K_{ATP} channel. In addition, channels comprising the fusion protein of SUR1 and a dimeric repeat of Kir6.2 (SUR1:Kir6.2=1:2) show less sensitivity to ATP than do the channels reconstituted from SUR1-Kir6.2 (1:1) fusion protein, and the properties of this triple fusion protein are restored by supplementation with monomeric wild-type SUR1 (48,49). This suggests that the Kir6.2 subunits and the SUR1 subunits assemble with a 4:4 stoichiometry to form the K_{ATP} channel (Figure 4).

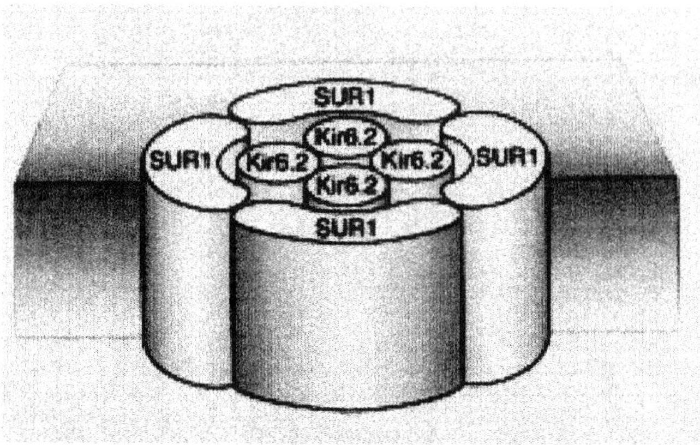

Figure 4. *A model of the stoichiometry of the pancreatic β-cell K_{ATP} channel. The channel is a hetero-octamer of four Kir6.2 subunits and four SUR1 subunits.*

The K_{ATP} Channel as ATP and ADP Sensor

In pancreatic β-cells, an increase in glucose metabolism increases the intracellular ATP concentration with a concomitant decrease in the ADP concentration (50), and the K_{ATP} channel in pancreatic β-cells is thought to act as an ATP and ADP sensor for glucose-induced insulin secretion (51). Regulation of the channel by adenine nucleotide is complex. Because SUR contains two nucleotide-binding folds while there is apparently no ATP binding site in Kir6.2, and both SUR and Kir6.2 are normally required for functional expression of K_{ATP} channels, it was initially assumed that the SUR subunits confer sensitivity to channel inhibition by ATP (32). However, electrophysiological studies have shown that mutations in NBF-1 and/or NBF-2 of SUR1 do not alter channel inhibition by ATP (52,53). In addition, Kir6.2 with a deletion of the last 26 amino acids (Kir6.2 ΔC26) or 36 amino acids (Kir6.2 ΔC36) in the C-terminus produces functional K_{ATP} channels in the absence of SUR1, although the ATP-sensitivity is reduced 10-fold (54). These findings suggest that ATP inhibition of the K_{ATP} channel is conferred primarily by Kir6.2 and that sensitivity to ATP is enhanced by SUR1. Electrophysiological studies have shown that MgADP-induced K_{ATP} channel activation is abolished by mutations in either NBF-1 or NBF-2 of SUR1 (53), indicating that SUR confers sensitivity to MgADP activation of the K_{ATP} channel. On the other hand, biochemical studies suggest that 8-azido-[γ-^{32}P] ATP strongly binds at NBF-1 of SUR1, and that MgADP, by either direct binding to NBF-2 or hydrolysis of bound MgATP at NBF-2, stabilizes prebound ATP at NBF-1 (55). In addition, Kir6.2 alone has been shown to be photo-labeled by 8-azido-[γ–^{32}P] ATP, although Kir6.2 has much lower affinity for 8-azido-[γ-^{32}P] ATP than SUR1 (56). A model of ATP and ADP regulation of the pancreatic β-cell K_{ATP} channel SUR1 subunit can be discerned, although the mechanisms are yet to be clarified. K_{ATP} channel activation is induced by cooperative binding of both ATP at NBF-1 and MgADP at NBF-2. ATP binding at NBF-1 is probably required for the action of SUR1 (Figure 4A). When the intracellular MgADP concentration is decreased, e.g. by an increase in glucose metabolism in pancreatic β-cells, MgADP dissociates from NBF-2. Thus, the intracellular concentration of MgADP may be the primary factor in alteration between the active state and the inactive state of SUR1 (Figure 5) (57). Although ATP and MgADP are primary determinants of the activity of the β-cell K_{ATP} channel, the sensitivity of the channel to ATP is affected by other cytosolic factors such as PIP2 (17,18).

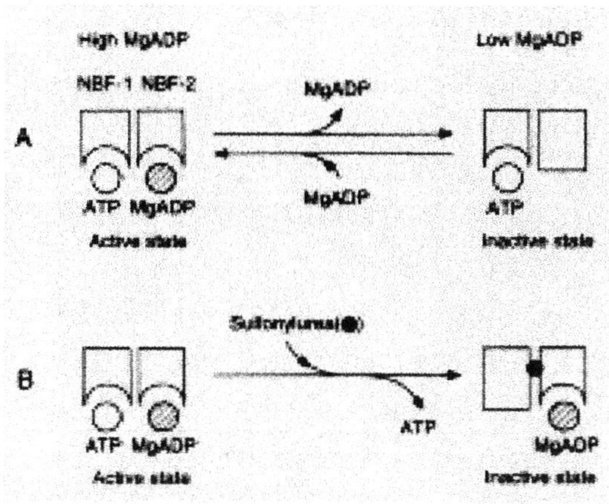

Figure 5. *Possible models of ATP and ADP regulation of the SUR1 subunit.* ***A)*** *K_{ATP} channel activation is induced by cooperative binding of ATP at NBF-1 and MgADP at NBF-2 of SUR1.* ***B)*** *Sulfonylureas dissociate ATP from NBF-1, in cooperation with MgADP at NBF-2, and may convert of the active state of SUR1 directly into the inactive state. These models are from reference 57 with modifications and reprinted with permission.*

Sulfonylurea Inhibition

It is clear from electrophysiological studies that SUR1 confers sensitivity to inhibition of the β-cell K_{ATP} channel by sulfonylureas (58,59). A biochemical study suggests that the sulfonylurea glibenclamide blocks both the cooperative binding of ATP and MgADP, and, in association with MgADP bound at NBF-2, causes ATP to be released from NBF-1 (55) (Figure 4B). Although the precise binding sites of glibenclamide are not known, an electrophysiological study suggests that the distinct binding sites for the various sulfonylureas might overlap, and that inhibition of the K_{ATP} channels by sulfonylureas is tissue-specific (60,61). The inhibitory effect of the sulfonylureas on the β-cell K_{ATP} channel is enhanced by MgADP (13,14).

PATHOPHYSIOLOGY OF THE PANCREATIC β-CELL K_{ATP} CHANNEL

Persistent Hyperinsulinemic Hypoglycemia of Infancy (PHHI) or Familial Hyperinsulinism (HI)

PHHI, also referred to as familial hyperinsulinism (HI) and formerly called pancreatic nesidioblastosis, is a rare metabolic disorder occurring in neonates and infants that is characterized by an excessive release of insulin despite severe hypoglycemia. Nesidioblastosis is a diffuse proliferation and budding of pancreatic islet cells from pancreatic ducts, and, often disorganized formation of new islets. Although this was once thought to be the pathological basis of insulin-mediated hypoglycemia in infants, quantitative immunohistochemical studies found the condition to occur also in normal infants. The finding of nesidioblastosis, therefore, is not sufficient to explain the excessive insulin release (62). PHHI or HI are now the proper names of this syndrome.

Clinical Description

Diagnosis usually follows multiple generalized convulsions, at age generally younger than 2 years old. Prompt diagnosis and treatment are indispensable to protect the brain from serious hypoglycemia. Not all patients, however, present with such severe symptoms - some present several weeks to several months of age with much milder symptoms. Most of these patients are managed with diet with or without addition of diazoxide, although some require treatment with octreotide, a more potent and longer lasting analogue of somatostatin. Treatment often requires partial or subtotal removal of the pancreas. The reason for variation in clinical severity is not known. The clinical symptoms of both severe and milder forms have been found to diminish with age. Remission from hypoglycemia occurs after months to years in most patients with PHHI independent of the mode of treatment in infancy. However, most patients continue to secrete some insulin, and fail to suppress endogenous secretion in induced hypoglycemia (63). Most of the PHHI patients who are in clinical remission and have undergone partial pancreatectomy developed overt diabetes around the age of puberty. An effort, therefore, should be made to treat PHHI patients medically to avoid pancreatectomy to reduce the incidence of diabetes at puberty (63-66). Nevertheless, due to the urgent and uncontrollable hypoglycemia, subtotal pancreatectomy still plays an important role in some cases.

Autosomal Recessive Trait and the Incidence

Glaser et al. (67) reported a total of 21 cases in 7 pedigrees which included a large Bedouin family, an Arab family, and 5 Jewish families of Eastern European origin (Ashkenazi). Consanguinity was evident in the Bedouin and Arab families. Woolf et al. (68) found consanguinity in 5 of 28 families. The sex ratio was close to 1. Thornton et al. (69) found the segregation ratio was 0.254, compatible with an autosomal recessive disorder. The great majority of PHHI cases are sporadic, with an estimated incidence of 1/50,000 live births (70), but in some Saudi Arabian populations with substantial inbreeding, the incidence may be as high as 1/2,500 (71).

Mutations in the SUR1 and Kir6.2 Genes

Glaser et al (72). mapped the PHHI locus to a 6.6 cM interval between the markers D11S926 and D11S928 on human chromosome 11p by linkage analysis in 15 families (12 of Ashkenazi-Jewish, 2 consanguineous Arab, 1 non-Jewish Caucasian origin). Thomas et al. (73) mapped the gene for this disorder to a region of 11p between markers D11S1334 and D11S899 in five consanguineous families of Saudi Arabian origin. Additional investigation further localized the gene between D11S419 and D11S1310, a region estimated to be 0.8 cM in length (74). The β-cell high-affinity SUR1 gene was mapped to the same chromosomal region as PHHI. Subsequently, cloning of the SUR1 and Kir6.2 genes led to the identification of various mutations in both genes of PHHI patients. Most cases of PHHI are inherited in an autosomal recessive pattern, and mutations of the sulfonylurea receptor (SUR1) gene or the closely linked Kir6.2 gene have been found in several families. Thomas et al. (33) found two mutations (G1400D(23)X and 3992-9 guanine→adenine) within or preceding the NBF-2 region in the SUR1 gene. The first mutation, G1400D(23)X, is a guanine to adenine mutation at the 3' end of exon 35, which causes skipping of exon 35 and results in a premature stop codon and lack of NBF-2. The second mutation (3992-9 guanine→adenine), which was found in another family, is a guanine to adenine homozygous mutation in the 3' splice site 9-bp upstream from exon 33 which could generate three abnormal cryptic splice sites: a 7-bp addition, a 20-bp deletion, or a 30-bp deletion in the NBF-2 region. After Thomas et al. described the first two mutations of the SUR1 gene in patients with PHHI, additional mutations in the SUR1 gene were identified (Figure 6). Two mutations of the NBF-1 region (G716V and 2292-1 guanine→adenine) were also described (75). The affected children were homozygous for an amino acid substitution in the Walker A motif of NBF-1 (G716V), and the other was found to be compound heterozygous for a mutation in intron, 20-bp upstream from exon 12 (1672-20 adenine→guanine). These mutations are thought to result in altered RNA processing in the NBF-1 region, suggesting the importance of NBF-1 in activity of the K_{ATP} channel. Other compound heterozygous mutations were found in Ashkenazi Jews – the combination of an in-frame deletion of phenylalanine at codon 1388 (ΔF 1388) and a 3' splice mutation in intron 32 (3992-9 guanine→adenine) were responsible for 88% of the PHHI chromosomes (76). A point mutation in exon 37 (G1479R), which is located between the Walker A and Walker B motifs in NBF-2 of SUR1, was found in a Sephardic Jewish proband by Nichols et al. (77). They introduced the analogous mutation into the hamster SUR1 and coexpressed it with mouse Kir6.2 in COSm6 cells. The mutant channel was activated by diazoxide but not by metabolic inhibition in $^{86}Rb^{+}$ efflux experiments. In inside-out patch-clamp experiments, the mutant channel had normal sensitivity to inhibition by ATP in the absence or presence of Mg^{2+}, but inhibition by ATP was not antagonized by ADP as in wild-type channels. An additional G1485D mutation in NBF-2 resulted in the same phenotype, whereas the equivalent G827D mutation in NBF-1 showed normal sensitivity to MgADP. Nichols et al. (77) concluded that stimulation by MgADP is necessary for activation of K_{ATP} channels in intact β-cells, and that MgADP is an intracellular regulator of insulin secretion through binding to NBF-2 of SUR1 and antagonizing ATP inhibition of K_{ATP} channels. In addition, no K_{ATP} channel activity was observed in the pancreatic β-cells of the patient with the other mutation, SUR1R1437Q(23)X, and reconstitution from a similarly truncated SUR1 and Kir6.2 in COS cells failed to elicit K_{ATP} channel currents (78), suggesting that MgADP does not activate the K_{ATP} channel due to the absence of NBF-2 or that the truncated SUR1 does not couple to Kir6.2. Other SUR1 mutations have been identified in PHHI patients including H125Q, N188S, F591L, T1139M, R1215Q, G1382S, and R1394H (79). R1394H and ΔF1388 SUR1 do not constitute functional channels when coexpressed with Kir6.2 in COS cells, while H125Q, N188S, F591L, T1139M, R1215Q, and G1382S SUR1 constitute functional channels in the absence of ATP. With the exception of N188S and H125Q, all mutants showed a reduced response to stimulation by MgADP. These results indicate that lack or reduction of K_{ATP} channel sensitivity to MgADP is a molecular defect commonly associated with the disease. The mutant channels also showed a varied response to activation by the potassium channel opener diazoxide. In 1998, Nestorowicz et al. (80) reported more mutations: a nonsense mutation, Q954X, occurring in NBF1 and a missense mutation, G1379R, within the Walker A motif of NBF2. Other missense mutations (R74Q and N406D) were also detected, and two novel deletions were identified. A 949ΔC mutation is predicted to result in a frameshift at codon 317, resulting in introduction of a stop codon at position 358, and a 1893ΔT mutation in exon 13 is predicted to result in a frameshift at codon 631 resulting in the introduction of a termination codon at position 645. Both deletions produce a truncated SUR1 lacking both NBFs. An in-frame insertion of 6 nucleotides in exon 37 also was found. Three novel splice site mutations, 3992-3C→G, 1630+1G→T, and 2117-1G→A also were identified, and are predicted to impair mRNA splicing. With the exception of the 3992-9G→A mutation, which was detected in 4.5% of disease chromosomes, the allelic frequencies for the identified mutations varied between 1.1 and 2.3%, indicating that each mutation was rare in the cohort. In contrast with those in the Ashkenazi Jewish patients, these findings suggest a large degree of allelic heterogeneity at the SUR1 locus in non-Ashkenazi Jewish patients.

Thomas et al. (85) screened genomic DNA from infants with PHHI for mutations in the Kir6.2 gene. They found a homozygous KCNJ11 gene mutation (L147P) in an affected individual with severe PHHI. The patient was the offspring of consanguineous mating and was homozygous for a 649T→C point mutation of the genomic sequence that resulted in the substitution of proline for leucine-147. The mutation resulted in a predicted disruption of the M2 alpha-helical transmembrane domain of the protein. Her parents were heterozygous for the mutation. Another homozygous nonsense mutation in the Kir6.2 gene, Y12X, was also identified in a proband from a consanguineous Palestinian Arab family. Reconstitution from SUR1 and Kir6.2Y12X in COS-1 cells results in the absence of functional K_{ATP} channel activity (86). Therefore, the finding of a mutation in the Kir6.2 gene indicates genetic heterogeneity of PHHI, but there are only two reports of mutations in the Kir6.2 gene (Figure 6), suggesting that most PHHI cases are not attributable to mutations in the coding region of the Kir6.2 gene. Despite similar clinical presentation of PHHI, there is a focal form and a diffuse form of the histopathological lesions associated with this disease. The focal form, in 30% of the reported cases, is characterized by focal hyperplasia of the islet-like cells, including the hypertrophied insulin cells with giant nuclei (81). In sporadic cases of the focal form, there was a specific loss of maternal alleles of the imprinted chromosome region 11p15 in cells of the hyperplastic area of the pancreas that did not appear in the diffuse form, as in normal pancreatic cells, providing the first molecular explanation of the heterogeneity of the sporadic form of PHHI (82, 83). Accordingly, to avoid iatrogenic diabetes, partial pancreatectomy limited to the focal somatic lesion, may be the more reasonable treatment in patients with focal adenomatous hyperplasia (66,84).

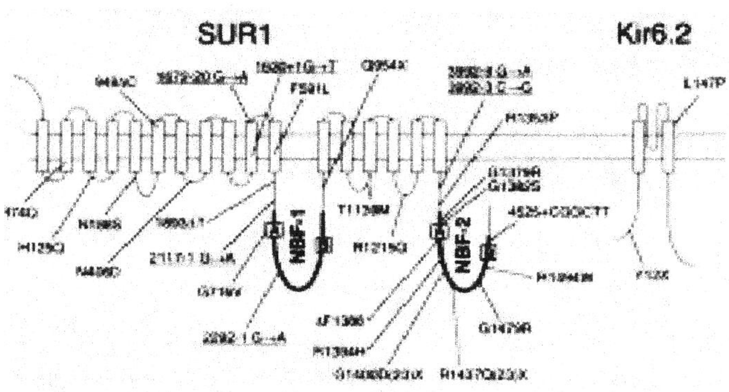

Figure 6. *Mutations of SUR1 and Kir6.2. Membrane topology is based on Tusnady et al. (38). Nonsense and missense mutations are shown with amino-acid number. Mutations in introns that cause the alteration of mRNA splicing and produce the truncated proteins are shown with nucleotide number according to Gonzalez et al. (GenBank accession number L78207) with underlines.*

Mutations in Genes other than *SUR1* and *Kir6.2*

In some families, recessive PHHI is not linked to the SUR1/Kir6.2 gene-locus on 11p15, suggesting genetic heterogeneity. Kukuvitis et al. (87) described an autosomal dominant form of PHHI in a French-Canadian family, and excluded linkage to SUR1 and Kir6.2 on 11p15. The PHHI phenotype can be produced by mutation of a gene other than *SUR1* or *Kir6.2* – recently, two novel mutations have been reported to associate with PHHI. One is a missense mutation (V455M) in the glucokinase gene in autosomal dominant familial hyperinsulinism (88); the other, in the glutamate dehydrogenase gene, was found in sporadic PHHI with hyperammonemia (89). However, many sporadic and familial cases of hyperinsulinism still remain unexplained.

Association and Linkage with Type 2 Diabetes Mellitus

Type 2 diabetes mellitus is characterized by impaired insulin secretion - the β-cells of type 2 diabetic patients contain insulin, but an inadequate amount is released in response to glucose. Because insulin secretion can be triggered in type 2 diabetic patients by sulfonylurea, it has generally been thought that regulation of the β-cell K_{ATP} channels is defective in the disease. In the Zucker diabetic fatty male rat, a model of type 2 diabetes mellitus, expression of Kir6.2 mRNA is reduced more than 70%, as compared to controls, but the levels of SUR1 mRNA remain constant, suggesting that decreased expression of Kir6.2 contributes to β-cell dysfunction in this animal model (90). Searching for variations in the human Kir6.2 gene, we found four polymorphic sites in Japanese normal subjects, in comparison with the amino acid sequence deduced from the Kir6.2 gene originally isolated from a genomic library, three of which cause amino acid replacements (Y. Yamada et al., unpublished observations). The first is a G to A substitution in codon 23 resulting in an E23K replacement. The second, S148I (Ile-148 substitution) may represent racial difference, the original Kir6.2 gene having been isolated from a genomic library constructed from a Caucasian foetus, because no Ser at this position in any of the Japanese examined was found. The third is an A to G substitution in codon 337 resulting in a V337I replacement. Iwasaki et al. (91) have identified two microsatellite DNA polymorphisms located near the Kir6.2 and SUR genes, and have typed these polymorphisms in 140 Japanese affected sib-pairs. They found no evidence for linkage between these markers and NIDDM, suggesting that genetic variation in the SUR and Kir6.2 genes does not play a major role in susceptibility to NIDDM in Japanese. Similar results were reported in white Caucasians by Sakura et al. (92), in two Northern European populations (Utah and the U.K.) by Inoue et al. (93) and in Danish Caucasians by Hansen et al. (94). However, in French Caucasians, Kir6.2 polymorphisms are frequently associated with type 2 diabetes (95). Moreover, a meta-analysis combining the different Caucasian groups reported by Sakura et al., Inoue et al., and Hansen et al., showed a significant association with type 2 diabetes, suggesting a possible role in the polygenic context of human type 2 diabetes (95). The molecular mechanisms associated with these observations are yet to be determined.

Several sequence variants have been found within the SUR1 gene, and these have been used in attempts to link the SUR1 gene with type 2 diabetes mellitus. In general, neither clear evidence of linkage in a Mexican-American population (96) and Japanese (91), nor a clear association between type 2 diabetes and the SUR1 gene in Japanese (97,98) or Caucasian populations has been established. However, data suggesting an association between the SUR1 locus and the inherited basis of type 2 diabetes in Northern European whites (99), Danish Caucasians (100), and French Caucasians (101), has been reported. In two Northern European populations (Utah and the U.K.), an ACC→ACT silent variant in exon 22 (T761T) was more common in patients than in control subjects. Moreover, an intronic t→c change located at position -3 of the exon 24 splice acceptor site also was more common in patients. The combined genotypes of exon 22 C/T or T/T and intron 24 -3c/-3c occurred in 8.9% of patients and 0.5% of control subjects. These results suggest that defects at the SUR locus may be a major contributor to the inherited basis of type 2 diabetes mellitus in Northern European Caucasians. The exon 22 T-allele also was associated with type 2 diabetes and morbid obesity in French Caucasians. A silent T775T polymorphism in exon 18 of the SUR1 gene has been associated with type 2 diabetes in a Danish Caucasian population. The association is higher in combination with the c→t intron variant in position -3 of exon 16, and young, healthy carriers of this intragenic combination have reduced serum C-peptide and insulin responses to a tolbutamide load, but not to a glucose load. Another finding by Goksel et al. (102) suggests that a variant in the SUR1 gene (G→A, R1272R in exon 31) is associated with high insulin concentrations in non-diabetic Mexican-Americans. These results suggest that genetic defects at the SUR1/Kir6.2 locus may account for a component of the inherited basis of type 2 diabetes in these racial groups.

LESSONS FROM GENETICALLY ENGINEERED MICE

Transgenic mice

The K^+ ion-permeable domain, H5, is highly conserved in K^+ channels, and the motif Gly-Tyr (or Phe)-Gly is thought to be critical for K^+ ion selectivity (103-105). Mutant Kir6.2 with a substitution of the first residue of the Gly-Phe-Gly motif with serine, Kir6.2G132S, was demonstrated to act as a dominant-negative inhibitor of K_{ATP} channels, probably by forming a heteromeric tetramer, by $^{86}Rb^+$ efflux measurement from COS-1 cells transfected with Kir6.2 and Kir6.2G132S at various ratios with SUR1. By patch-clamp recording, no significant potassium currents were detected in the COS-1 cells transfected with Kir6.2G132S alone with SUR1. Transgenic mice expressing the mutant Kir6.2G132S specifically in pancreatic β-cells under the regulation of the human insulin promoter (106) were generated. These transgenic mice exhibit severe hypoglycaemia in neonates, but the insulin levels remain relatively high, a phenotype that resembles PHHI in humans. However, blood glucose levels in transgenic mice at 4 weeks become markedly elevated and increase further with age. The glucose-induced insulin secretion is markedly reduced in these transgenic mice, as assessed by intraperitoneal glucose tolerance test, and the K_{ATP} channel conductance of the β-cells is significantly decreased. The resting membrane potential and basal intracellular calcium concentration ($[Ca^{2+}]_i$) of the β-cells are significantly higher than those of control mice. Histological analysis reveals the islets to be decreased in size and irregular in shape due to the loss of β-cells. Apoptotic β-cell death is frequently observed by the TUNEL method in these transgenic mice, suggesting that the loss of β-cells is due to increased apoptosis.

Knockout mice

The physiological role of K_{ATP} channels in insulin secretion was further analyzed in mice lacking K_{ATP} channels (K_{ATP} channel deficient mice) (107). Because the Kir6.2 subunits form the K^+ ion-selective pore (47,48,49), mice lacking K_{ATP} channels were generated by disruption of the Kir6.2 gene (Kir6.2$^{-/-}$). K_{ATP} channel activity was completely absent in pancreatic β-cells of mice lacking Kir6.2 (Kir6.2$^{-/-}$), indicating that the Kir6.2 subunit is essential for functional K_{ATP} channels. Kir6.2$^{-/-}$ mice showed a transient hypoglycaemia in neonates, similarly to the transgenic mice described above. Although the blood glucose levels of Kir6.2$^{-/-}$ mice in adults in the fed state were not significantly different from those of Kir6.2$^{+/+}$ mice, the insulin response to glucose *in vivo* also was impaired in Kir6.2$^{-/-}$ mice, as evaluated by intraperitoneal glucose tolerance test. Interestingly, the glucose-lowering effect of insulin, as assessed by insulin tolerance test, is increased significantly in Kir6.2$^{-/-}$, possibly accounting for the only mild impairment of glucose tolerance seen in Kir6.2$^{-/-}$. This also suggests how the K_{ATP} channels in skeletal muscle could be involved in glucose disposal *in vivo*. Intriguingly, Hansen et al. (94) found that young healthy Danish carriers of the maximal load of combined missense mutations in the Kir6.2 gene had an increase in insulin sensitivity index, suggesting that insulin action in peripheral tissues may be influenced by changes in the electrochemical state of the plasma membrane in peripheral tissues. Studies of Kir6.2$^{-/-}$ *in vitro* revealed the resting membrane potential and basal $[Ca^{2+}]_i$ of pancreatic β-cells to be determined primarily by the K_{ATP} channels: raising $[Ca^{2+}]_i$ in pancreatic β-cells requires closure of the K_{ATP} channels in response to glucose or sulfonylureas, and both glucose-induced and sulfonylurea-induced insulin secretion require the rapid rise in $[Ca^{2+}]_i$ that is caused by closure of the K_{ATP} channels. Histological examination shows that glucagon-positive α-cells, which are present primarily in the periphery in islets of normal mice, appear also in the central region in the islets of Kir6.2$^{-/-}$, similarly to those in the transgenic (Kir6.2G132S Tg) mice (Figure 7).

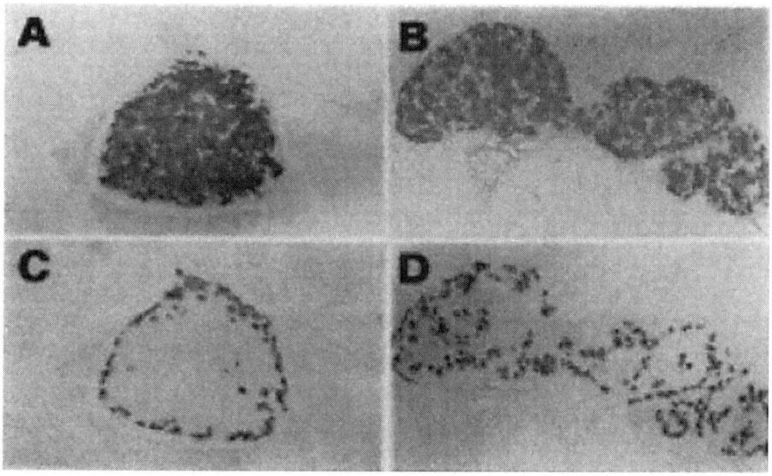

Figure 7. *Histological changes of pancreatic islets in K_{ATP} channel knockout mice. Pancreatic islets were from control mice (A and C) and from mice lacking K_{ATP} channels (B and D). Pancreatic β-cells (A and B) and α-cells (C and D) were immunostained with guinea pig antiinsulin and rabbit antiglucagon antibodies, respectively. Note the presence of glucagon-positive α-cells in the central region of islets from mice lacking Kir6.2 (The authors thank Dr. Iwanaga, Hokkaido University, for supplying these photomicrographs).*

ACKNOWLEDGEMENTS

Work in our laboratory has been supported by Grants in aid from the Ministry of Education, Science, Sports and Culture, Japan and by Research Grants from the Ministry of Health and Welfare, Japan.

REFERENCES

1. Noma A. ATP-regulated K+ channels in cardiac muscle. Nature 1983;305:147-8.
2. Ashcroft FM, Harrison DE, Ashcroft SJH. Glucose induces closure of single potassium channels in isolated rat pancreatic β-cells. Nature 1984;312:446-8.
3. Cook DL, Hales CN. Intracellular ATP directly blocks K+ channels in pancreatic β-cells. Nature 1984; 311: 271-3.
4. Findly I, Dunne MJ, Petersen OH. ATP-sensitive inward rectifier and voltage and calcium activated K+ channels in cultured pancreatic islet cells. J Memb Biol 1985;88:165-72.

5. Rorsman P, Trube G. Glucose dependent K^+ -channels in pancreatic β-cells are regulated by intracellular ATP. Pflügers Arch 1985;405:305-9.
6. Spruce AE, Standen NB, Stanfield PR. Voltage-dependent ATP-sensitive potassium channels of skeletal muscle membrane. Nature 1985;316:736-8.
7. Standen NB, Quayle JM, Davies NW, et al. Hyperpolarizing vasodilators activate ATP-sensitive K^+ Channels in arterial smooth muscle. Science 1989;245:177-80.
8. Ashford MLJ, Sturgess NC, Trout NJ, Gardner NJ, Hales CN. Adenosine-5'-triphosphate-sensitive ion channels in neonatal rat cultured central neurones. Pflügers Arch 1988;412:297-304.
9. Bernardi H, De Weille JR, Epelbaum J, et al. ATP-modulated K^+ channels sensitive to antidiabetic sulfonylureas are present in adenohypophysis and are involved in growth hormone release. Proc Natl Acad Sci USA 1993;90:1340-4.
10. Hunter M, Giebisch G. Calcium-activated K^+-channels of Amphiuma early distal tubule: inhibition by ATP. Pflügers Arch 1988;412:331-3.
11. Inoue I, Nagase H, Kishi K, Higuti T. ATP-sensitive K^+ channel in the mitochondrial inner membrane. Nature 1991;352:244-7.
12. Ashcroft FM. Adenosine 5'-triphosphate-sensitive potassium channels. Annu Rev Neurosci 1988;11:97-118.
13. Dunne MJ and Petersen MJ. Intracellular ADP activates K^+ channels that are inhibited by ATP in an insulin-secreting cell line. FEBS Lett 1986;208:59-62.
14. Kakei M, Kelly RP, Ashcroft AJH, Ashcroft FM. The ATP- sensitivity of K^+ channels in rat pancreatic β-cells is modulated by ADP. FEBS Lett 1986;208:63-6.
15. Misler S, Falke LC, Gillis K, McDaniel ML. A metabolite-regulated potassium channel in rat pancreatic β-cells. Proc Natl Acad Sci USA 1986;83:7119-23.
16. Hilgemann DW, Ball R. Regulation of cardiac Na^+, Ca^{2+} exchange and K_{ATP} potassium channels by PIP2. Science 1996;273:956-9.
17. Shyng SL, Nichols CG. Membrane phospholipid control of nucleotide sensitivity of K_{ATP} channels. Science 1998;282:1138-41.
18. Baukrowitz T, Schulte U, Oliver D, et al. PIP2 and PIP as determinants for ATP inhibition of K_{ATP} channels. Science 1998;282:1141-44.
19. Henquin JC. D-glucose inhibits potassium efflux from pancreatic islet cells. Nature 1978;271:271-3.
20. Terzic A, Jahangir A, Kurachi Y. Cardiac ATP-sensitive K^+ channels regulation by intracellular nucleotides and K^+ channel-opening drugs. Am J Physiol1995;269:C525-45.
21. Sturgess NC, Ashford NLJ, Cook DL, Hales CN. The sulphonylurea receptor may be an ATP-sensitive potassium channel. Lancet 1985;8453:474-5.
22. Trube G, Rorsman P, Ohno S. Opposite effects of tolbutamide and diazoxide in the ATP-dependent K^+ channel in mouse pancreatic β-cells. Eur J Physiol 1986;407:493-9.
23. Inagaki N, Tsuura Y, Namba N, et al. Cloning and functional characterization of a novel ATP-sensitive potassium channel ubiquitously expressed in rat tissues, including pancreatic islets, pituitary, skeletal muscle, and heart. J Biol Chem 1995;270:5691-4.
24. Yamada M, Isomoto S, Matsumoto S, et al. Sulphonylurea receptor 2B and Kir6.1 form a sulphonylurea-sensitive but ATP-insensitive K^+ channel. J Physiol (Lond) 1997;499:715-20.
25. Beech DJ, Zhang H, Nakao K, Bolton TB. Single channel and whole-cell K-currents evoked by levcromakalim in smooth muscle cells from the rabbit portal vein. Br J Pharmacol 1993;110:583-90.
26. Kajioka S, Kitamura K, Kuriyama H. Guanosine diphosphate activates an adenosine 5'-triphosphate-sensitive K^+ channel in the rabbit portal vein. J Physiol (Lond) 1991;444:397-418.
27. Nelson MT, Quayle JM. Physiological roles and properties of potassium channels in arterial smooth muscle. Am J Physiol 1995;268:C799-C822.
28. Suzuki M, Kotake K, Fujikura K, et al. Kir6.1: a possible subunit of ATP-sensitive K^+ channels in mitochondria. Biochem Biophys Res Commun 1998;241:693-97.
29. Inagaki N, Inazawa J, Seino S. cDNA sequence, gene structure, and chromosomal localization of human ATP-sensitive potassium channel, u K_{ATP}-1 gene (KCNJ8). Genomics 1995;30:102-4.
30. Inagaki N, Gonoi T, Clement IV JP, et al. Reconstitution of I_{KATP}: An inward rectifier subunit plus the sulfonylurea receptor. Science 1995;270:1166-70.
31. Suzuki M, Fujikura K, Inagaki N, Seino S, Takata K. Localization of the ATP-sensitive K^+ channel subunit Kir6.2 in mouse pancreas. Diabetes 1997;46:1440-4.
32. Aguilar-Bryan L, Nichols CG, Wechsler SW, et al. Cloning of the β-cells high affinity sulfonylurea receptor: A regulator of insulin secretion. Science 1995;268:423-6.
33. Thomas PM, Cote GJ, Wohllk N, et al. Mutations in the sulfonylurea receptor gene in familial persistent hyperinsulinemic hypoglycemia of infancy. Science 1995;268:426-9.
34. Evans GA, Athanasiou M, Aguayo P, et al. Homo sapiens Chromosome11p14.3 PAC clone pDJ239b22, complete sequence. GenBank accession number U90583 1998.
35. Faure C, Partiseti M, Gouhier C, Graham D. GenBank accession number X97279.
36. Higgins. ABC transporters: from microorganisms to man. Ann Rev Cell Biol 1992;8:67-113.

37. Walker JE, Saraste MJ, Runswick MJ, Gay NJ. Distantly related sequences in the A- and B-subunits of ATP synthase, myoson, kinase and other ATP-requiring enzymes and a common nucleotide binding fold. EMBO J;1:945-51.
38. Tusnady GE, Bakos E, Varadi A, Sarkadi B. Membrane topology distinguishes a subfamily of the ATP-binding cassette (ABC) transporters. FEBS Lett1997;402:1-3.
39. Suzuki M, Fujikawa K, Kotake K, Inagaki N, Seino S, Takata K. Immuno-localization of sulfonylurea receptor 1 in rat pancreas. Diabetologia 1999;42:1204-11.
40. Inagaki N, Gonoi T, Clement IV JP, et al. A family of sulfonylurea receptors determines the pharmacological properties of ATP-sensitive K^+ channels. Neuron 1996;16:1011-7.
41. Isomoto S, Kondo C, Yamada M, et al. A novel sulfonylurea receptor forms with BIR (Kir6.2) a smooth muscle type ATP-sensitive K^+ channel. J Biol Chem1996;271:24321-4.
42. Chutkow WA, Simon MC, Le Beau MM, Burant CF. Cloning, tissue expression, and chromosomal localization of SUR2, the putative drug-binding subunit of cardiac, skeletal muscle, and vascular K_{ATP} channels. Diabetes 1996;45:1439-45.
43. Aguilar-Bryan L, Clement IV JP, Gonzalez G, Kunjilwar K, Babenko A, Bryan J. Toward understanding the assembly and structure of K_{ATP} channels. Physiol Rev 1998;78:227-45.
44. Chutkow WA, Makielski JC, Nelson D, Burant CF, Fan Z. Alternative splicing of SUR2 exon 17 regulates nucleotide sensitivity of K_{ATP}. J Biol Chem 1999;274:13656-65.
45. Aguilar-Bryan L, Bryan J. ATP-sensitive potassium channels, sulfonylurea receptors, and persistent hyperinsulinemic hypoglycemia of infancy. Diabetes Review 1996;4:336-46.
46. Ueda K, Inagaki N, Seino S. MgADP antagonism to Mg^{2+} -independent ATP binding of the sulfonylurea receptor SUR1. J Biol Chem 1997;272:22983-6.
47. Clement IV JP, Kunjilwar K, Gonzales G, et al. Association and stoichiometry of K_{ATP} channel subunits. Neuron 1997;18:827-38.
48. Inagaki N, Gonoi T, Seino S. Subunit stoichiometry of the pancreatic β-cells ATP-sensitive K^+ channel. FEBS Lett 1997;409:232-6.
49. Shyng SL, Nichols CG. Octameric stoichiometry of the K_{ATP} channel complex. J Gen Physiol 1997;110:655-64.
50. Meglasson MD, Matschinsky FM. Pancreatic islet glucose metabolism and regulation of insulin secretion. Diabetes Metab Rev 1986;2:163-214.
51. Ashcroft FM, Ashcroft SJH, Harrison DE. Properties of single channels modulated by glucose in rat pancreatic β-cells. J Physiol (Lond) 1988;400:501-27.
52. Shyng S-L, Ferrigni T, Nichols CG. Regulation of K_{ATP} channel activity by diazoxide and MgADP distinct functions of the two nucleotide binding folds of the sulfonylurea receptor. J Gen Physiol 1997;110:643-54.
53. Gribble FM, Tucker SJ, Ashcroft FM. The essential role of the Walker A motifs of SUR1 in K_{ATP} channel activation by Mg-ADP and diazoxide. EMBO J 1997;16:1145-52.
54. Tucker SJ, Gribble FM, Zhao C, Trapp S, Ashcroft FM. Truncation of Kir6.2 produces ATP-sensitive K^+ channels in the absence of the sulphonylurea receptor. Nature 1997;387:179-83.
55. Ueda K, Inagaki N, Seino S. MgADP Antagonism to Mg^{2+}- independent ATP binding of the sulfonylurea receptor SUR1. J Biol Chem 1997;272:22983-86.
56. Tanabe K, Tucker SJ, Matsuo M, et al. Direct photoaffinity labelling of the Kir6.2 subunit of the ATP-sensitive K^+ channel by 8-azido-ATP. J Biol Chem 1999;274:3931-33.
57. Ueda K, Komine J, Matsuo M, Seino S, Amachi T. Cooperative binding of ATP and MgADP in the sulfonylurea receptor is mediated by glibenclamide. Proc Natl Acad Sci USA 1999;96:1268-72.
58. Seino S, Inagaki N, Namba N, Gonoi T. Molecular biology of the β-cells ATP-sensitive K^+ channel. Diabetes Rev 1996;4:177-90.
59. Ashcroft FM, Gribble FM. Correlating structure and function in ATP-sensitive K^+ channels. Trends Neurosci 1998;21:288-94.
60. Ashcroft FM, Ashcroft SJH. Properties and functions of ATP-sensitive K -channels. Cell Signal 1990;2:197-214.
61. Gribble F, Tucker SJ, Seino S, Ashcroft FM. Tissue specificity of sulfonylyreas: studies on cloned cardiac and β-cell K_{ATP} channels. Diabetes1998;47:1412-18.
62. Axelrod L, Levitsky LL. Nesidioblastosis in HYPOGLYCEMIA. In: Kahn CR, Weir GC eds. Joslin's Diabetes Mellitus, 13th ed. Malveern: Lea & Febiger. 1994;991.
63. Leibowitz G, Glaser B, Higazi AA, Salameh M, Cerasi E, Landau H. Hyperinsulinemic hypoglycemia of infancy (nesidioblastosis) in clinical remission: high incidence of diabetes mellitus and persistent β-cell dysfunction at long-term follow-up. J Clin Endocrinol Metab 1995;80:386-92.
64. Glaser B, Hirsch HJ, Landau H. Persistent hyperinsulinemic hypoglycemia of infancy: Long-term octreotide treatment without pancreatectomy. J Pediatr 1993;123:637-43.
65. Shilyansky J, Fisher S, Cutz E, Perlman K, Filler RM. Is 95% pancreatectomy the procedure of choice for treatment of persistent hyperinsulinemic hypoglycemia of the neonate? J Pediatr Surg 1997;32:342-6.
66. Dacou-Voutetakis C, Psychou F, Maniati-Christides M. Persistent hyperinsulinemic hypoglycemia of infancy: Long term result. J Pediatr Endocrinol Metab 1998;Suppl 11:131-41.

67. Glaser B, Phillip M, Carmi R, Lieberman E, Landau H. Persistent hyperinsulinemic hypoglycemia of infancy ("nesidioblastosis"): autosomal recessive inheritance in 7 pedigrees. Am J Med Genet 1990;37:511-5.
68. Woolf DA, Leonard JV, Trembath RC, Pembrey ME, Grant DB. Nesidioblastosis: evidence for autosomal recessive inheritance. Arch Dis Child 1991;66:529-30.
69. Thornton PS, Sumner AE, Ruchelli ED, Spielman RS, Baker L, Stanley CA. Familial and sporadic hyperinsulinism: histopathologic findings and segregation analysis support a single autosomal recessive disorder. J Pediat 1991;119:721-24.
70. Bruining GJ. Recent advances in hyperinsulinism and the pathogenesis of diabetes mellitus. Curr Opin Pediat 1990;2:758-65.
71. Mathew PM, Young JM, Abu-Osba YK, et al. Persistent neonatal hyperinsulinism. Clin Pediat 1988;27:148-51.
72. Glaser B, Chiu KC, Anker R, et al. Familial hyperinsulinism maps to chromosome 11p14-15.1, 30 cM centromeric to the insulin gene. Nature Genet 1994;7:185-8.
73. Thomas PM, Cote GJ, Hallman DM, Mathew PM. Homozygosity mapping, to chromosome 11p, of the gene for familial persistent hyperinsulinemic hypoglycemia of infancy. Am J Hum Genet 1995;56:416-21.
74. Glaser B, Chiu KC, Liu L, et al. Recombinant mapping of the familial hyperinsulinism gene to an 0.8 cM region on chromosome 11p15.1 and demonstration of a founder effect in Ashkenazi Jews. Hum Mol Genet1995;4:879-86.
75. Thomas PM, Wohllk N, Huang E, et al. Inactivation of the first nucleotide binding fold of the sulfonylurea receptor, and familial persistent hyperinsulinemic hypoglycemia of infancy. Am J Hum Genet 1996;59:510-8.
76. Nestorowicz A, Wilson BA, Schoor KP, et al. Mutations in the sulfonylurea receptor gene are associated with familial hyperinsulinism in Ashkenazi Jews. Hum Mol Genet 1996;5:1813-22.
77. Nichols CG, Shyng SL, Nestorowicz A, et al. Adenosine diphosphate as an intracellular regulator of insulin secretion. Science 1996;272:1785-7.
78. Dunne MJ, Kane C, Shepherd RM, et al. Familial persistent hyperinsulinemic hypoglycemia of infancy and mutations in the sulfonylurea receptor. New Engl J Med 1997;336:703-6.
79. Shyng SL, Ferrigni T, Shepard JB, et al. Functional analyses of novel mutations in the sulfonylurea receptor 1 associated with persistent hyperinsulinemic hypoglycemia of infancy. Diabetes 1998;47:1145-51.
80. Nestorowicz A, Glaser B, Wilson BA, et al. Genetic heterogeneity in familial hyperinsulinism. Hum Mol Genet 1998;7:1119-28.
81. Filler RM, Weinberg MJ, Cutz E, Wesson DE, Ehrlich RM. Current status of pancreatectomy for persistent idiopathic neonatal hypoglycemia due to islet cell dysplasia. Prog Pediatr Surg 1991;26:60-75.
82. Verkarre, V.; Fournet, J.-C.; de Lonlay, P.; Gross-Morand, M.-S.; Devillers. Paternal mutation of the sulfonylurea receptor (SUR1) gene and maternal loss of 11p15 imprinted genes lead to persistent hyperinsulinism in focal adenomatous hyperplasia. J Clin Invest 1998;102:1286-91.
83. de Lonlay P, Fournet JC, Rahier J, et al. Somatic deletion of the imprinted 11p15 region in sporadic persistent hyperinsulinemic hypoglycemia of infancy is specific of focal adenomatous hyperplasia and endorses partial pancreatectomy. J Clin Invest 1997;100:802-7.
84. Dubois J, Brunelle F, Touati G, et al. Hyperinsulinism in children: diagnostic value of pancreatic venous sampling correlated with clinical, pathological and surgical outcome in 25 cases. Pediatr Radiol 1995;25:512-6.
85. Thomas P, Ye Y, Lightner E. Mutation of the pancreatic islet inward rectifier Kir6.2 also leads to familial persistent hyperinsulinemic hypoglycemia of infancy. Hum Mol Genet 1996;5:1809-12.
86. Nestorowicz A, Inagaki N, Gonoi T, et al. A nonsense mutation in the inward rectifier potassium channel gene, Kir6.2, is associated with familial hyperinsulinism. Diabetes 1997;46:1743-8.
87. Kukuvitis A, Deal C, Arbour L, Polychronakos C. An autosomal dominant form of familial persistent hyperinsulinemic hypoglycemia of infancy, not linked to the sulfonylurea receptor locus. J Clin Endocrinol Metab 1997;82:1192-4.
88. Glaser B, Kesavan P, Heyman M, et al. Familial hyperinsulinism caused by an activating glucokinase mutation. N Engl J Med 1998;338:226-30.
89. Stanley CA, Lieu YK, Hsu BY, et al. Hyperinsulinism and hyperammonemia in infants with regulatory mutations of the glutamate dehydrogenase gene. N Engl J Med 1998;338:1352-7.
90. Tokuyama Y, Fan Z, Furuta H, et al. Rat inwardly rectifying potassium channel Kir6.2: cloning electrophysiological characterization, and decreased expression in pancreatic islets of male Zucker diabetic fatty rats. Biochem Biophys Res Commun 1996; 220:532-8.
91. Iwasaki N, Kawamura M, Yamagata K, et al. Identification of microsatellite markers near the human genes encoding the β-cells ATP-sensitive K^+ channel and linkage studies with NIDDM in Japanese. Diabetes 1996;45:267-9.
92. Sakura H, Wat N, Horton V, Millns H, Turner RC, Ashcroft FM. Sequence variations in the human Kir6.2 gene, a subunit of the beta-cell ATP-sensitive K-channel: no association with

NIDDM in while Caucasian subjects or evidence of abnormal function when expressed in vitro. Diabetologia 1996;39:1233-6.

93. Inoue H, Ferrer J, Warren-Perry M, et al. Sequence variants in the pancreatic islet β-cell inwardly rectifying K^+ channel Kir6.2 (Bir) gene: identification and lack of role in Caucasian patients with NIDDM. Diabetes 1997;46:502-7.
94. Hansen L, Echwald SM, Hansen T, Urhammer SA, Clausen JO, Pedersen O. Amino acid polymorphisms in the ATP-regulatable inward rectifier Kir6.2 and their relationships to glucose and tolbutamide-induced insulin secretion, the insulin sensitivity index, and NIDDM. Diabetes1997;46:508-12.
95. Hani EH, Boutin P, Durand E, et al. Missense mutations in the pancreatic islet β-cell inwardly rectifying K^+ channel gene (KIR6.2/BIR): a meta-analysis suggests a role in the polygenic basis of Type II diabetes mellitus in Caucasians. Diabetologia 1998;41:1511-5.
96. Stirling B, Cox NJ, Bell GI, Hanis CL, Spielman RS, Concannon P. Linkage studies in NIDDM with markers near the sulphonylurea receptor gene. Diabetologia 1995;38:1479-81.
97. Ohta Y, Tanizawa Y, Inoue H, et al. Identification and functional analysis of sulfonylurea receptor 1 variants in Japanese patients with NIDDM. Diabetes 1998;47:476-81.
98. Ishiyama-Shigemoto S, Yamada K, Yuan X, Koyama W, Nonaka K. Clinical characterization of polymorphisms in the sulphonylurea receptor 1 gene in Japanese subjects with Type 2 diabetes mellitus. Diabet Med 1998;15:826-9.
99. Inoue H, Ferrer J, Welling CM, Elbein SC, Hoffman M et al. Sequence variants in the sulfonylurea receptor (SUR) gene are associated with NIDDM in Caucasians. Diabetes 1996;45:825-31
100. Hansen T, Echwald SM, Hansen L, et al. Decreased tolbutamide-stimulated insulin secretion in healthy subjects with sequence variants in the high-affinity sulfonylurea receptor gene. Diabetes 1998;47:598-605.
101. Hani EH, Clement K, Velho G, et al. Genetic studies of the sulfonylurea receptor gene locus in NIDDM and in morbid obesity among French Caucasians. Diabetes 1997;46: 688-94
102. Goksel DL, Fischbach K, Duggirala R, et al. Variant in sulfonylurea receptor-1 gene is associated with high insulin concentrations in non-diabetic Mexican Americans: SUR-1 gene variant and hyperinsulinemia. Hum Genet 1998;103:280-5.
103. Heginbotham L, Abramson T, MacKinnon R. A functional connection between the pores of distantly related ion channels as revealed by mutant K^+ channels. Science 1992;258:1152-5.
104. Jan LY, Jan Y. Potassium channels and their evolving gates. Nature 1994;371:119-22.
105. Kerr ID, Sansom MS. Cation selectivity in ion channels. Nature 1995;373:112.
106. Miki T, Tashiro F, Iwanaga T, et al. Abnormalities of pancreatic islets by targeted expression of a dominant-negative K_{ATP} channel. Proc Natl Acad Sci USA 1997;94:11969-73.
107. Miki T, Nagashima K, Tashiro F, et al. Defective insulin secretion and enhanced insulin action in K_{ATP} channel-deficient mice. Proc Natl Acad Sci USA 1998;95:10402-6.

7

GLUCAGON-LIKE PEPTIDE-1: AN INSULINOTROPIC HORMONE WITH POTENT GROWTH FACTOR ACTIONS AT THE PANCREATIC ISLETS OF LANGERHANS

George G. Holz, Ph.D. and Colin A. Leech, Ph.D.
New York University School of Medicine, New York, NY, USA
Howard Hughes Medical Institute, Massachusetts General Hospital
Harvard Medical School, Boston, MA, USA

INTRODUCTION

Identification of chemical mediators that support pancreatic β-cell neogenesis, differentiation, growth, and survival offers the prospect for introduction of novel therapeutic strategies in the treatment of diabetes mellitus. One such chemical mediator is glucagon-like peptide-1 (GLP-1), an intestinally-derived blood glucose-lowering hormone that is a potential therapeutic agent for use in treatment of adult-onset diabetes mellitus (type 2 diabetes) (1-4). GLP-1 exerts a direct action at the pancreatic islets of Langerhans to stimulate biosynthesis and secretion of insulin, thereby lowering levels of blood glucose. Additional effects of GLP-1 at the islets include stimulation of DNA synthesis, increased cellular proliferation, and alterations in the pattern of gene expression that are critical to maintenance of a fully differentiated β-cell phenotype. Such growth factor-like effects of GLP-1 suggest its possible usefulness as a stimulus for *de novo* production of islets in diabetic subjects, or for *ex vivo* expansion of β-cells in islets isolated for purposes of transplantation. It is also appreciated that GLP-1 acts within the central nervous system as an appetite suppressant (5,6). This surprising finding suggests an additional beneficial action of GLP-1 for treatment of eating disorders, obesity, and/or adipogenic diabetes mellitus.

GLP-1 receptors are high affinity G protein-coupled receptors (GPCRs) expressed on insulin-producing β-cells. Receptor occupancy by GLP-1 stimulates production of cAMP, increases activity of mitogen-activated protein kinases (MAPK), raises levels of cytosolic Ca^{2+} concentration $[Ca^{2+}]_i$, and stimulates exocytosis of insulin-containing secretory granules (7-9). Insulin secretion is accompanied by increased transcriptional activity of the insulin gene, increased insulin biosynthesis, and a replenishment of the releasable pool of insulin. Such insulinotropic actions of GLP-1 are dependent on metabolism of D-glucose by the β-cells, thereby emphasizing the importance of intermediary metabolism as a necessary co-factor in support of GLP-1 signal transduction. Here we review the current status of GLP-1 from the standpoint of its novel signal transduction properties in the pancreatic islets. Emphasized are important modulatory influences of GLP-1 on β-cell glucose metabolism, gene expression, and stimulus-secretion coupling.

GLP-1 IS AN INCRETIN HORMONE AT THE ENTERO-INSULAR AXIS

Two biologically active isopeptides of GLP-1, namely GLP-1(7-37) and GLP-1(7-36)amide, are synthesized by enteroendocrine L-cells of the distal intestine and are derived by tissue-specific post-translational processing of proglucagon (10). Although the predominant circulating form of GLP-1 is GLP-1(7-36)amide, the signal transduction properties of the amidated peptide are indistinguishable from those of GLP-1(7-37). Secretion of GLP-1 into the bloodstream occurs postprandially and is triggered by 1) the autonomic nervous system, 2) stimulatory effects of intestinally-derived glucose-dependent insulinotropic peptide (GIP), and by 3) nutrient stimuli acting at the luminal surface of the gut following a meal. The half-life of biologically active GLP-1 is short (< 2 min) due in large measure to the enzymatic activity of circulating dipeptidyl peptidase IV (DPP IV) (4,8).

The timing of the secretion of GLP-1 is such that circulating levels of the hormone rise coincident with the postprandial increase of blood glucose concentration. Plasma concentrations of GLP-1 rise to pM levels, consistent with the empirically determined affinity constant of β-cell GLP-1 receptors. Receptor occupancy by GLP-1 leads to production of cAMP, a rise of $[Ca^{2+}]_i$, and a potentiation of glucose-dependent insulin secretion. The concentration of circulating insulin is then observed to increase to a level above that attributable to glucose alone. This augmentation of glucose-stimulated insulin secretion by the gut hormone GLP-1 is termed the incretin effect. It plays a critical role in the maintenance of systemic glucose homeostasis.

From a systems physiology standpoint, GLP-1 can be viewed as an incretin hormone within the enteroinsular axis (11). It mediates humoral communication between the intestine, the pancreas, and target sites of insulin action. In healthy individuals, the direct stimulatory influence of GLP-1 at the pancreatic islets enables β-cells to match the ambient blood glucose concentration to an appropriate insulin secretory response. Although this homeostatic glucose sensing mechanism is dysfunctional in type 2 diabetes, pharmacological concentrations of GLP-1 still produce a robust blood glucose lowering effect. GLP-1 restores the missing first phase component of postprandial insulin secretion and delays the rise of blood glucose concentration when administered to type 2 diabetic subjects concomitant with a meal (11-13). This remarkable finding indicates that GLP-1 corrects for a metabolic dysfunction of the diabetic pancreas. We refer to this compensatory phenomenon as the induction of glucose competence by GLP-1 (see below).

It is reasonable to conclude that the immediate blood glucose-lowering effect of GLP-1 is primarily a consequence of its action to stimulate secretion of insulin. It should be noted, however, that GLP-1 also inhibits secretion of a hyperglycaemic hormone - intra-islet glucagon. Long-term blood glucose-lowering effects of GLP-1 most likely involve alterations of β-cell gene expression. GLP-1 stimulates insulin gene promoter activity, stabilizes preproinsulin mRNA, and enhances translational biosynthesis of proinsulin. GLP-1 also up-regulates transcription of genes comprising the β-cell glucose signalling system. These include the type 2 glucose transporter (Glut2) and glucokinase (14). Such effects of GLP-1 might be mediated by PDX-1 (15,16), a homeodomain transcription factor that is reported to serve as a master regulator of the fully differentiated β-cell phenotype. Less well understood actions of GLP-1 include increased hepatic glycogenesis (17,18), stimulation of glycogen synthesis in skeletal muscle (17,19), alterations of fat cell lipid or cAMP metabolism, acceleration of glucose uptake in adipocytes (20,21), and delayed gastric emptying (22,23). Such extrapancreatic actions of GLP-1 may explain how it lowers levels of blood glucose in individuals with type 1 diabetes (24,25). Whether or not any of these extrapancreatic effects of GLP-1 are mediated by specific pancreatic-type GLP-1 receptors expressed on hepatocytes, myocytes, or adipocytes remains unproved.

GLP-1 is also reported to increase insulin receptor binding activity, as demonstrated in RINm5F insulinoma cells (26). This effect is achieved by an increase of the affinity and binding capacity of insulin autoreceptors located on β-cells. Insulin autoreceptors mediate stimulatory actions of insulin on insulin secretion, Ca^{2+} signalling, and insulin gene expression (27-32). A central hypothesis concerning the aetiology of type 2 diabetes is that there exists a defect of insulin signal transduction, such that target tissues of insulin action (liver, fat, and muscle) become resistant to insulin (peripheral insulin resistance). What has not been appreciated is the possibility that resistance to insulin is also manifest at the islets of Langerhans. Defects of β-cell insulin signalling might constitute a direct causative factor in the generation of type 2 diabetes (33). Therefore, the beneficial blood glucose-lowering actions of GLP-1 in type 2 diabetic subjects may arise not only from a stimulation of pancreatic insulin secretion, but also from a restoration of insulin signalling within β-cells.

GLP-1 AND THE GLUCOSE COMPETENCE CONCEPT

The role of GLP-1 as a regulator of pancreatic β-cell function can be viewed from the perspective of the glucose competence concept (34-37). We propose that GLP-1 corrects for a metabolic dysfunction of β-cell glucose signalling, thereby allowing islets from diabetic subjects to secrete insulin in response to a rise of blood glucose concentration. We view induction of glucose competence by GLP-1 as an ability of the hormone to act as a *glucose sensitizer*, thereby overcoming β-cell glucose-dependent resistance. Support for the glucose competence concept is provided by numerous reports that GLP-1 and stimulators of cAMP signal transduction restore glucose-dependent insulin secretion in β-cells, islets, insulinoma cells, and animal models of type 2 diabetes (38-43). Furthermore, as outlined above, GLP-1 restores glucose-dependent secretion of insulin in type 2 diabetic subjects (1,12,44,45). It should be noted that the glucose competence concept has been misconstrued by some to imply that normal β-cells require GLP-1 in order to secrete insulin. This confusion arose due to the observation that the glucose-dependent insulin secretory profile of normal islets is blunted in the absence of a conditioning hormonal stimulus. Stimulus-secretion coupling is delayed and the magnitude of the secretory response is a fraction of that obtained in the presence of GLP-1. However, normal islets, or islets from transgenic GLP-1-receptor knockout mice, can and do secrete insulin in the absence of GLP-1 (46). It is only in dysfunctional islets that glucose signalling is compromised, and under such conditions, GLP-1 is a fully effective glucose competence hormone.

THE INTERACTION OF GLP-1 WITH METABOLISM OF D-GLUCOSE

All reported insulinotropic actions of GLP-1 are known to be absolutely contingent on simultaneous exposure of β-cells to concentrations of D-glucose that meet or exceed levels commonly observed following ingestion of a meal. This requirement for postprandial metabolism of D-glucose is demonstrable *in vitro*. GLP-1-induced secretion of insulin from isolated pancreatic islets is blocked by mannoheptulose (47), an inhibitor of glycolysis, and is supported by succinic acid dimethyl ester (SAD), a non-glucidic nutrient that, once deesterified, becomes available for mitochondrial metabolism (48). Clearly, events intimately associated with mitochondrial metabolism are prerequisites for an effective insulinotropic response to GLP-1.

To understand the interaction of GLP-1 with β-cell intermediary metabolism, it is important to recognize this hormone's modulatory influence on glucose signalling (Figure 1). D-glucose triggers secretion of insulin, a process that requires uptake of glucose and aerobic glycolysis. This "fuel hypothesis" predicts that metabolism of glucose generates metabolic coupling factors necessary for exocytosis of insulin (49). Such factors are derived from glycolysis, the Krebs (TCA) cycle, NADH-dependent mitochondrial shuttles, or anaplerotic production of malonyl-CoA. Uptake of glucose and its conversion to glucose 6-phosphate constitute a glucose-sensing mechanism. Glucose uptake is mediated by the type 2 facilitative glucose transporter, whereas glucokinase (a type 4 hexokinase rate-limiting for glucose sensing) converts glucose to glucose 6-phosphate (50). An oscillatory burst of respiration ensues as a consequence of glycolytic and mitochondrial metabolism. It is accompanied by increased pyridine and flavin nucleotide reduction state, alkalinization, and an increased ratio of $[ATP]_i$ / $[ADP]_i$. Also observed is the generation of malonyl-CoA and synthesis of long-chain fatty acyl CoA esters. Each of these events constitutes a potential metabolic coupling factor for glucose-induced secretion of insulin. The glucose competence concept predicts that the conditioning influence of GLP-1 results from an ability of the hormone to stimulate the production and/or effectiveness of such coupling factors (Figure 1). This would then explain how GLP-1 increases the efficacy and potency of glucose as a stimulator of insulin secretion (51).

One hint as to how GLP-1 may act is provided by recent studies examining the interaction of glycolysis with mitochondrial metabolism. It was reported that NADH shuttle systems play a major role in the glucose-induced activation of mitochondrial metabolism and insulin secretion (52-55). NADH is generated by the glycolytic enzyme glyceraldehyde 3-phosphate dehydrogenase (GAPDH). It is transferred into mitochondria for oxidative metabolism and ATP production via two distinct NADH shuttle systems: 1) the glycerol phosphate shuttle, and 2) the malate-aspartate shuttle. A rate-limiting enzyme of the glycerol phosphate shuttle is mitochondrial glycerol 3-phosphate dehydrogenase (mGPDH). Mice homozygous for a targeted disruption of mGPDH are nomoglycaemic and secrete insulin in response to glucose (54,55). However, treatment of islets derived from mGPDH -/- mice with aminooxyacetate (AOA), an inhibitor of aspartate aminotransferase in the malate-aspartate shuttle, abrogates glucose-dependent secretion of insulin. This effect is positively correlated with disruption of glucose-dependent ATP production, and most likely explains why glucose fails to inhibit cell surface ATP-sensitive K^+ channels under these experimental conditions. Such findings suggest the possibility that the NADH shuttle systems constitute a potential locus at which GLP-1 regulates β-cell glucose metabolism.

GROWTH FACTOR-LIKE ACTIONS OF GLP-1

GLP-1 exerts growth factor-like actions on β-cells manifest as an induction of immediate early gene expression (c-*fos*, c-*jun*), increased DNA synthesis, and cellular proliferation (56,57). Exactly how such trophic effects are achieved is a new area of investigation for which limited information is available. It is known that GLP-1 stimulates phosphatidyl inositol 3-phosphate kinase (PI3 kinase), and promotes binding of AP-1 and PDX-1 transcription factors to *cis*-acting regulatory elements within specific gene promoters (15). By doing so, GLP-1 may allow for maintenance of the fully differentiated β-cell phenotype. PI3 kinase is a down stream effector of IRS-2, a signal transducer of insulin receptors, and of insulin receptor-related receptors, expressed on β-cells (27,28,58,59). PI3 kinase is also activated as a consequence of β-cell glucose metabolism (29), a process that may be reinforced by GLP-1. These observations provide a mechanistic explanation for the interaction of GLP-1, glucose, and insulin to regulate β-cell gene expression.

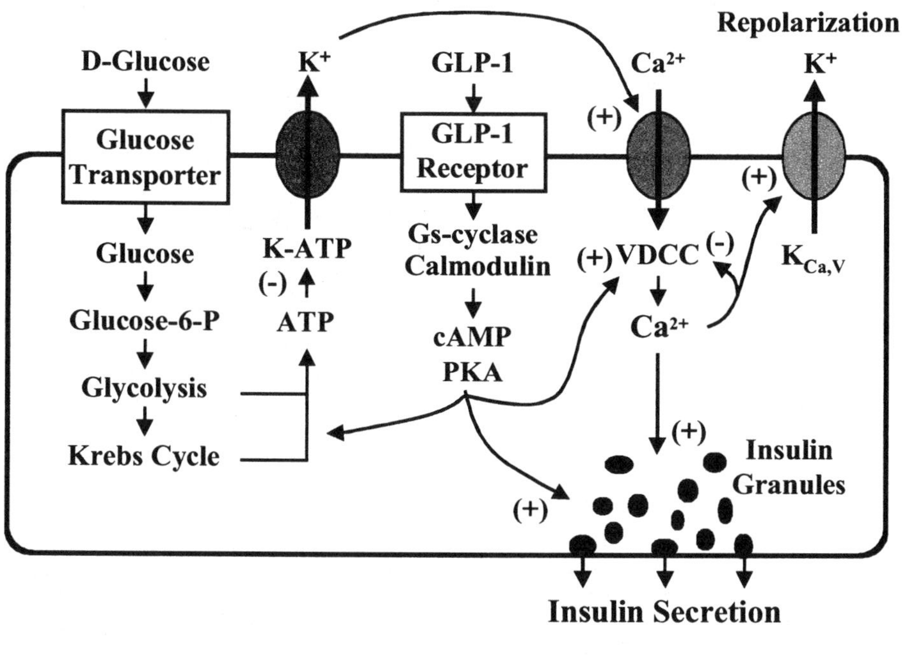

Figure 1. *Hormonal regulation of glucose-dependent insulin secretion from pancreatic β-cells. Uptake of glucose is facilitated by the type-2 glucose transporter, conversion of glucose to glucose-6-phosphate is then catalyzed by glucokinase. Aerobic glycolysis generates multiple signals, one of which is an increased ratio of cytosolic ATP relative to ADP. Binding of ATP to* K_{ATP} *induces closure of the channels. The resulting cellular depolarization activates voltage-dependent* Ca^{2+} *channels (VDCCs). Entry of* Ca^{2+} *across the plasma membrane triggers insulin secretion by* Ca^{2+}*-dependent exocytosis. Repolarization of the membrane results from the action of* Ca^{2+} *to activate* Ca^{2+}*-dependent* K^+ *channels* ($K_{-Ca,V}$) *which inhibits VDCCs. Each step in the pathway is viewed as a potential target for modulation by GLP-1. In this example, GLP-1 binds to cell surface receptors and activates* G_S*. Resulting production of cAMP by adenylyl cyclase activates protein kinase A (PKA) which catalyzes phosphorylation of multiple targets within the glucose-signalling cascade. These targets include enzymes of glycolysis or the Krebs cycle, ion channels, and components of the secretory apparatus that are responsible for exocytosis of insulin-containing granules. Figure 1 adapted from Holz and Habener, 1992.*

GLP-1 also stimulates mitogen-activated protein kinases (MAPK) including MEK (MAP kinase kinase), p38 (stress-activated protein kinase), ERK1 (p44) and ERK2 (p42) (60,61). MAPK activation is observed in response to CPT-cAMP (60), thereby implicating cAMP as an initiator of these events. Activation of MAPK by GLP-1 requires glucose metabolism, and is amplified by an increase of $[Ca^{2+}]_i$ resulting from opening of Ca^{2+} channels (60). Taken together, such findings provide evidence for a synergistic interaction of GLP-1, glucose, and Ca^{2+} to regulate gene expression by way of the MAPK signalling systems.

To investigate in greater detail how a cAMP-elevating hormone such as GLP-1 regulates gene expression; we examined whether β-cells express cAMP-activated guanine nucleotide exchange factors (cAMP-GEFs). The cAMP-GEFs bind cAMP, but act in a PKA-independent manner to stimulate Rap 1 (62). Rap 1 is a small molecular weight GTP-binding protein that activates B-Raf-dependent MAPK signalling (63). It also activates protein kinase C (64). Using reverse transcriptase-catalyzed synthesis of cDNA in combination with the polymerase chain reaction (RT-PCR), we observed expression of the type 1 and type 2 isoforms of cAMP-GEF mRNAs in INS-1 insulinoma cells and human islets (Holz & Leech, unpublished observations). Furthermore, we confirmed previous reports that Rap 1 protein is expressed in β-cells (65,66). Based on these observations, we propose that PKA-independent actions of GLP-1 to regulate gene expression might result from cAMP production and activation of a signalling complex comprised of cAMP-GEF, Rap 1 and B-Raf. It is interesting to note that such an action of GLP-1 may explain the antagonist interaction of cAMP and oncogenic Ras to regulate gene expression, as reported for βTC1 insulinoma cells (67).

PROXIMAL EVENTS IN GLP-1 SIGNAL TRANSDUCTION

The GLP-1 receptor located on β-cells is a GTP-binding protein-coupled receptor (GPCR) classified as a member of the Group III family of B-Type GPCRs (7,68,69). It shares structural homology with GPCRs for glucagon, parathyroid hormone (PTH), GIP, vasoactive intestinal polypeptide (VIP), pituitary adenylyl cyclase-activating polypeptide (PACAP), secretin, calcitonin, corticotropin releasing factor (CRF), and growth hormone releasing hormone (GHRH). The GLP-1 receptor binds with high affinity structurally-related peptides that include not only GLP-1, but also exendin-4 (an agonist) and exendin(9-39) (an antagonist) (70). Exendin-4 is derived from the salivary glands of the Gila monster *Heloderma suspectum*. It has attracted attention not only as a molecular probe of GLP-1 signal transduction pathways (71), but also as a possible antidiabetogenic agent or appetite suppressant. When compared with GLP-1, exendin-4 exhibits greater potency and a longer duration of action as a stimulator of insulin secretion or as a blood glucose-lowering agent (72,73).

The N-terminal ligand-binding domain of the GLP-1 receptor bears structural resemblance to CIRL, an orphan GPCR that binds α-latrotoxin (LTX; a toxin derived from the venom of the black widow spider *Latrodectus tredecimguttatus*). Sequence alignments of GPCRs for GLP-1, LTX, CRF, GHRH, PACAP, VIP, secretin, and glucagon demonstrated highly significant conservation of primary structure in a region of the receptors corresponding to amino acid residues 72-92 of the GLP-1 receptor (74). It was proposed that this region of the receptor is a ligand-binding domain, a conclusion strengthened by the observation that there exists a high degree of structural similarity when comparing the GLP-1, PACAP, VIP, secretin and glucagon peptide ligands. Surprisingly, LTX, itself, bears primary amino acid sequence homology with both GLP-1 and exendin-4. Recognizing this, we reported the characterization of a GLP-1/LTX synthetic peptide chimera (Black Widow GLP-1) that exhibits insulinotropic efficacy similar to that of GLP-1. Such observations prompt speculation that novel therapeutic agents might be derived by the synthesis of chimeric peptides in which functional domains of toxins and hormones are intermixed.

The third intracellular loop of GLP-1 receptors interacts with heterotrimeric G_S GTP-binding proteins and stimulates adenylyl cyclase (75-78). Multiple isoforms of adenylyl cyclases are expressed in β-cells, including those inhibited by Ca^{2+} (79-81). This is significant because GLP-1 produces an increase of $[cAMP]_i$ that drives Ca^{2+} influx and release of Ca^{2+} from intracellular stores (82-86). We propose the existence of an inhibitory feedback mechanism whereby oscillations of $[cAMP]_i$ and $[Ca^{2+}]_i$ are generated during continual exposure of β-cells to GLP-1. In this model, elevation of $[Ca^{2+}]_i$ suppresses cAMP production which in turn allows levels of $[Ca^{2+}]_i$ to return to baseline. A new round of cAMP production is then initiated whereupon the concentration of $[Ca^{2+}]_i$ increases, thus completing the cycle. Such oscillations of [cAMP] and $[Ca^{2+}]_i$ are proposed to contribute to the pulsatile secretion of insulin observed during a rise of blood glucose concentration.

Second messenger actions of cAMP in the β-cell are likely to be spatially restricted and selective for distinct effector molecules. This is because cAMP-dependent activation of protein kinase A (PKA) is accompanied by A-kinase anchoring protein (AKAP)-mediated targeting of PKA to specific subcellular compartments (87,88). Disruption of AKAP blocks stimulatory effects of GLP-1 on voltage-dependent Ca^{2+} channels and insulin secretion (87). This finding is consistent with the previously reported ability of GLP-1 to facilitate Ca^{2+} influx, to raise $[Ca^{2+}]_i$ and to augment insulin exocytosis. However, it is important to note that pharmacological inhibitors of PKA are ineffective when tested for their ability to block stimulation of insulin gene expression by GLP-1 or cAMP (89). These findings suggest the existence of an additional PKA-independent signalling pathway by which GLP-1 and cAMP influence β-cell function.

GLP-1 may also stimulate phospholipase C (PLC), activate protein kinase C (PKC), and raise intracellular levels of inositol trisphosphate (IP3) (90,91). GLP-1 increases inositol phosphate production in COS-7 cells transfected with the recombinant GLP-1 receptor (90), and in *Xenopus* oocytes injected with GLP-1 receptor mRNA (91). Studies of insulinoma cells also demonstrate inositol phosphate production in response to GLP-1 (92). However, the action of GLP-1 in isolated rat islets is much smaller in comparison. It is known that PLC expressed in β-cells is stimulated by Ca^{2+} (93), and that GLP-1 produces a cAMP-dependent increase of $[Ca^{2+}]_i$. Therefore, Ca^{2+} might mediate an indirect stimulatory action of GLP-1 on PLC. An unusual feature of this indirect effect is that stimulation of PLC by GLP-1 and glucose may be voltage-sensitive (94).

Alterations of $[Ca^{2+}]_i$ observed upon exposure of β-cells to GLP-1 are described as having transient (sec) or sustained (min) kinetics (84,95). The transient increase of $[Ca^{2+}]_i$ observed in response to GLP-1 is demonstrated to result from mobilization of intracellular Ca^{2+} stores (82,84). In contrast, the sustained rise of $[Ca^{2+}]_i$ results from influx of Ca^{2+} that is a consequence of three distinct mechanisms. GLP-1 potentiates glucose-induced closure of ATP-sensitive K^+ channels (36), thereby generating depolarization and activation of voltage-dependent Ca^{2+} channels. Second, GLP-1 exerts a direct stimulatory influence on the entry of Ca^{2+} through voltage-dependent Ca^{2+} channels (96-98). Third, GLP-1 stimulates the opening of Ca^{2+}-activated nonselective cation channels that are permeant to Ca^{2+} as well as to Na^+ (95,99). These multiple processes act in concert to augment oscillatory electrical activity, Ca^{2+} influx, and pulsatile secretion of insulin characteristic of whole islets of Langerhans.

ATP-SENSITIVE K⁺ CHANNELS AS MEDIATORS OF GLP-1 SIGNAL TRANSDUCTION

Pancreatic β-cells are excitable cells capable of generating electrical activity manifest as oscillations of membrane potential upon which are superimposed bursts of action potentials (100,101). Action potentials induce the influx of Ca^{2+} through voltage-dependent channels, and a rise of $[Ca^{2+}]_i$. This ionic mechanism interacts with metabolism of glucose and with protein kinase-mediated phosphorylation to stimulate exocytosis of insulin-containing secretory granules. Under normal conditions, the rate limiting step in exocytosis is the rise of $[Ca^{2+}]_i$ that triggers fusion of secretory granules with the plasma membrane. Low levels of glucose do not support insulin secretion whereas higher levels do. The effect of glucose is explained, at least in part, by glucose-induced closure of ATP-sensitive K^+ channels (K_{ATP}). K_{ATP} closes in response to the increased ratio of $[ATP]_i$ / $[ADP]_i$ that results from metabolism of glucose. A "spare channel hypothesis" (102) predicts that glucose-induced closure of K_{ATP} produces cellular depolarization necessary to allow Na^+ and Ca^{2+} channel activation, important events in the generation of action potentials. A seminal observation was that pharmacological activators of cAMP signalling potentiate the depolarizing action of glucose in β-cells (103). Although unappreciated at the time, this report was the first inkling that a synergistic interaction exists between β-cell cAMP and glucose signalling systems to inhibit K_{ATP}.

K_{ATP} is an integral membrane protein comprised of Kir6.2 (pore-forming subunit) and SUR1 (sulfonylurea receptor) (104-106). The β-cell K_{ATP} exhibits a single channel conductance of 60-80 pS, weak inward rectification, and flickery channel gating characterized by brief openings occurring in clusters (107). From an historical perspective, it was appreciated that permeation of K_{ATP} by K^+ is inhibited by glucose metabolism, by sulfonylureas, or by ATP applied directly to the cytosolic surface of the plasma membrane (108). K_{ATP} was also known to be activated by diazoxide or by Mg-ADP (108). What was not realized prior to our published studies (36) is that there exists a powerful synergistic interaction of GLP-1 and glucose to inhibit K_{ATP}. This effect is specific for a distinct subpopulation of β-cells and produces a decrease of whole cell conductance, depolarization, and generation of action potentials (Figures 2A through 2D).

Measurements of K_{ATP} single channel ionic currents in patches of β-cell plasma membrane demonstrated that GLP-1 potentiates the inhibitory effect of glucose metabolism on channel function (36). Application of GLP-1 to the surface of the cell produced an inhibition of K_{ATP} under conditions of cell-attached patch recording (Figure 2D). In this configuration of the patch clamp technique, access of GLP-1 to its receptors within the patch is obstructed by the glass wall of the recording electrode. Therefore, the action of GLP-1 must be mediated by a cytosolic signalling mechanism whereby activation of GLP-1 receptors outside of the patch influences K_{ATP} within the patch. This signalling system interacts with β-cell glucose metabolism because the action of GLP-1 was conditional on simultaneous exposure of cells to 10 mM glucose.

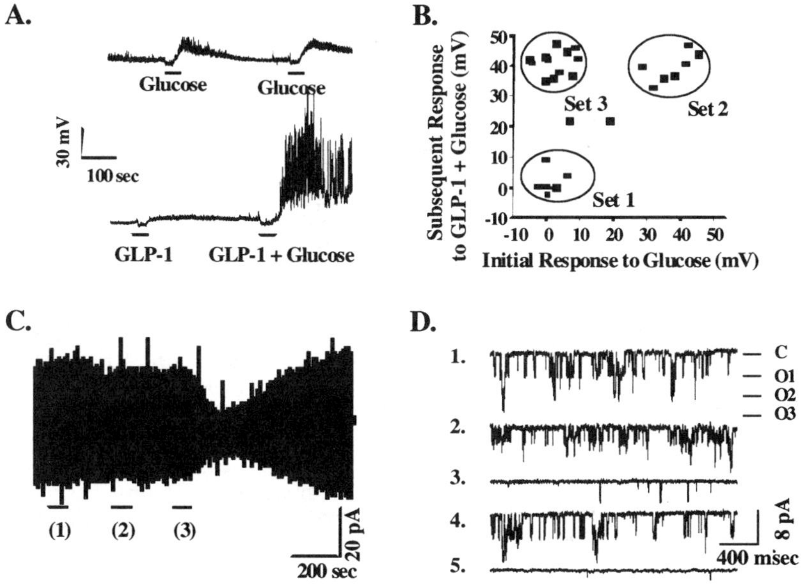

Figure 2. *A) Synergism of GLP-1 and glucose to depolarize rat β-cells. Measurement of the membrane potential was obtained from a single cell equilibrated in saline containing no glucose. Repeated 30 sec applications of 10 mM glucose produced small depolarizing responses (upper trace), whereas combined application of 10 nM GLP-1 and 10 mM glucose produced a large response accompanied by action potentials (lower trace, right). No effect of GLP-1 was observed in the absence of glucose (lower trace, left).* ***B)*** *Induction of glucose competence by GLP-1 is specific for a distinct subpopulation of rat β-cells. Scatter plot analysis (where each square represents observations obtained from a single cell) revealed that the majority of cells (Sets 1 and 3) exhibited little change in membrane potential when exposed to 10 mM glucose alone (x-axis). A subpopulation of cells (Set 3) exhibited a large response when challenged with 10 mM glucose and 10 nM GLP-1 (y-axis).* ***C)*** *GLP-1 and glucose synergize to decrease whole-cell conductance. The membrane conductance was monitored in the voltage clamp mode under conditions in which extracellular saline contained no added glucose. Application for 30 sec of 10 mM glucose (1) or 10 nM GLP-1 (2) was without effect on evoked current responses to ± 10 mV voltage steps from a holding potential of -80 mV. Evoked currents were reversibly inhibited by simultaneous application of 10 mM glucose and 10 nM GLP-1 (3). The conductance decreased 80% from 2.0 nS to 0.4 nS. Outward currents are indicated by upward deflections.* ***D)*** *Synergism of GLP-1 and glucose to inhibit K-ATP. Cell-attached patch recordings of unitary inward currents measured when the bath solution contained no added glucose (traces 1,4), 20 mM glucose (2), 20 mM glucose and 10 nM GLP-1 (3), or 10 nM glyburide (5), each applied for 30 sec. Inward currents are indicated by downward deflections from a closed level (C) to three superimposed levels of openings (O_{1-3}). Figure 2 A-D adapted from Holz et al., 1993.*

Using this methodology, we demonstrated that GLP-1 decreases the probability of K_{ATP} single channel openings while exerting no effect on single channel conductance. A role for cAMP in this process is implied by studies demonstrating inhibition of whole-cell K_{ATP} currents by a cAMP phosphodiesterase inhibitor (IBMX) (109,110). Furthermore, it was reported that a membrane-permeant analogue of cAMP (db-cAMP) inhibits K_{ATP} single channel currents measured in the cell-attached patch configuration (109). Such findings are noteworthy because they provide a clear explanation for the effects of cAMP as measured in isolated, whole islets. Studies of bursting activity in mouse islets demonstrated that glucagon, forskolin, IBMX, or theophylline synergize with metabolism of glucose to accelerate the interburst depolarization and to shorten the interburst interval (9). These alterations in the pattern of bursting activity are consistent with decreased K_{ATP} channel activity.

The findings summarized above suggest that K_{ATP} serves as a substrate for PKA-dependent phosphorylation. However, it was demonstrated that PKA *stimulates* K_{ATP} when tested in excised patches of plasma membrane (111). This observation appears to rule out an attractive hypothesis - that PKA increases the affinity of K_{ATP} for ATP generated by glucose metabolism. What then is the exact mechanism by which GLP-1 exerts its effects? One clue is provided by recent studies examining inhibition of K_{ATP} by glucagon (110). Glucagon produced an inhibition of K_{ATP} under conditions of cell-attached patch recording. The effect was blocked by inhibitors of calmodulin, and reproduced by db-cAMP. Interestingly, the actions of glucagon and db-cAMP were facilitated by an increase of $[Ca^{2+}]_i$. Such findings are notable in light of the previously reported action of glucagon to increase intracellular levels of NAD(P)H (112). This reduced pyridine nucleotide accumulates as a consequence of glucose metabolism. The action of glucagon to stimulate production of NAD(P)H was also shown to be blocked by antagonists of calmodulin. On the basis of these findings, it was proposed that glucagon stimulates Ca^{2+}-dependent glycogenolysis, thereby generating glucose for mitochondrial production of ATP. The resultant increase of $[ATP]_i$ / $[ADP]_i$ ratio would provide a necessary stimulus for closure of K_{ATP} (110). Although this too is an attractive hypothesis, it should be noted that important aspects of this proposal remain untested. In particular, it remains to be demonstrated that stimulation of β-cell glycogenolysis by glucagon requires activation of calmodulin by Ca^{2+}.

An alternative hypothesis exists that seeks to explain inhibitory actions of glucagon on K_{ATP}. It was reported that glucagon receptors couple to a membrane-delimited signalling system whereby GTP-binding proteins interact directly with the channel (113). However, these findings do not explain the glucose-dependent inhibitory action of glucagon, nor do they explain why inhibition of K_{ATP} is observed during exposure of β-cells to cAMP-elevating agents. Furthermore, a membrane-delimited mechanism of action might not be consistent with the observation that bath application of glucagon inhibits K_{ATP} under conditions of cell-attached patch recording (110,113). Still, it should be noted that there is ample precedent for direct effects of GTP-binding proteins on K^+ channel function in other cell types (114,115).

In conclusion, available evidence suggests that GLP-1 influences K_{ATP} via two different modes of action. GLP-1 may increase production of ATP, as suggested by the action of glucagon. Alternatively, GLP-1 may increase the effectiveness of ATP acting as an inhibitor of K_{ATP}. This latter effect appears not to be mediated by direct actions of PKA on the channel. Instead, recent findings suggest an alternative signalling mechanism. It was reported that phosphatidylinositol 4,5-bisphosphate (PIP2) stimulates K_{ATP} by reducing its sensitivity to ATP (116,117). This is significant because glucose produces a decrease of PIP2 levels in the β-cell (118). Such an effect of glucose on PIP2 levels might contribute to the inhibition of K_{ATP} by increasing channel sensitivity to ATP. It seems reasonable to speculate that an analogous process of PIP2 signal transduction might mediate inhibitory actions of GLP-1 on K_{ATP}.

INFLUENCES OF GLP-1 ON VOLTAGE-DEPENDENT Ca^{2+} CHANNEL FUNCTION

It is well established that voltage-dependent Ca^{2+} channels (VDCCs) are important determinants of oscillatory electrical activity in intact islets. VDCCs are integral membrane proteins that respond to cellular depolarization by allowing permeation of the plasma membrane by Ca^{2+}. This process of Ca^{2+} channel activation occurs in β-cells as a consequence of glucose metabolism and is facilitated by GLP-1. Opening of dihydropyridine-sensitive VDCCs is primarily responsible for the influx of Ca^{2+} that triggers insulin secretion. These channels are comprised of α1D subunits, are referred to as Class D channels, and generate L-type Ca^{2+} currents (119,120). L-type channels open in response to strong depolarizing stimuli and are thus high voltage-activated. The preferential role channels of this type play in insulin secretion is most likely explained by their close proximity to the readily releasable pool of secretory granules located at docking sites on the plasma membrane. Functional coupling of the channels to exocytotic proteins such as syntaxin or to intracellular Ca^{2+} release channels may also play a role in determining their effectiveness (121-125).

Ca^{2+} influx through dihydropyridine-sensitive Ca^{2+} channels is increased by β-cell glucose metabolism (126), an effect reported to result from inositol hexakisphosphate (IP6) production. IP6 inhibits serine and threonine protein phosphatases, thereby maintaining channels in a phosphorylated form that favours their opening in response to depolarization (127-129). Earlier studies of the effects of GLP-1 or cAMP on L-type Ca^{2+} channel current were less conclusive, although a slowing of current inactivation was noted (130-132). However, more recent reports suggest that short-term exposure of β-cells to GLP-1 increases peak L-type Ca^{2+} current by as much as two-fold, shifts the voltage-dependence of channel activation to more negative membrane potentials (96,97) and shifts the voltage-dependence of steady-state channel inactivation to more positive membrane potentials (78). Therefore, GLP-1 might exert two complementary effects: it augments Ca^{2+} influx associated with generation of action potentials, and 2) it allows a small but significant Ca^{2+} current to be active at membrane potentials close to the resting potential. This latter effect contributes to increased excitability and is postulated to be an initiator of Ca^{2+}-induced Ca^{2+} release from Ca^{2+} stores (84).

Actions of GLP-1 on Ca^{2+} channel function appear to be mediated by cAMP and PKA. L-type Ca^{2+} current is facilitated by exposure of β-cells to stimulators of cAMP signalling, and the action of GLP-1 is inhibited by a cAMP antagonist (Rp-cAMPS) or by an inhibitor of PKA (H-89) (98,133). It should be noted that PKC is also reported to maintain β-cell Ca^{2+} channels in a functional state (127). Such an action might be of relevance under conditions in which cells are stimulated with ligands that have dual signalling potential. An example is the neuropeptide PACAP. It is released from nerve endings that innervate the endocrine pancreas, and it is reported to activate PKA and PKC signalling in the β-cell (134-138).

An additional high voltage-activated Ca^{2+} channel that may underlie P/Q-type Ca^{2+} currents is the Class A channel. These channels are dihydropyridine-resistant and are blocked by omega-agatoxin IVA (139). Q-like Ca^{2+} currents (140) and Class A channels are expressed in β-cells and mediate glucose-dependent insulin secretion that is dihydropyridine-insensitive (141). This finding provides evidence for a functional overlap between Class A and D channels to support exocytosis. Class B and Class C channels are also expressed in various insulinoma cell lines (142,143). However, the low level of expression of these two types of Ca^{2+} channels in authentic β-cells indicates that they are unlikely to play a significant role in stimulus-secretion coupling. Finally, it should be noted that a low voltage-activated Ca^{2+} current is observed in β-cells (144,145). This T-type Ca^{2+} current is active at membrane potentials close to the resting potential, influences β-cell excitability, and may mediate cytokine-induced cell death.

MOBILIZATION OF INTRACELLULAR Ca^{2+} STORES BY GLP-1

Sequestration of Ca^{2+} within the β-cell occurs in mitochondria, secretory granules, and the endoplasmic reticulum. These sources of Ca^{2+} are implicated in the regulation of enzyme activity, stimulus-secretion coupling, and gene expression. Available evidence indicates that it is the endoplasmic reticular Ca^{2+} stores that are mobilized by GLP-1. This might be achieved by stimulatory effects of GLP-1 on IP3-gated Ca^{2+} release channels or ryanodine receptor Ca^{2+} release channels. Both types of channels are integral membrane proteins of the endoplasmic reticulum that form homotetrameric complexes allowing efflux of luminal Ca^{2+} to the cytosol. The type 3 isoform of IP3 receptor (IP3R-3) (146,147) and type 2 isoform of ryanodine receptor (RYR-2) (84,148) predominate in the β-cell. Mobilization of Ca^{2+} from endoplasmic reticular Ca^{2+} stores is a process of Ca^{2+}-induced Ca^{2+}release (CICR). IP3 acts as a co-agonist with cytosolic Ca^{2+} to gate IP3R-3, whereas CICR mediated by RYR2 is facilitated by combined actions of Ca^{2+} and possibly cyclic ADP-ribose (cADPR) (149-152). It is important to note that the filling state of endoplasmic reticular Ca^{2+} stores is dependent on metabolism of glucose (153-156). This is because mitochondrial production of ATP drives sequestration of Ca^{2+} mediated by SERCA-2b and SERCA-3 isoforms of Ca^{2+}-ATPases expressed in β-cells (157-159).

GLP-1 might mobilize IP-3-sensitive Ca^{2+} stores by stimulating production of IP3 or by promoting phosphorylation of IP3 receptors. This seems unlikely given that GLP-1 has only a small stimulatory effect on IP3 levels in isolated rat islets (47,51). Furthermore, there is no direct evidence for phosphorylation of β-cell IP3 receptors in response to GLP-1. Still, activators of cAMP signalling are reported to potentiate the IP3-mediated increase of $[Ca^{2+}]_i$ in β-cells (160,161). An alternative explanation for the action of GLP-1 at the IP3 receptor is provided by one recent study documenting "allosteric tuning" of the receptor by ATP (162). Facilitation of IP3 receptor/channel gating by ATP was observed, an action compatible with the hypothesized role of GLP-1 as a stimulator of mitochondrial ATP production.

A second type of intracellular Ca^{2+} release channel targeted by GLP-1 is the ryanodine receptor. Gromada and co-workers (82,85) proposed that PKA-mediated phosphorylation of ryanodine receptors explains how GLP-1 mobilizes ryanodine-sensitive Ca^{2+} stores in the βTC3 insulinoma cell line. Islam and colleagues (148) offered support for this hypothesis by demonstrating a synergistic interaction between cAMP and caffeine to trigger CICR in mouse β-cells. Caffeine is a methylxanthine that potentiates stimulatory actions of Ca^{2+} at RYR2 (163,164). To examine this hypothesis in greater detail, we performed studies using human and rat β-cells (84). Binding of ryanodine to its receptor in insulin-containing β-cells was visualized using a fluorescent derivative of ryanodine (BODIPY FL-X ryanodine).

The interaction of the BODIPY FL-X ryanodine with its receptors was shown to be saturable, reversible, and of high affinity. Furthermore, a perinuclear pattern of labelling was observed, consistent with the expected localization of ryanodine receptors at the endoplasmic reticulum. RT-PCR analyses of rat islet mRNA demonstrated that it is the RYR2 isoform that is preferentially expressed in these tissues. Consistent with the report of Islam and colleagues, caffeine was demonstrated to be an effective stimulator of CICR in these cells (84).

Figures 3A through 3D illustrate that the action of GLP-1 to trigger CICR is reproduced by stimulators of cAMP signalling (forskolin, 8-Br-cAMP) and by caffeine. Although the action of GLP-1 was blocked by the cAMP antagonist Rp-cAMPS (84), contrary findings were reported by Bode and co-workers who observed no such antagonist effect (165). Furthermore, a specific inhibitor of PKA was observed to be ineffective in this assay (165). Therefore, the postulated role of PKA as a mediator of CICR in response to GLP-1 remains in question. More detailed pharmacological studies also indicate that GLP-1 promotes CICR by augmenting influx of Ca^{2+} through L-type VDCCs, and by sensitizing RYR2 to stimulatory influences of cytosolic Ca^{2+} (84). The source of Ca^{2+} targeted for mobilization by GLP-1 was shown to be depleted by thapsigargin (84), an inhibitor of endoplasmic reticular Ca^{2+}-ATPase. It should be noted that a role of cADPR as a mediator of GLP-1 signal transduction has yet to be reported. This is an important issue to address because cADPR is a candidate second messenger that may serve as a coupling factor for glucose-dependent insulin secretion (149,151,166,167). A role for cADPR in GLP-1 signal transduction is suggested by one recent report that PKA stimulates CD38 (168), an ADP ribosyl cyclase that catalyzes synthesis of cyclic ADP ribose from β-NAD^+.

REGULATION OF NON-SELECTIVE CATION CHANNELS BY GLP-1

Stimulation of β-cells with GLP-1 is associated with the opening of Non-Selective Cation Channels (NSCCs) that allow permeation of the plasma membrane by Na^+, K^+, and Ca^{2+} (95, 99). One of several types of NSCC expressed in β-cells (169,170) is the Ca^{2+}-sensitive non-selective cation channel (Ca-NS). These channels are relatively voltage-insensitive and are activated by Ca^{2+} applied to the cytosolic face of the membrane in isolated patches (169,171). A potential role for Ca-NS channels as mediators of GLP-1 signal transduction is suggested by studies demonstrating that extracellular Na^+ is required for GLP-1 to generate membrane depolarization, to increase $[Ca^{2+}]_i$ and to stimulate insulin secretion (172-174). Such observations prompted us to test for an ability of GLP-1 to activate Ca-NS in rat β-cells equilibrated in saline containing 7.5 mM glucose (95). Under these conditions, GLP-1 produced an increase of whole cell conductance, depolarization, and an increase of $[Ca^{2+}]_i$. An inward current carried predominantly by Na^+ was observed at membrane potentials close to the resting potential. Figures 4A through 4C illustrate that the action of GLP-1 to stimulate opening of non-selective cation channels is reproduced by forskolin and 8-Br-cAMP. Importantly, the effect of GLP-1 was never observed when cells were equilibrated in a solution to which no glucose was added. However, combined application of GLP-1 and glucose resulted in a prompt inhibition of K_{ATP} (36). We propose that intermediate levels of glucose favor a dual mode of hormone action whereby inhibition of K_{ATP} is superimposed on activation of Ca-NS. Inhibition of K_{ATP} by GLP-1 produces a decrease of membrane resistance that serves to amplify cellular depolarization generated by an increased Na^+ conductance of the plasma membrane.

Ca-NS channels were first described by Sturgess and co-workers (169,171) in studies of CRI-G1 insulinoma cells. Ca-NS exhibits a 25-30 pS single channel conductance, is activated by Ca^{2+}, and is inhibited by intracellular adenine (ATP) or pyridine (β-NAD^+) nucleotides (175-177). Cyclic nucleotides (cAMP, cGMP) stimulate or inhibit channel activity depending on the concentrations used. A role for Ca-NS in the process by which GLP-1 generates inward Na^+ current is indicated because: 1) the current is activated not only by GLP-1, but also by 8-Br-cAMP, 2) the current exhibits a reversal potential (ca. -15 to -5 mV) consistent with its nonselective nature, and 3) reduction of Na^+_o from 142 mM to 14 mM shifts the reversal potential from -14 mV to -38 mV, as predicted for Ca-NS. Involvement of Ca-NS is also indicated because: 4) substitution of extracellular Na^+ with N-methyl-D-glucamine (NMG) inhibits the current, 5) intracellular application of Ca^{2+} chelators (EGTA, BAPTA) abolish current activation, and 6) activation of the current by GLP-1 is supported by an intracellular solution containing 160 nM Ca^{2+}. These effects of GLP-1 are independent of voltage-dependent Na^+ channels because current flow is voltage-insensitive and not blocked by tetrodotoxin (95,99).

The Na^+ current activated by GLP-1 might be a store-operated current (SOC) triggered by opening of Ca-NS channels in response to the mobilization of Ca^{2+} stores (178,179). This conclusion is consistent with the demonstrated ability of GLP-1 to stimulate CICR and to increase $[Ca^{2+}]_i$. It is also consistent with the established action of cytosolic Ca^{2+} to activate Ca-NS. Precedent for an interaction of NSCCs and Ca^{2+} stores exists because it was reported that a Na^+ current is activated during exposure of β-cells to thapsigargin. Thapsigargin blocks Ca^{2+} sequestration, produces an increase of $[Ca^{2+}]_i$, and stimulates capacitative Ca^{2+} influx that serves to refill Ca^{2+} stores (180,181). Depletion of Ca^{2+} stores by treatment of β-cells with thapsigargin or muscarinic agonists activates an inward current carried by Na^+ and Ca^{2+} (182). This current shares some similarities with capacitative Ca^{2+} currents as well as the inward current activated by GLP-1. One interpretation of these findings is that capacitative Ca^{2+} entry is mediated by stimulatory effects of GLP-1 on Ca-NS. Although this is an attractive hypothesis, no direct evidence currently exists to support it.

The molecular nature of NSCCs expressed in β-cells remains elusive. Analyses of βTC3 insulinoma cells revealed expression of trp-4 mRNA (183). Trp-4 is one of a family of trp-like proteins related to the *Drosophila* photoreceptor channel responsible for the transient receptor potential (184-191). It may play a role in forming thapsigargin-sensitive, store-operated Ca^{2+} channels. Experiments in which trp-4 was expressed, or in which cells were injected with trp-4 antisense oligonucleotides, suggest that trp-4 mediates capacitative Ca^{2+} entry (191,192).

Worley and colleagues (179) reported that NSCCs activated by β-cell Ca^{2+} store depletion are also activated by maitotoxin (MTX; a polyether isolated from dinoflagellates). Picomolar concentrations of MTX generate an inward current carried predominantly by Na^+, and to a lesser extent Ca^{2+}. Current flow through the channels activated by MTX is supported by extracellular Na^+, Li^+, K^+ or Cs^+. It is blocked by extracellular La^{3+}, by substitution of extracellular Na^+ with NMG, or by intracellular ATP. The whole cell current-voltage relationship for the MTX-induced current is linear and exhibits a reversal potential of -10 mV. Estimates of single channel conductance indicate a value of 25-30 pS. Therefore, available evidence suggests that the MTX-sensitive Na^+ current results from activation of Ca-NS channels also activated by GLP-1 (99,193).

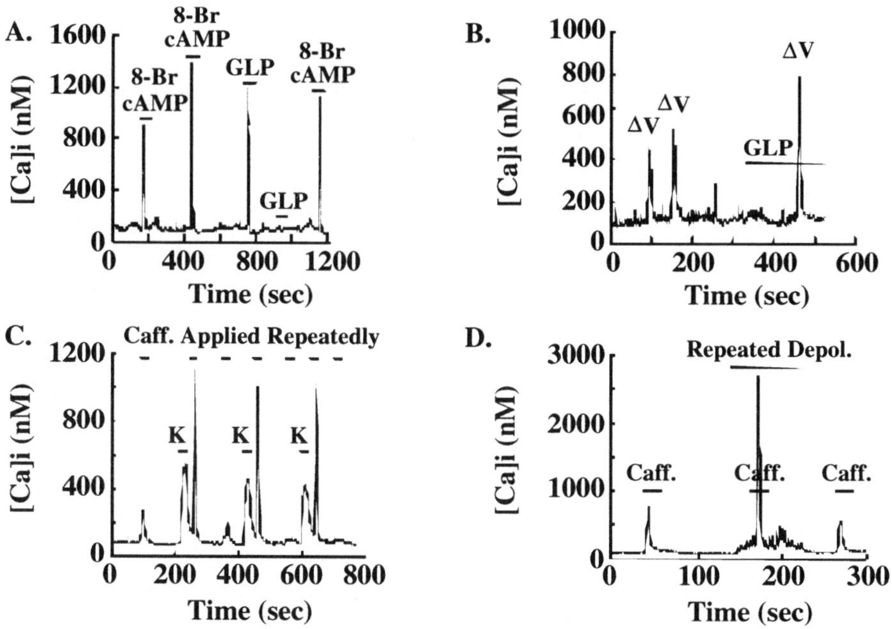

Figure 3. *A) Stimulation of CICR by 8-Br-cAMP and GLP-1. Measurements obtained from a rat β-cell loaded with fura-2 and exposed to successive 10 sec applications of 1 mM 8-Br-cAMP or 10 nM GLP-1. The action of GLP-1 exhibited desensitization.* ***B)*** *GLP-1 (10 nM) facilitates CICR induced by influx of Ca^{2+} through VDCCs in a fura-2 loaded rat β-cell. Activation of VDCCs was triggered by depolarizing voltage steps (ΔV_m) from -70 to 0 mV under conditions of voltage clamp in the perforated patch configuration.* ***C)*** *Stimulation of CICR by caffeine. Measurements obtained from a HIT-T15 cell loaded with fura-2 and exposed to successive 30 sec applications of 10 mM caffeine or 44 mM KCl. Prior application of KCl facilitated CICR induced by caffeine.* ***D)*** *Caffeine facilitates CICR induced by influx of Ca^{2+} through VDCCs. Measurements obtained from a fura-2 loaded HIT-T15 cell in which the membrane potential was shifted from -70 to 0 mV for 100 msec at 2 sec intervals using the perforated patch configuration. Depolarizing voltage steps produced a gradual increase of $[Ca^{2+}]_i$ upon which was superimposed a large transient increase of $[Ca^{2+}]_i$ due to CICR induced by caffeine. Figure 3 A,C,D adapted from Holz et al., 1999.*

Estimates of cell surface channel density and open channel probability indicate that the channels activated by GLP-1 and MTX are ideally suited to serve as a regulator of the membrane potential (193). This concept is incorporated in a mathematical model of β-cell electrical activity. In the model, NSCCs activated as a consequence of Ca^{2+} store depletion generate a steady-state inward SOC referred to as I_{CRAN} (194, 195). Ca^{2+} store depletion and activation of I_{CRAN} result from exposure of cells to a low concentration of glucose that does not support ATP-dependent Ca^{2+} sequestration. Subsequent exposure of cells to a high concentration of glucose results in a reduction of K_{ATP} outward current, thereby allowing I_{CRAN} to induce cellular depolarization. Therefore, the SOC is believed to be a critical determinant of β-cell excitability and glucose responsiveness.

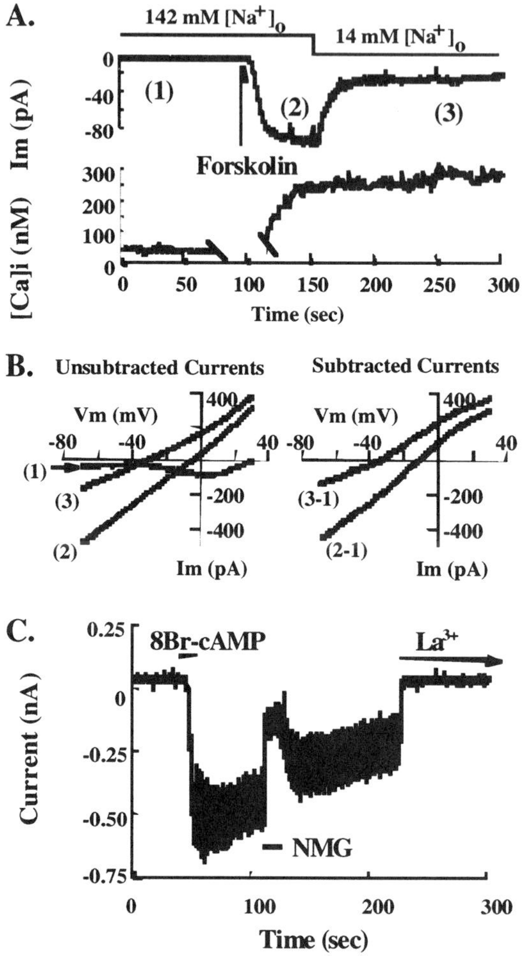

Figure 4. *A) Activation of a Na^+-sensitive membrane current by forskolin. A mouse β-cell was loaded with fura-2 and equilibrated in saline containing 7.5 mM glucose and 142 mM NaCl. Measurement of the whole-cell current was obtained in the voltage clamp mode using the perforated patch configuration (top trace, holding potential -70 mV) while simultaneously monitoring $[Ca^{2+}]_i$ (lower trace). Application of 10 μM forskolin (arrow) produced an inward shift of the holding current (2) and an increase of $[Ca^{2+}]_i$. The current was reduced by exchanging the extracellular saline for a solution containing 14 mM NaCl (3).* ***B)*** *Current as a function of voltage (I-V) relationships obtained under experimental conditions illustrated in (A). I-V relationships were determined using a ramp stimulus protocol (-70 to +30 mV). On the left is illustrated raw unsubtracted I-V relationships prior to (1) and during exposure to forskolin when the extracellular saline contained 142 mM NaCl (2) or 14 mM NaCl (3). On the right is illustrated the subtracted I-V relationships for determination of the reversal potential. Reducing the concentration of NaCl from 142 mM to 14 mM shifted the reversal potential from -14 mV to -38 mV.* ***C)*** *Activation of a Na^+-sensitive membrane current by 8-Br-cAMP. The whole-cell conductance of a HIT-T15 insulinoma cell equilibrated in saline containing 142 mM NaCl was monitored in the voltage clamp mode (holding potential -70 ± 10 mV). 8-Br-cAMP (1 mM) was applied for 10 sec. An inward shift of the holding current was accompanied by an increase of whole-cell conductance, as indicated by the increased amplitude of evoked currents (upward and downward deflections). Focal application of a Na^+-free solution containing N-methyl-glucamine (NMG) inhibited the current in a reversible fashion, whereas bath application of 100 μM La^{3+} blocked the current. Figure 4C adapted from Holz et al., 1995.*

DOES GLP-1 REGULATE CHLORIDE ION CHANNEL FUNCTION?

Kinard and Satin (196) reported a stimulatory action of cAMP on Cl^- channels expressed in mouse β-cells and HIT-T15 insulinoma cells. An increase of Cl^- conductance generated an outwardly rectifying Cl^- current designated as I-Cl^-, islet. Activation of I-Cl^-, islet was observed under conditions of whole-cell dialysis in which the Cl^- equilibrium potential was defined to be positive to the resting membrane potential. Using this approach, activation of I-Cl^-, islet by cAMP produced an inward current at membrane potentials close to the resting potential (196) (Figure 5). Therefore, it might be predicted that I-Cl^-, islet mediates cellular depolarization observed in response to cAMP-elevating agents such as GLP-1. One argument against such a role for I-Cl^-, islet is that chloride ions in β-cells are passively distributed with the Cl^- equilibrium potential being equal to the membrane potential (197). Under such conditions, alterations of Cl^- conductance are not expected to be accompanied by a change of membrane potential.

I-Cl^-, islet is not equivalent to the inward current we observed in response to GLP-1, 8-Br-cAMP, or MTX. Under conditions of perforated patch recording, GLP-1 activates a Na^+ current, the reversal potential of which is not sensitive to alterations of extracellular Cl^- concentration (99). We used the perforated patch technique (198) because it does not impede second messenger-mediated signal transduction, and does not disrupt intracellular Ca^{2+} homeostasis. This is significant because the Na^+ current activated by GLP-1 may be an SOC resulting from opening of Ca-NS. In contrast, Cl^- channels activated by cAMP are reported to be Ca^{2+} insensitive (196) though other studies have reported Ca^{2+}-sensitivity of chloride currents in insulinoma cells (199). Therefore, the failure of Satin and colleagues (196) to observe Na^+ current activation in response to cAMP may be related to their use of whole-cell dialysis in which the pipette solution contained a Ca^{2+} chelator (EGTA). Chelation of Ca^{2+} depletes Ca^{2+} stores and lowers levels of cytosolic Ca^{2+} to concentrations that do not favor activation of Ca-NS.

A significant role for Cl^- channels in β-cell function is suggested by reports that I-Cl^-, islet is activated by cell swelling in response to osmotic stress. Figure 5 shows the effects of hypotonic solutions on INS-1 rat insulinoma cells and also on human islet cells. Hypotonic solutions induce an increase in $[Ca^{2+}]_i$ consistent with the activation of a depolarizing anion current. Hypotonic solutions do not produce an increase of $[Na^+]_i$, in contrast to activation of non-selective cation channels, consistent with the volume-sensitive currents in β-cells being anion-selective. Cell swelling is observed in response to an increase of extracellular glucose concentration, and is accompanied by the appearance of a cell volume-activated Cl^- current (196,200-203). Surprisingly, I-Cl^-, islet is also reported to be activated by the sulfonylurea glyburide. It was suggested that β-cell Cl^- channels may be coupled to high affinity sulfonylurea receptors (SUR) that act as transmembrane conductance regulators and that the channel itself may be formed by a low affinity SUR (196). Tolbutamide binding to granular SUR is also reported to stimulate Ca^{2+}-dependent exocytosis in β-cells through effects mediated by a 65 kDa mdr-like P-glycoprotein that activates a Cl^- conductance (204). It is interesting to note that sulfonylureas are also reported to stimulate a glycosyl-phosphatidylinositol (GPI)-specific PLC (205). GPI-PLCs generate diacylglycerol (DAG), activate PKC, and both PKC and PKA phosphorylate P-glycoproteins that play a role in regulating volume-activated Cl^- currents (206). P-glycoproteins are members of the ATP-binding cassette family of integral membrane proteins (ABC proteins) that also include the high affinity sulfonylurea receptor. Preliminary data indicate expression of P-glycoprotein in HIT-T15 cells (C.A.L., unpublished observations). It seems possible, therefore, that a yet to be characterized member of the ABC protein family mediates activation of I-Cl^-, islet by cAMP and/or sulfonylureas.

DIRECT INFLUENCES OF GLP-1 ON EXOCYTOSIS

GLP-1 facilitates insulin exocytosis by promoting fusion of secretory granules with the β-cell plasma membrane (9,98,133). This effect occurs at a distal step in stimulus-secretion coupling, is reproduced by cAMP (109,131,207), and is independent of more proximal actions of the hormone on ion channel function. The secretagogic action of GLP-1 amplifies Ca^{2+}-dependent exocytosis of insulin. Using single cell measurements of exocytosis, Gromada and co-workers reported that the action of GLP-1 is reproduced by intracellular application of cAMP under conditions in which $[Ca^{2+}]_i$ is fixed at a concentration (340 nM) sufficient to support Ca^{2+}-dependent exocytosis (98). An interpretation of these findings is that GLP-1 facilitates insulin secretion by sensitizing a readily releasable pool of secretory granules to the increase of $[Ca^{2+}]_i$ that triggers exocytosis (131). More recent findings suggest that GLP-1 also mobilizes a reserve pool of secretory granules, thereby increasing the size of the readily-releasable pool (98,207,208). Whatever the exact mechanism of action, it can be concluded that GLP-1 potentiates insulin secretion by stimulating phosphorylation of as yet to be identified regulatory proteins that comprise the exocytotic secretory apparatus (209).

The stimulation of insulin secretion by GLP-1 is absolutely dependent on simultaneous exposure of β-cells to concentrations of glucose that support oxidative phosphorylation. This phenomenon is understandable if the exocytotic secretory apparatus functions as an ATP-sensor. Kasai and colleagues (210) proposed that ATP generated by metabolism of glucose acts as: 1) a precursor for adenylyl cyclase-catalyzed cAMP production and, 2) a phosphate donor for PKA-mediated phosphorylation. Consistent with this concept, intracellular administration of ATP facilitates Ca^{2+}-dependent exocytosis, an action blocked by antagonists of cAMP signal transduction (Rp-cAMPS, H-89). The action of ATP is mimicked by ATP-γ-S, a nucleotide that supports phosphorylation, but not insulin granule transport or priming. On the basis of these findings, it was suggested that an exocytotic ATP sensor promotes cAMP production and PKA-mediated phosphorylation, thereby facilitating Ca^{2+}-dependent exocytosis. Should this prove to be the case, it can be predicted that in the absence of glucose, cytosolic concentrations of ATP drop to levels that do not support cAMP production. Under these conditions, GLP-1 is expected to be an ineffective insulin secretagogue.

A substantial body of evidence also exists demonstrating that secretion of insulin can occur under conditions in which β-cells are treated with pharmacological agents that bypass proximal events in GLP-1 signal transduction. These "K_{ATP} independent" actions of GLP-1 result from stimulatory effects of the hormone on an unusual process of glucose-dependent insulin secretion (211-213). In this alternative model, K_{ATP}-independent actions of glucose result from direct effects of metabolic coupling factors at the exocytotic secretory apparatus. One such coupling factor is ATP, and it can be speculated that distal effects of glucose metabolism on insulin secretion result from adenylyl cyclase-catalyzed conversion of ATP to cAMP, as outlined above (210). Therefore, the insulin secretagogic action of GLP-1 appears to involve the participation of two distinct signalling pathways, both of which constitute β-cell ATP sensors. By promoting glucose-dependent closure of K_{ATP}, GLP-1 targets an ATP sensor that is an ion channel and which regulates the complex process of cellular depolarization, electrical bursting activity, and Ca^{2+} influx deemed necessary for exocytosis. This action of GLP-1 is supported by its direct effect at the exocytotic ATP sensor where conversion of ATP to cAMP acts locally to promote stimulatory effects of Ca^{2+} on insulin granule exocytosis.

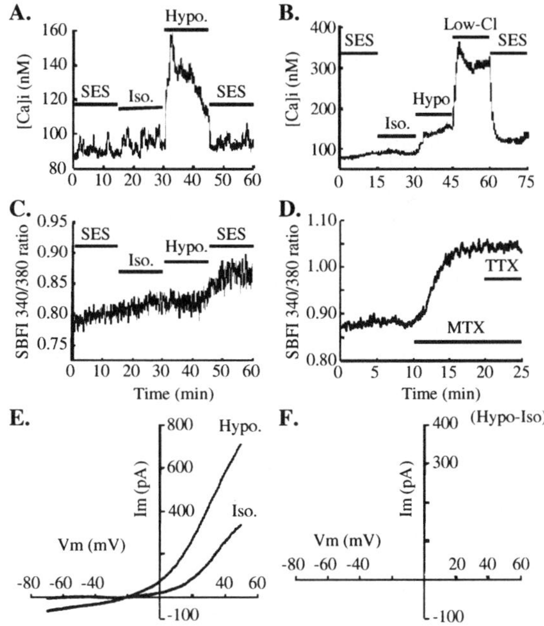

Figure 5. *The effect of hypotonic solutions on intracellular Ca^{2+}, Na^{+} and membrane currents of β-cells. Cell swelling induced by glucose or by hypotonic solutions activates a chloride conductance in β-cells. Hypotonic solutions produce a small increase of $[Ca^{2+}]_i$ in both INS-1 insulinoma cells (A) and human islets cells (B), transfer to a hypotonic, low-Cl^- (Low-Cl) solution produced a further rapid rise of $[Ca^{2+}]_i$ (B), as would be predicted from a positive shift in the chloride reversal potential producing membrane depolarization and opening voltage-dependent Ca^{2+} channels. Hypotonic (Hypo.) solution was made by reducing the NaCl concentration and was measured to be 12% hypotonic using a vapour pressure osmometer. Isotonic (Iso.) solution, to control for the reduced NaCl concentration in hypotonic solution, was made by adding mannitol to hypotonic solution. The hypotonic, low-Cl^- (Low-Cl) solution was made by substituting NaAspartate for NaCl. The same experimental protocol as in (A) was used to investigate whether changes of $[Na^{+}]_i$ occur in INS-1 cells under these conditions. Changing from SES to isotonic and hypotonic solutions had no significant effect on $[Na^{+}]_i$ which increased on re-introduction of SES (C) as a consequence of extracellular Na^{+} increasing. In contrast to hypotonic solutions, activation of non-selective cation channels by MTX results in a marked increase of $[Na^{+}]_i$ (D), this increase is not blocked by tetrodotoxin (TTX) confirming that Na^{+} influx is through cation channels, and not through voltage-dependent Na^{+} channels. These observations indicate that hypotonic solutions activate a different type of current to the GLP-1- and MTX-sensitive current. (E,F) Volume-activated membrane currents in an INS-1 cell held under whole cell voltage clamp. Voltage ramps from –70 mV to +50 mV were applied with the cell bathed in isotonic solution and after exchanging the bath solution to hypotonic solution (E). To obtain the volume-sensitive current, the current in isotonic solution was subtracted from that obtained in hypotonic solution and is shown in (F). This current reverses close to the calculated Cl^- equilibrium potential and shows outward rectification. In contrast, the current-voltage relation of non-selective cation currents is linear (Figure 4B) further distinguishing these two currents.*

THE INTERACTION OF GLP-1 AND LEPTIN TO REGULATE β-CELL FUNCTION

We provided evidence that there exists a counter-regulatory relationship between GLP-1 and the obesity hormone leptin to control pancreatic insulin secretion and insulin gene expression. Physiological concentrations of leptin (1-100 ng/ml) activate β-cell K_{ATP}, lower $[Ca^{2+}]_i$, and inhibit insulin exocytosis (214,215). The anti-insulinotropic action of leptin is also manifest as an inhibition of insulin gene expression (216,217). On the basis of these findings, we proposed the existence of an "adipo-insular axis" (214,218). In our model, insulin stimulates adipogenesis and leptin production, whereas leptin inhibits insulin secretion and insulin gene expression. Insulin secretion and insulin biosynthesis are therefore regulated by competing influences of leptin, GLP-1, and nutrient stimuli acting at the β-cells. It seems possible that an imbalance of the leptin - GLP-1 interaction might be an important predisposing factor for development of type 2 diabetes.

Leptin (*ob* protein) is a 16 kDa 146 amino acid protein synthesized and secreted by adipocytes (219). It acts to suppress appetite and to increase energy expenditure. Leptin is encoded by the obesity (*ob*) gene that is mutated in the *ob/ob* strain of obese mice. Blood levels of leptin are proportionate to adipose mass, therefore leptin is a hormonal indicator of adiposity. The secondary structure of leptin characterizes this protein as a member of the long-chain helical bundle family of cytokine signalling molecules. Leptin binds to a cell surface receptor (Ob-R) first identified by the screening of a cDNA library derived from choroid plexus (220, 221). Ob-R is encoded by the diabetes (*db*) gene mutated in the *db/db* strain of obese mice and in Zucker diabetic fatty (*fa/fa*) rats. The structure of Ob-R indicates it is a member of the class I family of cytokine receptors. It resembles the gp130 component of the interleukin-6 receptor. Ligand binding to receptors of this type promotes Janus kinase (JAK)-mediated phosphorylation, and the transcriptional activity of the Signal Transducers and Activators of Transcription (STAT) family of DNA binding proteins. *In vitro* assays demonstrate that Ob-Rb homodimerizes in response to ligand binding, activates JAK2, and stimulates the DNA binding activity of STATs 1,3, and 5.

The Ob-R gene encodes multiple splice variants (Ob-Ra – Ob-Rf), and the longest form of Ob-R (Ob-Rb) was first shown to be responsible for activation of JAK/STAT signalling. Recently, it has been suggested that the short form of the leptin receptor can also activate JAK2 and insulin receptor substrate 2 (IRS-2)/PI-3 kinase signalling pathways in myotubes (222). Mutations of *ob* and Ob-R genes result in leptin deficiency, as in *ob/ob* mice, or leptin-resistance, as in *db/db* mice and *fa/fa* rats. Mutations of the *ob* gene are also observed, albeit rarely, in severe early-onset obesity in humans. Since the *ob/ob*, *db/db*, and *fa/fa* phenotypes are also hyperinsulinemic and hyperglycaemic, they are useful models for analysis of the interaction of obesity with a syndrome resembling that of type 2 diabetes.

Initial reports indicated that Ob-Rb is expressed in hypothalamic satiety centers where leptin suppresses appetite. This appeared to explain fully the ability of leptin to induce profound weight-loss when administered to *ob/ob* mice. However, an additional action of leptin is indicated by its ability to stimulate expression of uncoupling protein (UCP-2) and to reduce triglyceride (TG) content in pancreatic islets (223). Such peripheral effects of leptin are accompanied by hypoinsulinemia and hypoglycaemia, indicative of improved insulin sensitivity. Decreased levels of plasma insulin are likely to be a consequence of a direct inhibition by leptin of insulin secretion. In cultured islets, leptin stimulated expression of UCP-2, reduced ATP production, and inhibited glucose-dependent insulin secretion. Leptin also reduced islet TG content, diminished TG synthesis, and increased free fatty acid (FFA) oxidation. Effects of leptin on islet lipid metabolism were associated with increased levels of islet mRNAs coding for enzymes of FFA oxidation, and decreased expression of an enzyme of FFA esterification. Such observations suggest that leptin might exert anti-insulinotropic actions by regulating the balance between TG synthesis and breakdown in the β-cell.

Actions of leptin on β-cells are likely to be mediated by the long (Ob-Rb) isoform of the leptin receptor. RT-PCR demonstrated expression of Ob-Rb in rat islets and insulinoma cell lines (218). A polyclonal antiserum raised against the leptin receptor detected its immunoreactivity on insulin-containing rat β-cells, and binding of a fluorescent derivative of leptin (Cy3-leptin) was visualized on insulin-immunoreactive rat and human β-cells (214, 216). Leptin receptors labeled with Cy3-leptin appeared as punctate aggregates, as expected if binding of leptin stimulates clustering of leptin receptors.

Whether leptin exerts a direct inhibitory effect on insulin secretion was initially a matter of some controversy. No such action was observed in the perfused pancreas, whereas two groups reported a stimulation of insulin secretion by leptin. However, physiological concentrations (1-100 ng/ml) of leptin can, under appropriate conditions, inhibit glucose-dependent secretion of insulin from islets of *ob/ob* mice, rats, and humans (214,216,224). The action of leptin exhibits a U-shaped dose-response relationship, inhibiting at low concentrations but being less effective at higher concentrations of the hormone (225). It has been suggested that leptin inhibits second phase insulin secretion by reducing the activity of Ca^{2+}-dependent PKC isoforms in rat and *ob/ob* mouse islets (226, 227). Of particular interest are additional reports that leptin reverses the stimulatory effect of GLP-1 on insulin secretion. A mechanistic explanation for this interaction was provided by Beavo and co-workers (225) who reported that leptin lowers levels of cAMP in β-cells. This is achieved by PI3-kinase-mediated activation of cAMP phosphodiesterase 3B. An ability of leptin to inhibit β-cell cAMP signal transduction is noteworthy because it reinforces our central hypothesis that leptin and GLP-1 are counter-regulatory hormones.

Figures 6A through 6D demonstrate a physiological role for leptin in the regulation of β-cell ion channel function. We observed that leptin produced cellular hyperpolarization and a reduction of $[Ca^{2+}]_i$ when applied to wild-type or *ob/ob* mouse β-cells (214). These effects of leptin were associated with an increase of membrane conductance, and were reversed by GLP-1 or by the sulfonylurea tolbutamide. Cell-attached patch measurements demonstrated that the increase of membrane conductance resulted from opening of K_{ATP}. Leptin increased the probability of K_{ATP} single channel openings while exerting no effect on mean open time or single channel conductance. A remarkable aspect of this action of leptin is that its time course is biphasic. A fast activation of K_{ATP} occurred within 60-120 sec followed by a larger response occurring after a 7-10 min delay. A delayed action of the hormone was also reported for stimulatory effects of leptin on K_{ATP} in CRI-G1 insulinoma cells (215).

These observations indicate that K_{ATP} is activated by leptin, a hormone that stimulates phosphodiesterase and which lowers levels of cAMP in the β-cell (225). In marked contrast, K_{ATP} is inhibited by GLP-1, a stimulator of cAMP production. It should be noted that Ashford and colleagues (228) provided an alternative explanation for the action of leptin in CRI-G1 insulinoma cells. Stimulation of K_{ATP} by leptin was shown to be blocked by orthovanadate, an inhibitor of tyrosine phosphatases. In contrast, K_{ATP} was activated by the tyrosine kinase inhibitors genistein and herbimycin A. These observations imply that leptin stimulates K_{ATP} by inhibiting tyrosine kinase-mediated phosphorylation and/or or by promoting dephosphorylation. Exactly how tyrosine kinase signalling interacts with cAMP to regulate K_{ATP} remains to be elucidated.

The interaction of GLP-1 and leptin to regulate β-cell function is also measurable at the level of insulin gene expression (216,217). GLP-1 stimulates preproinsulin mRNA biosynthesis in primary cultures of human or rodent islets, an action blocked by physiologically relevant concentrations of leptin. The inhibitory action of leptin is also observed *in vivo* where intraperitoneal administration of leptin to *ob/ob* mice decreases levels of islet preproinsulin mRNA by 40%. Luciferase reporter gene assays conducted using transfected INS-1 insulinoma cells demonstrate that GLP-1 up regulates transcriptional activity of the rat insulin gene 1 promoter (RIP1), an effect opposed by leptin. This is as expected given that leptin lowers levels of cAMP, thereby reducing stimulatory effects of GLP-1 mediated by the cAMP response element (CRE). However, it should be noted that truncation of RIP1 from -410 bp to -307 bp reduces inhibitory effects of leptin while leaving CRE-mediated signal transduction intact. Electrophoretic mobility shift assays (EMSA) of INS-1 cellular lysates demonstrate further that leptin promotes formation of specific nuclear protein-RIP1 DNA binding complexes. These include a complex formed by the interaction of a STAT5b-like protein with the STAT5b recognition element of RIP1 located between -410 bp and -307 bp of the promoter (217). This is surprising given that the STAT5b recognition element of RIP1 is reported to mediate transactivation of the promoter in response to growth hormone. Perhaps of additional significance is a report that leptin activates STAT3 but not STAT5 DNA binding in RINm5F insulinoma cells (229,230), an effect opposed by stimulators of intracellular Ca^{2+} signalling (acetylcholine, ionomycin) or cAMP signalling (forskolin, IBMX). The action of leptin at STAT3 is also associated with stimulation of ERK1 and ERK2 MAP kinases (229). Therefore, the relative importance of JAK/STAT and MAP kinase signalling in the regulation of insulin gene expression by leptin remains to be evaluated more fully.

CONCLUSION

The findings summarized herein reinforce a central hypothesis - that GLP-1, an intestinally-derived hormone, serves as a competence factor for glucose-dependent secretion of insulin at the pancreatic islets of Langerhans. GLP-1 is a glucose sensitizing hormone because it increases the efficacy and potency of glucose as an insulin secretagogue. Induction of glucose competence by GLP-1 results from increased production and/or effectiveness of glucose derived metabolic coupling factors. Such actions of GLP-1 are likely to be a consequence of increased cAMP production with concomitant activation of PKA. GLP-1 is also shown to upregulate insulin gene expression and proinsulin biosynthesis, actions that enhance its usefulness as a blood glucose-lowering agent. Insulinotropic effects of GLP-1 are opposed by the counter-regulatory hormone leptin acting as an anti-insulinotropic agent. Growth factor-like effects of GLP-1 include stimulation of islet cell neogenesis, differentiation, and survival. MAP kinase and PI3 kinase signaling systems may mediate such novel actions of the hormone. GLP-1 also targets a transcription factor (PDX-1) that is a master regulator of the β-cell phenotype. PDX-1 confers expression of important components of the β-cell glucose signaling system. In conclusion, the interplay of intermediary metabolism and second messenger signal transduction is necessary for induction of glucose competence and is viewed as a natural consequence of co-ordinate gene expression.

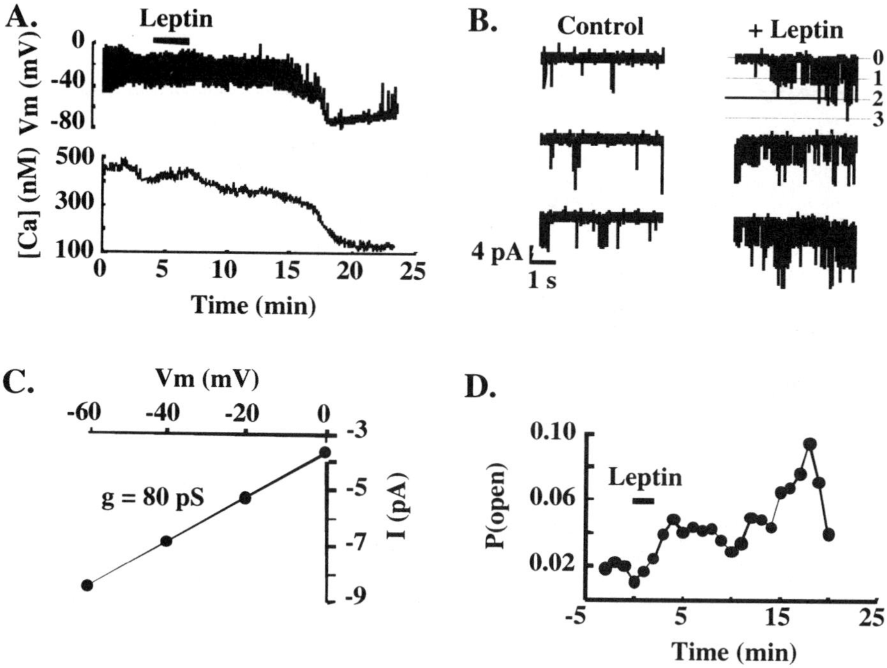

Figure 6. *A) Cellular hyperpolarization and a reduction of $[Ca^{2+}]_i$ in response to leptin. Measurements were obtained from a fura-2 loaded mouse β-cell using the perforated patch configuration under conditions in which cells were equilibrated in saline containing 5.5 mM glucose. Leptin (100 ng/ml) was applied for 3 min as indicated.* ***B)*** *Activation of K_{ATP} by leptin. Cell-attached patch recordings of unitary inward currents were obtained from an ob/ob mouse β-cell equilibrated in saline containing 5.5 mM glucose. Currents shown in the left and right panel sets are continuous stretches of data. Control K_{ATP} currents are shown on the left, and currents beginning 4 min after the start of a 3 min application of leptin (100 ng/ml) are shown on the right. Channel openings are downward current deflections indicated by the opening of 1, 2, or 3 channels (O_{1-3}) from a closed state (C).* ***C)*** *Single channel I-V relationship for K_{ATP} activated by leptin. The slope of the I-V relationship indicates a unitary conductance of 80 pS, as expected for K_{ATP}.* ***D)*** *The single channel open probability (P open) for K_{ATP} determined prior to, during, and following exposure to leptin (100 ng/ml). Values are averages for 6 cell-attached patches (pipette potential 0 mV) from ob/ob mouse β-cells equilibrated in 5.6 mM glucose. Figure 6 adapted from Kieffer et al., 1997.*

ACKNOWLEDGEMENT

This work was supported in part by grants to GGH from the National Institutes of Health (R01-DK42817, R01-DK52166) and the American Diabetes Association (Research Award).

REFERENCES

1. Habener JF. The incretin notion and its relevance to diabetes. Endocrinol Metabol Clin N Am 1993;22:775-794.

2. Thorens B, Waeber G. Glucagon-like peptide-1 and the control of insulin secretion in the normal state and in NIDDM. Diabetes 1993;42:1219-1225.
3. Holst JJ. Glucagon-like peptide-1: A newly discovered gastrointestinal hormone. Gastroenterology 1994;107:1848-1855.
4. Drucker DJ. Glucagon-like peptides. Diabetes 1998;47:159-169.
5. Turton MD, O'Shea D, Gunn I, Beak SA, Edwards CM, Meeran K, Choi SJ, Taylor GM, Heath MM, Lambert PD, Wilding JP, Smith DM, Ghatei MA, Herbert J, Bloom SR. A role for glucagon-like peptide-1 in the central regulation of feeding. Nature 1996;379:69-72.
6. Blazquez E, Alvarez E, Navarro M, Roncero I, Rodriguez-Fonseca F, Chowen JA, Zueco JA. Glucagon-like peptide-1(7-36)amide as a novel neuropeptide. Mol Neurobiol 1998;18:157-173.
7. Thorens B. Expression cloning of the pancreatic β cell receptor for the gluco-incretin hormone glucagon-like peptide-1. Proc Natl Acad Sci USA 1992;89:8641-8645.
8. Fehmann HC, Goke R, Goke B. Cell and molecular biology of the incretin hormones glucagon-like peptide-1 and glucose-dependent insulin releasing polypeptide. Endocrine Rev 1995;16:390-410.
9. Gromada J, Holst JJ, Rorsman P. Cellular regulation of islet hormone secretion by the incretin hormone glucagon-like peptide-1. Pflugers Arch 1998;435:583-594.
10. Holst JJ. Enteroglucagon. Ann Rev Physiol 1997;59:257-271.
11. Kreymann B, Ghatei MA, Williams G, Bloom SR. Glucagon-like peptide-1(7-36): A physiological incretin in man. Lancet 1987;2:1300-1304.
12. Nathan DM, Schreiber E, Fogel H, Mojsov S, Habener JF. Insulinotropic action of glucagon-like peptide-1(7-37) in diabetic and nondiabetic subjects. Diabetes Care 1992;15:270-276.
13. Gutniak M, Orskov C, Holst JJ, Ahren B, Efendic S. Antidiabetogenic effect of glucagon-like peptide-1(7-36)amide in normal subjects and patients with diabetes mellitus. N Engl J Med 1992;326:1316-1322.
14. Wang Y, Perfetti R, Greig NH, Holloway HW, DeOre KA, Montrose-Rafizadeh C, Elahi D, Egan JM. Glucagon-like peptide-1 can reverse the age-related decline in glucose tolerance in rats. J Clin Invest 1997;99:2883-2889.
15. Buteau J, Roduit R, Susini S, Prentki M. Glucagon-like peptide-1 promotes DNA synthesis, activates phosphatidylinositol 3-kinase and increases transcription factor pancreatic and duodenal homeobox gene 1 (PDX-1) DNA binding in beta (INS-1)-cells. Diabetologia 1999;42:856-864.
16. Wang X, Cahill CM, Pineyro MA, Zhou J, Doyle ME, Egan JM. Glucagon-like peptide-1 regulates the β-cell transcription factor, PDX-1, in insulinoma cells. Endocrinology 1999;140:4904-4907.
17. Alcantara AI, Morales M, Delgado E, Lopez-Delgado MI, Clemente F, Luque MA, Malaisse WJ, Valverde I, Villanueva-Penacarrillo ML. Exendin-4 agonist and exendin(9-39)amide antagonist of the GLP-1(7-36)amide effects in liver and muscle. Arch Biochem Biophys 1997;341:1-7.
18. Trapote MA, Clemente F, Galera C, Morales M, Alcantara AI, Lopez-Delgado MI, Villanueva-Penacarrillo ML, Valverde I. Inositolphosphoglycans are possible mediators of the glucagon-like peptide-1(7-36)amide action in the liver. J Endocrinol Invest 1996;19:114-118.
19. Yang H, Egan JM, Wang Y, Moyes CD, Roth J, Montrose MH, Montrose-Rafizadeh C. GLP-1 action in L6 myotubes is via a receptor different from the pancreatic GLP-1 receptor. Am J Physiol 1998;275:C675-C683.
20. Egan JM, Montrose-Rafizadeh C, Wang Y, Bernier M, Roth J. Glucagon-like peptide-1(7-36)amide (GLP-1) enhances insulin-stimulated glucose metabolism in 3T3-L1 adipocytes: One of several potential extrapancreatic sites of GLP-1 action. Endocrinology 1994;135:2070-2075.
21. Perea A, Vinambres C, Clemente F, Villanueva-Panacarrillo ML, Valverde I. GLP-1(7-36)amide: effects on glucose transport and metabolism in rat adipose tissue. Horm Metab Res 1997;29:417-421.
22. Tolessa T, Gutniak M, Holst JJ, Hellstrom PM. Glucagon-like peptide-1 retards gastric emptying and small bowel transit in the rat: effect mediated through central or enteric nervous mechanisms. Dig Dis Sci 1998;43:2284-2290.
23. Imereyuz N, Yegen BC, Bozkurt A, Coskun T, Villanueva-Penacarrillo ML, Ulusoy NB. Glucagon-like peptide-1 inhibits gastric emptying via vagal afferent-mediated central mechanisms. Am J Physiol 1997;273:G920-G927.
24. Dupre J, Behme MT, Hramiak IM, McFarlane P, Williamson MP, Zabel P, McDonald TJ. Glucagon-like peptide-1 reduces postprandial glycemic excursions in IDDM. Diabetes 1995;44:626-630.
25. Creutzfeldt WO, Kleine N, Willms B, Orskov C, Holst JJ, Nauck MA. Glucagonostatic actions and reduction of fasting hyperglycemia by exogenous glucagon-like peptide-1(7-36)amide in type-1 diabetic patients. Diabetes Care 1996;19:580-586.
26. Jehle PM, Jehle D, Fussganger RD, Adler G. Effects of glucagon-like peptide-1 (GLP-1) in RINm5F insulinoma cells. Stimulation of insulin secetion, insulin content, and insulin receptor binding. Exp. Clin. Endocrinol. Diabetes 1995;103:31-36.
27. Harbeck MC, Louie DC, Howland J, Wolf BA, Rothenberg PL. Expression of insulin receptor mRNA and insulin receptor susbstrate 1 in pancreatic islet β-cells. Diabetes 1996;45:711-717.

28. Velloso LA, Carneiro EM, Crepaldi SC, Boschero AC, Saad MJA. Glucose- and insulin-induced phosphorylation of the insulin receptor and its primary substrates IRS-1 and IRS-2 in rat pancreatic islets. FEBS Lett 1995;377:353-357.
29. Hugl SR, White MF, Rhodes CJ. Insulin-like growth factor 1 (IGF-1)-stimulated pancreatic β-cell growth is glucose-dependent. Synergistic activation of insulin receptor substrate-mediated signal transduction pathways by glucose and IGF-1 in INS-1 cells. J Biol Chem 1998;273:17771-17779.
30. Kulkarni RN, Bruning JC, Winnay JN, Postic C, Magnuson MA, Kahn CR. Tissue-specific knockout of the insulin receptor in pancreatic β cells creates an insulin secretory defect similar to that in type-2 diabetes. Cell 1999;96:329-339.
31. Xu GG, Gao Z, Borge PD, Wolf BA. Insulin receptor substrate 1-induced inhibition of endoplasmic reticulum Ca^{2+} uptake in β cells. Autocrine regulation of intracellular Ca^{2+} homeostasis and insulin secretion. J Biol Chem 1999;274:18067-18074.
32. Aspinwall CA, Lakey JR, Kennedy RT. Insulin-stimulated insulin secretion in single pancreatic β cells. J Biol Chem 1999;274:6360-6365.
33. Withers DJ, Gutierrez JS, Towery H, Burks DJ, Ren JM, Previs S, Zhang Y, Bernal D, Pons S, Shulman GI, Bonner-Weir S, White MF. Disruption of IRS-2 causes type-2 diabetes in mice. Nature 1998;391:900-904.
34. Holz GG, Kuhtreiber WM, Habener JF. Induction of glucose competence in pancreatic β cells by glucagon-like peptide-1(7-37). Trans Assoc Amer Phys 1992;105:260-267.
35. Holz GG, Habener JF. Signal transduction crosstalk in the endocrine system: Pancreatic β cells and the glucose competence concept. Trends in Biochem Sci 1992;17:388-393.
36. Holz GG, Kuhtreiber WM, Habener JF. Pancreatic β-cells are rendered glucose competent by the insulinotropic hormone GLP-1(7-37). Nature 1993;361:362-365.
37. Holz GG, Leech CA. Glucagon-like peptide-1 and the glucose competence concept of pancreatic beta-cell function. In: The insulinotropic hormone glucagon-like peptide 1. Eds. Fehmann, HC and Goke, B 1997;13:171-193.
38. Dachicourt N, Serradas P, Bailbe D, Kergoat M, Doare L, Portha B. Glucagon-like peptide-1(7-36)amide confers glucose sensitivity to previously glucose-incompetent β-cells in diabetic rats: *in vivo* and *in vitro* studies. J Endocrinol 1997;155:369-376.
39. Abdel-Halim SM, Guenifi A, Khan A, Larsson O, Berggren PO, Ostenson CG, Efendic S. Impaired coupling of glucose signal to the exocytotic machinery in diabetic GK rats: a defect ameliorated by cAMP. Diabetes 1996;45:934-40.
40. Byrne MM, Gliem K, Wank U, Arnold R, Katschinski M, Polonsky KS, Goke B. Glucagon-like peptide 1 improves the ability of the β-cell to sense and respond to glucose in subjects with impaired glucose tolerance. Diabetes 1998;47:1259-65.
41. Linn T, Schneider K, Goke B, Federlin K. Glucagon-like-peptide-1(7-36)amide improves glucose sensitivity in beta-cells of NOD mice. Acta Diabetol 1996;33:19-24.
42. Montrose-Rafizadeh C, Wang Y, Janczewski AM, Henderson TE, Egan JM. Overexpression of glucagon-like peptide-1 receptor in an insulin- secreting cell line enhances glucose responsiveness. Mol Cell Endocrinol 1997;130:109-17.
43. Otonkoski T, Hayek A. Constitution of a biphasic insulin response to glucose in human fetal pancreatic beta-cells with glucagon-like peptide 1. J Clin Endocrinol Metab 1995;80:3779-83.
44. Nauck MA, Heimesaat MM, Orskov C, Holst JJ, Ebert R, Creutzfeldt W. Preserved incretin activity of glucagon-like peptide-1(7-36)amide but not of synthetic human gastric inhibitory peptide in patients with type-2 diabetes mellitus. J Clin Invest 1993;91:301-307.
45. Nauck MA, Kleine N, Orskov C, Holst JJ, Willms B, Creutzfeldt W. Normalization of fasting hyperglycaemia by exogenous glucagon-like peptide-1 (7-36 amide) in type 2 (non-insulin dependent) diabetic patients. Diabetologia 1993;36:741-744.
46. Flamez D, Breusegem AV, Scrocchi LA, Quartier E, Pipeleers D, Drucker DJ, Schuit F. Mouse pancreatic β cells exhibit preserved glucose competence after disruption of the glucagon-like peptide-1 receptor gene. Diabetes 1998;47:646-652.
47. Zawalich WS, Zawalich KC, Rasmussen H. Influence of glucagon-like peptide-1 on β-cell responsiveness. Regul Pept 1993;44:277-283.
48. Leclercq-Meyer V, Malaisse WJ. Potentiation of GLP-1 insulinotropic action by a nonglucidic nutrient in the pancreas of diabetic GK rats. Biochem Mol Med 1996;59:87-90.
49. Newgard CB, McGarry JD. Metabolic coupling factors in pancreatic β-cell signal transduction. Ann Rev Biochem 1995;64:689-719.
50. Matschinsky FM, Glaser B, Magnuson MA. Pancreatic β-cell glucokinase. Closing the gap between theoretical concepts and experimental realities. Diabetes 1998;47:307-315.
51. Fridolf T, Ahren B. GLP-1(7-36)amide stimulates insulin secretion in rat islets: studies on the mode of action. Diabetes Res 1991;16:185-191.
52. Dukes ID, McIntyre MS, Mertz RJ, Philipson LH, Roe MW, Spencer B, Worley JF. Dependence on NADH produced during glycolysis for β-cell glucose signaling. J Biol Chem 1994;269:10979-10982.

53. Mertz RJ, Worley JF, Spencer B, Johnson JH, Dukes ID. Activation of stimulus-secretion coupling in pancreatic β cells by specific products of glucose metabolism. Evidence for privileged signaling by glycolysis. J Biol Chem 1996;271:4838-4845.
54. Eto K, Tsubamoto Y, Terauchi Y, Sugiyama T, Kishimoto T, Takahashi N, Yamauchi N, Kubota N, Murayama S, Aizawa T, Akanuma Y, Kasai H, Yazaki Y, Kadowaki T. Role of NADH shuttle system in glucose-induced activation of mitochondrial metabolism and insulin secretion. Science 1999;283:981-985.
55. Eto K, Suga S, Wakui M, Tsubamoto Y, Terauchi Y, Taka J, Aizawa S, Noda M, Kimura S, Kasai H, Kadowaki T. NADH shuttle system regulates K_{ATP} channel-dependent pathway and steps distal to cytosolic Ca^{2+} concentration elevation in glucose-induced insulin secretion. J Biol Chem 1999;274:15386-25392.
56. Susini S, Roche E, Prentki M, Schlegel W. Glucose and glucoincretin peptides synergize to induce c-fos, c-jun, junB, zif-268, and nur-77 gene expression in pancreatic β(INS-1) cells. FASEB J 1998;12:1173-1182.
57. Edvell A, Lindstrom P. Initiation of increased pancreatic islet growth in young normoglycemic mice (Umea +/?). Endocrinology 1999;140:778-783.
58. Rothenberg PL, Willison D, Simon J, Wolf BA. Glucose-induces insulin receptor tyrosine phosphorylation in insulin-secreting β-cells. Diabetes 1995;44:802-809.
59. Hirayama I, Tamemoto H, Yokata H, Kubo SK, Wang J, Kuwano H, Nagamachi Y, Takeuchi T, Izumi T. Insulin receptor-related receptor is expressed in pancreatic β-cells and stimulates tyrosine phosphorylation of insulin receptor substrate-1 and -2. Diabetes 1999;48:1237-1244.
60. Frodin M, Sekine N, Roche E, Filloux C, Prentki M, Wollheim CB, Van Obberghen E. Glucose, other secretagogues, and nerve growth factor stimulate mitogen-activated protein kinase in the insulin-secreting β-cell line, INS-1. J Biol Chem 1995;270:7882-7889.
61. Montrose-Rafizadeh C, Avdonin P, Garant MJ, Rodgers BD, Kole S, Yang H, Levine MA, Schwindinger W, Bernier M. Pancreatic glucagon-like peptide-1 receptor couples to multiple G proteins and activates mitogen-activated protein kinase pathways in Chinese hamster ovary cells. Endocrinology 1999;140:1132-1140.
62. Kawasaki H, Springett GM, Mochizuki N, Toki S, Nakaya M, Matsuda M, Housman DE, Graybiel AM. A family of cAMP-binding proteins that directly activate Rap1. Science 1998;282:2275-2279.
63. Ohtsuka T, Shimizu K, Yamamori B, Kuroda S, Takei Y. Activation of brain B-Raf protein kinase by Rap1B small GTP-binding protein. J Biol Chem 1996;271:1258-1261.
64. Labadia ME, Bokoch GM, Huang CK. The Rap1A protein enhances protein kinase C activity *in vitro*. Biochem Biophys Res Comm. 1993;195:1321-1328.
65. Leiser M, Efrat S, Fleischer N. Evidence that Rap1 carboxymethylation is involved in regulated insulin secretion. Endocrinology 1995;136:2521-2530.
66. Kowluru A, Seavey SE, Li G, Sorenson RL, Weinhaus AJ, Nesher R, Rabaglia ME, Vadakekalam J, Metz SA. Glucose- and GTP-dependent stimulation of the carboxyl methylation of CDC42 in rodent and human pancreatic islets and pure β-cells. Evidence for an essential role of GTP-binding proteins in nutrient-induced insulin secretion. J Clin Invest 1996;98:540-555.
67. Gherzi R, Briata P, Fehmann HC, Goke B. Ras antagonizes cAMP stimulated glucagon gene transcription in pancreatic islet cell lines. FEBS Lett 1994;353:277-280.
68. Widmann C, Burki E, Dolci W, Thorens B. Signal transduction by the cloned Glucagon-like peptide-1 receptor: Comparison with signalling by the endogenous receptors of β cell lines. Mol Pharmacol 1994;45:1029-1035.
69. Thorens B, Widmann C. Molecular and functional characterization of the pancreatic β cell glucagon-like peptide-1 receptor. Diabetes 1994 1995;Excerpta Medica Int Congress Series 1100:184-186.
70. Thorens B, Porret A, Buhler L, Deng SP, Morel P, Widmann C. Cloning and functional expression of the human islet GLP-1 receptor. Demonstration that exendin-4 is an agonist and exendin-(9-39) an antagonist of the receptor. Diabetes 1993;42:1678-1682.
71. Goke R, Fehmann HC, Linn T, Schmidt H, Krause M, Eng J, Goke B. Exendin-4 is a high potency agonist and truncated exendin-(9-39)amide an antagonist at the glucagon-like peptide-1 receptor of insulin-secreting β-cells. J Biol Chem 1993;268:19650-19655.
72. Greig NH, Holloway HW, DeOre KA, Jani D, Wang Y, Zhou J, Garant MJ, Egan JM. Once daily injection of exendin-4 to diabetic mice achieves long-term beneficial effects on blood glucose concentrations. Diabetologia 1999;42:45-50.
73. Young AA, Gedulin BR, Bhavsar S, Bodkin N, Jodka C, Hansen B, Denaro M. Glucose-lowering and insulin-sensitizing actions of exendin-4: studies in obese diabetic (*ob/ob, db/db*) mice, diabetic fatty Zucker rats, and diabetic rhesus monkeys (*Macaca mulatta*). Diabetes 1999;48:1026-1034.
74. Holz GG, Habener JF. Black widow spider α-latrotoxin: a presynaptic neurotoxin that shares structural homology with the glucagon-like peptide-1 family of insulin secretagogic hormones. Comp Biochem Physiol B 1998;121:177-184.
75. Heller RS, Kieffer TJ, Habener JF. Point mutations in the first and third intracellular loops of the glucagon-like peptide-1 receptor alter intracellular signaling. Biochem Biophys Res Comm 1996;223:624-632.

76. Takhar S, Gyomorey S, Su RC, Mathi SK, Li X, Wheeler MB. The third cytoplasmic domain of the GLP-1(7-36)amide receptor is required for coupling to the adenylyl cyclase system. Endocrinology 1996;137:2175-2178.
77. Mathi SK, Chan Y, Li X, Wheeler MB. Scanning of the glucagon-like peptide-1 receptor localizes G protein-activating determinants primarily to the N-terminus of the third intracellular loop. Mol Endocrinol 1997;11:424-432.
78. Salapatek AM, MacDonald PE, Gaisano HY, Wheeler MB. Mutations to the third cytoplasmic domain of the glucagon-like peptide-1 (GLP-1) receptor can functionally uncouple GLP-1-stimulated insulin secretion in HIT-T15 cells. Mol Endocrinol 1999;13:1305-1317.
79. Abdel-Halim SM, Guenifi A, He B, Yang B, Mustafa M, Hojeberg B, Hillert J, Bakhiet M, Efendic S. Mutations in the promoter of adenylyl cyclase (AC)-III gene, overexpression of AC-III mRNA, and enhanced cAMP generation in islets from the spontaneously diabetic GK rat model of type 2 diabetes. Diabetes 1998;47:498-504.
80. Leech CA, Castonguay MA, Habener JF. Expression of adenylyl cyclase subtypes in pancreatic β cells. Biochem. Biophys. Res. Comm. 1999;254:703-706.
81. Yang B, He B, Abdel-Halim SM, Tibell A, Brendel MD, Bretzel RG, Efendic S, Hillert J. Molecular cloning of a full length cDNA for human type 3 adenylyl cyclase and its expression in human islets. Biochem Biophys Res Comm 1999;254:548-551.
82. Gromada J, Dissing S, Bokvist K, Renstrom E, Frokjaer-Jensen J, Wulff BS, Rorsman P. Glucagon-like peptide-1 increases cytoplasmic calcium in insulin-secreting βTC-3-cells by enhancement of intracellular calcium mobilization. Diabetes 1995;44:767-774.
83. Gromada J, Rorsman P, Dissing S, Wulff BS. Stimulation of cloned human glucagon-like peptide-1 receptor expressed in HEK 293 cells induces cAMP-dependent activation of calcium-induced calcium release. FEBS Lett 1995;373:182-186.
84. Holz GG, Leech CA, Heller RS, Castonguay MA, Habener JF. cAMP-dependent mobilization of intracellular Ca^{2+} stores by activation of ryanodine receptors in pancreatic β-cells. A Ca^{2+} signaling system activated by the insulinotropic hormone glucagon-like peptide-1(7-37). J Biol Chem 1999;274:14147-14156.
85. Gromada J, Rorsman P. Molecular mechanism underlying glucagon-like peptide-1 induced calcium mobilization from internal stores in insulin-secreting βTC3 cells. Acta Physiol Scand 1996;157:349-351.
86. Yaekura K, Yada T. $[Ca^{2+}]_i$-reducing action of cAMP in rat pancreatic β-cells: involvement of thapsigargin-sensitive stores. Am J Physiol 1998;274:C513-C521.
87. Lester LB, Langeberg LK, Scott JD. Anchoring of protein kinase A facilitates hormone-mediated insulin secretion. Proc Natl Acad Sci USA 1997;94:14942-14947.
88. Gray PC, Tibbs VC, Catterall WA, Murphy BJ. Identification of a 15-kDa cAMP-dependent protein kinase-anchoring protein associated with skeletal muscle L-type Calcium channels. J Biol Chem 1997;272:6297-6302.
89. Holz GG, Hussain MA, Skoglund GS. Rat insulin gene promoter activity stimulated by picomolar concentrations of GLP-1. Abst American Diabetes Assoc Meeting, San Diego. 1999;
90. Wheeler MB, Lu M, Dillon JS, Leng XH, Chen C, Boyd AE. Functional expression of the rat glucagon-like peptide-1 receptor, evidence for coupling to both adenylyl cyclase and phospholipase C. Endocrinology 1993;133:57-62.
91. Gromada J, Anker C, Bokvist K, Knudsen LB, Wahl P. Glucagon-like peptide-1 receptor expression in *Xenopus* oocytes stimulates inositol trisphosphate-dependent intracellular Ca^{2+} mobilization. FEBS Lett 1998;425:277-280.
92. Lu M, Wheeler MB, Leng XH, Boyd AE. The role of free cytosolic calcium level in β cell signal transduction by gastric inhibitory polypeptide and glucagon-like peptide-1(7-37). Endocrinol 1993;132:94-100.
93. Rasmussen H, Isales CM, Calle R, Throckmorton D, Anderson M, Gassalla-Herraiz J, McCarthy R. Diacylglycerol production, Ca^{2+} influx, and protein kinase C activation in sustained cellular responses. Endocrine Rev 1995;16:649-681.
94. Gromada J, Frokjaer-Jensen J, Dissing S. Glucose stimulates voltage- and calcium-dependent inositol trisphosphate production and intracellular calcium mobilization in insulin-secreting βTC3 cells. Biochem J 1996;314:339-345.
95. Holz GG, Leech CA, Habener JF. Activation of a cAMP-regulated Ca^{2+}-signalling pathway in pancreatic β cells by the insulinotropic hormone glucagon-like peptide-1. J Biol Chem 1995;270:17749-17757.
96. Suga S, Kanno T, Nakano K, Takeo T, Dobashi Y, Wakui M. GLP-1(7-36)amide augments Ba^{2+} current through L-type Ca^{2+} channel of rat pancreatic β-cell in a cAMP-dependent manner. Diabetes 1997;46:1755-1760.
97. Suga S, Kanno T, Dobashi Y, Wakui M. GLP-1(7-36)amide activates L-type Ca^{2+} channels of pancreatic β-cells through cAMP signaling. Jap J Physiol 1997;47:S13-S14.
98. Gromada J, Bokvist K, Ding WG, Holst JJ, Nielsen JH, Rorsman P. Glucagon-like peptide-1(7-36)amide stimulates exocytosis in human pancreatic beta-cells by both proximal and distal regulatory steps in stimulus-secretion coupling. Diabetes 1998;47:57-65.

99. Leech CA, Habener JF. Insulinotropic glucagon-like peptide-1-mediated activation of non-selective cation currents in insulinoma cells is mimicked by maitotoxin. J Biol Chem 1997;272:17987-17993.
100. Cook DL, Satin LS, Hopkins WF. Pancreatic β cells are bursting, but how? Trends in Neurosci 1991;14:411-414.
101. Cook DL. Isolated islets of Langerhans have slow oscillations of electrical activity. Metabolism 1983;32:681-685.
102. Cook DL, Satin LS, Ashford MLJ, Hales CN. ATP-sensitive K^+ channels in pancreatic β-cells. Spare channel hypothesis. Diabetes 1988;37:495-498.
103. Eddlestone GT, Oldham SB, Lipson LG, Premdas FH, Biegelman PM. Electrical activity, cAMP concentration, and insulin release in mouse islets of Langerhans. Am J Physiol 1985;248:C145-C153.
104. Inagaki N, Gonoi T, Seino S. Subunit stoichiometry of the pancreatic β-cell ATP-sensitive K^+ channel. FEBS Lett 1997;409:232-236.
105. Clement JP, Kunjilwar K, Gonzalez G, Schwanstecher M, Panten U, Aguilar-Bryan L, Bryan J. Association and stoichiometry of K_{ATP} channel subunits. Neuron 1997;18:827-838.
106. Shyng SL, Nichols CG. Octameric stoichiometry of the K_{ATP} channel complex. J Gen Physiol 1997;110:655-664.
107. Alekseev AE, Kennedy ME, Navarro B, Terzic A. Burst kinetics of co-expressed Kir6.2/SUR1 clones: Comparison of recombinant with native ATP-sensitive K^+ channel behaviour. J Membrane Biol 1997;159:161-168.
108. Ashcroft FM, Rorsman P. Electrophysiology of the pancreatic β-cell. Prog Biophys Molec Biol 1989;54:87-143.
109. Barnett DW, Pressel DM, Chern HT, Scharp DW, Misler S. cAMP-enhancing agents permit stimulus-secretion coupling in canine pancreatic islet β cells. J Membrane Biol 1994;138:113-120.
110. He LP, Mears D, Atwater I, Kitasato H. Glucagon induces suppression of ATP-sensitive K^+ channel activity through a Ca^{2+}/calmodulin-dependent pathway in mouse pancreatic β-cells. J Membrane Biol 1998;166:237-244.
111. Ribalet B, Ciani S, Eddlestone GT. ATP mediates both activation and inhibition of K(ATP) channel via cyclic-AMP dependent protein kinase in insulin secreting cell lines. J Gen Physiol 1989;94:693-717.
112. He LP, Kitasato H. Glucagon induces Ca^{2+} dependent increase of reduced pyridine nucleotides in mouse pancreatic _-cells. Biochim Biophys Acta 1996;1310:325-333.
113. Ribalet B, Ciani S. Characterization of the G-protein coupling of a glucagon receptor to the K-ATP channel in insulin secreting cells. J Membrane Biol 1994;142:395-408.
114. Sui JL, Petit-Jacques J, Logothetis DE. Activation of the atrial KACh channel by the __ subunits of G proteins or intracellular Na^+ ions depends on the presence of phosphatidylinositol phosphates. Proc Natl Acad Sci USA 1998;95:1307-1312.
115. Huang CL, Feng S, Hilgemann DW. Direct activation of inward rectifier potassium channels by PIP_2 and its stabilization by Gβγ. Nature 1998;391:803-806.
116. Shyng SL, Nichols CG. Membrane phospholipid control of nucleotide sensitivity of K_{ATP} channels. Science 1998;282:1138-1141.
117. Baukrowitz T, Schulte U, Oliver D, Herlitze S, Krauter T, Tucker SJ, Ruppersberg JP, Fakler B. PIP2 and PIP as determinants for ATP inhibition of K_{ATP} channels. Science 1998;282:1141-1144.
118. Laychock SG. Identification and metabolism of polyphosphoinositides in isolated islets of Langerhans. Biochem J 1983;216:101-106.
119. Seino S, Chen L, Seino M, Blondel O, Takeda J, Johnson JH, G.I. B. Cloning of the α_1 subunit of a voltage-dependent calcium channel expressed in pancreatic β-cells. Proc Natl Acad Sci USA 1992;89:584-588.
120. Seino S. CACN4, the major alpha 1 subunit isoform of voltage-dependent calcium channels in pancreatic β-cells: a minireview of current progress. Diabetes & Clin Practice 1995;28:s99-s103.
121. Satin LS, Tavalin SJ, Kinard TA, Teague J. Contribution of L- and non-L-type calcium channels to voltage-gated calcium current and glucose-dependent insulin secretion in HIT-T15 cells. Endocrinology 1995;136:4589-4601.
122. Bokvist K, Eliasson L, Ammala C, Renstrom E, Rorsman P. Co-localization of L-type Ca^{2+} channels and insulin-containing secretory granules and its significance for the initiation of exocytosis in mouse pancreatic β-cells. EMBO J 1995;14:50-57.
123. Kindmark H, Kohler M, Larsson O, Khan A, Berggren PO. Dissociation between exocytosis and Ca^{2+}-channel activity in mouse pancreatic β-cells stimulated with calmidazolium (compound R24571). FEBS Lett 1995;315-320.
124. Wiser O, Trus M, Hernandez A, Renstrom E, Barg S, Rorsman P, Atlas D. The voltage sensitive Lc-type Ca^{2+} channel is functionally coupled to the exocytotic machinery. Proc Natl Acad Sci USA 1999;96:248-253.
125. Yang SN, Larsson O, Branstrom R, Bertorello AM, Leibiger B, Leibiger IB, Moede T, Kohler M, Meister B, P.O. B. Syntaxin 1 interacts with the L_D subtype of voltage-gated Ca^{2+} channel in pancreatic β cells. Proc Natl Acad Sci USA 1999;96:10164-10169.

126. Smith PA, Rorsman P, Ashcroft FM. Modulation of dihydropyridine-sensitive Ca^{2+} channels by glucose metabolism in mouse pancreatic β-cells. Nature 1989;342:550-553.
127. Arkhammer P, Juntti-Berggren L, Larrson O, Welch M, Nanberg E, Sjoholm A, Kohler M, Berggren PO. Protein kinase C modulates the insulin secretory process by maintaining a proper function of the β-cell voltage-activated Ca^{2+}-channels. J Biol Chem 1994;269:2743-2749.
128. Haby C, Larsson O, Islam MS, Aunis D, Berggren PO, Zwiller J. Inhibition of serine/threonine protein phosphatases promotes opening of voltage-activated L-type Ca^{2+} channels in insulin-secreting cells. Biochem J 1994;298:341-346.
129. Larsson O, Barker CJ, Sjoholm A, Carlqvist H, Michell RH, Bertorello A, Nillson T, Honkanon RE, Mayr GW, Zwiller J, Berggren PO. Inhibition of phosphatases and increased Ca^{2+} channel activity by inositol hexakisphosphate. Science 1997;278:471-474.
130. Leech CA, Holz GG, Habener JF. Signal Transduction of PACAP and GLP-1 in pancreatic β-cells. Ann NY Acad Sci 1996;805:81-93.
131. Ammala C, Ashcroft FM, Rorsman P. Calcium-independent potentiation of insulin release by cyclic AMP in single β-cells. Nature 1993;363:356-358.
132. Britsch S, Krippeit-Drews P, Lang F, Gregor M, Drews G. Glucagon-like peptide-1 modulates Ca^{2+} current but not K^{+}ATP current in intact mouse pancreatic β cells. Biochem Biophys Res Comm 1995;207:33-39.
133. Gromada J, Ding WG, Barg S, Renstrom E, Rorsman P. Multisite regulation of insulin secretion by cAMP-increasing agonists: evidence that glucagon-like peptide-1 and glucagon act via distinct receptors. Pflugers Arch 1997;434:515-524.
134. Yada T, Sakurada M, Nakata M, Ihida K, Yaekura K, Shioda S, Kikuchi M. Current status of PACAP as a regulator of insulin secretion in pancreatic islets. Ann NY Acad Sci 1996;805:329-342.
135. af Klinteberg K, Karlsson S, Ahren B. Signaling mechanisms underlying the insulinotropic effect of pituitary adenylate cyclase-activating polypeptide in HIT-T15 cells. Endocrinology 1996;137:2791-2798.
136. af Klinteberg K, Karlsson S, Moller K, Sundler F, Ahren B. Pituitary adenylate cyclase activating polypeptide (PACAP) and insulin secretion: Effects and mechanisms. Ann NY Acad Sci 1996;805:543-548.
137. Filipsson K, Ahren B. Protein kinase A inhibition and PACAP-induced insulin secretion in HIT-T15 cells. Ann NY Acad Sci 1998;865:441-444.
138. Filipsson K, Sundler F, Ahren B. PACAP is an islet neuropeptide which contributes to glucose-stimulated insulin secretion. Biochem Biophys Res Comm 1999;256:664-667.
139. Moreno Davila H. Molecular and functional diversity of voltage-gated calcium channels. Ann NY Acad Sci 1999;868:102-117.
140. Magnelli V, Grassi C, Parlatore E, Sher E, Carbone E. Down-regulation of non-L, non-N-type (Q-like) Ca^{2+} channels by Lambert-Eaton myasthenic syndrome (LEMS) antibodies in rat insulinoma RINm5F cells. FEBS Lett 1996;387:47-52.
141. Ligon B, Boyd AE, Dunlap K. Class A calcium channel variants in pancreatic islets and their role in insulin secretion. J Biol Chem 1998;273:13905-13911.
142. Yaney GC, Wheeler MB, Wei X, Perez-Reyes E, Birmbaumer L, Boyd AE, Moss LG. Cloning of a novel α_1-subunit of the voltage-dependent calcium channel from the β-cell. Mol Endo 1992;6:2143-2152.
143. Safayhi H, Haase H, Kramer U, Bihlmayer A, Roenfeldt M, Ammon HPT, Froschmayr M, Cassidy TN, Morano I, Ahlijanaian MK, Striessnig J. L-type calcium channels in insulin-secreting cells: biochemical characterization and phosphorylation in RINm5F cells. Mol Endo 1997;11:619-629.
144. Wang L, Bhattacharjee A, Zuo Z, Hu F, Honkanen RE, Berggren PO, Li M. A low voltage-activated Ca^{2+} current mediates cytokine-induced pancreatic β-cell death. Endocrinology 1999;140:1200-1204.
145. Bhattacharjee A, Whitehurst RM, Zhang M, Wang L, Li M. T-type calcium channels facilitate insulin secretion by enhancing general excitability in the insulin-secreting beta cell line, INS-1. Endocrinology 1997;138:3735-3740.
146. Blondel O, Takeda J, Janssen H, Seino S, Bell GI. Sequence and functional characterization of a third inositol trisphosphate receptor subtype, IP3R-3, expressed in pancreatic islets, kidney, gastrointestinal tract, and other tissues. J Biol Chem 1994;268:11356-11363.
147. Lee B, Bradford PG, Laychock SG. Characterization of inositol 1,4,5-trisphosphate receptor isoform mRNA expression and regulation in rat pancreatic islets. J Mol Endocrinol 1998;21:31-39.
148. Islam MS, Leibiger I, Leibiger B, Rossi D, Sorrentino V, Ekstrom TJ, Westerblad H, Andrade FH, Berggren PO. *In situ* activation of the type 2 ryanodine receptor in pancreatic beta cells requires cAMP-dependent phosphorylation. Proc Natl Acad Sci USA 1998;95:6145-6150.
149. Takasawa S, Nata K, Yonekura H, Okamoto H. Cyclic ADP-ribose in insulin secretion from pancreatic β-cells. Science 1993;259:370-373.
150. Noguchi N, Takasawa S, Nata K, Tohgo A, Kato I, Ikehata F, Yonekura H, Okamoto H. Cyclic-ADP-ribose binds to FK506-binding protein 12.6 to release Ca^{2+} from islet microsomes. J Biol Chem 1997;272:3133-3136.

151. Takasawa S, Akiyama T, Nata K, Kuroki M, Tohgo A, Noguchi N, Kobayashi S, Kato I, Katada T, Okamoto H. Cyclic ADP-ribose and inositol 1,4,5-trisphosphate as alternative second messengers for intracellular Ca^{2+} mobilization in normal and diabetic β-cells. J Biol Chem 1998;273:2497-2500.
152. Takasawa S, Ishida A, Nata K, Nakagawa K, Noguchi N, Tohgo A, Kato I, Yonekura H, Fujisawa H, Okamoto H. Requirement of calmodulin-dependent protein kinase II in cyclic ADP-ribose-mediated intracellular Ca^{2+} mobilization. J Biol Chem 1995;270:30257-30259.
153. Roe MW, Philipson LH, Frangakis CJ, Kuzetsov A, Mertz RJ, Lancaster ME, Spencer B, Worley JF, Dukes ID. Defective glucose-dependent endoplasmic reticulum Ca^{2+} sequestration in diabetic mouse islets of Langerhans. J Biol Chem 1994;269:18279-18282.
154. Roe MW, Mertz RJ, Lancaster ME, Worley JF, Dukes ID. Thapsigargin inhibits the glucose-induced decrease of intracellular Ca^{2+} in mouse islets of Langerhans. Am J Physiol 1994;266:E852-E862.
155. Gilon P, Arredouani A, Gailly P, Gromada J, Henquin JC. Uptake and release of Ca^{2+} by the endoplasmic reticulum contribute to the oscillations of the cytosolic Ca^{2+} concentration triggered by Ca^{2+} influx in the electrically excitable pancreatic β-cell. J Biol Chem 1999;274:20197-20205.
156. Maechler P, Kennedy ED, Sebo E, Valeva A, Pozzan T, Wollheim CB. Secretagogues modulate the calcium concentration in the endoplasmic reticulum of insulin-secreting cells. Studies in aequorin-expressing intact and permeabilized INS-1 cells. J Biol Chem 1999;274:12583-12592.
157. Varadi A, Molnar E, Ashcroft SJ. Characterization of endoplasmic reticulum and plasma membrane Ca^{2+}-ATPases in pancreatic β-cells and in islets of Langerhans. Biochim Biophys Acta 1995;1236:119-127.
158. Varadi A, Molnar E, Ostenson CG, Ashcroft SJ. Isoforms of endoplasmic reticulum Ca^{2+}-ATPase are differentially expressed in normal and diabetic islets of Langerhans. Biochem J 1996;319:521-527.
159. Varadi A, Lebel L, Hashim Y, Mehta Z, Ashcroft SJH, Turner R. Sequence variants of the saco(endo)plasmic reticulum Ca^{2+} transport ATPase 3 gene (SERCA3) in caucasian type II diabetic patients (UK prospective diabetes study 48). Diabetologia 1999;42:1240-1243.
160. Schofl C, Rossig L, Mader T, Von Zur Muhlen A, Brabant G. Cyclic adenosine 3',5'-monophosphate potentiates Ca^{2+} signaling and insulin secretion by phospholipase C-linked hormones in HIT cells. Endocrinology 1996;137:3026-3032.
161. Liu YJ, Grapengiesser E, Gylfe E, Hellman B. Crosstalk between cAMP and inositol trisphosphate-signalling pathways in pancreatic β-cells. Arch Biochem Biophys 1996;334:295-302.
162. Mak DOD, McBride S, Foskett JK. ATP regulation of type-1 inositol 1,4,5-trisphosphate receptor channel gating by allosteric tuning of Ca^{2+} activation. J Biol Chem 1999;274:22231-22237.
163. Islam MS, Rorsman P, Berggren PO. Ca^{2+}-induced Ca^{2+} release in insulin-secreting cells. FEBS Lett 1992;296:287-291.
164. Gamberucci A, Fulceri R, Pralong W, Banhegyi G, Marcolongo P, Watkins SL, Benedetti A. Caffeine releases a glucose-primed endoplasmic reticulum Ca^{2+} pool in the insulin secreting cell line INS-1. FEBS Lett 1999;446:309-312.
165. Bode HP, Moorman B, Dabew R, Goke B. Glucagon-like peptide-1 elevates cytosolic calcium in pancreatic β-cells independently of protein kinase A. Endocrinology 1999;140:3919-3927.
166. Kato I, Takasawa S, Akabane A, Tanaka O, Abe H, Takamura T, Suzuki Y, Nata K, Yonekura H, Yoshimoto T, Okamoto H. Regulatory role of CD38 (ADP-ribosyl cyclase/cyclic ADP-ribose hydrolase) in insulin secretion by glucose in pancreatic β-cells. Enhanced insulin secretion in CD38-expressing transgenic mice. J Biol Chem 1995;270:30045-30050.
167. Li Q, Yamada Y, Yasuda K, Ihara Y, Okamoto Y, Kaisaki PJ, Watanabe R, Ikeda H, Tsuda K, Seino Y. A cloned rat CD-38-homologous protein and its expression in pancreatic islets. Biochem Biophys Res Comm 1994;202:629-636.
168. Morita K, Kitayama S, Dohi T. Stimulation of cyclic ADP-ribose synthesis by acetylcholine and its role in catecholamine release in bovine adrenal chromaffin cells. J Biol Chem 1997;272:21002-21009.
169. Sturgess NC, Hales CN, Ashford MLJ. Inhibition of a calcium-activated non-selective cation channel, in a rat insulinoma cell line, by adenine derivatives. FEBS Lett 1986;208:397-400.
170. Herson PS, Ashford MLJ. Activation of a novel non-selective cation channel by alloxan and H_2O_2 in the rat insulin-secreting cell line CRI-G1. J Physiol 1997;501:59-66.
171. Sturgess NC, Hales CN, Ashford MLJ. Calcium and ATP regulate the activity of a non-selective cation channel in a rat insulinoma cell line. Pflugers Arch 1987;409:607-615.
172. Fridolf T, Ahren B. GLP-1(7-36)amide-stimulated insulin secretion in rat islets is sodium-dependent. Biochem Biophys Res Commun 1991;179:701-706.
173. Fridolf T, Ahren B. Effects of glucagon-like peptide-1(7-36)amide on the cytoplasmic Ca^{2+}-concentration in rat islet cells. Mol Cell Endocrinol 1993;96:85-90.
174. Kato M, Ma HT, Tatemoto K. GLP-1 depolarizes the rat pancreatic β–cell in a sodium-dependent manner. Regulatory Peptides 1996;62:23-27.
175. Reale V, Hales CN, Ashford MLJ. Nucleotide regulation of a calcium activated cation channel in the rat insulinoma cell line, CRI-G1. J Membrane Biol 1994;141:101-112.

176. Reale V, Hales CN, Ashford MLJ. The effects of pyridine nucleotides on the activity of a calcium-activated non-selective cation channel in the rat insulinoma cell line, CRI-G1. J Membrane Biol 1994;142:299-307.
177. Reale V, Hales CN, Ashford MLJ. Regulation of calcium-activated nonselective cation channel activity by cyclic nucleotides in the rat insulinoma cell line, CRI-G1. J Membrane Biol 1995;145:267-278.
178. Worley JF, McIntyre MS, Spencer B, Mertz RJ, Roe MW, Dukes ID. Endoplasmic reticulum calcium store regulates membrane potential in mouse islet β-cells. J Biol Chem 1994;269:14359-14362.
179. Worley JF, McIntyre MS, Spencer B, Dukes ID. Depletion of intracellular Ca^{2+} stores activates a maitotoxin-sensitive nonselective cationic current in β–cells. J Biol Chem 1994;269:32055-32058.
180. Miura Y, Henquin JC, Gilon P. Emptying of intracellular Ca^{2+} stores stimulates Ca^{2+} entry in mouse pancreatic β-cells by both direct and indirect mechanisms. J Physiol 1997;503:387-398.
181. Liu YJ, Gylfe E. Store-operated Ca^{2+} entry in insulin-releasing pancreatic β-cells. Cell Calcium 1997;22:277-286.
182. Henquin JC, Garcia MC, Bozem M, Hermans MP, Nenquin M. Muscarinic control of pancreatic β-cell function involves sodium-dependent depolarization and calcium influx. Endocrinology 1988;122:2134-2142.
183. Roe MW, Worley JF, Qian F, Tamarina N, Mittal AA, Dralyuk F, Blair NT, Mertz RJ, Philipson LH, Dukes ID. Characterization of a Ca^{2+} release-activated nonselective cation current regulating membrane potential and $[Ca^{2+}]_i$ oscillations in transgenically derived beta cells. J Biol Chem 1998;273:10402-10410.
184. Vaca L, Sinkins WG, Hu Y, Kunze DL, Schilling WP. Activation of recombinant *trp* by thapsigargin in Sf9 insect cells. Am J Physiol 1994;267:C1501-C1505.
185. Zhu X, Jiang M, Peyton M, Boulay G, Hurst R, Stefani E, Birnbaumer L. *trp*, a novel mammalian gene family essential for agonist-activated capacitative Ca^{2+} entry. Cell 1996;85:661-671.
186. Sinkins WG, Vaca L, Hu Y, Kunze DL, Schilling WP. The COOH-terminal domain of *Drosophila* TRP channels confers thapsigargin sensitivity. J Biol Chem 1996;271:2955-2960.
187. Philipp S, Cavalie A, Freichel M, Wissenbach U, Zimmer S, Trost C, Marquart A, Murakami M, Flockerzi V. A mammalian capacitative calcium entry channel homologous to *Drosophila* Trp and Trpl. EMBO J 1996;15:6166-6171.
188. Gillo B, Chorna I, Cohen H, Cook B, Manistersky I, Chorev M, Arnon A, Pollock JA, Selinger Z, Minke B. Coexpression of *Drosophila* TRP and TRP-like proteins in *Xenopus* oocytes reconstitutes capacitative Ca^{2+} entry. Proc Natl Acad Sci USA. 1996;93:14146-14151.
189. DasGupta S, Qian F, Miller RJ, Philipson LH. Expression of MTrpb-1 a mammalian *Trp* homologue in neuronal and non-neuronal cells. Neurosci Abst 1996;22:1028.
190. Boulay G, Zhu X, Peyton M, Jiang M, Hurst R, Stefani E, Birnbaumer L. Cloning and expression of a novel mammalian homolog of *Drosophila Transient Receptor Potential* (Trp) involved in calcium entry secondary to activation of receptors coupled by the G_q class of G protein. J Biol Chem 1997;272:29672-29680.
191. Birnbaumer L, Zhu X, Jiang M, Boulay G, Peyton M, Vannier B, Brown D, Platano D, Sadeghi H, Stefani E, Birnbaumer M. On the molecular basis and regulation of cellular capacitative calcium entry: Roles for Trp proteins. Proc Natl Acad Sci USA. 1996;93:15195-15202.
192. Petersen CCH, Berridge MJ, Borgese MF, Bennett DL. Putative capacitative calcium entry channels: expression of *Drosophila trp* and evidence for the existence of vertebrate homologues. Biochem J 1995;311:41-44.
193. Leech CA, Habener JF. A role for Ca^{2+}-dependent non-selective cation channels in regulating the membrane potential of pancreatic β-cells. Diabetes 1998;47:1066-1073.
194. Bertram R, Smolen P, Sherman A, Mears D, Atwater I, Martin F, Soria B. A role for calcium release-activated current (CRAC) in cholinergic modulation of electrical activity in pancreatic β cells. Biophys J 1995;68:1-10.
195. Mears D, Sheppard NF, Atwater I, Rojas E, Bertram R, Sherman A. Evidence that calcium release-activated current mediates the biphasic electrical activity of mouse pancreatic β-cells. J Membrane Biol 1997;155:47-59.
196. Kinard TA, Satin LS. An ATP-sensitive Cl^- channel current that is activated by cell swelling, cAMP, and glyburide in insulin-secreting cells. Diabetes 1995;44:1461-1466.
197. Eddleston GT, Beigelman PM. Pancreatic β-cell electrical activity: the role of anions and the control of pH. Am J Physiol 1983;244:C188-C197.
198. Horn R, Marty A. Muscarinic activation of ionic currents measured by a new whole-cell recording method. J Gen Physiol 1988;92:145-159.
199. Kozak JA, Logothetis DE. A calcium-dependent chloride current in insulin-secreting βTC-3 cells. Pflugers Arch 1997;433:679-690.
200. Best L. Glucose and α-ketoisocaproate induce transient inward currents in rat pancreatic beta cells. Diabetologia 1997;40:1-6.
201. Miley HE, Sheader EA, Brown PD, Best L. Glucose-induced swelling in rat pancreatic β-cells. J Physiol 1997;504:191-198.

202. Best L, Sheader EA, Brown PD. A volume-activated anion conductance in insulin-secreting cells. Pflugers Arch 1996;431:363-370.
203. Miley HE, Brown PD, Best L. Regulation of a volume-sensitive anion channel in rat pancreatic β-cells by intracellular adenine nucleotides. J Physiol 1999;515:413-417.
204. Barg S, Renstrom E, Berggren PO, Bertorello A, Bokvist K, Eliasson L, Holmes WE, Kohler M, Rorsman P, Thevenod F. The stimulatory action of tolbutamide on Ca^{2+}-dependent exocytosis in pancreatic β cells is mediated by a 65-kDa mdr-like P-glycoprotein. Proc Natl Acad Sci USA 1999;96:5539-5544.
205. Muller G, Geisen K. Characterization of the molecular mode of action of the sulfonylurea, glimeprimide, at adipocytes. Horm Metab Res 1996;28:469-487.
206. Vanoye CG, Castro AF, Pourcher T, Reuss L, Altenberg GA. Phosphorylation of P-glycoprotein by PKA and PKC modulates swelling-activated Cl^- currents. Am J Physiol 1999;276:C370-C378.
207. Renstrom E, Eliasson L, Rorsman P. Protein kinase A-dependent and -independent stimulation of exocytosis by cAMP in mouse pancreatic β-cells. J Physiol 1997;502:105-118.
208. Hisatomi M, Hidaka H, Niki I. Ca^{2+}/calmodulin and cyclic 3',5' adenosine monophosphate control movement of secretory granules through protein phosphorylation/dephosphorylation in the pancreatic β-cell. Endocrinology 1996;137:4644-4649.
209. Lang J. Molecular mechanisms and regulation of insulin exocytosis as a paradigm of endocrine secretion. Eur J Biochem 1998;259:1-16.
210. Takahashi N, Kadowaki T, Yazaki Y, Ellis-Davies GCR, Miyashita Y, Kasai H. Post-priming actions of ATP on Ca^{2+}-dependent exocytosis in pancreatic beta cells. Proc Natl Acad Sci USA 1999;96:760-765.
211. Sato Y, Anello M, Henquin JC. Glucose regulation of insulin secretion independent of the opening or closure of adenosine triphosphate-sensitive K^+ channels in β-cells. Endocrinology 1999;140:2252-2257.
212. Aizawa T, Komatsu M, Asanuma N, Sato Y, Sharp GW. Glucose action "beyond ionic events" in the pancreatic β cell. Trends Pharmacol Sci 1998;19:496-499.
213. Aizawa T, Sato Y, Ishihara F, Taguchi N, Komatsu M, Suzuki N, Hashizume K, Yamada T. ATP-sensitive K^+ channel-independent glucose action in rat pancreatic β cell. Am J Physiol 1994;266:C622-C627.
214. Kieffer TJ, Heller RS, Leech CA, Holz GG, Habener JF. Leptin suppression of insulin secretion by the activation of ATP-sensitive K^+ channels in pancreatic β-cells. Diabetes 1997;46:1087-1093.
215. Harvey J, McKenna F, Herson PS, Spanswick D, Ashford MLJ. Leptin activates ATP-sensitive potassium channels in the rat insulin-secreting cell line, CRI-G1. J Physiol 1997;504:527-535.
216. Seufert JR, Kieffer TJ, Leech CA, Holz GG, Moritz W, Ricordi C, Habener JF. Leptin suppression of insulin secretion and gene expression in human pancreatic islets: Implications for the development of adipogenic diabetes mellitus. J Clin Endo Metab 1999;84:670-676.
217. Seufert J, Kieffer TJ, Habener JF. Leptin inhibits insulin gene transcription and reverses hyperinsulinemia in leptin-deficient *ob/ob* mice. Proc Natl Acad Sci USA 1999;96:674-679.
218. Kieffer TJ, Heller RS, Habener JF. Leptin receptors expressed on pancreatic β-cells. Biochem Biophys Res Comm 1996;224:522-527.
219. Zhang Y, Proenca R, Maffei M, Barone M, Leopold L, Friedman JM. Positional cloning of the mouse obese gene and its human homologue. Nature 1995;372:425-432.
220. Tartaglia LA, Dembski M, Weng X, Deng N, Culpepper J, Devos R, Richards GJ, Campfield LA, Clark FT, Deeds J, Muir C, Sanker S, Moriarty A, Moore KJ, Smutko JS, Mays GG, Woolf EA, Monroe CA, Tepper RI. Identification and expression cloning of a leptin receptor, OB-R. Cell 1995;83:1263-1271.
221. Tartaglia LA. The leptin receptor. J Biol Chem 1997;272:6093-6096.
222. Kellerer M, Koch M, Metzinger E, Mushack J, Capp E, Haring HU. Leptin activates PI-3 kinase in C2C12 myotubes via janus kinase-2 (JAK-2) and insulin receptor substrate-2 (IRS-2) dependent pathways. Diabetologia 1997;40:1358-1362.
223. Zhou YT, Shimabukuro M, Koyama K, Lee Y, Wang MY, Trieu F, Newgard CB, Unger RH. Induction by leptin of uncoupling protein-2 and enzymes of fatty acid oxidation. Proc Natl Acad Sci USA 1997;94:6386-6390.
224. Emilsson V, Liu YL, Cawthorne MA, Morton NM, Davenport M. Expression of the functional leptin receptor mRNA in pancreatic islets and direct inhibitory action of leptin on insulin secretion. Diabetes 1997;46:313-316.
225. Zhao AZ, Bornfeldt KE, Beavo JA. Leptin inhibits insulin secretion by activation of phosphodiesterase 3B. J Clin Invest 1998;102:869-873.
226. Ookuma M, Ookuma K, York DA. Effects of leptin on insulin secretion from isolated rat pancreatic islets. Diabetes 1998;47:219-223.
227. Chen NG, Swick AG, Romsos DR. Leptin constrains acetylcholine-induced insulin secretion from pancreatic islets of *ob/ob* mice. J Clin Invest 1997;100:1174-1179.
228. Harvey J, Ashford MLJ. Role of tyrosine phosphorylation in leptin activation of ATP-sensitive K^+ channels in the rat insulinoma cell line CRI-G1. J Physiol 1998;510:47-61.

229. Morton NM, Emilsson V, deGroot P, Pallet AL, Cawthorne MA. Leptin signalling in pancreatic islets and clonal insulin-secreting cells. J Mol Endocrinol 1999;22:173-184.
230. Wang MY, Koyama K, Shimabukuro M, Mangelsdorf D, Newgard CB, Unger RH. Overexpression of leptin receptors in pancreatic islets of Zucker diabetic fatty rats restores GLUT-2, glucokinase, and glucose-stimulated insulin secretion. Proc Natl Acad Sci USA 1998;95:11921-11926.

8
COMMUNICATION OF ISLET CELLS: MOLECULES AND FUNCTIONS

Paolo Meda, M.D. and Domenico Bosco, Ph.D.
University of Geneva Medical School, CH-1211 Geneva 4, Switzerland

INTRODUCTION

The appearance of multicellular systems, approximately 800 million years ago, was dependent on the ability of cells to develop mechanisms for adhesion to neighbours and to components of an extracellular matrix, as well as mechanisms for exchange of signals between adjacent and distant cells. With evolution, such mechanisms diversified and have been progressively integrated into a complex regulatory network, whereby individual cells sense the state of activity of their neighbours and adapt their own level of function.

Like most other types of vertebrate cells, islet cells communicate in a variety of ways that differ in the types of structures and mechanisms used to establish cellular cross-talk, as well as in the nature of signals exchanged by the communicating cells (1-4). A widespread mechanism for intercellular communication is by way of diffusion in the extracellular space of hormones and neuromediators that are sensed by cells bearing cognate receptors. A second form of cell-to-cell communication is provided by the diffusion in the extracellular space of ions and molecules that enter cells either by free diffusion through the lipid membrane bi-layer or by way of specific channels and transporters. Co-ordination is then achieved by the simultaneous activation of specific metabolic and effector steps in several cells. A common feature of these pathways of communication is that they require signals to diffuse through extracellular spaces. Since these spaces mediate the transfer of information from one cell to another, these forms of cell-to-cell communications are referred to as "indirect." Most cell types also communicate in a "direct" way, i.e. by mechanisms that do not involve the passage of signals through the extracellular space, but require a contact between the interacting cells or between the cells and the extracellular matrix. These mechanisms are dependent on the expression of several families of membrane proteins that have become specialized for cell-to-cell adhesion (Cell Adhesion Molecules and junctional proteins), sealing of the membrane and of the extracellular space (occludins, claudins), direct intercellular exchanges of cytoplasmic ions and molecules (connexins) and cell-to-matrix adhesion (integrins). Most, if not all of these molecules also allow for the reciprocal transmission of signals between the cell membrane and the nucleus, thus linking extracellular signals to gene expression, and *vice versa*. The same molecules also exchange intercellular signals, thereby integrating individual cells into co-ordinated multicellular units.

The secretory cells of pancreatic islets communicate in a variety of ways that include all the indirect and direct mechanisms listed above. Thus, insulin-producing β-cells regulate their functions through interactions with hormones, neuromediators and other signals that reach the pancreas from outside or that are generated within the gland itself (5-8). However, insulin secretion is still a regulated event under *in vitro* conditions that perturb the native blood supply, innervation and flux of extracellular fluid, indicating that islets need not be embedded in their native environment to exhibit regulated secretion. Insulin secretion is altered after β-cells are dispersed, and rapidly improves after re-aggregation of β-cells or their interaction with components of the extracellular matrix (9-16). This circumstance suggests that insulin secretion depends on proper cell-to-cell and cell-to-matrix contact. Here, we briefly summarize the indirect communications that take place between β-cells (5-7). We discuss in more detail the direct communication in the control of islet development and function, particularly in insulin secretion.

INTEGRATING CELLS INTO PANCREATIC ISLETS

In vitro, isolated islets of Langerhans retain most of the secretory characteristics of the intact pancreas, and still acutely respond to natural stimuli of the gland, including glucose. Although quantitatively reduced, the pattern of insulin release and biosynthesis observed during this stimulation is analogous to that observed *in situ*, indicating that islets actually represent functional subunits of the endocrine pancreas. Because each islet releases amounts of insulin that largely exceed those produced by individual β-cells, proper function of an islet implies an adequate co-ordination of its β-cells. This co-ordination is likely to be achieved by multiple mechanisms, involving both indirect and direct intercellular communication.

Indirect Islet Cell Communication

Individual islets of Langerhans respond to most of the neuromediators and hormones that affect the endocrine secretion of the intact pancreas, including the four main islet hormones (5,6,17). Thus, insulin inhibits glucagon secretion, and maybe also the secretion of somatostatin, pancreatic polypeptide; glucagon stimulates insulin and somatostatin secretion; pancreatic polypeptide inhibits somatostatin secretion; somatostatin inhibits the release of all islet hormones (5,6,17). Some of these effects can be prevented by antibodies to specific hormones, suggesting that they are elicited *in vivo* after release of endogenous islet products (5,6,17). Since islet cells are influenced by hormone levels much lower than those found in the venous effluent of the pancreas, it is unlikely that any paracrine effect occurs by diffusion of hormones from the producing cell to nearby targets, through a continuous extracellular space. If this were the case, might islet cell receptors be downregulated by the sustained exposure to high hormone concentrations (5,6,17)? However, it is possible that islet hormones are channelled to specific membrane domains, either by restricted diffusion in the extracellular islet space or by vectorial transport via the islet microcirculation (5-7,17,18). Microvessels originate from afferent arterioles in the centre of the islets that predominantly comprise insulin-producing β-cells, and direct blood flow to the islet periphery (19), a region comprising β-, α-, δ- and PP-cells (20). Comparison of arterial and venous infusions in the presence and absence of hormone-neutralizing antibodies, suggests that blood flow reaches β-cells first, then α-cells and finally δ-cells (17,19). According to this scheme, high concentrations of insulin should almost continuously bath the islet periphery, whereas glucagon and somatostatin reach β-cells after first passing through the systemic circulation. However, whether and how islet hormones actually have any intraislet effect *in vivo* is still the subject of debate, since we still do not know the actual concentration of hormones in the interstitial islet fluid, the flux and direction of this fluid and the distribution of islet cell receptors. Recent studies suggest that insulin signalling is important for islet function. Knockout of the insulin receptors of pancreatic β-cells leads to mice that exhibit loss of insulin secretion in response to glucose and, thus, impaired glucose tolerance (21).

Autonomic ganglia are not found in isolated islets (7), indicating that basal and stimulated insulin secretion may be sustained in the absence of innervation. Nevertheless, interruption of neural input modifies islet function, as revealed by an increased frequency in the oscillations of insulin secretion (22). The rapid oscillations of individual, isolated islets are probably driven by periodic fluctuations of intracellular free Ca^{2+} levels and/or in the glycolytic activity of β-cells (23). *In vivo*, these oscillations may be masked by the longer cycle pulses that result from the neural co-ordination of multiple islets.

In addition to hormones and neuromediators, numerous signals flowing through extracellular spaces co-ordinate β-cell behaviour. For example, electrophysiological characteristics of single β-cells are quite variable and become uniform and stable when β-cells form clusters (23-25). Within intact islets, virtually all β-cells show a high degree of electrical synchronization during both silent and burst periods of electrical activity (23-28), implying an almost immediate intercellular co-ordination of levels of current-carrying ions. This co-ordination is reflected by intracellular Ca^{2+}, whose oscillatory levels appear to be determined collectively by groups of synchronised β-cells rather than by individual β-cells (23), and may rapidly equilibrate across entire islets (29,30). The mechanism responsible for this electrical synchronisation remains to be elucidated. Connexin-dependent coupling is involved (see below), other mechanisms may also contribute. Further, the occurrence in the extracellular islet fluid of K^+ waves that regularly precede the bursts of electrical activity (31) may provide a rapid and efficient way for coordinating membrane depolarization, as well as the subsequent Ca^{2+} oscillations and insulin release in distant β-cells (8). Still other islet cell interactions may involve signalling by cytokines and nitric oxide (32-35).

Direct Islet Cell Communication

Regulated secretion is dependent on preservation of at least some of the contacts cells establish within the islets of Langerhans. Disruption of such contacts markedly perturbs the secretory response of β-cells (9-16). This observation, and the rapid recovery of a qualitatively normal secretory response with cell reaggregation, suggest an important role for direct communications mediated by cell-to-cell and/or cell-to-matrix contact. Islet cells express a variety of membrane proteins that allow for such communications (Figure 1), including integrins, cadherins, connexins and other junctional proteins (Table 1).

Integrins

Integrins are dimers of two glycoprotein chains, broadly divided into α- and β-subtypes that associate as non-covalent dimers (Figure 1). Approximately twenty different combinations of various α- and β-chains have been described. Regardless of the subunit composition, α- and β-chains function as receptors that bind with their amino terminal region to specific ligand molecules of the basal lamina. This binding is dependent on Mn^{2+} and Mg^{2+} ions, while dissociation is dependent on extracellular Ca^{2+}. In cell-matrix interactions, integrins function as receptors for molecules, such as collagen, laminin, fibronectin and vitronectin. Most cells express multiple integrin dimers, each with its own affinity for specific extracellular molecules and, conversely, distinct components of the extracellular matrix may be bound by several integrin isoforms (36). This adjustable system allows epithelial cells to adhere firmly to the basal lamina, while preserving their ability to crawl along its surface (37). The carboxyl terminal tail of α- and especially β-integrin chains are connected to cytoplasmic microfilaments via adapter proteins, such as talin or α-actinin (Figure 1 and Table 1).

This organization leads to a system in which the cytoskeleton regulates the concentration of integrins in the plasma membrane, whereas the molecular composition of the basal lamina modulates, through integrin binding, cellular functions such as secretion of metalloproteases, apoptosis, cell cycle and gene expression (38-42).

Integrins also function as centers to sort and dispatch cellular messages for both intracellular and intercellular signalling (39,43,44). Thus, binding of integrins to their extracellular ligand transfers a signal that may alter attachment to the cytoskeleton and, therefore, cell anchorage, whereas stimulation of intracellular messenger pathways may alter integrin affinity for proteins of the extracellular matrix and, hence, cell adherence. Upon ligand binding, integrins acquire the ability to interact with cytoskeletal proteins, a step that, in hemidesmosomes, requires tyrosine phosphorylation of the β_4 subunit (45). This phosphorylation event appears to be necessary to activate signalling pathways dependent on Ras and Rho. These two members of the superfamily of small GTPases transduce signals from tyrosine kinase receptors to both nucleus (Ras) and cytoskeleton (Rho), and initiate a cascade of phosphorylations that activates the mitogen-activated protein kinases. Central elements in the co-ordination of this bi-directional transfer of information are focal adhesion kinase, a multifunctional tyrosine kinase that directly interacts with several β integrin subunits, and integrin-linked kinase (46-49).

Integrins containing a β_1 chain are expressed in undifferentiated pancreatic cells that may comprise progenitors of islet cells (Table 1) (50). These progenitors are initially located within the epithelium of pancreatic ducts and form islets, by clustering around a capillary network, after migration into the pancreatic mesenchyme (51). Integrins may be important molecules in directing migration of these cells. Ductal cells of foetal pancreas express $\alpha_v\beta_3$ and $\alpha_v\beta_5$, two integrins also found at high levels in cell clusters budding out from the ducts but less so in differentiated hormone-containing cells of organised islets (52). Adult islet cells express low levels of $\alpha_v\beta_3$ and $\alpha_v\beta_5$ integrins (52-54).

Fully differentiated β- and non β-cells express $\alpha_3\beta_1$ and $\alpha_6\beta_1$ and low levels of $\alpha_v\beta_3$ and $\alpha_v\beta_5$ integrins (52-54). When cultured on a matrix containing laminin, primary and immortalized β-cells strongly adhere to the substratum and spread out on it within a few hours (Figure 2). Antibodies against the β_1 chain of integrins inhibit the spreading out of cells, indicating that this, *in vitro*, is important for β-cell attachment (53,54). Whether integrins have the same function *in vivo* is unknown. Integrins are not confined to regions of contact between the basal portion of the cell membrane and the matrix, but are also localised at cell-cell interfaces (53,54). This suggests that, as it is the case in other cell types (55,56), integrins may also mediate β-to-β-cell interaction in addition to ensuring cell-matrix interaction. This possibility is further supported by the finding that integrin $\alpha_6\beta_1$ is expressed heterogeneously between β-cells (54), in a pattern reminiscent of - if not correlated with - the heterogeneity in the secretory response of individual β-cells (15,16). Glucose concentrations that enhance insulin release by decreasing the heterogeneous behaviour of single cells selectively upregulate the expression of $\alpha_6\beta_1$ as well as the attachment and spreading of β-cells on laminin V (54).

Extracellular Ligands of Integrins

Epithelial cells are dependent on an underlying extracellular matrix that serves both as a selective filter for passage of nutrients and as a site for binding of growth factors and other signalling molecules that control cell motility, proliferation and differentiation during both morphogenetic development and adult life. Changes in type and concentration of these signal molecules are sensed by integrins that act as surface receptors for different extracellular ligands (Figure 1). The signal molecules are in the basal lamina, which is a layer of extracellular material produced by the epithelial cells. It is typically subdivided into a superficial region, referred to as the lamina lucida, that is mainly composed of laminin and perlecan, and a deeper region, the lamina densa, where proteoglycans and glycoproteins are intermingled with type IV collagen and fibronectin. The latter components are synthesized by cells of the underlying connective tissues. The combination and prevalence of each signal molecule differs depending on the type of epithelial cell (57-59).

Neonatal and adult rat pancreatic cells cultured in a collagen matrix form three-dimensional aggregates similar to islets embedded in the pancreas (60-62). Whether components of the extracellular matrix are also important for the ontogeny of pancreatic islets *in vivo*, remains to be assessed. In human pancreas, fibronectin and vitronectin colocalize around endocrine cells budding out of the ducts, and collagen IV as well as laminin are present in more organized islets (52). Rat pancreatic islets produce matrix metalloproteinases that are involved in the turnover of extracellular matrix and tissue remodelling (63). Morphogenesis of rat islets is associated with an activation of metalloproteinases, and is inhibited under conditions that inhibit activity of these enzymes (64). Thus, changes in the composition of the extracellular matrix, possibly as a result of its remodelling, are involved in the migration of duct cells and/or in their subsequent differentiation into mature islet cells.

In adult vertebrates, most pancreatic islets are surrounded by a capsule of connective tissue whose thickness varies in different animal species (65). Collagen, laminin and fibronectin are major constituents of this capsule (65-67). Different components of the extracellular matrix form basal laminas that separate islet cells from the endothelial cells of capillaries. While the molecules of the basal lamina remain to be fully identified, some of these molecules also influence β-cell function.

Some extracellular molecules also appear to enhance the life span (61) and proliferation rates (70-72,75) of adult β-cells. Adult human islet cells (76) and pancreatic ductal cells (77) proliferate faster when exposed to a matrix produced by a rat-bladder carcinoma cell line. Levels of insulin, glucagon and somatostatin mRNAs are increased in both rat islets (78) and a rat insulinoma cell line when cultured on extracellular matrices (79).

Cell Adhesion Molecules

Epithelial cells strongly adhere to each other via numerous types of surface molecules that are generally cadherins and cell adhesion molecules (CAMs). Cadherins operate in Ca^{2+}-dependent cell adhesion (81,82), whereas other CAMs belonging to the immunoglobulin family are involved in Ca^{2+}-independent cell adhesion (3,80). CAMs tightly link adjacent cells, ensuring the physical cohesiveness of an epithelium. They are crucial for epithelial morphogenesis. By controlling the migration and sorting of different cell types as well as their precise topographic arrangement within tissues (3,80), CAMs also influence the final differentiation of epithelial cells (81,82).

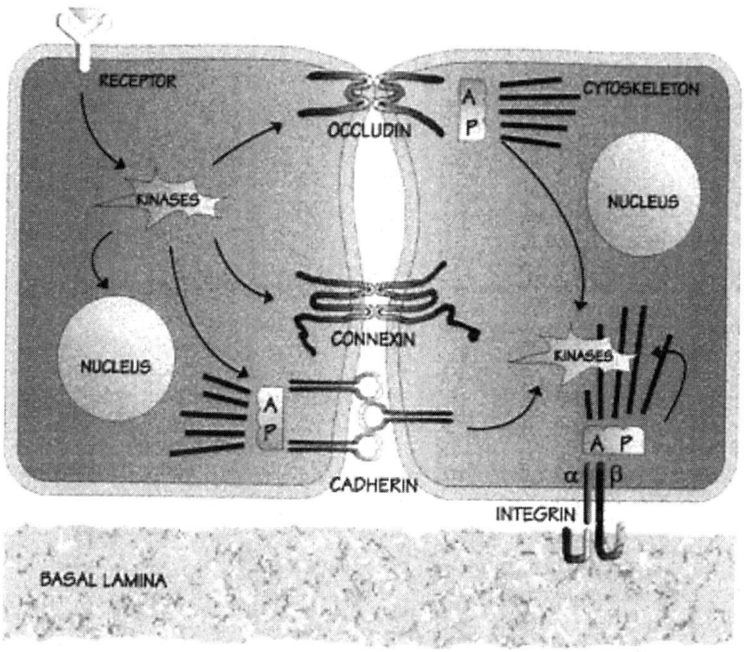

Figure 1. *Topography of the membrane molecules that mediate direct interactions between epithelial cells. Integrins are dimers of* α *and* β *chains, whose amino termini bind to components of the basal lamina. The carboxyl termini of integrins extend in the cytoplasm where they interact with actin microfilaments, via various intracellular attachment proteins (AP). Integrins may concentrate to form hemidesmosomes that are associated to intermediate filaments of keratins. Cadherins are single pass, transmembrane glycoproteins, whereas other CAMs, such as N-CAM, are usually attached to the membrane by a glycosylphosphatidylinositol anchor. In the presence of* Ca^{2+}, *dimers of two cadherin molecules interdigitate in the extracellular space with two analogous structures of an adjacent cell, as in a zipper. The carboxy termini of cadherins extend in the cytoplasm where they interact, via various attachment proteins, with actin microfilaments. Cadherins may concentrate in the lateral portion of the cell membrane to form adherens junctions or desmosomes. In the latter case, attachment proteins link cadherins to intermediate filaments of keratins. Connexins are integral proteins with four transmembrane regions. At gap junctions, hexamers of these proteins interact in the extracellular space with similar structures made by an adjacent cell to form an intercellular channel that permits the exchange of ions and molecules between the cytoplasm of adjacent cells. The termini of connexins, which extend in the cytoplasm, do not interact with cytoskeletal elements. Occludins and claudins also feature four transmembrane regions. At focal sites, these molecules interact to closely link adjacent cells and to establish a barrier that separates the apical from the basolateral region of the membrane. Both molecules are connected, through multiple intracellular attachment proteins, to actin microfilaments. Several membrane proteins that ensure cell interactions also serve as integration and sorting centers for signals that regulate the activity of individual cells and co-ordinate it within tissues. These effects are mediated via a cascade of events, including the phosphorylation of multiple substrates by various kinases, that affects, in series, the attachment proteins of cytoplasm and elements of cytoskeleton. This chain of events transfers membrane signals to the nucleus and vice versa.*

integral membrane proteins	junctions	cytoplasmic attachment proteins	cytoskeletal structure	functions	presence in β-cells
integrins		talin, vinculin, paxillin, α-actinin	microfilaments (actin)	cell movement, adhesion to basal lamina, cell communication, gene expression	$\alpha_3\beta_1$ $\alpha_6\beta_1$ $\alpha_v\beta_3$ $\alpha_v\beta_5$
$\alpha_6\beta_4$, BPA1, BPA2	hemidesmosome	desmoplakins	intermediate filaments (keratins)	adhesion to basal lamina, gene expression, cell communication	
cell adhesion molecules		catenins	microfilaments (actin)	cell-to-cell adhesion, cell recognition, cell communication, gene expression	cadherins Ep-CAM N-CAM
E,N and P cadherins	intermediate	catenins, vinculin	microfilaments (actin)	cell movement, cell communication, gene expression	
desmocollins desmogleins	desmosome	desmoplakins, catenins ZO-1 ZO-2 ZO-3 Cingulin	intermediate filaments (keratins)	cell-to-cell adhesion, cell communication, gene expression	yes
connexins	gap		α-spectrin ?	cell communication, gene expression	Cx43 ? Cx36 Cx45 ?
occludins, claudins	tight	ZOs, cingulin	microfilaments (actin)	maintenance of membrane polarity, sealing of extracellular space, cell-to-cell adhesion, gene expression	yes

Table 1. *Mediators of direct interactions between epithelial cells*

The molecules involved in Ca^{2+}-independent adhesion belong to the superfamily of immunoglobulins, which is characterized by the presence of immunoglobulin-like repeats. The most abundant and best studied member of this family is neural cell adhesion molecule (N-CAM). This protein occurs in at least 20 different isoforms that result from alternative RNA splicing of a single gene transcript. Some of these isoforms are soluble, others are attached to the plasma membrane via a glycosylphosphatidylinositol anchor, but the majority are glycosylated integral membrane proteins. Immunoglobulin-dependent intercellular adhesion is mechanically weaker than that mediated by cadherins and may be mainly responsible for a fine modulation of specific cell-cell interactions (81,82).

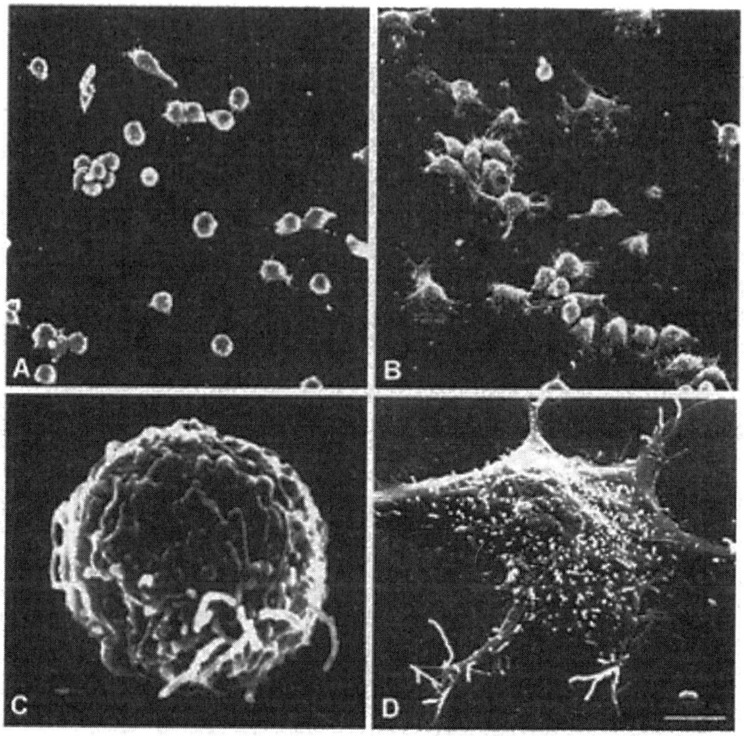

Figure 2. *Function of integrins in pancreatic β-cells. Several proteins of the integrin group ensure adherence of β-cells to components of the extracellular matrix.* ***A)*** *The function of these molecules may be demonstrated by comparing the shape and adherence of cells to different substrates. Under scanning electron microscopy, most cells grown on glass feature a round shape irrespective of whether they are single or form small clumps.* ***B)*** *Coating of glass with an extracellular ligand, causes the rapid spreading of most cells, which acquire a polygonal outline.* ***C*** *and* ***D*** *) Higher magnification views clearly reveal the different appearance of plasma membrane in cells grown in the absence (**C**) and presence of laminin (**D**). The different phenotype presumably results from the rearrangement of cytoplasmic microfilaments that takes place once integrins have bound an extracellular ligand. The bar represents 60 μm in A and B and 7 μm in C and D.*

The cadherin family includes at least twelve different proteins; each encoded by a distinct gene. All cadherins are glycoproteins and share a common structure with one transmembrane domain, a short cytoplasmic carboxyl terminal tail and a large extracellular portion (Figure 1) that consists of five homologous regions that contain Ca^{2+}-binding sites (83). The presence of extracellular Ca^{2+} is essential for the adhesive properties of cadherins. When Ca^{2+} is removed, the extracellular portion is cleaved by proteases and the function of cadherins is lost (Figure 3). Cadherins of adjacent cells interact with each other to form a sort of intercellular "zipper" (83). The strength of interaction between cells is determined by the number of adhesion molecules and not their affinity, which is usually low (84).

Cadherins play a major role in the aggregation of β-cells into islet-like structures (Table 1). Transgenic mice expressing a truncated form of E-cadherin that lacks all extracellular amino acids, β-cells are dispersed throughout pancreas that contains islets formed solely by α-cells (85). Truncated E-cadherin functions as a dominant negative mutant that displaces native E- and N-cadherins, possibly by interfering with their binding to β-catenin, thus preventing their normal function in pancreatic β-cells (85). Other Ca^{2+}-dependent cell adhesion molecules that have been identified in the developing pancreas may also play a morphoregulatory role. In human foetuses, clusters of islet cells budding out from pancreatic ducts express high levels of Ep-CAM (86). The abundance of this cell adhesion molecule decreases as the differentiation of islet cells progresses. Remarkably, antibodies directed against Ep-CAM promote the endocrine differentiation of pancreatic epithelial cells *in vitro* (86).

When cultured in an artificial matrix or on a dish that lacks the coat necessary for the adherence of animal cells, dissociated islet cells spontaneously reaggregate into tridimensional structures that, like native islets, have a centre made of insulin-producing β-cells and a periphery of a mixture of α-, β-, δ- and PP-cells (60,87,88). This segregation of cell phenotypes is controlled by Ca^{2+} independent adhesion molecules (89-91). Topographic arrangement of the different types of islet cells within newly formed aggregates is markedly perturbed *in vitro*, when cells reaggregate in the presence of antibodies against N-CAM (91). *In vivo*, an analogous perturbation is observed in transgenic mice that are N-CAM deficient (92). In this model, α-cells were not located as usual at the periphery of the islets and E-cadherin, P-cadherin and actin are abnormally concentrated in regions of cell-cell contact, and Na^+/K^+-ATPase is not colocalized with cadherins as in control islets. The islet cell nuclei have an unusual location at the periphery of the cell bodies. All these alterations suggest that N-CAM is required for establishing and/or maintaining islet cell polarity (92).

E-, N- and R-cadherins (85,93-95), as well as N- and Ep-CAM are also expressed in adult islets (86,96) (Table 1). It is unlikely that these molecules have the same functions during development as in adult islets, inasmuch as under physiological conditions, adult islets undergo fewer morphogenetic changes than those that take place prenatally. As in other systems, the main function of CAMs in adult islets is to tightly link together adjacent cells.

Connexins

Multicellular organisms co-ordinate the activity of groups of cells under different functional conditions. For example, the response to an external signal may be amplified by recruiting neighbouring cells and, conversely, cells undergoing deleterious changes need to be isolated to preserve the integrity of the group. In either case, a system is required to permit cells to review and shape the functional state of their neighbours by the exchange of signalling molecules. Such a system of communication should also be rapidly modulated, to continuously adapt to the changing needs of coupled cells. These features are met by the intercellular channels that are located at distinct regions of the plasma membrane, known as gap junctions, that are found in all metazoans, regardless of their phylogenetic position. Each of these channels spans two adjacent plasma membranes and is formed by the association of two half channels, or connexons, contributed separately by each of the two participating cells. Connexons are products of a multigene family of highly conserved proteins, called connexins. These molecules feature four transmembrane domains, two extracellular loops and extend both their amino- and their carboxyl-terminus in the cytoplasm. The cytoplasmic domains distinguish different connexin isoforms and are thought to be involved in the regulation of channel permeability. Each connexin isoform conveys a particular set of signals, so that channels made of different connexins may be endowed with distinct biophysical and regulatory properties. Intercellular channels may be homotypic, when the connexons contributed by each cell are composed of the same connexin, or heterotypic, when the connexins are different. Most cell types express more than one connexin and the same connexin may be found expressed by several cell types (4,99,100).

The interaction of two connexons in the extracellular space establishes a direct communication between the cytoplasm of two adjacent cells. Through this pathway, cells rapidly exchange cytoplasmic ions and molecules of less than 900 Daltons that otherwise cannot permeate the cell membrane (ionic and metabolic, cell-to-cell or junctional coupling) (4,99,100). Connexins do not form ion-selective channels in the classical sense, but nevertheless exhibit a certain degree of selectivity for cations and anions. Since connexin channels are also permeable to cyclic nucleotides and inositol trisphosphate that are negatively charged at normal intracellular pH, this selectivity allows for discrimination between different second messengers and, hence, for differential modulation of their intercellular exchange (101). Connexins can discriminate between molecules of 400 and 600 Daltons, thus favouring the passage of a distinct set of signals (101). Intercellular channels are regulated by both covalent and non-covalent modifications of connexins, such as phosphorylation that results in changes in channel permeability depending on the connexin isoform and the cell type involved (101).

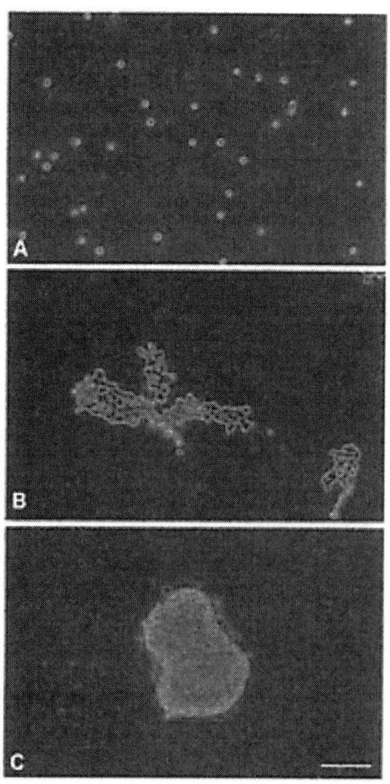

Figure 3. *Function of cadherins between pancreatic β-cells. Ca^{2+}-dependent cell adhesion molecules of the cadherin family are abundantly expressed by pancreatic cells.* **A**) *The function of these proteins may be demonstrated after Ca^{2+} depletion. Under this condition, FACS-purified β-cells dissociate from each other and feature a spherical shape.* **B**) *Addition of a medium containing mM concentrations of Ca^{2+} allows for restoration of the homophilic cadherin interactions, leading to a rapid and spontaneous reaggregation of β-cells into tridimensional clusters. Under these conditions, cells changed their initially spherical shape and featured a linear interface with nearby cells.* **C**) *In a few hours, clusters grow and merge to form compact, tridimensional assemblies in which β-cells feature topographical relationships and distributions alike those observed within native pancreatic islets. The bar represents 100 μm.*

Connexin-dependent cell communication participates in controlling early embryogenetic events, as revealed by drastic alterations in development after functional blockade of connexin channels or aberrant coupling between groups of cells that are usually segregated (100). Connexins have also been implicated in the control of cell division, *in vitro* and *in vivo* (102).

Pancreatic β-cells are connected to each other by numerous gap junctions comprised of the Cx43, Cx36 and Cx45 isoforms of the connexin family (103-106). A normal β-cell contains 800-2000 connexin channels that allow it to exchange ions (23,26,27,30,104,107,108) as well as molecules such as cytoplasmic nucleotides, glycolytic intermediates and exogenous fluorescent probes with nearby β- and non β-cells (104,109-112). Not all cells within an islet consistently exchange molecules, and communication is somewhat spatially redirected to small groups of β-cells (104,107-110,112,104,108-110,113). Hence, the 10-6000 β-cells that may form a pancreatic islet appear to be functionally grouped in multiple communication territories (8,98) rather than in a single syncytial unit.

Single β-cells show decreased secretion and reduced expression of the insulin gene. Isolated β-cells poorly respond to stimulation by glucose and other secretagogues in terms of both insulin release and biosynthesis (9-13,15,16,114-116). Restoration of β-cell contacts is paralleled by a rapid improvement in all these parameters (9-13,15,16,114-116). Connexin channels rapidly form during β-cell reaggregation (10,11) and blocking these channels prevents the increase in insulin secretion that normally occurs as β-cells interact in pairs (16,117). This indicates that coupling may acutely control the recruitment of secreting β-cells as well as their individual level of activity. Sustained stimulation of insulin release increases β-cell coupling *in vivo* and *in vitro* (104,188-121). As yet, there is much less evidence for a more acute regulation of β-cell coupling, resulting from changes in the conductance and/or permeability of existing connexin channels.

Conditions that inhibit insulin release decrease or abolish β-cell coupling (109). *In vivo*, an opposite change is seen whenever the inhibition of β-cell secretion results in hyperglycaemia (121), suggesting that the level of circulating glucose and the ability of β-cells to properly recognise hyperglycemia independently influences junctional coupling. The acute pharmacological blockade of gap junction channels increases basal insulin release and is associated with the loss of stimulated insulin secretion from both isolated islets of Langerhans and islets of an intact pancreas (117,122). These functional changes that cannot be accounted for by concomitant changes in the main second messengers controlling insulin secretion, are rapidly and fully reversible after washing out the uncoupling drugs, and are not observed in single β-cells. This indicates that intact gap junctions are central in the functional coordination of islets (117).

Transformed insulin-producing cell lines show abnormal glucose sensitivity and do not express connexins and gap junctions and are thus uncoupled (123). These defects cannot be explained by the *in vitro* downregulation of gap junctional channels since primary β-cells in monolayer culture retain connexin-dependent coupling (112,123), and cannot be ascribed solely to the proliferative capacity of the cell lines, since the glucose-sensitive cells of a rat insulinoma, from which at least two of the communication-deficient lines were derived, still express connexins and coupling *in vivo* (104,124). Hence, coupling defects appear to be a common feature among cell lines with abnormal sensitivity to glucose. Cell lines that are stably transfected with the gene coding for Cx43, and express gap junctions and coupling similar to primary β-cells, display enhanced expression of the insulin gene, a markedly increased insulin content, and preserved ability of increasing insulin release when stimulated by physiologically relevant concentrations of glucose (123). When implanted in rats, the transfected cells form insulinomas that grow at a slower rate than those formed by wild-type controls lacking connexins, but still induce a faster lethal hypoglycaemia, due to the release of much higher levels of circulating, biologically active insulin (124). In contrast, several clones of the same cells that express unusually high levels of Cx43, gap junctions and coupling, do not show any improvement of these secretory characteristics. Most of these cells show loss of the major features that characterize primary β-cells (123).

To test whether connexins are relevant for the function of non-tumoral β-cells, a number of mouse lines with changes in pancreatic expression of connexins have been generated. Complete deletion of Cx43, Cx32, and of these two proteins in combination, as well as the ectopic expression of Cx32 in β-cells, does not alter pancreatic islet development, the differentiation of β-cells, storage of insulin, and does not lead to metabolic defects. However, mice that express half the amount of Cx43 as compared to controls, develop with age a marked glucose intolerance that is also observed in animals with transgenic overexpression of Cx32 (105,113). The latter animals are hyperinsulinaemic and completely lack responsiveness to physiological glucose levels.

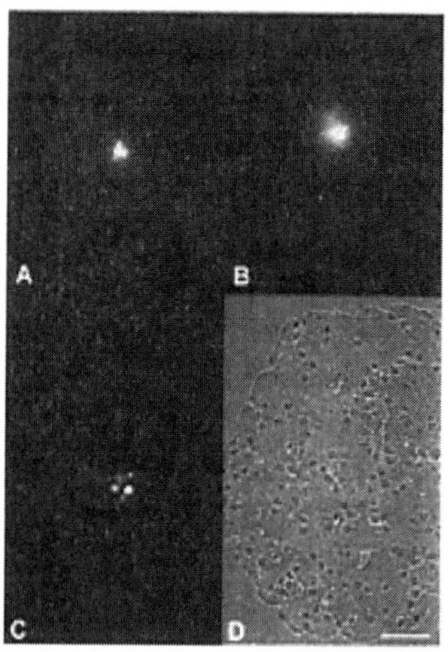

Figure 4. *Function of connexins between pancreatic β-cells. Several connexin isoforms form membrane channels for the direct exchange of cytoplasmic ions and molecules between adjacent β-cells.* ***A)*** *Their function may be demonstrated by microinjecting one β-cell within an isolated islet of Langerhans with a small, hydrophilic and fluorescent tracer molecule (Lucifer Yellow CH in this case) which does not permeate the cell membrane. When connexin channels are opened, the tracer is rapidly transferred from the injected cell into adjacent cells, revealing territories of intercommunicating cells.* ***B)*** *The size of such territories enlarges in islets of animals treated with glibenclamide to stimulate the release of insulin.* ***C)*** *Analysis of sections cut throughout the microinjected islets reveals that, under control conditions, communicating territories comprise 3-8 β-cells. About six of such coupled cells are identified in this section, observed under fluorescence illumination.* ***D)*** *Phase-contrast view of the section shown in C. The bar represents 80 μm in A and B and 50 μm in C and D.*

Transgenic mice with β-cells expressing Cx32 also feature unusually large islets (125), indicating that coupling may also participate in the control of islet cell growth *in vivo*. Because the animals over expressing Cx32 feature increased levels of junctional communication, the data also implicate that connexin-dependent communication needs to be maintained within precise limits for proper β-cell secretion and growth.

Other Junctions

Tight junctions are focal points of cell-to-cell contact that prevent the movement of proteins and lipids between the apical and the basolateral regions of the plasma membrane. These structures thus lead to a structural and functional polarization of epithelial cells (126). By preventing free diffusion of fluids, solutes and cells across the paracellular space, tight junctions also contribute to a selective permeability of epithelial cells. A tight junction consists of an extracellular, a transmembrane and a cytoplasmic portion made of claudins and occludins (Figure 1). Within the cytoplasm, the carboxyl terminus of an occludin interacts with various intracellular attachment proteins (of the ZO and the cingulin family), each of which functionally links claudins to occludins and to the actin microfilaments of the cytoskeleton. Tight junctions are functionally heterogeneous and plastic structures whose selective permeability may be modulated by various kinase-dependent mechanisms, triggered by both CAMs and intracellular signals (127,128). Structures similar to tight junctions have been documented between the insulin-producing β-cells (20). However, contrary to what is observed in most other types of adult epithelia, the islet fibrils do not form a continuous belt around cells and, hence, do completely seal the intercellular spaces of islets. No study has actually assessed the presence of tight junction proteins in the islets.

In a variety of epithelial cells, specific cadherin isoforms accumulate in discrete regions of the lateral cell membrane to form adherens, or intermediate junctions. Via cytoplasmic catenins, the carboxyl terminal tail of cadherins interacts with actin filaments (127), thus functionally connecting the cytoskeleton of adjacent cells into an intercellular network. Such connections confer mechanical strength to tissues, and permits cells to retain their specific tridimensional shape (127,131). Contraction of the intercellular cytoskeletal network further enables sheets of epithelial cells to fold and to undergo a variety of other tridimensional reorganisations that are essential for tissue morphogenesis. Adherens junctions also function as signalling centres by a mechanism that is presumably triggered by changes in the phosphorylation status of catenins. Several tyrosine kinases accumulate in the vicinity of adherens junctions where they act on substrate junctional molecules, thereby modulating cellular adhesion and morphology (40,132). Whether adherens junctions also connect islet cells remains to be investigated.

Desmosomes provide adjacent cells with mechanically strong adhesive and anchoring junctions that give strength and resistance to sheets of epithelial cells. These junctions consist of adhesion molecules of the cadherin family whose cytoplasmic carboxyl tails are anchored, via multiple adapter proteins, to the various isoforms of keratin molecules that form intermediate filaments (131). This arrangement establishes an intercellular network that links and stabilizes the membranes of adjacent cells, and is continuously altered for modulation of cell shape, differentiation and mobility (127,131). Small desmosomes are found between islet cells (129). However, the function of these structures remains hypothetical, since pancreatic islets are not exposed to major mechanical constraints.

INTEGRATING ISLETS INTO THE ENDOCRINE PANCREAS

Insulin secretion is a multicellular event, resulting from the co-ordinated activation of numerous β-cells that form the bulk of pancreatic islets. Hence, some mechanism should functionally link the numerous islets that collectively form the endocrine pancreas. Furthermore, since insulin secretion normally undergoes cyclic fluctuations (18,22) and should be continuously adapted to the changing needs of the organism, the mechanisms coordinating the function of individual islets should also allow a dynamic, moment-to-moment modulation of β-cell function.

Co-ordination of distinct islets must rely on mechanisms of indirect communication, since most islets are separated from each other by basal laminae, connective tissue constituents and exocrine acini. Experimentally, stimulation of insulin secretion is induced by gastric inhibitory peptide, thyrotropin-releasing hormone, glucagon-like peptide 1, β-adrenergic agonists, acetylcholine, cholecystokinin, gastrin-releasing peptide and vasoactive intestinal peptide. Conversely, inhibition is induced by corticotropin-releasing factor, peptide YY, atrial natriuretic peptide, pancreastatin, α_2-adrenergic agonists, galanin, and neuropeptide Y. Which of these factors actually control insulin secretion *in vivo* remains to be determined. The current view is that the secretory response of β-cells that is initiated by circulating nutrients, is essentially modulated by gut hormones, and particularly by gastric inhibitory peptide, glucagon-like peptide-1 and cholecystokinin (5-7,18,133).

No physiological stimulus increases the levels of glucose, other nutrients and gut hormones, with the speed and magnitude required to induce an almost immediate and synchronous activation of all pancreatic islets. Such a massive, all or none signal may be inappropriate to ensure the long-term pulsatility of insulin secretion, which is observed *in vivo* and *in vitro* (18,22). Hence, fine tuning of islet co-ordination requires an additional connection between these micro-organs. The observation that pulsatility of insulin secretion is preserved in the absence of hormonal circulation (18,22) suggests that this connection is ensured by the intrapancreatic nervous system. Since insulin pulses are perturbed by tetrodotoxin but not by drugs blocking cholinergic and adrenergic receptors, islet co-ordination most likely involves autonomous intrapancreatic ganglia that serve both as pacemakers and as integration centers (18). These ganglia receive adrenergic, cholinergic and peptidergic inputs, and their postganglionic fibres are seen to interconnect endocrine islets (7).

FUNCTIONS OF ISLET CELL COMMUNICATION

The studies summarized above demonstrate that the insulin-producing β-cells, and presumably also other types of islet cells, directly interact with each other in multiple ways, via a number of different surface molecules. These proteins are specialized to couple events taking place outside the cell to changes in gene expression, via a series of intermediate proteins that form a functional continuum between the plasma membrane and the nucleus, across the cytoplasm. These proteins also transfer signals between adjacent cells across a tissue. The network of communication that these proteins establish contributes in multiple ways to control the major functions of pancreatic islets. It appears that, as in other epithelial systems, different mechanisms contribute to a specific islet function. Whereas cadherins appear prominent in governing islet development, together with integrins they also control islet cell growth. Connexins co-ordinate islet cell function, particularly the regulated biosynthesis and release of insulin. However, a substantial degree of overlap and interdependence of function exists between these intercellular connections. For example, cell communication via connexins depends on the preliminary contact of cells that is mediated by cell adhesion molecules, and is also influenced by integrins and other types of junctional contacts (102).

ISLET CELL DEVELOPMENT AND GROWTH

Development of islets from endocrine stem cells that are thought to be located in pancreatic ducts, involves a series of morphogenetic events including cell migration, growth, sorting and differentiation. These events are predominantly controlled by CAMs, including several cadherins, as well as the Ca^{2+}-independent N- and Epi-CAM (85,86,91,92). Integrins may also be involved in these processes (50,52-54).

The growth capacity of primary islet cells markedly decreases with their postnatal, final differentiation, even though adult, fully differentiated β-cells retain a limited potential to proliferate throughout life. This potential appears to be enhanced by molecules of the extracellular matrix that are presumably recognised by specific integrins (61,70-72,75-77). Recent observations further suggest that β-cell growth is also promoted by changes in connexins, particularly when Cx36 and Cx43 are replaced or complemented by Cx32, a connexin isoform that provides the channels with conductance and permeability characteristics different from those of the channels that natively connect β-cells (125).

In contrast to primary β-cells, transformed insulin-producing cells grow almost continuously. This change appears to be controlled by cell adhesion molecules, inasmuch as insulinomas develop in transgenic mice that lack E-cadherin (135). Furthermore, whereas normal islets express a 120-kDa isoform of N-CAM that is linked to the membrane via a glycophosphatidylinositol anchor, insulinomas have two transmembrane isoforms of this protein of 140 and 180 kDa, respectively (136). When N-CAM knockout mice are crossed with transgenic mice expressing the SV40 T antigen under control of an insulin promoter, the insulinomas metastasise. Metastasis is prevented by crossing mice with transgenic mice whose β-cells express the 120 kDa isoform of N-CAM (135). The data clearly indicate that CAMs play an important role in controlling the growth and spatial dissemination of islet tumours. Still, other mechanisms may also contribute to this control. Inverse correlation exists between the extent of connexin-dependent communication and tumorigenesis (137). In fact, connexins have been regarded as tumour suppressors, inasmuch as they allow for the passage of growth regulatory signals that inhibit cell division (102). Enhanced coupling after connexin overexpression leads to reduced growth of multiple types of tumour cells (137), including an experimental insulinoma (124).

CONCLUSIONS AND PERSPECTIVES

Epithelial cells use multiple systems to recognise and adhere to each other and to the extracellular matrix, via the expression of specific combinatorial sets of surface molecules that transduce signals within and between cells. Once adhesion molecules have ensured cell recognition, migration and adhesion, that are essential initial events in the building plan of a tissue, they become necessary for both the formation of junctions and for the interaction with the cytoskeleton elements that stabilise tissue structure. As a result of these interactions, epithelial cells become polarised and develop specialised functions in distinct membrane domains, whose maintenance depends on the contact with other cells and the extracellular matrix. Among these membrane domains, junctional complexes play a pivotal role in generating, receiving, and integrating extracellular as well as intracellular and intercellular signals. Abnormal function of these systems is responsible for several human diseases.

Insulin secretion results from the activity of numerous and functionally heterogeneous cells, whose integration depends on proper communication. As the mechanisms of this communication are unravelled, it becomes evident that full control of β-cell function is dependent on the interactions between multiple mechanisms that involve cell-to-cell signalling by nutrients, intrinsic and extrinsic neural inputs, local and circulating hormones, as well as direct interactions between adjacent cells and between these cells and their surrounding extracellular matrix. A major problem in unravelling the regulation of insulin secretion stems from the complexity of the interactions between these signals, which converge at the islet level. The mechanisms ensuring communication of islet cells functionally overlap to some extent and, hence, may partly or totally replace each other in case one mechanism is disturbed.

The precise contribution of different communication mechanisms to the net response of pancreatic islets remains to be fully understood, as does their hierarchic organization. In this respect, CAMs appear to play a central role during islet development and, together with integrins, in the control of islet cell growth. In contrast, the influence of these molecules is less evident in modulating the function of primary, fully differentiated islets. In this context, connexins appear to have a predominant role. In view of the functional heterogeneity of β-cells, the communication mediated by these proteins provides the most direct way for compensation of intrinsic metabolic and effector differences of secretory cells. By equilibrating ions and molecules across domains of coupled cells, junctional communication allows rapid changes in secretory function, appropriate output of insulin. Junctional communication is tightly linked to the ability of β-cells to appropriately release and synthesize insulin, and that abnormal coupling participates in the loss of β-cell responsiveness to secretagogues.

ACKNOWLEDGEMENTS

I wish to thank my coworkers J. Bauquis, L. Burkhardt, D. Caille, A. Calabrese, D. Caton, A. Charollais, F. De Leon, C. Devenoges, P. Fruleux, V. Serre, E. Sutter, L. Wiszniewski and A. Wonkam for their essential implication in these studies. Our work was supported by grants from the Swiss National Science Foundation (3100-053720), the Juvenile Diabetes Foundation International (197124), the European Union (QLG1-CT-1997-00516), and the programme commun de recherche en genie biomedical (1999-2002).

REFERENCES

1. LeRoith D. Are all cells "endocrine"? In: Becker KL, ed. Principles and Practice of Endocrinology and Metabolism. Philadelphia: JB Lippincott Company, 1990:10-3.
2. Greenwald I, Rubin GM. Making a difference: the role of cell-to-cell interactions in establishing separate identities for equivalent cells. Cell 1992;68:271-81.
3. Edelman GM, Crossin KL. Cell adhesion molecules: implications for a molecular histology. Ann Rev Biochem 1991;60:155-90.
4. Kumar NM, Gilula NB. Molecular biology and genetics of gap junction channels. Sem Cell Biol 1992;3:3-16.
5. Samols E, Stagner JI. Intraislet and islet-acinar portal systems and their significance. In: Samols E, ed. The Endocrine Pancreas. New York: Raven Press, 1991:93-124.
6. Marks V, Samols E, Stagner J. Intra-islet interactions. In: Flatt PR, ed. Nutrient Regulation of Insulin Secretion. London: Portland Press 1992:41-57.

7. Berggren PO, Rorsman P, Efendic S, et al. Mechanisms of action of entero-insular hormones, islet peptides and neural input on the insulin secretory process. In: Flatt PR, ed. Nutrient Regulation of Insulin Secretion. London: Portland Press, 1992;289-318.
8. Meda P. Junctional coupling of pancreatic β-cells. In: Huizinga JD, ed. Pacemaker activity and intercellular communication. Boca Raton, Florida: CRC Press, 1995:275-91.
9. Pipeleers D. Islet cell interactions with pancreatic β-cells. Experientia 1984;40:1114-26.
10. Chertow BS, Baranetsky NG, Sivitz WI, et al. Cellular mechanisms of insulin release. Effects of retinoids on rat islet cell-to-cell adhesion, reaggregation, and insulin release. Diabetes 1983;32:568-74.
11. Halban PA, Wollheim CB, Blondel B, et al. The possible importance of contact between pancreatic islet cells for the control of insulin release. Endocrinology 1982;111:86-94.
12. Maes E, Pipeleers D. Effects of glucose and 3',5'-cyclic adenosine monophosphate upon reaggregation of single pancreatic B-cells. Endocrinology 1984;114:2205-9.
13. Lernmark A. The preparation of, and studies on, free cell suspensions from mouse pancreatic islets. Diabetologia 1974;10:431-8.
14. Pipeleers D. Heterogeneity in pancreatic β-cell population. Diabetes 1992;41:777-81.
15. Salomon D, Meda P. Heterogeneity and contact-dependent regulation of hormone secretion by individual β-_cells. Exp CellRes 1986;162:507-20.
16. Bosco D, Orci L, Meda P. Homologous but not heterologous contact increases the insulin secretion of individual pancreatic β-cells. Exp Cell Res 1989;184:72-80.
17. Kawai K, Ipp E, Orci L, et al. Circulating somatostatin acts on the islets of Langerhans by way of a somatostatin-poor compartment. Science 1982;218:477-8.
18. Stagner JI. Pulsatile secretion from the endocrine pancreas: metabolic, hormonal, and neural modulation. In: Samols E, ed. The Endocrine Pancreas. New York: Raven Press, 1991:283-302.
19. Samols E, Stagner JI, Ewart RBL, Marks V. The order of islet cellular perfusion is B-A-D in the perfused rat pancreas. J Clin Invest 1988;82:1715-21.
20. Orci L, Unger RH, Renold AE. Structural coupling between pancreatic islet cells. Experientia 1973;29:1015-8.
21. Kulkarni, RN, Bruning JC, Winnay JN, et al. Tissue-specific knockout of the insulin receptor in pancreatic β-cells creates an insulin secretory defect similar to that in type 2 diabetes. Cell 1999;96:329-339.
22. Bergsten P, Hellman B. Glucose-induced amplitude regulation of pulsatile insulin secretion from individual pancreatic islets. Diabetes 1993;42:670-4.
23. Hellman B, Gylfe E, Grapengiesser E, et al. Cytoplasmic Ca^{2+} oscillations in pancreatic β-cells. Biochem Biophys Acta 1992;1113:95-305.
24. Rorsman P, Trube G. Calcium and delayed potassium currents in mouse pancreatic β-cells under voltage clamp conditions. J Physiol 1986;374:531-50.
25. Falke LC, Gillis KD, Pressel DM, Misler S. Perforated patch recording allows long-term monitoring of metabolite-induced electrical activity and voltage-dependent Ca^{2+} currents in pancreatic β–cells. FEBS Lett 1989;251:167-72.
26. Meissner HP. Electrophysiological evidence for coupling between pancreatic β–cells of pancreatic islets. Nature 1976;262:502-4.
27. Eddlestone GT, Gonçalves A, Bangham JA, Rojas E. Electrical coupling between cells in islets of Langerhans from mouse. J Membr Biol 1984;77:1-14.
28. Meda P, Atwater I, Gonçalves A, et al. The topography of electrical synchrony among β-cells in the mouse islets of Langerhans. Quart J Exp Physiol 1984;69:719-35.
29. Valdeolmillos M, Nadal A, Soria B, Garcia-Sancho J. Fluorescence digital image analysis of glucose-induced $[Ca^{2+}]_i$ oscillations in mouse pancreatic islets of Langerhans. Diabetes 1993;42:1210-4.
30. Valdeolmillos M, Santos RM, Contreras D, et al. Glucose-induced oscillations of intracellular Ca^{2+} concentration resembling bursting electrical activity in single mouse islets of Langerhans. FEBS Lett 1989;259:19-23.
31. Pérez-Armendariz E, Atwater I, Rojas E. Glucose-induced oscillatory changes in extracellular ionized potassium concentration in mouse islets of Langerhans. Biophys J 1985;48:741-9.
32. Bleich D, Chen S, Gu JL, Nadler JL. The role of 12-lipoxygenase in pancreatic β-cells. Int J Mol Med 1998;1:265-72.
33. McDaniel ML, Corbett JA, Kwon G, Hill JR. A role for nitric oxide and other inflammatory mediators in cytokine-induced pancreatic beta-cell dysfunction and destruction. Adv Exp Med Biol 1997;426:313-9.
34. Eizirik DL, Flodstrom M, Karlsen AE, Welsh N. The harmony of the spheres: inducible nitric oxide synthase and related genes in pancreatic beta cells. Diabetologia 1996; 39:875-90.
35. Argiles JM, Lopez-Soriano J, Ortiz MA, et al. Interleukin-1 and beta-cell function: more than one second messenger? Endocr Rev 1992; 13: 515-24.
36. Schwartz MA, Schaller MD, Ginsberg MH. Integrins: emerging paradigms of signal transduction. Annu Rev Cell Dev Biol 1995;11:549-99.
37. Sheppard D. Epithelial integrins. BioEssays 1996;18:655-60.

38. Ruoslahti E, Reed JC. Anchorage dependence, integrins and apoptosis. Cell 1994;77:477-8.
39. Clark EA, Brugge JS. Integrin and signal transduction pathways: the road taken. Science 1995;268:233-9.
40. Yamada KM, Geiger B. Molecular interactions in cell adhesion complexes. Curr Opin Cell Biol 1997;9:76-85.
41. Albelda SM, Buck CA. Integrins and other cell adhesion molecules. Faseb J 1990;4: 2868-80.
42. Hynes RO. Integrins: versatility, modulation, and signalling in cell adhesion. Cell 1992;69:11-25.
43. Schwartz MA, Denninghoff K. αv integrins mediate the rise in the intracellular calcium in endothelial cells on fibronectin even though they play a minor role in adhesion. J Biol Chem 1994;269:11133-7.
44. Meredith JE, Winitz S, Lewis JM, et al. The regulation of growth and intracellular signalling by integrins. Endocrine Reviews 1996;17:207-20.
45. Mainiero F, Pepe A, Wary KK, et al. Signal transduction by the α6/β4 integrin: distinct β4 subunit sites mediate recruitment of Shc/Grb2 and association with the cytoskeleton of hemidesmosomes. EMBO J 1995;14:4470-81.
46. Hannigan GE, Leung-Hagesteijn C, Fitz-Gibbon L, et al. Regulation of cell adhesion and anchorage-dependent growth by a new beta 1-integrin-linked protein kinase. Nature 1996;379:91-6.
47. Schaller MD, Otey CA, Hildebrand JD, Parsons JT. Focal adhesion kinase and paxillin bind to peptides mimicking beta integrin cytoplasmic domains. J Cell Biol 1995;130:1181-7.
48. Burridge K, Fath K, Kelly T, et al. Focal Adhesions: transmembrane junctions between the extracellular matrix and the cytoskeleton. Annu Rev Cell Biol 1988;4:487-525.
49. Hildebrand JD, Schaller MD, Parsons JT. Paxillin. A tyrosine phosphorylated focal adhesion-associated protein binds to the carboxyl terminal domains of focal adhesion kinase. Mol Biol Cell 1995;6:637-47.
50. Levine F, Beattie GM, Hayek A. Differential integrin expression facilitates isolation of human fetal pancreatic epithelial cells. Cell Transplant 1994;3:307-13.
51. Pictet RL, Rutter WJ. Development of embryonic endocrine pancreas. In: Handbook of physiology. Section 8, vol 1. The endocrine pancreas. Steiner D, Freinkel N, eds. Baltimore: Williams and Wilkins Company, 25-66.
52. Cirulli V, Beattie GM, Klier G, et al. Expression and function of αvβ3 and αvβ5 integrins in the developing pancreas: roles in the adhesion and migration of putative endocrine progenitor cells. 1999;*in press*.
53. Kantengwa S, Baetens D, Sadoul K, et al. Identification and characterization of alpha 3 beta 1 integrin on primary and transformed rat islet cells. Exp Cell Res 1997;237:394-402.
54. Bosco D, Meda P, Halban PA, Rouiller D. Importance of cell-matrix interactions in rat β-cell secretion in vivo. Role of $\alpha_6\beta_1$ integrin. Diabetes 2000;233-43.
55. Hynes RO. Integrins: a family of cell surface receptors. Cell 1987;48:549-54.
56. Lenter M, Uhlig H, Hamann A, et al. A monolonal antibody against an activation epitope on mouse integrin chain-β1 blocks adhesion of lymphocytes to the endothelial integrin α6β1. Proc Natl Acad Sci USA 1993;90:51-5.
57. Timpl R. Macromolecular organization of basement membranes. Curr Opin Cell Biol 1996;8:1451-5.
58. Yancey KB. Adhesion molecules. II: interactions of keratinocytes with epidermal basal membrane. J Invest Dermatol 1995;104:1008-14.
59. Fuchs E. Of mice and men: genetic disorders of the cytoskeleton. Mol Biol Cell 1997;8:189-203.
60. Montesano R, Mouron P, Amherdt M, Orci L. Collagen matrix promotes reorganization of pancreatic endocrine cell monolayers into islet-like organoids. J Cell Biol 1983;97:935-9.
61. Lucas-Clerc C, Massart C, Campion JP, et al. Long-term culture of human pancreatic islets in an extracellular matrix: morphological and metabolic effects. Mol Cell Endocrinol 1993;94:9-20.
62. Amory B, Mourmeaux JL, Remacle C. *In vitro* cytodifferentiation of perinatal rat islet cells within a tridimensional matrix of collagen. *In Vitro* Cell Dev Biol 1988;24:91-9.
63. Barro C, Zaoui P, Morel F, Benhamou P. Matrix metalloproteinase expression in rat pancreatic islets. Pancreas 1998;17:378-82.
64. Miralles F, Battelino T, Czernichow P, Scharfmann R. TGF-beta plays a key role in morphogenesis of the pancreatic islets of Langerhans by controlling the activity of the matrix metalloproteinase MMP-2. J Cell Biol 1998;143:827-36.
65. Van Deijnen Jh, Hulstaert Ce, Wolters Gh, Van Schilfgaarde R. Significance of the peri-insular extracellular matrix for islet isolation from the pancreas of rat, dog, pig, and man. Cell Tissue Res 1992;267:139-46.
66. Meyer T, Czub S, Chodnewska I, et al. Expression pattern of extracellular matrix proteins in the pancreas of various domestic pig breeds, the goettingen minipig and the wild boar. Ann Transplant 1997;2:17-26.
67. Van Deijnen Jh, Van Suylichem Pt, Wolters Gh, Van Schilfgaarde R. Distribution of collagens type I, type III and type V in the pancreas of rat, dog, pig and man. Cell Tissue Res 1994;277:115-21.

68. Kaiser N, Corcos Ap, Sarel I, Cerasi E. Monolayer culture of adult rat pancreatic islets on extracellular matrix: modulation of β-cell function by chronic exposure to high glucose. Endocrinology 1991;129:2067-76.
69. Kaiser N, Corcos AP, Tur-Sinai A, et al. Monolayer culture of adult rat pancreatic islets on extracellular matrix: long term maintenance of differentiated β-cell function. Endocrinology 1988;123:834-40.
70. Hulinsky I, Cooney S, Harrington J, Silink M. *In vitro* growth of neonatal rat islet cells is stimulated by adhesion to matrix. Horm Metab Res 1995;27:209-15.
71. Beattie GM, Lappi DA, Baird A, Hayek A. Functional impact of attachment and purification in the short term culture of human pancreatic islets. J Clin Endocrinol Metab 1991;73:93-8.
72. Thivolet Ch, Chatelain P, Nicoloso H, et al. Morphological and functional effects of extracellular matrix on pancreatic islet cell cultures. Exp Cell Res 1985;159:313-22.
73. Schuppin Gt, Bonner-Weir S, Montana E, et al. Replication of adult pancreatic-beta cells cultured on bovine corneal endothelial cell extracellular matrix. *In Vitro* Cell Dev Biol Anim 1993;29a:339-44.
74. Hulinsky I, Harrington J, Cooney S, Silink M. Insulin secretion and DNA synthesis of cultured islets of Langerhans are influenced by the matrix. Pancreas 1995;11:309-14.
75. Beattie GM, Rubin JS, Mally MI, et al. Regulation of proliferation and differentiation of human fetal pancreatic islet cells by extracellular matrix, hepatocyte growth factor, and cell-cell contact. Diabetes 1996;45:1223-8.
76. Hayek A, Beattie GM, Cirulli V, et al. Growth factor/matrix-induced proliferation of human adult beta-cells. Diabetes 1995;44:1458-60.
77. Lefebvre VH, Otonkoski T, Ustinov J, et al. Culture of adult human islet preparations with hepatocyte growth factor and 804G matrix is mitogenic for duct cells but not for beta-cells. Diabetes 1998;47:134-7.
78. Perfetti R, Henderson TE, Wang Y, et al. Insulin release and insulin mRNA levels in rat islets of Langerhans cultured on extracellular matrix. Pancreas 1996;13: 47-54.
79. Muschel R, Khoury G, Reid LM. Regulation of insulin mRNA abundance and adenylation: dependence on hormones and matrix substrata. Mol Cell Biol 1986;6:337-41.
80. Edelman GM, Cunningham BA, Thiery J-P, eds. Morphoregulatory molecules. New York: John Wiley & Sons, 1990.
81. Takeichi M. Cadherin cell adhesion receptors as a morphogenetic regulator. Science 1991;251:1451-5.
82. Gumbiner BM. Cell adhesion: the molecular basis of tissue architecture and morphogenesis. Cell 1996;84:345-57.
83. Shapiro L, Fannon AM, Kwong PD, et al. Structural basis of cell-cell adhesion by cadherins. Nature 1995;374:327-33789.
84. Huber O, Bierkamp C, Kemler R. Cadherins and catenins in development. Curr Opin Cell Biol 1996;8:685-91.
85. Dahl U, Sjodin A, Semb H. Cadherins regulate aggregation of pancreatic beta-cells in vivo. Development 1996;122 2895-902.
86. Cirulli V, Crisa L, Beattie GM, et al. Ksa Antigen Ep-Cam Mediates Cell-Cell Adhesion of Pancreatic Epithelial Cells: Morphoregulatory Roles in Pancreatic Islet Development. J Cell Biol 1998;140:1519-34.
87. Hopcroft DW, Mason DR, Scott RS. Insulin secretion from perifused rat pancreatic pseudoislets. *In vitro* Cell Dev Biol 1985;21:421-7.
88. Halban PA, Powers SL, George KL, Bonner-Weir S. Spontaneous reassociation of dispersed adult rat pancreatic islet cells into aggregates with three-dimensional architecture typical of native islets. Diabetes 1987;36:783-90.
89. Rouiller DG, Cirulli V, Halban PA. Differences in aggregation properties and levels of the neural cell adhesion molecule (NCAM) between islet cell types. Exp Cell Res 1990;191:305-12.
90. Rouiller DG, Cirulli V, Halban PA. Uvomorulin mediates calcium-dependent aggregation of islet cells, whereas calcium-independent cell adhesion molecules distinguish between islet cell types. Dev Biol 1991;148:233-42.
91. Cirulli V, Baetens D, Rutishauser U, et al. Expression of neural cell adhesion molecule (n-cam) in rat islets and its role in islet cell type segregation. J Cell Sci 1994;107:1429-36.
92. Esni F, Taljedal IB, Perl AK, et al. Neural cell adhesion molecule (N-cam) is required for cell type segregation and normal ultrastructure in pancreatic islets. J Cell Biol 1999;144:325-37.
93. Begemann M, Tan SS, Cunningham BA, Edelman GM. Expression of chicken liver cell adhesion molecule fusion genes in transgenic mice. Proc Natl Acad Sci USA 1990;87:9042-6.
94. Moller CJ, Christgau S, Williamson MR, et al. Differential expression of neural cell adhesion molecule and cadherins in pancreatic islets, glucagonomas, and insulinomas. Mol Endocrinol 1992;6:1332-42.
95. Hutton JC, Christofori G, Chi WY, et al. Molecular cloning of mouse pancreatic islet R-cadherin: differential expression in endocrine and exocrine tissue. Mol Endocrinol 1993;7:1151-60.

96. Langley OK, Aletsee-Ufrecht MC, Grant NJ, Gratzl M. Expression of the neural cell adhesion molecule Ncam in endocrine cells. J Histochem Cytochem 1989;37:781-91.
97. Cirulli V, Halban PA, Rouiller DG. Tumor necrosis factor-alpha modifies adhesion properties of rat islet β-cells. J Clin Invest 1993;91:1868-76.
98. Meda P. The role of gap junction membrane channels in secretion and hormonal action. J Bioenerg Biomembr 1996;28:369-78.
99. Paul DL. New functions for gap junctions. Curr Opin Cell Biol 1995;7:665-72.
100. Bruzzone R, White TW, Scherer SS, et al. Null mutations of connexin32 in patients with X-linked Charcot-Marie-Tooth disease. Neuron 1994;13:1253-60.
101. Meda P. Probing the function of connexin channels in primary tissues. Methods 2000; 20:232-44.
102. Meda P, Spray DC. Gap junction function. Adv Mol Cell Biol 2000;30:263-322.
103. Meda P, Pepper M, Traub O, et al. Differential expression of gap junction connexins in endocrine and exocrine glands. Endocrinology 1993;133:2371-8.
104. Meda P, Chanson M, Pepper M, et al. *In vivo* modulation of connexin 43 gene expression and junctional coupling of pancreatic β-cells. Exp Cell Res 1991;192:469-80.
105. Charollais A, Serre V, Mock C, et al. Loss of α1 connexin does not alter the prenatal differentiation of pancreatic β-cells and leads to the identification of another islet cell connexin. Dev Genet 1999;24:13-26.
106. Serre-Beinier V, Le Gurun S, Belluardo N, et al. Cx36 preferentially connects β-cells within pancreatic islets. 2000 abstr, *in press.*
107. Pérez-Armendariz M, Roy C, Spray DC, Bennett MVL. Biophysical properties of gap junctions between freshly dispersed pairs of mouse pancreatic beta cells. Biophys J 1991;59:76-92.
108. Meda P, Amherdt M, Perrelet A, Orci L. Metabolic coupling between cultured pancreatic β-cells. Exp Cell Res 1981;133:421-30.
109. Kohen E, Kohen C, Rabinovitch A. Cell-to-cell communication in rat pancreatic islet monolayer cultures is modulated by agents affecting islet cell secretory activity. Diabetes 1983;32:95-8.
110. Kohen E, Kohen C, Thorell B, et al. Intercellular communication in pancreatic islet monolayer cultures: a microfluorometric study. Science 1979;204:862-5.
111. Michaels RL, Sheridan JD. Islets of Langerhans: dye coupling among immunocytochemically distinct cell types. Science 1981;214:801-3.
112. Meda P, Kohen E, Kohen C, et al. Direct communication of homologous and heterologous endocrine islet cells in culture. J Cell Biol 1982;92:221-6.
113. Meda P, Charollais A, Gjnovci A, et al. Altered β-cell coupling results in abnormal insulin secretion and glucose tolerance in vivo. Diabetologia 1999;42,Suppl. 1:A46.
114. Pipeleers D, In't Veld P, Maes E, Van de Winkel M. Glucose-induced insulin release depends on functional cooperation between islet cells. Proc Natl Acad Sci USA 1982;79:7322-5.
115. Bosco D, Meda P. Actively synthesizing β-cells secrete preferentially during glucose stimulation. Endocrinology 1992;129:3157-66.
116. Philippe J, Giordano E, Gjinovci A, Meda P. cAMP prevents the glucocorticoid-mediated inhibition of insulin gene expression in rodent islet cells. J Clin Invest 1992;90:2228-33.
117. Meda P, Bosco D, Chanson M, et al. Rapid and reversible secretion changes during uncoupling of rat insulin-producing cells. J Clin Invest 1990;86:759-68.
118. Meda P, Denef J-F, Perrelet A, Orci L. Nonrandom distribution of gap junctions between pancreatic β-cells. Am J Physiol 1980;238:C114-9.
119. Meda P, Halban P, Perrelet A, et al. Gap junction development is correlated with insulin content in the pancreatic β-cell. Science 1980;209:1026-8.
120. Meda P, Perrelet A, Orci L. Increase of gap junctions between pancreatic β-cells during stimulation of insulin secretion. J Cell Biol 1979;82:441-8.
121. Meda P, Michaels RL, Halban PA, et al. *In vivo* modulation of gap junctions and dye coupling between β-cells of the intact pancreatic islet. Diabetes 1983;32:858-68.
122. Bruzzone R, Trimble ER, Gjinovci A, et al. Regulation of pancreatic exocrine function: a role for cell-to-cell communication? Pancreas 1987;2:262-71.
123. Vozzi C, Ullrich S, Charollais A, et al. Adequate connexin expression is required for proper insulin production. J Cell Biol 1995;131:1561-72.
124. Vozzi C, Bosco D, Dupont E, et al. Hyperinsulinemia-induced hypoglycemia is enhanced by overexpression of Cx43. Endocrinology 1997;138:2879-85.
125. Wonkam A, Charollais A, Meda P. Expression of Cx32 in β-cells leads to hypertrophy of pancreatic islets. 2000;abstr. *in press*
126. Drubin DG, Nelson WJ. Origins of cell polarity. Cell 1996;84:335-44.
127. Kirkpatrick C, Peifer M. Not just glue: cell-cell junctions as cellular signalling centers. Curr Opin Genet Dev 1995;5:56-65.
128. Kim SK. Tight junctions, membrane-associated guanylate kinase and cell signalling. Curr Opin Cell Biol 1995;7:641-9.
129. Orci L, Perrelet A. Morphology of membrane systems in pancreatic islets. In: Volk BW, Wellmann KF, eds. The diabetic pancreas. New York: Plenum Press, 1977:171-210.

130. In't Veld PA, Pipeleers DG, Gepts W. Evidence against the presence of tight junctions in normal endocrine pancreas. Diabetes 1984;33:101-4.
131. Garrod D, Chidgey M, North, A. Desmosomes: differentiation, development, dynamics and diseases. Curr Opin Cell Biol 1996;8:670-8.
132. Adams JC. Cell adhesion - spreading frontiers, intricate insights. Trends Cell Biol 1997;7:107-10.
133. Thorens B. Glucagon-like peptide-1 and control of insulin secretion. Diab Metab 1995;21:311-8.
134. Chanson M, Fanjul M, Bosco D, et al. Enhanced secretion of amylase from exocrine pancreas of connexin32-deficient mice. J Cell Biol 1998;141:1267-75.
135. Perl AK, Wilgenbus P, Dahl U, et al. A causal role for E-Cadherin in the transition from adenoma to carcinoma. Nature 1998;39:190-3.
136. Perl AK, Dahl U, Wilgenbus P, et al. Reduced expression of neural cell adhesion molecule induces metastatic dissemination of pancreatic β tumor cells. Nature Medicine 1999;5:286-91.
137. Yamasaki H, Naus CCG. Role of connexin genes in growth control. Carcinogenesis 1996;17:1199-213.

9

SOLUBLE FACTORS IMPORTANT FOR PANCREAS DEVELOPMENT

Raphael Scharfmann, Ph.D., and Paul Czernichow, M.D.
INSERM U457, Hospital R. Debré, 48 Bd Sérurier, 75019 Paris, France

INTRODUCTION

The pancreas belongs to a family of organs such as the kidney, the lung and the mammary gland, whose development depends on inductive interactions between an epithelium and a mesenchyme. These interactions control proliferation, branching and differentiation of the epithelial cells. Interactions between mesenchymal and epithelial cells are mediated, at least in part, by soluble, diffusible factors. While some of soluble factors that control development of epithelial cells of the lung or the kidney have been identified (1,2), the soluble factors implicated in pancreatic development are less well known. From a theoretical point of view, soluble factors could control different crucial events during pancreatic development: 1) proliferation of immature epithelial cells, 2) their differentiation into endocrine or exocrine cells, and 3) the association of endocrine cells to form islets of Langerhans. These different events are summarized in Figure 1. In the present review, we concentrate on three families of soluble factors that are implicated in pancreatic development. These soluble factors are: ligands for tyrosine kinase receptors such as members of the Fibroblast Growth Factor (FGF) family or members of the Epidermal Growth Factor (EGF) family and members of the Transforming Growth Factor (TGF) superfamily.

IMPLICATION OF MEMBERS OF THE FIBROBLAST GROWTH FACTOR FAMILY IN PANCREATIC DEVELOPMENT

FGFs and epithelial cell development

At least nineteen members of the FGF family have been identified to date (3). They bind receptors encoded by four different genes (FGFR1 - FGFR4). An additional level of complexity is brought by the fact that FGFRs give rise to a large number of alternatively spliced forms (4). The specificity of the different FGFs for their receptors has been studied in detail (5,6). While some ligands such as FGF1 appear to be universal FGFR ligands, other ligands bind specific FGFR isoforms. This is the case for FGF7, which binds and signals only through FGFR2b isoform (6). FGFRs and their ligands are expressed in a large number of tissues that develop by way of interaction between the epithelium and the mesenchyme. Indeed, FGFR2b is expressed by a large number of epithelial cell types including cells of the salivary gland, the mammary gland, the trachea, the lung, and the kidney (7,8). On the other hand, ligands for FGFR2b are expressed in the mesenchyme that surrounds such epithelia. This is the case for FGF7 that is found in the mesenchyme of the salivary gland, mammary gland, trachea, lung, and kidney (7). This is also the case for FGF10, another ligand of FGFR2b (5) that is detected in the lung (9,10), specifically in the mesenchyme adjacent to the distal buds during embryonic life (11).

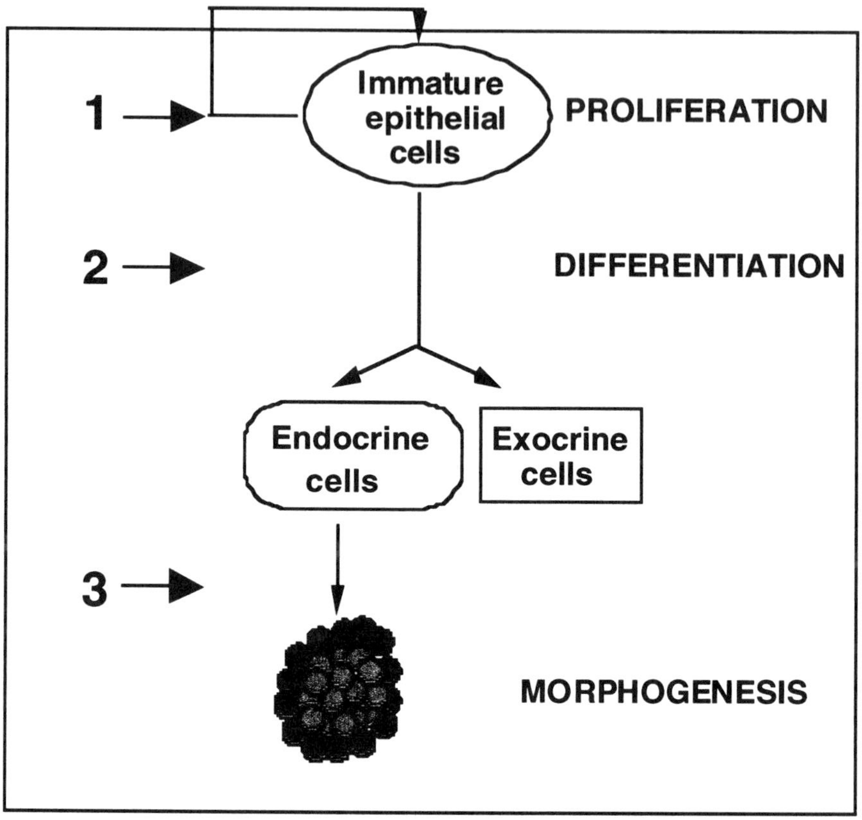

Figure 1. *Control of pancreatic development by soluble factors. Such factors can regulate pancreatic development at different steps. 1. Control of immature epithelial cell proliferation; 2. control of immature epithelial cell differentiation into endocrine or exocrine pancreatic cell; 3. control of islet morphogenesis.*

Perturbing experiments further demonstrate the implication of signals mediated by FGFR in epithelial mesenchymal interactions. In *in vitro* systems that recapitulate lung development, ligands of FGFR2b (FGF7 and FGF10) regulate lung branching (11-14). Moreover, *in vivo*, when a dominant negative FGFR2 is expressed in the lung, both branching morphogenesis and epithelial differentiation of the lung are repressed (15). Abnormal epithelium development also occurs in transgenic mice expressing a secreted kinase-deficient FGFR2b mutant, which disturbs the function of FGF1, FGF3, FGF7, and FGF10. In those mice, agenesis, or dysgenesis of the lung, salivary glands, or kidney are observed (16). Further, FGF10-deficient mice have recently been generated. In these mice, limb bud initiation is abolished and the lung is completely absent (17,18). Taken together, these data demonstrate that different FGF family members, specially the ligands for FGFR2b, are important for co-ordinated development of epithelial tissues.

FGFs and pancreatic development

A possible implication of FGFs in pancreatic development has recently been proposed based on the facts 1) that different FGFs and their receptors are expressed during pancreas development, and 2) that pancreas development is disturbed when the FGF/FGFR axis is perturbed in different experimental systems.

Expression of FGFs and their receptors in the pancreas

Different FGF receptors are expressed during pancreatic development. FGFR1 is found in the rat embryonic pancreas (19,20). FGFR2 is expressed in epithelial cells of the developing mouse pancreas (7,8). The expression of FGFR4 has been demonstrated in the embryonic mouse pancreatic ducts (21) and in the rat embryonic pancreas (19). Some of these receptors have been shown to be functional in terms of signal transduction (20).

Ligands of FGFR are also expressed during pancreatic development. FGF1 and FGF10 are found in the rat embryonic pancreas (22) FGF2 expression is localized to ductal epithelial cells and to small developing islets in both the rat and mid-trimester human foetus (23,24). FGF7 is expressed in the pancreas of mouse and rat during foetal life (7,22,25).

Perturbations of signals transduced via FGFR2b

In vivo, expression of FGF7 in the liver of transgenic mice leads to - among other phenotypes – an increased number of peri-ductular islets and a marked increase in insulin expression by ductule epithelial cells. This suggests that FGF7 plays a role in the proliferation and differentiation of pancreatic epithelial cells (26). Transgenic mice expressing FGF7 under control of the insulin promoter, develop hepatocytes in their islets and have an increased proliferation rate of pancreatic duct cells suggesting that FGF7 can modulate pancreatic cell differentiation (27). When signals mediated by FGFR2b are blocked in transgenic mice expressing a dominant negative soluble receptor, the pancreas consists of a greatly reduced number of morphologically aberrant acinar cells. Most importantly, no islets are found (16). Taken together, these *in vivo* experiments demonstrate that signals transduced via FGFR2b are important for pancreatic development.

In vitro, it has been shown that the proper development of the pancreatic embryonic epithelium into exocrine tissue requires signals derived from the surrounding mesenchyme. The exocrine pancreatic tissue, which derives from the pancreatic epithelium, develops properly when it is grown in the presence of its surrounding mesenchyme. On the other hand, development of exocrine pancreatic tissue is repressed when the epithelium is grown in the absence of mesenchyme (28-31). One working hypothesis is that FGF family members could be produced by the pancreatic mesenchyme and induce the development of the pancreatic epithelium into exocrine tissue. It has been shown that FGF7 and FGF10, two specific ligands of FGFR2b (5), influence the development of pancreatic epithelial cells. *In vitro*, FGF7 and FGF10 are strong inducers of rat embryonic pancreatic epithelial cell proliferation (22). These factors are also involved in pancreatic morphogenesis. Indeed, when embryonic pancreatic epithelium is grown in Matrigel, known to be permissive in different models for morphogenesis (11,13), morphogenesis does not occur in the absence of FGFs. In contrast, addition of both FGF7 and FGF10 causes bud-like branching (22). Finally, FGF7 and FGF10 are implicated in pancreatic exocrine cell differentiation *in vitro*. Indeed, while those factors do not modify the number of endocrine cells that develop, they induce a twenty-fold increase in the number of amylase-expressing cells that develop. The increase in exocrine cell number is paralleled by an increase in amylase activity (22).

The current hypothesis is thus the following one: as in other tissues that develop via interaction between the epithelium and the surrounding mesenchyme, the embryonic and/or foetal pancreatic mesenchyme produces FGF7 or FGF10, which act on the epithelium to induce both cell proliferation and differentiation into exocrine cells.

Implication of signals mediated by other FGFRs

In addition to FGF7 and FGF10, other FGFs have been shown to be expressed in the pancreas (22-24). FGF1, but also FGF2 which binds weakly to FGFR2b, induce embryonic pancreatic epithelial cell proliferation (19) and stimulate the development of the exocrine tissue (22). There are different ways to explain how FGF1 and FGF2 could control pancreatic development. The simplest hypothesis would be that FGF1 and FGF2 act directly on pancreatic epithelium to induce its development into exocrine tissue. However, another hypothesis would be that FGF1 and FGF2 act indirectly by inducing the production of additional soluble factors by their target cells. One factor whose production is induced by FGF1 or FGF2 is Hepatocyte Growth Factor (HGF). Both during lung development and in osteoblasts, FGFs stimulate HGF (14,32). Moreover, in the lung, both FGF1 and HGF stimulate branching morphogenesis. However, the effect of FGF1 almost completely disappears when it is tested in the presence of anti-HGF antibody (14). These results strongly suggest that FGF1 acts, at least in part, by inducing HGF production in mesenchyme. FGF thus acts indirectly on lung epithelium with HGF acting downstream of FGF. Because HGF is expressed by pancreatic mesenchymal cells, and its cognate receptor, c-Met, is expressed by pancreatic epithelial cells (33), it would be interesting to test whether exogenous HGF can mimic the effects of FGFs on pancreatic development and whether the effects of FGFs can be blocked by an anti-HGF antibody.

In conclusion, at least in rat and mice, FGFs are strong inducers of pancreatic development.

IMPLICATION OF MEMBERS OF THE EPIDERMAL GROWTH FACTOR FAMILY IN PANCREATIC DEVELOPMENT

The Epidermal Growth Factor family

The EGF family is a large family that includes EGF, Transforming Growth Factor-α (TGFα), amphiregulin, betacellulin, Heparin-binding EGF (HB-EGF), and several differentially spliced variants of neuregulin. These factors transduce their signals via tyrosine kinase receptors that belong to the ErbB family. The ErbB family consists of four members: ErbB1 (also called EGFR), ErbB2, ErbB3 and ErbB4. A large number of different signals can be transduced by such receptors that can form functionally distinct homodimers and heterodimers (34,35).

Expression of Epidermal Growth Factor family members and their receptors in the pancreas

Expression of EGF family members in the pancreas

Various members of the EGF family and their receptors are expressed in the pancreas. TGF-α is expressed in the human foetal pancreas (36). Betacellulin was first identified in the conditioned medium of cell lines derived from mouse pancreatic beta cell tumours (37), and was found to be expressed mainly in the pancreas and small intestine in humans (38). HB-EGF is present in the developing pancreas in rats. It was detected in the primitive ducts or ductular cells in the pancreas at embryonic day 14, in the islet-like endocrine cell clusters at embryonic day 20, and in the endocrine cells in the adult pancreas (39).

Expression of Receptors for EGF family members in the pancreas
ErbB1 expression has been detected in β-cell lines such as INS-1 and RINm5F (40), in the rat embryonic pancreas (19) and in the human embryonic pancreas (36). The expression of ErbB2 has been found in RINm5F cells (40), in the rat embryonic pancreas (20), and in the human foetal pancreas (41). ErbB3 expression has been found in RIN cells (40), in pancreatic mesenchymal cells in embryonic mice (42) and in the adult rat pancreas (40).

EGFS, THEIR RECEPTORS AND PANCREATIC DEVELOPMENT

Pancreatic development in ErbB knockout mice
Abnormal pancreatic development is found in at least two types of ErbB family member knockout mice. When ErbB1 is inactivated by homologous recombination, epithelial organs that undergo branching morphogenesis during development remain somewhat undeveloped and immature. This is the case for the lung, the kidney, the mammary gland, the prostate, and the pancreas. An abnormal morphogenesis correlates well with the fact that EGF family members are important growth factors for epithelial cells (43).

Abnormal pancreatic development has also been described in mice lacking ErbB3. In these mice, the pancreas develops poorly and has a thin mesenchyme. However, some endocrine differentiation does occur in those mice, and islet cell markers are detectable, albeit at a strikingly reduced level. This suggests that in the pancreas, EGF family members could either have a paracrine role, or that a cascade of mesenchymal factors is required for pancreatic differentiation (42).

Overexpression of EGF members and pancreatic development
Abnormal pancreatic development has been described in different types of transgenic mice overexpressing EGF family members. When TGFα, either under the control of the metallothionein promoter or under the control of the elastase promoter, is overexpressed in transgenic mice, abnormal proliferation of both pancreatic acinar cells and fibroblasts and altered acinar cell differentiation occurs (44,45). Moreover, numerous insulin-positive cells are found in the metaplastic pancreatic ducts from the TGFα transgenic adult mice, whereas pancreatic ducts from non-transgenic mice show virtually no such staining (46). Taken together, these results demonstrate that TGFα overexpression modifies pancreatic development.

***In vitro* effects of EGF family members on the pancreas**
Some effects of EGF family members have also been shown in different *in vitro* models of pancreatic development. In a model of a ductal epithelial cell line derived from the developing pancreatic bud of 12-day-old embryos, EGF, betacellulin, and heregulin induce cell growth (47). When pancreatic rudiments from E12.5 mouse embryos are cultured in the presence of EGF, the proportion of the tissue occupied by duct cells increases at the expense of the acinar structures, while the proportion of endocrine cells remains unchanged (48). EGF family members are thus inducers of ductal tissue.

Betacellulin is important for endocrine cell differentiation. Betacellulin converts a small proportion of AR42J cells, which possess exocrine and neuroendocrine properties, into insulin-expressing cells (49). Such an effect of betacellulin seems to be neither mimicked by EGF or TGFα, nor fully transduced via known ErbB family members. A specific, yet unidentified betacellulin binding protein has been postulated to be involved in the differentiation-inducing effects of betacellulin (50). Moreover, in contrast to EGF, betacellulin potently induces proliferation of INS-1 cells (40).

HB-EGF is also implicated in early pancreatic development. As described above, HB-EGF is found in pancreatic duct cells, with a pattern of expression identical to the one of Pdx1. Moreover, the regulatory region of the HB-EGF gene contains potential binding sites for Pdx1 and Pdx1 can activate HB-EGF gene expression in transient transfection assays (39). Thus, Pdx1 induces expression of HB-EGF, which activates pancreatic epithelial cell proliferation. In that case, the lack of pancreatic development in rodent deficient in Pdx1 expression (28,51,52) would be because of reduced HB-EGF expression.

IMPLICATION OF MEMBERS OF THE TGFβ SUPERFAMILY IN PANCREATIC DEVELOPMENT

Introduction

The TGFβ superfamily represents a very large family of soluble factors that contains factors that belong to subfamilies such as TGFβ, Activins, or Bone Morphogenetic Proteins (BMPs) (53). These factors have been implicated in many important events in development (54). Their possible implication in pancreatic development will be discussed.

Activins in pancreatic development

During early development, activin induces early expression of pancreatic genes. At early stages, the dorsal pancreas is in direct contact with the notochord and notochord to endoderm signalling is required for pancreas development (55). At those early stages, the notochord expresses activin-βB mRNA. Moreover, *in vitro*, exogenous activin-βB induces pancreatic gene expression in cultures from chick embryos (56)

Activins can also be implicated later during pancreatic development, when pluripotent pancreatic precursor cells have the capacity to differentiate into endocrine or exocrine cells. AR42J cells represent somewhat pluripotent precursor cells of the pancreas. Activin, in combination with either betacellulin, or with HGF converts AR42J cells into insulin-secreting cells (57,58). Such a simple *in vitro* experimental system will be useful to further dissect the mechanisms implicated in such an effect of activin on cell differentiation (58). Follistatin, a known inhibitor of activin (59), regulates the relative proportion of endocrine versus exocrine tissue during pancreatic development (60). In fact, follistatin increases the development of immature pancreatic epithelial cells into amylase-expressing cells, while repressing the development of insulin-expressing cells. Finally, when the formation of exocrine tissue is induced during pancreas development, both follistatin and activin are expressed in the pancreatic anlagen (60,61).

Transgenic mice expressing activin receptor mutants under the control of the insulin promoter (62) or the β-actin promoter (63) have hypoplastic pancreatic islets. It is interesting to note that in the work of Yamaoka et al. (62), pancreatic islet hypoplasia is also found in transgenic mice expressing either a dominant negative form of an activin receptor or a constitutively active form of such a receptor. This seems to indicate that a precisely regulated activin signalling intensity is necessary for the normal development of islets (62).

When 11-day embryonic pancreatic anlagen are cultured with activin, normal epithelial lobulation is abolished. Such perturbing effects of activin on epithelial branching is also found in other tissues, suggesting that activin is an intrinsic regulator of epithelial branching morphogenesis (61).

Activin is also implicated in the regulation of insulin secretion. Activin is present both in glucagon- and somatostatin-secreting cells (64). Moreover, activin-A which does not stimulate insulin secretion by itself, enhances glucose-stimulated insulin secretion, raising the possibility, that activin produced by glucagon- and somatostatin-secreting cells, could act on insulin-producing cells, acting as an important and physiological regulator of insulin secretion (64). Glucose-induced insulin secretion is severely impaired in transgenic mice expressing a dominant-negative form of activin receptor in β-cells.

Implication of TGFs in pancreatic development

TGFβ1-3 are expressed during the developing (31,48) and in the adult pancreas (65). Different experimental systems have been used to define whether TGFs could be implicated in pancreatic development. TGFβ1-3 knockout mice have no pancreatic abnormality (66,67). However, in other experimental models, both *in vivo* and *in vitro*, perturbation of TGFβs action induces a pancreatic phenotype. Transgenic mice overexpressing TGFβ1 in β-cells accumulate excessive amounts of extracellular matrix (68,69). Moreover, in transgenic mice expressing a dominant-negative mutant TGF-β type II receptor, proliferation of pancreatic acinar cells is increased, while acinar cell differentiation is perturbed (70).

When pancreatic rudiments from E12.5 mouse embryos are grown in the presence of exogenous TGFβ1, the development of acinar cells is repressed, while the development of the endocrine tissue is stimulated (48). This suggests that TGFβ1 regulates the balance between the acinar and the endocrine portion of the pancreas. Furthermore, TGFβ is implicated in islet morphogenesis. This hypothesis is derived from data obtained in a model of culture of E12.5 pancreatic epithelium, which is thought to recapitulate endocrine pancreas development (30,31). When E12.5 rat pancreatic epithelium is cultured *in vitro* in collagen gel in the absence of mesenchyme, the majority of the epithelial cells differentiate into insulin-containing cells. These insulin-containing cells resemble mature β-cells. They express the homeodomain protein Nkx6.1, a transcriptional factor that is characteristic of adult mature β-cells. Electron microscopy shows that these insulin-positive cells contain granules that resemble the ones found in mature β-cells. The maturity of these granules is further undermined by the fact that they contain Rab3A and SNAP25, 2 proteins associated with the insulin secretory pathway. Moreover, these insulin-positive cells express Glut-2 (71) and secrete insulin upon glucose stimulation. Finally, these insulin-containing cells, which develop *in vitro*, form cell clusters with a core of insulin-positive cells surrounded by glucagon-positive cells (30,31). In this model, TGFβ accelerates the morphogenesis of these islet-like clusters. This effect of TGFβ is associated with an induction of matrix metalloproteinase MMP2. However, as described above, islet morphogenesis does also occur in the absence of exogenous TGFβ. This suggests that pancreatic embryonic epithelial cells could produce TGFβ, which induces MMP2 activity, a step necessary for islet morphogenesis. Such a working hypothesis is further supported by the fact that when pancreatic embryonic epithelium is cultured in the presence of a pan-specific TGFβ neutralizing antibody, both MMP2 activity and islet morphogenesis are abolished (31). A schematic illustration of the role of TGFβ in islet morphogenesis in presented in Figure 2.

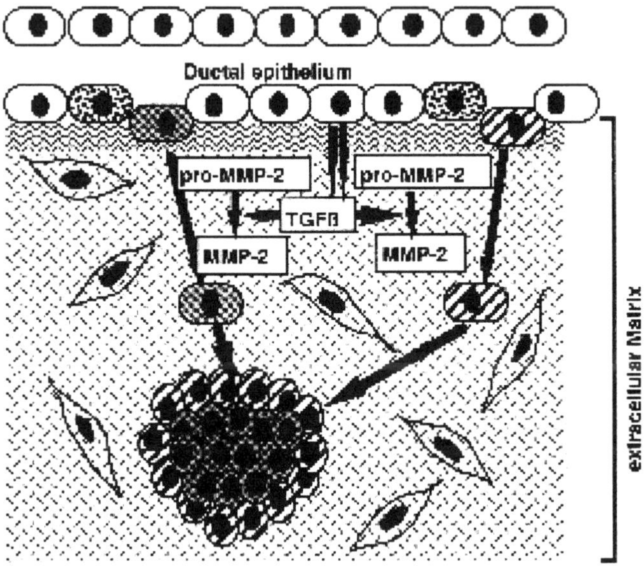

Figure 2. *Implication of TGFβ in islet morphogenesis. Precursor cells (dotted) located in the ductal epithelium differentiate into insulin- (grey) or glucagon (hatched)-expressing cells. These differentiated cells have to migrate and to degrade the extracellular matrix to associate and form islets of Langerhans. This degradation requires the activation by TGFβ of the matrix metalloproteinase pro-MMP-2 to its active form MMP-2.*

REFERENCES

1. Hogan BL. Morphogenesis. Cell 1999;96:225-33.
2. Vainio S and Müller U. Inductive tissue interactions, cell signaling, and the control of kidney organogenesis. Cell 1997;90:975-978.
3. Nishimura T, Utsunomiya Y, Hoshikawa M, Ohuchi H, and Itoh N. Structure and expression of a novel human FGF, FGF-19, expressed in the foetal brain. Biochim Biophys Acta 1999;1444:148-51.
4. Johnson D, and Williams L. Structural and functional diversity in the FGF receptor mutigene family. Adv Cancer Res 1993;60:1-41.
5. Igarashi M, Finch P, and Aaronson S. Characterization of recombinant human fibroblast growth factor (FGF)-10 reveals functional similarities with keratinocytes growth factor (FGF-7). J Biol Chem 1998;273:13230-13235.
6. Ornitz D, Xu J, Colvin J, McEwen D, McArthur C, Coulier F, Gao G, and Goldfarb M. Receptor specificity of the fibroblast growth factor family. J Biol Chem 1996;271:15292-15297.
7. Finch P, Cunha G, Rubin J, Wong J, and Ron D. Pattern of keratinocyte growth factor and keratinocyte growth factor receptor expression during mouse foetal development suggests a role in mediating morphogenetic mesenchymal-epithelial interactions. Dev Dynam 1995;203:223-240.

8. Orr-Urtreger A, Bedford M, Burakowa T, Arman E, Zimmer Y, Yayon A, Givol D, and Lonai P. Developmental localization of the splicing alternatives of fibroblast growth factorreceptor-2 (FGFR2). Dev Biol 1993;158:475-486.
9. Beer HD, Florence C, Dammeier J, McGuire L, Werner S, and Duan DR. Mouse fibroblast growth factor 10: cDNA cloning, protein characterization, and regulation of mRNA expression. Oncogene 1997;15:2211-8.
10. Yamasaki M, Miyake A, Tagashiri S, and Itoh N. Structure and expression of the rat mRNA encoding a novel member of the fibroblast growth factor family. J Biol Chem 1996;71:1518-1521.
11. Bellusci S, Grindley J, Emoto H, Itoh N, and Hoga BL. Fibroblast growth factor 10 (FGF10) and branching morphogenesis in the embryonic mouse lung. Development 11997;24:4867-78.
12. Cardoso WV, Itoh A, Nogawa H, Mason I, and Brody JS. FGF-1 and FGF-7 induce distinct patterns of growth and differentiation in embryonic lung epithelium. Dev Dyn 1997;208:398-405.
13. Nogawa H, and Ito T. Branching morphogenesis of embryonic mouse lung epithelium in mesenchyme-free culture. Development 1995;121:1015-1022.
14. Ohmichi H, Koshimizu U, and Matsumoto K. Hepatocyte growth factor acts as a mesenchyme-derived morphogenic factor during foetal lung development. Development 1998;125:1315-1324.
15. Peters K, Werner S, Liao X, Wert S, Whittset J, and Williams L. Targeted expression of a dominant negative FGF receptor blocks branching morphogenesis and epithelial differentiation of the mouse lung. Development 1994;114:233-243.
16. Celli G, LaRochelle W, Mackem S, Sharp R, and Merlino G. Soluble dominant-negative receptor uncovers essential roles for fibroblast growth factors in multi-organ induction and patterning. Embo J 1998;17:1642-1655.
17. Min H, Danilenko D, Scully S, Bolon B, Ring B, Tarpley J, DeRose M, and Simonet W. FGF-10 is required for both limb and lung development and exhibits striking functional similaruty to drosophila branchless. Genes & Dev 1998;12:3156-3161.
18. Sekine K, Ohuchi H, Fujiwara M, Yamasaki M, Yoshizawa T, Sato T, Yagishita N, Matsui D, Koga Y, Itoh N, and Kato S. Fgf10 is essential for limb and lung formation. Nat Genet 1999;21:138-41.
19. Le Bras S, Miralles F, Basmaciogullari A, Czernichow P, and Scharfmann R. Fibroblast growth factor 2 promotes pancreatic epithelial cell proliferation via functional fibroblast growth factor receptors during embryonic life. Diabetes 1998;47:1236-42.
20. LeBras S, Czernichow P, and Scharfmann R. A search for tyrosine kinase receptors expressed in the rat embryonic pancreas. Diabetologia 1998;41:1474-81.
21. Stark KL, McMahon JA, and McMahon AP. FGFR-4, a new member of the fibroblast growth factor receptor family, expressed in the definitive endoderm and skeletal muscle lineages of the mouse. Development 1991;113:641-51.
22. Miralles F, Czernichow P, Ozaki K, Itoh N, and Scharfmann R. Signaling through Fibroblast Growth Factor 2b plays a key role in the development of the exocrine pancreas. Proc Natl Acad Sci USA 1999;96:6267-6272.
23. Gonzalez AM, Buscaglia M, Ong M, and Baird A. Distribution of basic fibroblast growth factor in the 18-day rat fetus: localization in the basement membranes of diverse tissues. J Cell Biol 1990;110:753-65.
24. Gonzalez AM, Hill DJ, Logan A, Maher PA, and Baird A. Distribution of fibroblast growth factor (FGF)-2 and FGF receptor-1 messenger RNA expression and protein presence in the mid-trimester human fetus. Pediatr Res 1996;39:375-85.
25. Mason I, Fuller-Pace F, Smith R, and Dickson C. FGF-7 (keratinocyte growth factor) expression during mouse development suggests roles in myogenesis, forebrain regionalization and epithelial-mesenchymal interactions. Mech Dev 1994;45:15-30.
26. Nguyen H, Danilenko D, Bucay N, DeRose M, Van G, Thomason A, and Simonet W. Expression of keratinocyte growth factor in embryonc liver of transgenic mice causes changes in epithelial growth and differentiation resulting in polycystic kidneys and other organ malformations. Oncogene 1996;12:2109-2119.
27. Krakowski ML, Kritzik MR, Jones EM, Krahl T, Lee J, Arnush M, Gu D, and Sarvetnick N. Pancreatic expression of keratinocyte growth factor leads to differentiation of islet hepatocytes and proliferation of duct cells. Am J Pathol 1999;154:683-91.
28. Ahlgren U, Jonsson J, and Edlund H. The morphogenesis of the pancreatic mesenchyme is uncoupled from that of the pancreatic epithelium in IPF1/PDX1-deficient mice. Development 1996;122:1409-1416.
29. Gittes G, Galante P, Hanahan D, Rutter W, and Debas H. Lineage specific morphogenesis in the developing pancreas: role of mesenchymal factors. Development 1996;122:439-447.
30. Miralles F, Serup P, Cluzeaud F, Vandewalle A, Czernichow P, and Scharfmann R. Characterization of beta cells developed in vitro from rat embryonic pancreatic epithelium. Dev Dyn 1999;214:116-26.
31. Miralles F, Battelino T, Czernichow P, and Scharfmann R. TGF-beta plays a key role in morphogenesis of the pancreatic islets of Langerhans by controlling the activity of the matrix metalloproteinase MMP-2. J Cell Biol 1998;143:827-36.

32. Blanquaert F, Delany AM, and Canalis E. Fibroblast growth factor-2 induces hepatocyte growth factor/scatter factor expression in osteoblasts. Endocrinology 1999;140:1069-74.
33. Sonnenberg E, Meyer D, Weidner K, and Birchmeier C. Scatter factor/hepatocyte growth factor and its receptor, the c-met tyrosine kinase, can mediate a signal exchange between mesenchyme and epithelia during mouse development. J Cell Biol 1993;123:223-235.
34. Alroy I, and Yarden Y. The ErbB signaling network in embryogenesis and oncogenesis: signal diversification through combinatorial ligand-receptor interactions. FEBS Letters 1997;410:83-86.
35. Riese D, and Stern D. Specificity within the EGF family/ErbB receptor family signaling network. BioEssays 1998;20:41-48.
36. Miettinen PJ, and Heikinheimo K. Transforming growth factor-alpha (TGF-alpha) and insulin gene expression in human foetal pancreas. Development 1992;114:833-40.
37. Shing Y, Christofori G, Hanahan D, Ono Y, Sasada R, Igarashi K, and Folkman J. Betacellulin: a mitogen from pancreatic β cell tumors. Science 1993;259:1604-1607.
38. Seno M, Tada H, Kosaka M, Sasada R, Igarashi K, Shing Y, Folkman J, Ueda M, and Yamada H. Human betacellulin, a member of the EGF family dominantly expressed in pancreas and small intestine, is fully active in a monomeric form. Growth Factors 1996;13:181-91.
39. Kaneto H, Miyagawa J-I, Kajimoto Y, Yamamoto K, Watada H, Umayahara Y, Hanafusa T, Matsuzawa Y, Yamasaki Y, Higashiyama S, and Taniguchi N. Expression of heparin-binding epidermal growth factor-like growth factor during pancreas development. J Biol Chem 1997;46:29137-29143.
40. Huotari MA, Palgi J, and Otonkoski T. Growth factor-mediated proliferation and differentiation of insulin-producing INS-1 and RINm5F cells: identification of betacellulin as a novel beta-cell mitogen. Endocrinology 1998;139:1494-9.
41. Mori S, Akiyama T, Yamada Y, Morishita Y, Sugawara I, Toyoshima K, and Yamamoto T. C-erbB-2 gene product, a membrane protein commonly expressed on human foetal epithelial cells. Lab Invest 1989;61:93-7.
42. Erickson S, O'Shea K, Ghaboosi N, Loverro L, Frantz G, Bauer M, Lu L, and Moore M. ErbB3 is required for normal cerebellar and cardiac development: a comparison with ErbB2- and heregulin-deficient mice. Development 1997;124:4999-5011.
43. Miettinen PJ. Epidermal growth factor receptor in mice and men--any applications to clinical practice? Ann Med 1997;29:531-4.
44. Jhappan C, Stahle C, Harkins RN, Fausto N, Smith GH, and Merlino GT. TGF alpha overexpression in transgenic mice induces liver neoplasia and abnormal development of the mammary gland and pancreas. Cell 1990;61:1137-46.
45. Sandgren EP, Luetteke NC, Palmiter RD, Brinster RL, and Lee DC. Overexpression of TGF alpha in transgenic mice: induction of epithelial hyperplasia, pancreatic metaplasia, and carcinoma of the breast. Cell 1990;61:1121-35.
46. Wang T, Bonner-Weir S, Oates P, Chulack M, and Simon B. Pancreatic gastrin stimulates islet differentiation of transforming growth factor alpha-induced ductular precursor cells. J Clin Invest 1993;92:1349-1356.
47. Sundaresan S, Roberts PE, King KL, Sliwkowski MX, and Mather JP. Biological response to ErbB ligands in nontransformed cell lines correlates with a specific pattern of receptor expression. Endocrinology 1998;139:4756-64.
48. Sanvito F, Herrera P, Huarte J, Nichols A, Montesano R, Orci L, and Vassali J. TGF-β1 influences the relative development of the exocrine and endocrine pancreas in vitro. Development 1994;120:3451-3462.
49. Mashima H, Ohnishi H, Wakabayashi K, Mine T, Miyagawa J, Hanafusa T, Seno M, Yamada H, and Kojima I. Betacellulin and activin A coordinately convert amylase-secreting pancreatic AR42J cells into insulin-secreting cells. J Clin Invest 1996;97:1647-54.
50. Ishiyama N, Kanzaki M, Seno M, Yamada H, Kobayashi I, and Kojima I. Studies on the betacellulin receptor in pancreatic AR42J cells. Diabetologia 1998;41:623-8.
51. Offield M, Jetton T, Laborsky P, Ray M, Stein R, Magnuson M, Hogan B, and Wright C. PDX-1 is required for pancreatic outgrowth and differentiation of the rostral duodenum. Development 1996;122:983-995.
52. Ohlsson H, Thor S, and Edlund T. Novel insulin promoter- and enhancer-binding proteins that discriminate between pancreatic alpha and beta cells. Mol Endocrinol 1991;5:897-904.
53. Kingsley D. The TGF-β superfamily: new members, new receptors, and new genetic tests of function in different organisms. Genes & Dev 1994;8:133-146.
54. Hogan B. Bone morphogenic proteins: multifunctional regulators of vertebrate development. Genes & Dev 1996;10:1580-1594.
55. Kim S, Hebrok M, and Melton D. Notochord to endoderm signaling is required for pancreas development. Development 1997;124:4243-4252.
56. Hebrok M, Kim S, and Melton D. Notochord repression of endodermal sonic hedgehog permits pancreas development. Genes & Dev 1998;12:1705-1713.
57. Mashima H, Shibata H, Mine T, and Kojima I. Formation of insulin-producing cells from pancreatic acinar AR42J cells by hepatocyte growth factor. Endocrinology 1996;137:3969-76.

58. Mashima H, Yamada S, Tajima T, Seno M, Yamada H, Takeda J, and Kojima I. Genes expressed during the differentiation of pancreatic AR42J cells into insulin-secreting cells. Diabetes 1999;48:304-309.
59. Nakamura T, Takio K, Eto Y, Shibai H, Titani K, and Sugino H. Activin-binding protein from rat ovary is follistatin. Science 1990;247:836-838.
60. Miralles F, Czernichow P, and Scharfmann R. Follistatin regulates the relative proportions of endocrine versus exocrine tissue during pancreatic development. Development 1998;125:1017-24.
61. Ritvos O, Tuuri T, Eramaa M, Sainio K, Hildén K, Saxén L, and Gilbert S. Activin disrupts epithelial branching morphogenesis in developing glandular organs of the mouse. Mechanisms of Development 1995;50:229-245.
62. Yamaoka T, Idehara C, Yano M, Matsushita T, Yamada T, Li S, Moritani M, Hata J, Sugino H, Noji S, and Itakura M. Hypoplasia of pancreatic islets in transgenic mice expressing activin receptor mutants. J Clin Invest 1998;102:294-301.
63. Shiozaki S, Tajima T, Zhang YQ, Furukawa M, Nakazato Y, and Kojima I. Impaired differentiation of endocrine and exocrine cells of the pancreas in transgenic mouse expressing the truncated type II activin receptor. Biochim Biophys Acta 1999;1450:1-11.
64. Yasuda H, Inoue K, Shibata H, Takeuchi T, Eto Y, Hasegawa Y, Sekine N, Totsuka Y, Mine T, Ogata E, and Kojima I. Existence of activin-A in A- and D-cells of rat pancreatic islet. Endocrinology 1993;133:624-30.
65. Yamanaka Y, Friess H, Buchler M, Beger H, Gold L, and Korc M. Synthesis and expression of transforming growth factor β-1, β-2, and β-3 in the endocrine and exocrine pancreas. Diabetes 1993;42:746-756.
66. Kaartinen V, Voncken J, Shuler W, Warburton C, Bu D, Heisterkamp D, and Groffen J. Abnormal lung development and cleft palate in mice lacking TGF-beta 3 indicates defects of epithelial-mesenchymal interaction. Nature Genet 1995;11:415-421.
67. Sanford L, Ormsby I, Groot AG-d, Sariola H, Friedman R, Boivin G, Cardell E, and Doetschmann T. TGFβ2 knockout mice have multiple developmental defects that are non-overlapping with other TGFβ knockout phenotypes. Development 1997;124:2659-2670.
68. Lee M-S, Gu D, Feng L, Curriden S, Arnush M, Krahl T, Gurushanthaiah D, Wilson C, Loskutoff D, Fox H, and Sarvetnick N. Accumulation of extracellular matrix and developmental dysregulation in the pancreas by transgenic production of transforming growth factor-β1. Am J Pathol 1995;147:42-52.
69. Sanvito F, Nichols A, Herrer P, Huarte J, Wohlvend A, Vassali, J, and Orci L. TGF-ß1 overexpression in murine pancreas induces chronic pancreatitis and, together with TNF-α, triggers insulin-dependent diabetes. Biochem Biophys Res Commun 1995;217:1279-1286.
70. Böttinger EP, Jakubczak JL, Robets ISD, Mumy M, Hemmati P, Bagnall K, Merlino G, Wakefield LM. Expression of a dominant-negative mutant TGF-β type II receptor in transgenic mice reveals essentil roles for TGF-β in regulation of growth and differentiation in the exocrine pancreas. EMBO 1997;16:2621-2633.
71. Thorens B, Sarkar H, Kaback H, and Lodish H. Cloning and functional expression in bacteria of a novel glucose transporter present in liver, intestine, kidney, and β-pancreatic islet cells. Cell 1988;55:281-290.

10

ROLE OF MESENCHYMAL-EPITHELIAL INTERACTIONS IN PANCREAS DEVELOPMENT

Thomas S. Maldonado, M.D., Christopher A. Crisera, M.D.
Alan S. Kadison, M.D., Michael T. Longaker, M.D.
George K. Gittes, M.D.
New York University Medical Center, New York, N.Y., 10016, USA

HISTORICAL PERSPECTIVE

Mesenchyme is traditionally defined as a network of loosely organized mesodermal cells derived from the embryonic primitive streak with the potential to differentiate and give rise to structures such as connective tissue, blood and blood vessels, lymphatics, cartilage, muscle, bone, and stromal tissues of all glands. More recently, the mesenchyme has been found to play an increasingly sophisticated role in organogenesis through its interactions with other germ layers, specifically the endoderm. Mesenchymal-epithelial interactions have been shown to be important in the development of many organs including kidney, intestine, mammary, chick feathers, and salivary gland (1-5). The prepancreatic endoderm, originating in the duodenal anlage, requires its surrounding mesenchyme in order to differentiate into mature pancreas with acinar, ductal, and endocrine components (6-10).

A role for mesenchymal-epithelial interactions in pancreatic development was originally proposed in a landmark article by Golosow and Grobstein in 1962, (6) which characterized the growth of mouse pancreatic rudiments using *in vitro* conditions and demonstrated that epithelial morphogenesis and cytodifferentiation are promoted by mesenchyme. These classic experiments showed that isolated pancreatic epithelium, without its surrounding mesenchyme, failed to grow, demonstrating for the first time that a mesenchymal-epithelial interaction is essential for proper development of the pancreas. Furthermore, transfilter experiments, in which the epithelium was separated from the mesenchyme by a porous barrier, suggested that physical contact was not necessary for mesenchyme to promote epithelial growth and differentiation. Interestingly, salivary gland mesenchyme also induced these processes, suggesting the existence of a common soluble "mesenchymal factor" important for pancreatic development. Notably, Golosow and Grobstein's use of rooster plasma and "embryo juice" (20% 9-day chick embryo extract) to secure the epithelium to the undersurface of the filter, and as a component of their media, may have confounded the interpretation of these results by introducing potential unknown inductive factors, or even homogenized mesenchyme itself. Subsequent experiments showed that chick embryo extract can replace the mesenchyme as a factor necessary for the morphogenesis and cytodifferentiation (7,8). Membrane filters did not preclude that mesenchymal-epithelial contacts were necessary since cell extensions could have traversed through pores of adequate size. Indeed, analysis of millipore filters using electron microscopy reveals that, occasionally, epithelial "cell processes extend(ed) into the filter substance" (9). Nonetheless, the early work by Golosow and Grobstein initiated research on the role of mesenchymal-epithelial interactions in pancreatic development.

The embryonic pancreas forms as an evagination of the foregut epithelium into its surrounding mesenchyme, at approximately the 22- to 25-somite stage (gestational day 11 in the rat, day 10 in mouse), which subsequently gives rise to pancreatic islets, acini, and ducts. Pancreatic mesoderm gradually accumulates in the region of this evagination prior to its emergence and is followed by outgrowth of the pancreatic diverticulum in less than two hours (10). A region of the midgut endoderm isolated on the eighth gestational day (E8), approximately the 7-12-somite stage, is able to form pancreas tissue *in vitro*. Interestingly, salivary gland mesenchyme is capable of inducing early epithelium at the 15-somite stage to form acini, suggesting that epithelium is committed towards pancreas development at stages before the condensed pancreatic mesenchyme appears. The fact that mesenchymal accumulation immediately precedes the evagination of gut epithelium is consistent with the need for a mesenchymal signal to induce pancreatic morphogenesis.

The supportive role of mesenchyme in epithelial morphogenesis was corroborated in experiments by Spooner and Cohen (11). They showed that mouse gestational day 10 epithelium grown *in vitro* without its mesenchyme retained its cellular morphology, but was unable to form acini. Same-age epithelium grown with intact mesenchyme, however, went on to form mature-appearing acini. Interestingly, electron microscopy as well as amylase assays showed that individual cells within the disorganized epithelial monolayer grown *in vitro* in the absence of mesenchyme achieved some level of cytodifferentiation. Thus, while these experiments showed that mesenchyme is important for generating and maintaining acinar architecture, they also led to the notion that cytodifferentiation may occur independently of mesenchymal influence.

SEARCHING FOR THE MESENCHYMAL FACTOR

The evidence for the existence of a pancreatic mesenchymal factor (MF), whether permissive or instructive for epithelial differentiation, prompted Rutter and others (12,13) to isolate this factor from chick embryonic extracts, which had previously been shown to have effects similar to mesenchyme on developing epithelia (8). Interestingly, the MF was found to be neither species nor tissue specific since chicken embryo homogenates successfully replaced rat mesenchyme. Using the rate of ^{3}H-thymidine incorporation into DNA as an assay for activity, Ronzio and Rutter found that the addition of exogenous MF increased 10-20 fold the DNA precursor uptake by exposed epithelia from rat E12 epithelium (12). This effect was similar, if not greater, to that found when whole, intact pancreatic rudiments were grown. Exposure of epithelia to a variety of known growth factors, including insulin, epithelial growth factor, phytohaemoagglutinin, and hydrocortisone, failed to substitute for MF activity. Interestingly, while collagen had been implicated in morphogenesis of other branched epithelial organs (14), purified collagen (obtained from fibroblast cultures) was unable to replace MF in stimulating ^{3}H-thymidine incorporation by the epithelium. The absence of MF activity in other embryonic tissues such as heart, brain, liver, and thyroid, and its strong activity present in gut mesenchyme and cultured fibroblasts, demonstrated a wide but specific distribution limited to certain mesodermal derivatives. Extracts from older embryos and adults showed lower MF activity, presumably because these contained little or no mesenchyme, compared with younger embryos. Biochemical characterization of the chick embryo extracts revealed that the MF was sensitive to trypsin digestion. Furthermore, MF activity was also destroyed by oxidation with sodium periodate, which suggested that a carbohydrate moiety was required. Finally, fractionation of embryo extracts revealed that MF was a high molecular weight, non-lipid containing complex; most likely a composite of various protein factors (12).

Subsequent experiments by Levine et al. (15) showed that the MF acts at the cell membrane level, and that it may not necessarily be soluble, as proposed by Grobstein's millipore filter experiments (6). Mesenchymal factor bound to cyanogen bromide-activated Sepharose beads allowed pancreatic epithelial buds to adhere to the beads at their basal surface, the surface domain that normally interacts with mesenchymal cells *in vivo* (Figure 1). Moreover, rapid incorporation of DNA precursors, as well as the eventual appearance of acini-specific zymogen granules, occurred in cells directly in contact with the MF-coated beads (15). In addition to localizing the site of action of MF to the cell membrane, these experiments raised the exciting possibility that, contrary to Spooner and Cohen's findings (11), cytodifferentiation cannot proceed independently of mesenchymal signals. Mesenchyme may in fact play an instructive rather than a permissive role in epithelial growth and differentiation.

Perhaps most convincing in this regard, is the finding that when E12 rat pancreatic epithelia were grown in the presence of albumin, very few acini developed although a greater number of cells containing alpha granules was apparent by EM (13,16). Moreover, when MF was added to such rudiments, a large number of acinar cells containing characteristic zymogen granules was apparent, suggesting that mesenchyme might induce a commitment to the exocrine lineage, and could even have a suppressive effect on glucagon expressing cells.

MESENCHYMAL-EPITHELIAL INTERACTIONS: IMPLICATIONS FOR LINEAGE SELECTION

Although purification of the elusive "mesenchymal factor" by Rutter and associates was unsuccessful, their demonstration of a role for mesenchymal components in inducing epithelial gene expression encouraged others (17,18) to attempt to define the mechanisms by which mesenchyme may control exocrine versus endocrine differentiation. Implicit in this new approach was the prospect that a common pancreatic precursor cell exists whose developmental fate can be directed towards either endocrine or exocrine differentiation.

By growing E11 epithelia without its mesenchyme in various environments, Gittes et al. (18) were able to attribute lineage-specific responses of pancreatic epithelia to various signals generated by the mesenchyme. Epithelia cultured alone on a transparent filter were stunted in growth and showed no evidence of differentiation by histologic or immunohistochemical criteria. While consistent with other transfilter studies (6,10), these results contradicted the findings by Spooner and Cohen in the 1970's (11) that suggested that cytodifferentiation can proceed without mesenchyme. These discrepancies may have resulted from limitations in microscopy and microdissection that led to mesenchymal contamination of "isolated" epithelia in those early transfilter studies. Gittes et al. cultured epithelia in collagen gels and demonstrated that a three-dimensional scaffolding was not sufficient to induce differentiation. In contrast, when cultured in a matrix rich in basement membrane components, epithelia were able to form ducts with some loosely associated endocrine cells but no acini (Figure 2). Perhaps most significant, was the finding that epithelia, without mesenchyme, grown under the renal capsule for 10 days yielded a dense aggregate of mature islets (Figure 3) (18). These mature islets represent the first successful growth of embryonic pancreatic precursor cells into islets and suggested that the basement membrane component of mesenchyme drives ductal differentiation and that the endocrine lineage develops by a default pathway.

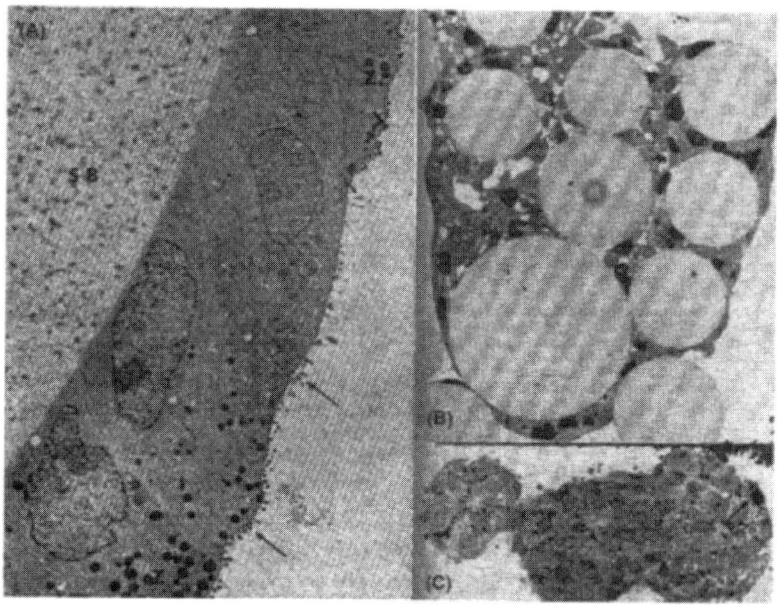

Figure 1. *A) EM radiograph of E12 epithelia bound to a sepharose bead (SB) at its basal cell membrane domain. Note apical microvilli (arrows) and zymogen granules (z)* ***B)*** *MF-sepharose stimulates DNA activity in E12 epithelia as shown by marked ^{3}H-thymidine nuclear uptake* ***C)*** *BSA-sepharose beads failed to attach to epithelia and only an occasional cell (arrow) showed evidence of ^{3}H-thymidine uptake (with permission, reference 15).*

The ability of mesenchyme to instruct epithelia towards exocrine cell commitment was first noted in 1966 by Wessells and Cohen (10). Early endoderm (0-6-somite stage) when recombined with older E11 mesenchyme, resulted in expression of acinar tissue in 6 of 52 recombinants. More than 30 years later, using an organ culture "mix-and-match" strategy with different-aged embryonic pancreatic epithelium and mesenchyme, Rose et al. (19) obtained strikingly similar results: E11 mouse epithelia grown *in vitro* with E12 mesenchyme developed a more mature appearing exocrine cell type than when grown with E11 or E10 mesenchyme (Figure 4). Moreover, acini formed exclusively at the mesenchymal-epithelial interface, while endocrine differentiation was confined to epithelia distant from mesenchyme.

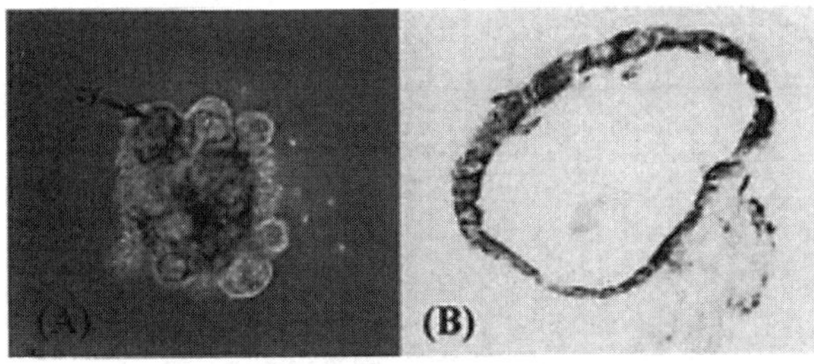

Figure 2. *E11.5 pancreatic epithelium grown in matrigel (rich in basement membrane components) for 7 days.* ***A)*** *Note the fluid filled cysts (cy) representing early ducts, seen here under phase contrast microscopy.* ***B)*** *Immuno-histochemistry of cysts seen in A, stained for cytokeratin 7, a ductal marker (with permission, reference 18).*

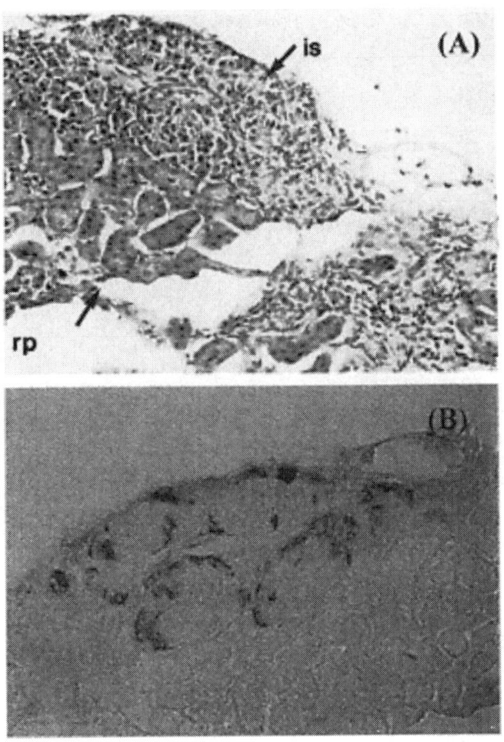

Figure 3. *E11.5 pancreatic epithelium grown in vivo under the renal capsule of an adult mouse.* ***A)*** *Hematoxylin and eosin staining shows clusters of islets (is) on top of the renal parenchyma (rp).* ***B)*** *Immunohisotchemistry for glucagon reveals mature islets with alpha cells located peripherally in a typical mantle distribution (with permission, reference 18).*

This polarized distribution of epithelial cells is consistent with the hypothesis that endocrine lineage selection occurs by default. Indeed, the same cells not exposed to mesenchyme may be unable to undergo exocrine differentiation, and thus become endocrine cells in the absence of a mesenchymal signal. Alternatively, while non-diffusible molecules, such as basement membrane components, may be necessary for exocrine differentiation, diffusible molecules, such as cytokines and growth factors, may play a role in pancreatic endocrine differentiation. In this case, the signal to form exocrine structures would have to override the signal for endocrine differentiation, since no endocrine cells were found in contact with the mesenchyme.

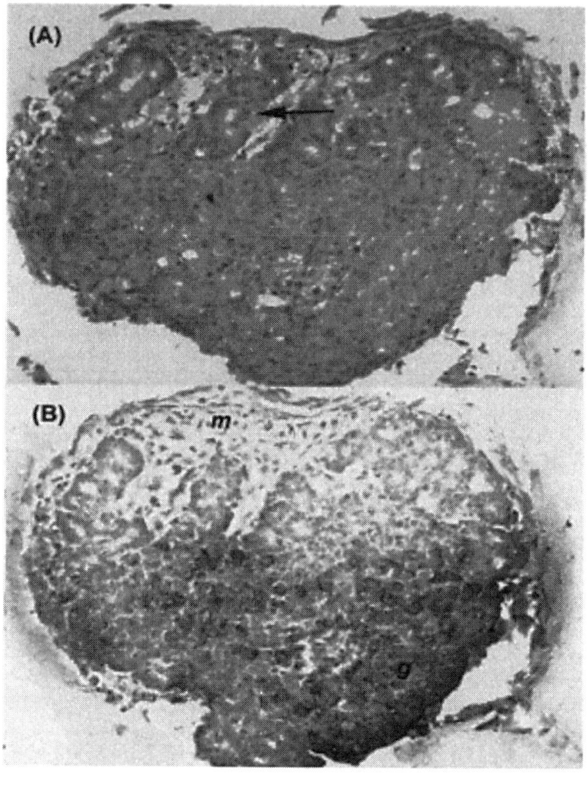

Figure 4. *E11.5 pancreas epithelium recombined with E12.5 mesenchyme and grown in vitrogen for 7 days.* ***A)*** *Hematoxylin and eosin staining showing polarization of endocrine and exocrine compartments. Note acini (arrow) developing at interface with mesenchyme.* ***B)*** *Immunohistochemistry of similar section to A. Staining for glucagon (g) shows glucagon positive cells confined to epithelial areas distant from mesenchyme (with permission, reference 19).*

Isl-1, a member of the LIM homeodomain family of transcription factors known to be important in cell-fate determination, is expressed in all islet cell types as well as in the mesenchyme enveloping the dorsal but not the ventral pancreatic anlage (20,21). Mice which lack isl-1 do not develop beyond embryonic day 9. They fail to develop dorsal mesenchyme as well as α-, β- and δ-cells in dorsal pancreatic epithelium (Figure 5).

Although exocrine cells appear to be relatively unaffected by the lack of isl-1 signal, closer examination shows that these amylase-positive cells are derived entirely from the ventral pancreas. Moreover, amylase-positive cells are only present in cultured ventral half-gut explants from isl-1 (-/-) mice and are absent from cultured dorsal half-gut explants. Thus, the dorsal pancreas, bereft of its mesenchyme, is unable to undergo exocrine differentiation, unlike its ventral counterpart. Interestingly, recombining isl-1 (-/-) dorsal half-gut with wild type dorsal mesenchyme *in vitro* restores development of the exocrine lineage but the wild type mesenchyme was unable to rescue the endocrine lineage, suggesting that *epithelial* isl-1 expression is necessary for endocrine lineage commitment. Nonetheless, these experiments provide definitive genetic evidence that pancreatic mesenchyme is necessary for exocrine lineage selection.

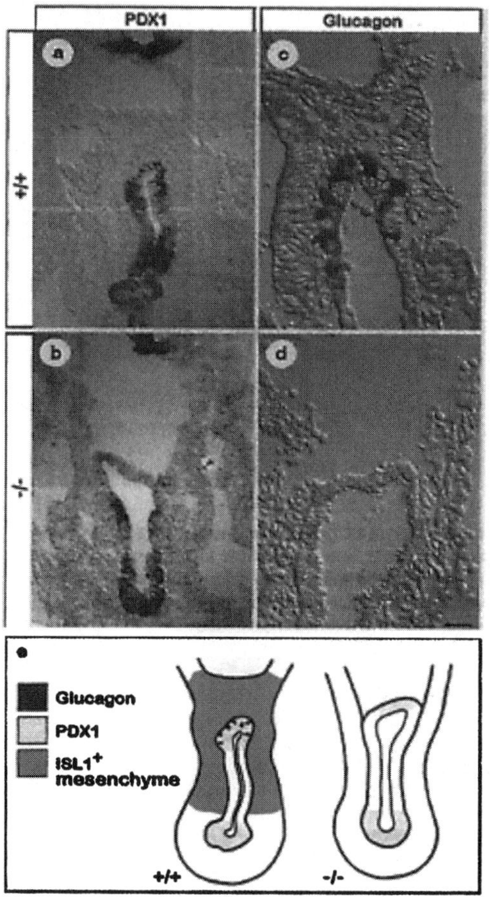

Figure 5. *Loss of dorsal pancreatic mesenchyme and glucagon+ cells in isl1(-/-). Photomicrographs of transverse sections of isl1(+/+) (A,C) and isl1(-/-) (B,D) at the level of the pancreas. In* ***A****) and* ***B****), in situ hybridization (dark blue) using a Shh probe was done to visualize the lateral endoderm.* ***A****), Transverse section of an E9.5 isl1(-/-) embryo labelled with pdx1 antibodies. The dorsal pancreatic mesenchyme is absent, whereas the ventral pancreatic epithelium with its associated mesenchyme appears normal.* ***C****), At the 25-somite stage, glucagon+ cells have appeared in the dorsal pancreatic epithelium in isl1(+/+) embryos, whereas in isl1(-/-) embryos* ***D****), no glucagon+ cells are detected.* ***E****) Comparison of E9.5 wild-type and isl1 mutant phenotype (with permission, reference 21).*

p48, the DNA-binding subunit of the hetero-oligomeric exocrine gene transcription factor PTF1, represents the only factor known to be specifically required for exocrine pancreas differentiation. The p48 subunit has been shown to be cell-specific, found exclusively in exocrine cells as early as E12 by RT-PCR and E15 by *in situ* hybridization (24). Mice lacking p48 (25) have an early post-natal lethal phenotype, characterized by the absence of an exocrine pancreas, with sparing of endocrine elements. In embryos of these p48-null mice, ranging in ages from E12 to E16, clusters of endocrine cells are detected in close association with the epithelial lining of duct-like structures in a primitive mesentery, where the pancreas normally would form. By age E18 these endocrine cells relocate to the spleen, a mesoderm-derived organ (Figure 6). Immunolocalization of pdx-1, a known epithelial-marker, refuted the possibility that these splenic-islets are generated *de novo* by crossing germ layers from splenic mesoderm, supporting the notion that they have migrated to colonize the spleen.

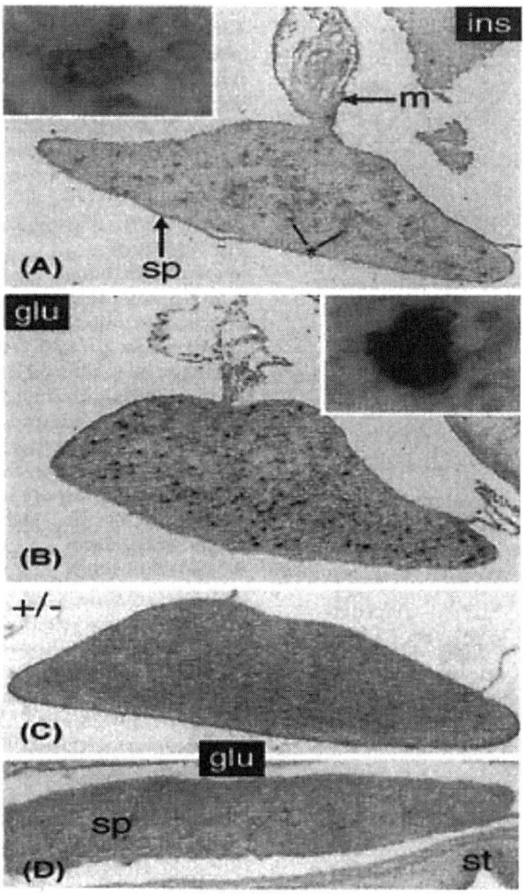

Figure 6. *Glucagon+ and insulin+ cells appear in the spleen of p48-deficient mice. (**A,B**), Immunohistochemistry performed on E18 intestinal tracts from p48 (-/-) embryos showed staining for insulin and glucagon in the spleen (sp). Note the absence of insulin or glucagon in the mesentery (m) at this age. (**C,D**), Spleens from E16 p48 (-/-) embryos and E18 (+/-) embryos did not stain for either endocrine marker. (Insets) Single intrasplenic cells positive for the respective endocrine markers at a higher magnification (with permission, reference 25).*

Thus, proper endocrine organization may require the presence of pancreatic mesenchyme, as well as an exocrine framework. Furthermore, it is important to note that while the lack of an exocrine pancreas in p48 (-/-) mice seems to confirm the essential function of this exocrine–specific transcription factor in exocrine lineage selection, the absence of normal pancreatic mesenchyme in isl-1 (-/-) mice has been shown to lead to absence of exocrine cells (21). Thus, the lack of normal pancreatic mesenchyme in p48 (-/-) mice, resulting from absence of an exocrine pancreas, could also contribute to their stunted exocrine differentiation.

The effect of mesenchymal-epithelial interactions on endocrine lineage commitment is less well understood. Gittes et al. (18) have suggested that endocrine cells differentiate by a default pathway, when mesenchymal contact is absent. However, the existence of a mesenchymal factor that influences endocrine differentiation cannot be excluded. Miralles and associates (17) were able to demonstrate a suppressive effect of mesenchyme on endocrine cell commitment in epithelia in addition to its suspected inductive effect on exocrine determination. Rat E12.5 epithelia isolated from its surrounding mesenchyme [M (-)] and grown in culture for seven days has a 4.8-fold increase in insulin-positive cells versus cultured whole pancreatic rudiments [M (+)] (Figure 7).

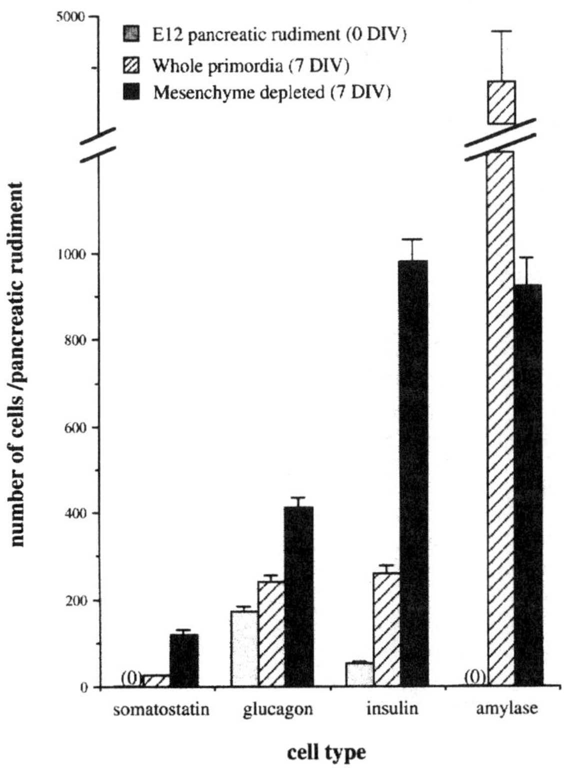

Figure 7. *Quantitative analysis of endocrine markers in M+ and M- rudiments. Gray bars: E12.5 rudiment before culture; hatched bar: M+ rudiments after 7 days in vitro; black bars: M- rudiments after 7 days in culture. Note that after 7 days in culture more endocrine cells have developed from M- rudiments than from M+ rudiments grown in the same conditions. On the contrary, the exocrine tissue developed more from M+ rudiments than from M- rudiments. Each data point represents the mean +/- s.e.m. of 10 pancreatic rudiments (with permission, reference 17).*

Moreover, endocrine cells grown without mesenchyme appear more differentiated than endocrine cells from cultured whole pancreas epithelia. These more differentiated endocrine cells express differentiation markers such as Glut-2 and Rab3A, a protein associated with secretory granules. Furthermore, while endocrine cells from M (+) cultured epithelia tend to be dispersed as individual cells, M (-) cultured epithelia form islets with a characteristic mantle distribution of glucagon cells around a core of insulin cells. Cells co-expressing insulin and glucagon (the purported endocrine progenitor cells), are abundant in M (+) and absent in M (-) cultured epithelia, further suggesting that an epithelium relieved of the suppressive effects of its mesenchyme develops more differentiated endocrine cells. An epithelium without its surrounding mesenchyme shows significantly fewer exocrine cells and fails to develop the proper acinar architecture seen in whole pancreatic rudiments with intact mesenchyme.

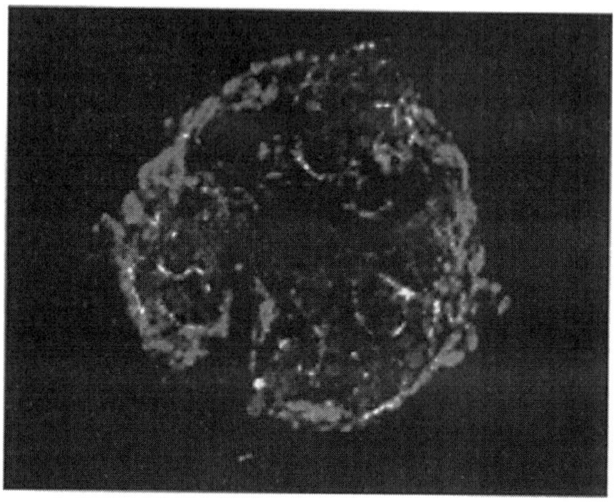

Figure 8. *Immuno-histochemical analysis of pancreatic rudiments grown in vitro for 7 days in the absence of mesenchyme. Acinar cells (stained for amylase) are confined to a central sphere. Note the residual mesenchyme (stained for vimentin) enveloping the exocrine tissue (with permission, reference 17).*

WHAT IS THE "MESENCHYMAL FACTOR" ? : A CANDIDATE APPROACH

Recognition of the mesenchyme's instructive, rather than permissive, role in determining pancreatic epithelial cell fate, has rekindled interest in characterizing the mesenchymal factor, or factors, responsible for lineage selection. Specifically, sonic hedgehog, activin / follistatin, hepatocyte growth factor, and laminin have each been implicated as important contributors to the mesenchymal-epithelial interactions guiding endocrine and exocrine commitment.

Sonic Hedgehog

Sonic hedgehog (Shh), a secreted protein and potent patterning signal implicated in cell-cell interactions in various developing organ systems, is expressed throughout the early embryonic gut endoderm (26). Curiously, neither ventral nor dorsal pancreatic endoderm express Shh at any point in its development. In order to better define the significance of absent Shh signalling in pancreatic endoderm, Apelqvist et al. (27) developed transgenic mice which selectively express Shh in the pancreatic endoderm, under the control of the ipf1/pdx1 promoter. Mesoderm from these ipf/pdx1-Shh pups developed into smooth muscle and interstitial cells of Cajal, thought to control pacemaker activity in the intestine, rather than into pancreatic mesenchyme and spleen. Furthermore, when Shh was added *in vitro* to wild type E10 dorsal pancreas grown seven days in culture, the mesenchyme was converted to smooth muscle and behaved functionally like intestine, as evidenced by its rhythmic peristalsis. Unexpectedly, however, the pancreatic epithelium in the ipf1/pdx1-Shh pups express glucagon, insulin, and amylase, although without acinar or islet structure. The appearance of any differentiated epithelial cells in the absence of normal pancreatic mesenchyme would suggest that either the conversion of mesenchyme to intestinal smooth muscle in their transgenic model progresses gradually, thus permitting some pancreatic mesenchymal-epithelial interaction to occur early on, or that the mutant mesenchyme retains some limited instructive properties towards pancreatic epithelium despite the conversion. Additionally, the use of the ipf1/pdx1 promoter to drive Shh expression may still allow some early inductive events to occur. It is well known that ipf1/pdx1 expression is not required for initial bud formation, and the appearance of a few insulin and glucagon positive cells is noted in ipf/pdx1 (-/-) mice (22). In any case, repression of Shh late in pancreatic development appears critical for normal pancreatic morphogenesis.

Early regulation of Shh appears to come from the notochord, which lies in close proximity to the dorsal embryonic pancreas prior to the fusion of the paired dorsal aortas in the midline (13-somite stage in mice, 22-somite stage in chicken) (28). Notochord ablation in Stage 11 chicken embryos prevents subsequent expression of important genes in dorsal pancreas development, such as isl-1 and pdx1, presumably as a result of unopposed Shh in this pancreatic endoderm. Indeed, following one day in culture, *in situ* hybridization for Shh in stage 11 notochord-deleted embryos shows increased expression of Shh in dorsal and ventral pancreatic endoderm. Recombining pancreatic endoderm with notochord *in vitro* is capable of restoring Shh suppression. In addition, cultured pancreatic endoderm from notochord-deleted embryos exposed to anti-Shh antiserum expresses pdx1 and insulin at similar levels to age-matched controls. Hebrok and colleagues have identified two proteins, activin βB and fibroblast growth factor-2 (FGF-2), present in notochord which appear to be important inhibitors of Shh (29). Adding either exogenous activin βB or FGF-2 induces expression of pdx1 and insulin while suppressing endodermal Shh and its receptor, patch (ptc). Notably, ventral pancreatic endoderm is unaffected by notochord deletion. Thus, there may exist sources of suppressive factors, similar to notochord, in the vicinity of the ventral bud which prevent Shh from interfering with ventral epithelial differentiation and mesenchymal development. Epithelial Shh expression later in gestation (> E10) causes a mesenchymal intestinalization and associated disruption of islet and acinar architecture (27). Therefore, the notochord's inhibitory effect on Shh observed early in gestation must persist in other forms later in gestation, after the notochord has been sequestered from the developing pancreas. One intriguing possibility is that inhibition of Shh results from the presence of activin βB in mid-gestation (E11) epithelium (Maldonado et al. unpublished data, discussed below).

ACTIVIN AND FOLLISTATIN

Activin, a member of the TGF-beta superfamily, is known to regulate the growth and differentiation of a variety of cell types. Data is beginning to accumulate that implicate activin signaling in exocrine and endocrine pancreas differentiation. Exogenous activin added to E11 pancreatic anlagen completely blocks exocrine formation (Maldonado et al. unpublished data) as well as ductal branching (30). This inhibitory effect is prevented by co-incubation with follistatin, a known inhibitor of activin, indicating that the effect of activin is specific and not toxic. The fate of endocrine cells was not specifically examined in these studies. However, activin signalling is clearly important for endocrine cell differentiation, as demonstrated in studies using transgenic mice expressing a dominant negative form of activin receptor (dn-ActR) (31). Mice with blocked activin signalling developed hypoplasia of pancreatic islets late in gestation (Figure 9).

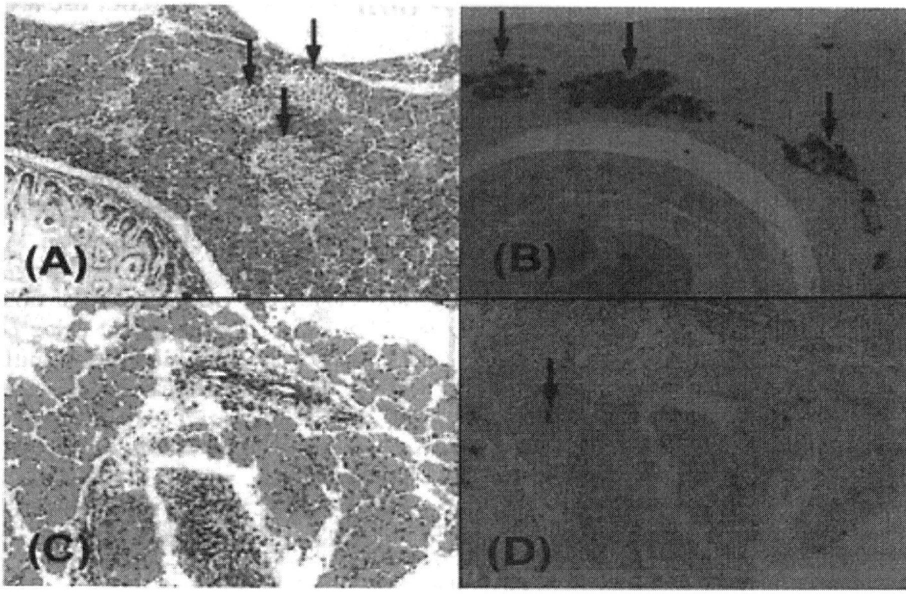

Figure 9. *Hematoxylin and eosin staining and immunostaining for insulin of E19.5 pancreas in a transgenic mouse with intact ActR,* ***(A,B)*** *and in a dnActR transgenic mouse* ***(C,D)****. Several normally developed islets are indicated by arrows in A and B, but almost no obvious islets were observed in C and D (with permission, reference 31).*

In addition, the dnActR pups had a severely impaired insulin response to glucose, as well as a decreased 15-week survival rate. Interestingly, transgenic mice with a constitutively active activin receptor also develop hypoplastic islets, suggesting that an activin signal of the appropriate intensity is necessary for proper endocrine cell differentiation. Activin exists in two isoforms, activin βA and βB. Activin βA has been shown to be co-expressed with glucagon as early as E11 in mouse embryonic pancreas and continues to be expressed in α-cells of the adult islet (32). Activin βB is also co-expressed with glucagon in these ages (Maldonado et al., unpublished data). The presence of activin exclusively in α-cells and its apparent inductive effect on other endocrine cells implies that it acts in a paracrine and autocrine fashion to regulate endocrine differentiation.

Follistatin is present in mesenchyme early in gestation. Unlike other known inhibitors of growth factors that are able to transiently attach to their specific ligands, follistatin neutralizes the biologic activity of activin by binding to it in an irreversible complex (30,33). Exogenous follistatin mimics the effect of mesenchyme on developing epithelia, driving exocrine and simultaneously suppressing endocrine differentiation (17). When added to *in vitro* developing E12.5 rat epithelium without its mesenchyme, follistatin results in a significant overgrowth of exocrine cells and a dramatic reduction in endocrine cells. Thus follistatin is likely to be an active component of the 'mesenchymal factor' mediating mesenchymal-epithelial interactions.

A delicate balance exists between activin and follistatin in the developing pancreas. Early in embryonic life mesenchymal follistatin inhibits epithelial activin, resulting in unimpeded exocrine differentiation and relative suppression of endocrine lineage. However, as gestation proceeds and mesenchyme represents a smaller proportion of the total pancreas, follistatin may no longer be able to inhibit activin's pro-endocrine effect, resulting in increased proliferation of endocrine tissue that occurs at day 14-15. Not surprisingly, compensatory or redundant regulatory mechanisms for dictating lineage selection must exist. Indeed, transgenic mice deficient in follistatin, while suffering multiple defects as well as perinatal death, appear to have normal pancreata (20,34). Furthermore, although dnActR pups do have a decreased survival rate compared to littermate controls, lack of activin signalling does not result in a lethal phenotype as might be expected if endocrine lineage selection were entirely dependent on activin.

In addition to their potential role in mesenchymal-epithelial interactions and lineage selection, activin and follistatin may play a part in maintaining endocrine homeostasis in the adult. Activin βA stimulates insulin secretion, even in the absence of glucose (35). Interestingly, while follistatin is found predominantly in the mesenchyme at early embryonic ages, it is also expressed in adult β-cells (36). This apparent inconsistency may reflect the paracrine or autocrine mechanisms necessary for maintaining appropriate glucose levels in the adult.

HEPATOCYTE GROWTH FACTOR

Another growth factor with potential paracrine effects which has been implicated in mesenchymal-epithelial interactions in pancreas organogenesis is hepatocyte growth factor (HGF). Also known as scatter factor (SF) for its ability to cause the dispersion and migration of epithelial cells in culture (37), HGF was first purified from rat platelets and shown to be a potent mitogen for mature hepatocytes (38). In addition to its mitogenic and cell-scattering effects on various cultured epithelial cell lines, HGF has striking morphogenic effects *in vitro,* such as the induction of lumen formation in breast carcinoma cells and tubule formation in kidney tubular cells (39,40). However, the functions of HGF and its tyrosine kinase cell-surface receptor, c-met, *in vivo* are less well characterized. While the distribution of c-met expression is confined to the epithelium of various embryonic organs, including the pancreas (41,42), localisation of HGF expression is more controversial. Mouse pancreas expressed HGF mRNA only in mesenchymal cells (42). Interestingly, HGF positive mesenchymal cells concentrate in areas of mesenchymal-epithelial interface, consistent with the notion that HGF may be signalling to epithelial receptor. Furthermore, HGF expression has been identified in a variety of foetal fibroblast cell lines, as well as adult mesenchyme derivatives such as Kupffer cells and Ito cells, suggesting a mesenchymal source for the growth factor (37,43-45). However, HGF expression is also found in the epithelium of various adult and embryonic organs (41,46-50). Localization studies in the pancreas that show epithelial expression of HGF looked exclusively for HGF protein and not for mRNA. One explanation for the discrepancies in HGF localization might be that HGF is secreted from the mesenchyme to the epithelium, where it binds to its receptor. Thus, HGF might not be made *de novo* in the epithelium and yet may be detected there by immunohistochemistry.

Although the precise distribution of HGF in adult and embryonic tissues may be a source of debate, numerous studies have corroborated the inductive effect of HGF on both exocrine and endocrine pancreatic cells. In primary organ cultures from mid-gestational human foetal pancreata exogenous HGF markedly stimulates the *in vitro* development of epithelial cell clusters containing increased numbers of β-cells (51). When these same organ cultures are exposed to media conditioned by foetal pancreatic fibroblasts (mesenchymal derivatives) for 4 days, a 2.3-fold increase in epithelial proliferation and a 1.5-fold increase in DNA content is found (52). This effect is blocked by anti-HGF antiserum. HGF from foetal fibroblast-conditioned media leads to a significant decrease in insulin content in proliferating epithelial cells. This is not due to a decrease in β-cell number but rather to a decrease in insulin content of individual β-cells, suggesting that HGF stimulates endocrine growth, but not differentiation. The potential role of HGF in endocrine lineage selection is further supported by the expression of its receptor, c-met, in early islets, with most intense localization in β-cells. Furthermore, HGF may serve to direct early epithelial cells, or even exocrine cells, towards endocrine commitment. *In vitro* experiments in which pancreatic AR42J cells, derived from acinar cells, are cultured with recombinant HGF, resulted in a reduction in amylase content and other acinar cell-like properties, and occasional conversion to insulin-producing cells (53). Moreover, when HGF was supplemented with activin βA, the conversion to insulin producing cells is increased. The additive effect of HGF and activin βA is particularly intriguing given that activin βA is expressed in embryonic α-cells (32) and HGF presumably binds to its receptor in β-cells. The potential paracrine effect of α-cell activin on its neighboring β-cell may in fact serve to augment the latter's response to HGF. Thus activin and HGF may act synergistically *in vivo* to induce β-cell differentiation.

In addition to its inductive effects on pancreatic endocrine cells, HGF appears to be important for exocrine growth and differentiation as well. Small multipotent epithelial stem cells known as oval cells, found in the embryonic and adult pancreas and liver, express c-met receptor *in vitro* and *in vivo* (54). These oval cells exhibit a proliferative response to exogenous HGF, forming branching tubular structures resembling ducts on electron microscopy, even in the absence of a surrounding extracellular matrix. In addition, when nude mice are injected subcutaneously with oval cells they develop focal ductal adenocarcinomas at the site of injection. Interestingly, while these oval cells express c-met they do not produce HGF and thus an autocrine effect cannot exist. Rather, HGF produced by nude mice themselves may be acting on the injected oval cells to produce the observed effect.

Further evidence that HGF has an instructive role in the growth and differentiation of exocrine cells comes from studies that show that HGF has a potent mitogenic effect on human exocrine pancreas cell cultures, containing both adult ductal and acinar cells (55). Proliferating cells exposed to HGF display a ductal phenotype, as shown by specific staining for characteristic ductal cell markers, such as cytokeratins, but lack acinar markers, such as amylase. c-met, the HGF receptor, has in adult pancreas an apical distribution, i.e. is confined to the luminal cell membrane domain (Figure 10). It is thus possible that HGF reaches its target, c-met, in adult or developing exocrine cells via existing ducts, causing growth and further differentiation during development, or uncontrolled proliferation as in pancreatic carcinoma. Indeed, the c-met receptor is detectable only at low levels in the normal adult exocrine pancreas, but has been noted to be upregulated in human pancreatic ductal carcinoma as well as numerous pancreatic cancer cell lines (56).

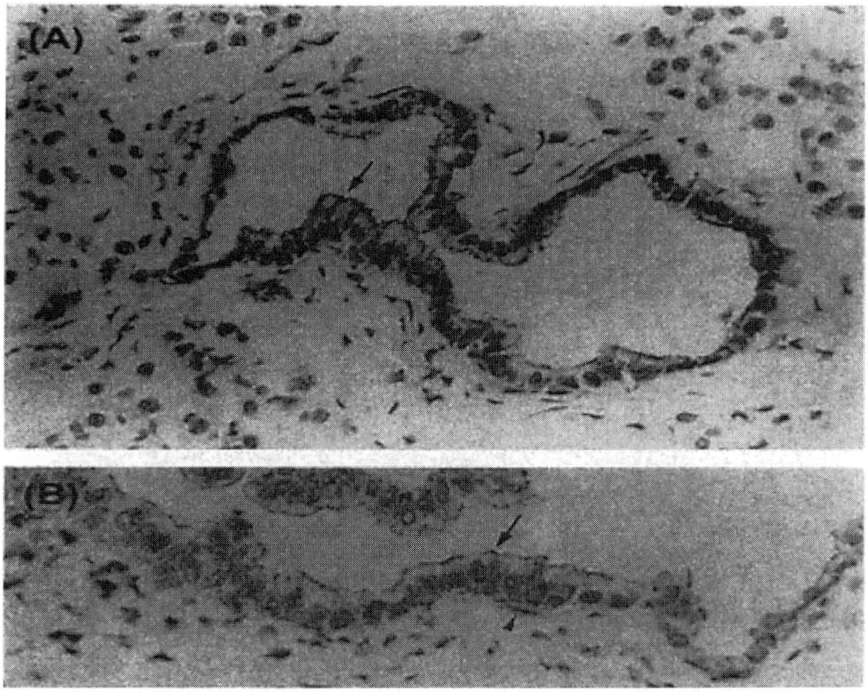

Figure 10. *Immunohistochemical analysis of c-met expression in normal pancreas tissue. The HGF receptor is exclusively detected in normal ductal cells **A**) and shows a predominantly apical distribution **B**). Arrows indicate apical reactivity in ductal cells. Arrowhead indicates weak basolateral reactivity (with permission, reference 55).*

Although the exact role of HGF *in vivo* remains to be defined, the mesenchymal expression of HGF and the epithelial expression of c-met, as well as the observed inductive effects of HGF on endocrine and exocrine cell growth and differentiation *in vitro*, suggest that this factor may have an important function in mesenchymal-epithelial interactions in the developing pancreas. Importantly, c-met and HGF mRNA expression appear to be upregulated in rats late in gestation and immediately after birth (57). Levels drop precipitously after post-natal day 20 and are almost undetectable in the adult. The upregulation of HGF and c-met expression coincides with the rapid proliferation of duct, islet, and acinar cells at birth and is consistent with the notion that HGF signaling is important in growth and differentiation of embryonic pancreas (58,59).

LAMININ

While Shh, activin, follistatin, and HGF represent potential regulatory molecules that do not require cell-cell contact to exert their effects, non-diffusible proteins found in basement membrane have also been implicated in mesenchymal-epithelial interactions. Basement membrane (lamina) contains type IV collagen, proteoglycans such as heparin sulfate and chondroitin sulfate, and non-collagenous proteins, like laminin and fibronectin (60,61). The laminins are a large family of glycoproteins consisting of more than 10 members, of which laminin-1 is best characterized. It is a heterotrimer composed of $\alpha_1\beta_1$ and γ chains arranged in a cross with three short arms and one long arm, as shown by EM of rotary shadowed molecules (61). In kidney, lung, and the submandibular gland, laminin appears to be the major basement membrane component responsible for tubule formation and branching (62-64). In all these organs, as in the pancreas, branching morphogenesis is the major developmental motif. Laminin mediates cell-cell and cell-substrate adhesion, cell movement and cell proliferation, all of which are important for normal branching morphogenesis to occur (65-67). Kidney tubule development is blocked by adding anti-laminin-1 antibodies to day 12 embryonic kidneys in culture (62) and anti-laminin-1 antibodies inhibit epithelial branching when added to day 13 lung explants in culture (63). A similar effect of the antibody is found on branching epithelia in day 13 submandibular explants (64).

E11.5 epithelia cultured in a basement membrane-rich gel incubated with polyclonal anti-laminin-1 antibodies fails to form ductal structures (Crisera et al., unpublished data). Similarly, monoclonal antibodies against the cross-region of the laminin-1 heterotrimer or against an $\alpha6$-containing integrin (which is known to bind laminin-1 (68)) also block the induction of duct formation. These studies demonstrate that the exocrine-inhibitory effects seen with the addition of the various antibodies are specifically attributable to the neutralization of laminin-1. Early in gestation, at E10.5, laminin-1 expression is diffuse in the pancreatic mesenchyme, but the epithelium is spared (Crisera et al. unpublished data). Two days later, at E12.5, laminin-1 remains expressed throughout the mesenchyme. However, in addition to the expression within the mesenchymal cells at this age, a strong extracellular deposition of laminin-1 is also apparent, forming a rim around the developing epithelial cells at the interface between the epithelium and the mesenchyme. The general mechanism of recruitment and organization of soluble laminin into an organized lattice adjacent to the epithelium has recently been elucidated and appears to involve α-dystroglycan (69). As pancreatic organogenesis progresses, laminin-1 expression localizes to developing exocrine structures. Laminin-1 becomes tightly associated with the acini, forming a rim around each developing acinus. It is also notably adjacent to the epithelial cells of the developing ductules. Interestingly, clusters of proliferating pancreatic cells that lack intimate contact with laminin-1 seem to select the endocrine lineage and organize into islets by E18.5.

CONCLUSION

Basement membrane laminin, through direct contact, as well as diffusible factors, such as activin, follistatin, Shh, and HGF, each appear to be important "mesenchymal factors" that individually or together influence cell lineage commitment of the epithelium during pancreatic development. Mesenchyme is more than a germ layer that gives rise to its derivative organs, tissues, and cell types. Rather it represents a sophisticated regulator of epithelium, essential for permitting organogenesis and capable of instructing cell lineage selection. The frustrating search for an elusive "mesenchymal factor" culminates with an appreciation that this factor is most likely a composite of many factors. Finally, using an educated candidate approach to identifying factors involved in mesenchymal-epithelial interactions, we have begun to assemble a growing list of growth factors, receptors, and inhibitors, each most likely acting through paracrine or autocrine routes to chart development and maintain homeostasis. Using these growth factors *in vitro* to drive a pluripotential stem cell towards a pre-determined differentiated state remains the ultimate goal of the study of pancreas development, and may someday provide a potential cure for diseases such as diabetes mellitus and ductal adenocarcinoma.

REFERENCES

1. Wallner EI, Yang Q, Peterson DR, Wada J, Kanwar YS. Relevance of extracellular matrix, its receptors, and cell adhesion molecules in mammalian nephrogenesis. Am J Physiol 1998;275:F467-77.
2. Kedinger M, Duluc I, Fritsch C, Lorentz O, Plateroti M, Freund JN. Intestinal epithelial-mesenchymal cell interactions. Ann NY Acad Sci 1998;859:1-17.
3. Cunha GR, Battle E, Young P, et al. Role of epithelial-mesenchymal interactions in the differentiation and spatial organization of visceral smooth muscle. Epithelial Cell Biol 1992;1:76-83.
4. Mizuno T, Yasugi S. Susceptibility of epithelia to directive influences of mesenchymes during organogenesis: uncoupling of morphogenesis and cytodifferentiation. Cell Differ Dev 1990;31:151-9.
5. Cutler LS, Gremski W. Epithelial-mesenchymal interactions in the development of salivary glands. Crit Rev Oral Biol Med 1991;2:1-12.
6. Golosow N, Grobstein C. Epitheliomesenchymal Interaction in Pancreatic Morphogenesis. Dev Biol 1962;4:242-255.
7. Rutter WJ, Wessells NK, Grobstein C. Control of specific synthesis 1964;13:51-65.
8. Fell PE, Grobstein C. The influence of extra-epithelial factors on the growth of embryonic mouse pancreatic epithelium. Exp Cell Res 1968;53:301-4.
9. Kallman F, Grobstein C. Fine structure of differentiating mouse pancreatic exocrine cells in transfilter culture. J Cell B 1964;20:399-413.
10. Wessells N, Cohen J. Early Pancreatic Organogenesis: Morphogenesis, Tissue Interactions, and Mass Effects. Dev Biol 1966;15:237-270.
11. Spooner BS, Cohen HI, Faubion J. Development of the embryonic mammalian pancreas: the relationship between morphogenesis and cytodifferentiation. Dev Biol 1977;61:119-30.
12. Ronzio RA, Rutter WJ. Effects of a partially purified factor from chick embryos on macromolecular synthesis of embryonic pancreatic epithelia. Dev Biol 1973;30:307-20.
13. Rutter WJ, Pictet RL, Harding JD, Chirgwin JM, MacDonald RJ, Przybyla AE. An analysis of pancreatic development: role of mesenchymal factor and other extracellular factors. Symp Soc Dev Biol 1978;35:205-27.
14. Grobstein C, Cohen J. Collagenase: effect on the morphogenesis of embryonic salivary epithelium in vitro. Science 1965;150:626-8.
15. Levine S, Pictet R, Rutter WJ. Control of cell proliferation and cytodifferentiation by a factor reacting with the cell surface. Nature New Biology 1973;246:49-52.
16. Pictet R, Rall L, de Gasparo M, Rutter WJ. Regulation of Differentiation of Endocrine Cells during Pancreatic Development In Vitro. In: Camerini-Davalos RA, Cole HS, eds. Early Diabetes in Early Life. New York: Academic Press, 1975:25-39.
17. Miralles F, Czernichow P, Scharfmann R. Follistatin regulates the relative proportions of endocrine versus exocrine tissue during pancreatic development. Development 1998;125:1017-24.
18. Gittes GK, Galante PE, Hanahan D, Rutter WJ, Debase HT. Lineage-specific morphogenesis in the developing pancreas: role of mesenchymal factors. Development 1996;122:439-47.
19. Rose M, Crisera C, Colen K, Longaker M, Gittes G. Epithelio-mesenchymal interactions in the developing pancreas: morphogenesis of the adult architecture. Journal of Pediatric Surgery 1999:(in press).
20. Edlund H. Transcribing pancreas. Diabetes 1998;47:1817-23.
21. Ahlgren U, Pfaff SL, Jessell TM, Edlund T, Edlund H. Independent requirement for ISL1 in formation of pancreatic mesenchyme and islet cells. Nature 1997;385:257-60.
22. Ahlgren U, Jonsson J, Edlund H. The morphogenesis of the pancreatic mesenchyme is uncoupled from that of the pancreatic epithelium in IPF1/PDX1-deficient mice. Development 1996;122:1409-16.
23. Offield MF, Jetton TL, Labosky PA, et al. PDX-1 is required for pancreatic outgrowth and differentiation of the rostral duodenum. Development 1996;122:983-95.
24. Krapp A, Knofler M, Frutiger S, Hughes GJ, Hagenbuchle O, Wellauer PK. The p48 DNA-binding subunit of transcription factor PTF1 is a new exocrine pancreas-specific basic helix-loop-helix protein. Embo J 1996;15:4317-29.
25. Krapp A, Knofler M, Ledermann B, et al. The bHLH protein PTF1-p48 is essential for the formation of the exocrine and the correct spatial organization of the endocrine pancreas. Genes Dev 1998;12:3752-63.

26. Bitgood MJ, McMahon AP. Hedgehog and Bmp genes are coexpressed at many diverse sites of cell- cell interaction in the mouse embryo. Dev Biol 1995;172:126-38.
27. Apelqvist A, Ahlgren U, Edlund H. Sonic hedgehog directs specialised mesoderm differentiation in the intestine and pancreas [published erratum appears in Curr Biol 1997 Dec 1;7(12):R809]. Curr Biol 1997; 7:801-4.
28. Kim SK, Hebrok M, Melton DA. Notochord to endoderm signaling is required for pancreas development. Development 1997;124:4243-4252.
29. Hebrok M, Kim SK, Melton DA. Notochord repression of endodermal Sonic hedgehog permits pancreas development. Genes Dev 1998;12:1705-13.
30. Ritvos O, Tuuri T, Eramaa M, et al. Activin disrupts epithelial branching morphogenesis in developing glandular organs of the mouse. Mech Dev 1995;50:229-45.
31. Yamaoka T, Idehara C, Yano M, et al. Hypoplasia of pancreatic islets in transgenic mice expressing activin receptor mutants. J Clin Invest 1998;102:294-301.
32. Furukawa M, Eto Y, Kojima I. Expression of immunoreactive activin A in fetal rat pancreas. Endocr J 1995;42:63-8.
33. Schneyer AL, Rzucidlo DA, Sluss PM, Crowley WF, Jr. Characterization of unique binding kinetics of follistatin and activin or inhibin in serum. Endocrinology 1994;135:667-74.
34. Matzuk MM, Lu N, Hannes V, Sellheryer K, Roop DR, Bradley A. Multiple defects and perinatal death in mice deficient in follistatin. Nature 1995;374:360-363.
35. Furukawa M, Nobusawa R, Shibata H, Eto Y, Kojima I. Initiation of insulin secretion in glucose-free medium by activin A. Mol Cel Endocrinol 1995;113:83-7.
36. Ogawa K, Abe K, Kurosawa N, et al. Expression of alpha, beta A and beta B subunits of inhibin or activin and follistatin in rat pancreatic islets. FEBS Lett 1993;319:217-20.
37. Stoker M, Gherardi E, Perryman M, Gray J. Scatter factor is a fibroblast-derived modulator of epithelial cell mobility. Nature 1987;327:239-42.
38. Nakamura T, Teramoto H, Ichihara A. Purification and characterization of a growth factor from rat platelets for mature parenchymal hepatocytes in primary cultures. Proc Natl Acad Sci USA 1986;83:6489-93.
39. Tsarfaty I, Resau JH, Rulong S, Keydar I, Faletto DL, Vande Woude GF. The met proto-oncogene receptor and lumen formation. Science 1992;257:1258-61.
40. Montesano R, Matsumoto K, Nakamura T, Orci L. Identification of a fibroblast-derived epithelial morphogen as hepatocyte growth factor. Cell 1991;67:901-8.
41. Kermorgant S, Walker F, Hormi K, Dessirier V, Lewin MJ, Lehy T. Developmental expression and functionality of hepatocyte growth factor and c-Met in human fetal digestive tissues. Gastroenterology 1997;112:1635-47.
42. Sonnenberg E, Meyer D, Weidner KM, Birchmeier C. Scatter factor/hepatocyte growth factor and its receptor, the c-met tyrosine kinase, can mediate a signal exchange between mesenchyme and epithelia during mouse development. J Cell Biol 1993;123:223-35.
43. Rubin JS, Chan AM, Bottaro DP, et al. A broad-spectrum human lung fibroblast-derived mitogen is a variant of hepatocyte growth factor. Proc Natl Acad Sci USA 1991;88:415-9.
44. Noji S, Tashiro K, Koyama E, et al. Expression of hepatocyte growth factor gene in endothelial and Kupffer cells of damaged rat livers, as revealed by in situ hybridization. Biochem Biophys Res Commun 1990;173:42-7.
45. Schirmacher P, Geerts A, Pietrangelo A, Dienes HP, Rogler CE. Hepatocyte growth factor/hepatopoietin A is expressed in fat-storing cells from rat liver but not myofibroblast-like cells derived from fat- storing cells. Hepatology 1992;15:5-11.
46. Zarnegar R, Muga S, Rahija R, Michalopoulos G. Tissue distribution of hepatopoietin-A: a heparin-binding polypeptide growth factor for hepatocytes. Proc Natl Acad Sci USA 1990;87:1252-6.
47. Wang Y, Selden C, Farnaud S, Calnan D, Hodgson HJ. Hepatocyte growth factor (HGF/SF) is expressed in human epithelial cells during embryonic development; studies by in situ hybridisation and northern blot analysis. J Anat 1994;185:543-51.
48. Wolf HK, Zarnegar R, Michalopoulos GK. Localization of hepatocyte growth factor in human and rat tissues: an immunohistochemical study. Hepatology 1991;14:488-94.
49. Defrances MC, Wolf HK, Michalopoulos GK, Zarnegar R. The presence of hepatocyte growth factor in the developing rat. Development 1992;116:387-95.
50. Tsuda H, Iwase T, Matsumoto K, et al. Immunohistochemical localization of hepatocyte growth factor protein in pancreas islet A-cells of man and rats. Jpn J Cancer Res 1992;83:1262-6.
51. Otonkoski T, Beattie GM, Rubin JS, Lopez AD, Baird A, Hayek A. Hepatocyte growth factor/scatter factor has insulinotropic activity in human fetal pancreatic cells. Diabetes 1994;43:947-53.
52. Otonkoski T, Cirulli V, Beattie M, et al. A role for hepatocyte growth factor/scatter factor in fetal mesenchyme-induced pancreatic beta-cell growth. Endocrinology 1996;137:3131-9.
53. Mashima H, Shibata H, Mine T, Kojima I. Formation of insulin-producing cells from pancreatic acinar AR42J cells by hepatocyte growth factor. Endocrinology 1996;137:3969-76.

54. Jeffers M, Rao MS, Rulong S, et al. Hepatocyte growth factor/scatter factor-Met signaling induces proliferation, migration, and morphogenesis of pancreatic oval cells. Cell Growth Differ 1996;7:1805-13.
55. Vila MR, Nakamura T, Real FX. Hepatocyte growth factor is a potent mitogen for normal pancreas cells in vivo. Lab Invest 1995;73:409-18.
56. Di Renzo MF, Poulsom R, Olivero M, Comoglio PM, Lemoine NR. Expression of the Met/hepatocyte growth factor receptor in human pancreatic cancer. Cancer Res 1995; 55:1129-38.
57. Calvo EL, Boucher C, Pelletier G, Morisset J. Ontogeny of hepatocyte growth factor and c-met/hgf receptor in rat pancreas. Biochem Biophys Res Commun 1996;229:257-63.
58. Parsa I, Marsh WH, Fitzgerald PJ. Pancreas acinar cell differentiation. II. Comparative DNA and protein synthesis of the embryonic rat pancreas and the pancreatic anlage grown in organ culture. Am J Pathol 1969;57:489-521.
59. Parsa I, Marsh WH, Fitzgerald PJ. Pancreas acinar cell differentiation. I. Morphologic and enzymatic comparisons of embryonic rat pancreas anlage grown in organ culture. Am J Pathol 1969;57:457-87.
60. Kleinman HK, McGarvey ML, Hassell JR, et al. Basement membrane complexes with biological activity. Biochemistry 1986;25:312-8.
61. Aumailley M, Smyth N. The role of laminins in basement membrane function. J Anat 1998;193(Pt. 1):1-21.
62. Klein G. Role of laminin A chain in the development of epithelial cell polarity. Cell 1988;55:331-341.
63. Schuger L, O'Shea S, Rheinheimer J, Varani J. Laminin in lung development: effects of anti-laminin antibody in murine lung morphogenesis. Dev Biol 1990;137:26-32.
64. Kadoya Y. Antibodies against domain E3 of laminin-1 and integrin alpha 6 subunit perturb branching epithelial morphogenesis of submandibular gland, but by different modes. J Cell Biol 1995;129(2):521-534.
65. Kleinman HK, Cannon FB, Laurie GW, et al. Biological activities of laminin. J Cell Biochem 1985;27:317-25.
66. Durbeej M, Ekblom P. Dystroglycan and laminins: glycoconjugates involved in branching epithelial morphogenesis. Exp Lung Res 1997;23:109-18.
67. Ekblom M, Falk M, Salmivirta K, Durbeej M, Ekblom P. Laminin isoforms and epithelial development. Ann N Y Acad Sci 1998;857:194-211.
68. Aumailley M, Timpl R, Sonnenberg A. Antibody to integrin alpha 6 subunit specifically inhibits cell-binding to laminin fragment 8. Exp Cell Res 1990;188:55-60.
69. Henry M, Campbell K. A role for dystroglycan in basement membrane assembly. Cell 1988;95:859-870.

11
HOMEODOMAIN PROTEINS IN PANCREAS DEVELOPMENT

Ulf Ahlgren, Ph.D. and Helena Edlund, Ph.D.
University of Umeå, S-90187 Umeå, Sweden

INTRODUCTION

The pancreas derives from the upper, duodenal part of the foregut via a dorsal and ventral protrusion of the epithelium directly posterior to the developing stomach, and in the mouse, the early pancreatic buds become evident on embryonic day 9 (e9) (Figure 1). The part of the gut from which the pancreas originates becomes committed to a pancreatic fate already at the ~10 somites stage, i.e. at e8.5 (1). A few somites later these regions of the duodenal epithelium will begin to evaginate, thus forming the dorsal and ventral pancreatic buds. During embryogenesis the pancreatic epithelium proliferates and invades the surrounding mesenchyme and the epithelial cells differentiate and segregate into duct, acinar and endocrine cells. As the stomach and duodenum rotates, the ventral bud will move around until it eventually comes in contact and fuses with its dorsal counterpart around e13-14 (Figure 1).

Over the past four decades, our understanding of the fundamental aspects that regulate these processes has been based on some few but major landmarks. In the 1960s the classical embryological experiments performed by Golosow and Grobstein (1) and Wessels and Cohen (2) described the morphogenesis of the pancreas and the epithelio-mesenchymal interactions that are required for proper pancreatic development. During the 1970s the groups of Le Douarin and Rutter showed that, despite their similarities with neurones, the pancreatic endocrine cells, like the exocrine and duct cells, are of an endodermal origin (3-5) and in the 1980s, Rutter and others identified various transcription factors that regulate both endocrine and exocrine gene expression (6,7). During the last decade the cloning of various transcription factors together with the development of the technology for generating transgenic animals, allowing "gain-of-function" and "loss-of-function" analysis have provided useful information regarding the function of some of these transcription factors during pancreas development. Thus, several homeodomain and basic-helix-loop-helix class transcription factors, notably IPF1/Pdx1, ISL1, *HB9*, Nkx2.2, Nkx6.1 Pax4, Pax6, and NeuroD/Beta2 have been shown to exert important functions in the control of pancreatic endocrine cell differentiation (8-18). The role of the Pax-genes are discussed elsewhere (see chapter 14 by Zhou & Gruss) and this chapter will focus predominantly on the role of the homeodomain proteins IPF1/Pdx1, ISL1 and *HB9*.

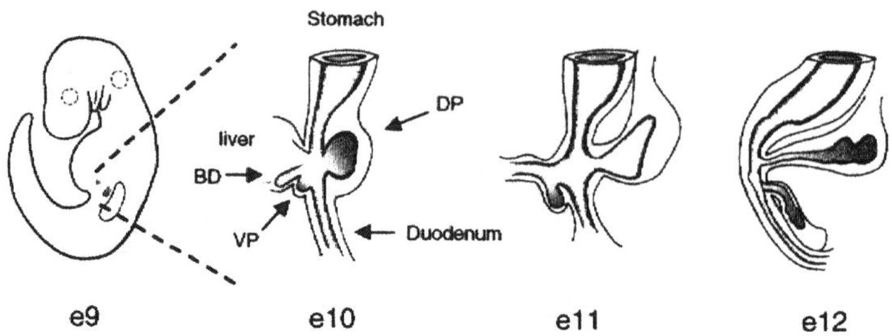

Figure 1. *Schematic drawing illustrating the morphological movements of the pancreatic anlagen during mouse development. The pancreatic buds form as a dorsal and ventral evagination of the foregut endoderm. The rotation of the stomach and duodenum positions the pancreatic buds at the same side of the duodenum where they will eventually fuse around e13-14. In all drawings, green fields correspond to the pancreatic epithelium. Abbreviations; DP, dorsal pancreas; VP, ventral pancreas; BD, bile duct (Illustration by U. Ahlgren/S. Sandström).*

More than a century has passed since homeotic mutations were first named and described (19). The homeobox was first described in genes controlling segment identity in Drosophila less than two decades ago (20,21). The protein region encoded by the homeobox, the DNA binding homeodomain, defines an important family of transregulatory factors that control developmental processes in organisms spanning from yeast and plants to insects and mammals. They are phylogenetically characterized, by a high degree of sequence similarities and chromosomal organization, although their numbers appear much greater in vertebrates than in insects due to successive duplication and chromosomal distribution events. The actual homeodomain is a conserved 60 amino acid domain, having three α-helical parts that creates an internal hydrophobic core. One of these helices, the recognition helix, inserts into the major groove of the DNA and makes base-specific contacts while the N-terminal arm makes contact with the minor groove, thereby stabilising the association with the DNA (22). The DNA motif most commonly associated with homeodomain binding is the 5'-TAAT-3' motif, although many other homeodomain binding consensus sequences have been identified. Perhaps the functionally best-conserved group of homeobox genes are a cluster of genes, which control segment identity along the anterior-posterior (A-P) axis, known as *HOM-C* in insects and nematodes and *Hox* in mammals (23). The HOM-C/Hox cluster is present in all animals studied to date and is ordered along the chromosome in the same order as they are expressed and function. Indeed, the functional relationship between the *HOM* and vertebrate *Hox* genes is so conserved that ubiquitous expression of certain mammalian *Hox* genes causes homeotic transformations in embryos that are similar to those produced by ectopic expression of related *HOM* genes (24). Within the homeodomain group, classes and families can be defined on the basis of primary sequence and/or unique regions outside the homeodomain; some of which themselves have DNA binding properties needed to determine binding specificity. Examples of such homeodomain proteins come from the pit-oct-unc (POU) and paired-homeobox (Pax) groups (25,26). The POU domain family of transcription factors was defined following the observation that the products of three mammalian genes, Pit-1, Oct-1, and Oct-2, and the protein encoded by the C. elegans gene unc-86, shared a region of homology, known as the POU domain (25). This is an approximately 75 amino acid domain capable of weak DNA binding in the absence of the homeodomain. However, no gene has yet been identified containing a POU specific domain only (27,28). Thus, POU proteins contain two autonomous DNA binding domains that work together to bind DNA, giving the interaction greater discriminatory capabilities (22). The *Pax* genes also include a second DNA-binding domain, encoded by the paired box motif, with variable sequence and organization. As with the POU domain, the paired domain can act synergistically with the homeodomain to increase the binding affinity to the DNA (29). In addition to monomer formation, some homeodomain proteins can bind to their target site as homodimer or heterodimer complexes. For example the Pit-1 POU domain can bind DNA as a homodimer (30). In contrast, the drosophila cofactor extradenticle, and its mammalian homologues the Pbx homeodomain proteins, bind co-operatively to DNA with members of the HOM-C/Hox family as well as with other homeodomain proteins (31,32) and as a consequence the DNA-binding specificity is modulated. A third group of homeodomain proteins sharing conserved regions outside the homeodomain are the LIM homeodomain proteins. The LIM motif was first identified in three developmentally important transcription factors, C. elegans Lin-11, rat Isl1 and C. elegans Mec-3 from which the acronym LIM is derived (33,34). The LIM domain is a cysteine-rich domain composed of two zinc-finger motifs that are joined by a 2 amino acid spacer. The LIM domain appears to be a protein-protein dimerization domain that enables interaction between identical or different LIM domains as well as with proteins lacking LIM-domains (35). Hence, in general terms homeodomain proteins constitute an array of conserved regulators of development, involved in anything from lineage determination and differentiation pathways to the mode of organ formation.

IPF1/PDX1 IN PANCREATIC DEVELOPMENT

IPF1/Pdx1, also known as IDX-1, STF-1 (36,37), an orphan homeodomain protein, was originally identified by its ability to interact with the insulin promoter, thereby being able to stimulate insulin gene transcription (38). IPF1/Pdx1 starts to be expressed around the 10-12 somite stage in the part of the dorsal and ventral gut epithelium that will later develop into a pancreas, i.e. prior to hormone gene expression. A few somites later these IPF1/Pdx1 expressing regions of the duodenal epithelium will begin to evaginate, thus forming the dorsal and ventral pancreatic buds in which the majority of the cells are IPF1/Pdx1+ (38)(Figure 2A). High level IPF1/Pdx1 expression is maintained in the majority of the epithelial cells of the buds until around e10.5, after which it is down regulated (38)(Figure 2B). The early glucagon cells and the majority of the insulin cells do not express IPF1/Pdx1 when they first appear, but later IPF1/Pdx1 is up-regulated in the differentiated β-cells (38)(Figures 2B and 2C). The pattern of IPF1/Pdx1 expression and its ability to stimulate insulin gene transcription suggested that IPF1/Pdx1 function both in the regionalization of the primitive gut endoderm and in the maturation of the pancreatic β-cell. Homozygosity for mutations in the *Ipf1/Pdx1* gene in mice and humans results in agenesis of the pancreas (8,39,40). *Ipf1/Pdx1* however, does not seem to be required for the evagination and initial bud formation but rather it appears to specify the early pancreatic epithelium, permitting its proliferation, branching and subsequent differentiation (9,39)(compare Figures 2D and 2E).

Thus, the initial stages of pancreas ontogeny involving the early inductive events leading to the formation of the pancreatic buds and the appearance of a few early insulin and glucagon cells, still occurs in the *Ipf1/Pdx1* deficient embryos (compare

Figures 2D and 2E)(9). These results suggest that additional transcriptional factors exist which act upstream of IPF1/Pdx1 in the initial specification of the pancreatic endoderm. However, the subsequent morphogenesis of the pancreatic epithelium and the progression of differentiation of the endocrine cells are arrested in the *Ipf1/Pdx1* (-/-) embryos. In contrast, the pancreatic mesenchyme in the IPF1/Pdx1 mutants grows and develops both morphologically and functionally independently of the epithelium (9). The pancreatic epithelium is, however, unable to respond to the mesenchymal-derived signal(s) that normally promote pancreatic morphogenesis (1,2). Together these data provide evidence that IPF1/Pdx1, despite its early pancreatic expression pattern, is not instrumental in the specification of the foregut endoderm to a pancreatic fate, but rather is required after the pancreatic program has been initiated by acting cell autonomously within the epithelium where it is expressed. IPF1/Pdx1 may function during the early phase of pancreas development by transcriptionally regulating the expression of a component(s) involved in a signal transduction machinery. This may act at a receptor level or by allowing the transmission of mesenchymal signal(s) to the nucleus, thereby promoting the morphogenesis of the pancreatic epithelium. Alternatively, IPF1/Pdx1 may control the expression of morphogens, adhesion molecules or growth factors, all of which could be required for the morphogenesis and differentiation of the pancreas. It has been proposed that the early IPF1/Pdx1 expressing cells represent a common endocrine and exocrine stem cell population (41). The apparent lack of IPF1/Pdx1 expression in the glucagon and early insulin expressing cells combined with the presence of both these cell types in the *Ipf1/Pdx1 -/-* mice indicates that if such a stem cell exists, it is not dependent on IPF1/Pdx1 function. Together these data provide evidence that IPF1/Pdx1 acts cell-autonomously and that the lack of a pancreas in the *Ipf1/Pdx1 -/-* mice is due to a defect in the pancreatic epithelium.

IPF1/PDX1 IN THE DIFFERENTIATED β-CELLS

The arrested development of the pancreatic epithelium in the *Ipf1/Pdx1* mutants obviously precluded a loss of function analysis of any later contribution of IPF1/Pdx1 to β-cell development and function in such animals. However, The bacteriophage P1 derived *Cre-loxP* system for targeted recombination allows the temporal and spatial excision of chromosomal DNA segments flanked by *LoxP* sequences (42-44). This system is based on the ability of the bacteriophage P1 Cre recombinase to separate phage genomes that have become joined to one another during phage infection. The Cre recombinase works by lining up *LoxP* sequences and excising the intervening DNA. Mice in which the *Ipf1/Pdx1* gene has been disrupted specifically in β-cells using the *Cre-loxP* system, *Rip1/Ipf1t* (Figure 3A) initially appear healthy but on ageing develop diabetes as marked by elevated blood and urine glucose levels (45).

Analysis of *Rip1/Ipf1*▲ mice revealed that the Cre-*LoxP*-mediated recombination deletion of *Ipf1/Pdx1* is a progressive event, resulting in an overt diabetic (OD) phenotype when IPF1/Pdx1 has been excised in ~80% of the insulin expressing (ins+) cells (Figures 3B and 3C). As a consequence of *Ipf1/Pdx1* inactivation the hormone cell ratio was perturbed in the *Rip1/Ipf1*▲ mice, as shown by a 40% decrease in the number of ins+ cells together a concomitant two-fold increase in the number glucagon expressing cells (45 and Figures 3D and 3E). In addition, a substantial number of cells co expressed the two hormones (insulin and glucagon) (45)(Figures 3D and 3E). Also, in contrast to the normal distribution, co-expression of glucagon and insulin and a segregation of insulin/IAPP expression were detected

(45). These results show that IPF1/Pdx1 is required to maintain the hormone producing phenotype of the β-cell by positively regulating insulin and IAPP expression and possibly by repressing glucagon expression in the β-cells. The homeodomain protein Nkx6.1 is expressed in β-cells (46) but in the *Rip1/Ipf1*▲ mutants virtually no Nkx6.1+ cells were detected (45). Interestingly, Nkx6.1 is homologous to the homeodomain protein, Gtx that can act as a transcriptional repressor (47). The loss of Nkx6.1 in the mutants may therefore suggest that IPF1/Pdx1 positively regulates the expression of Nkx6.1, which in turn might repress glucagon expression in β-cells.

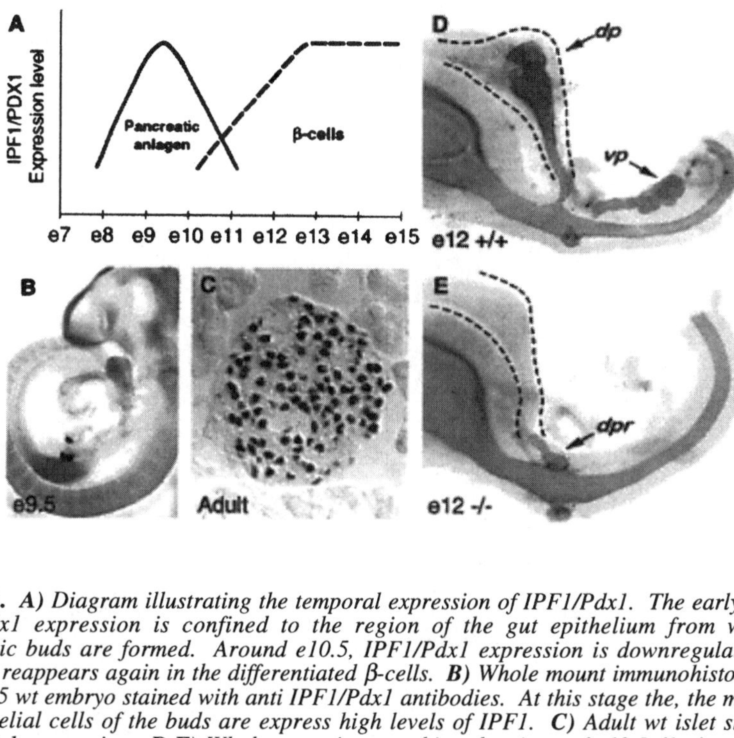

Figure 2. *A) Diagram illustrating the temporal expression of IPF1/Pdx1. The early phase of IPF1/Pdx1 expression is confined to the region of the gut epithelium from which the pancreatic buds are formed. Around e10.5, IPF1/Pdx1 expression is downregulated in the buds but reappears again in the differentiated β-cells.* ***B)*** *Whole mount immunohistochemistry of an e9.5 wt embryo stained with anti IPF1/Pdx1 antibodies. At this stage the, the majority of the epithelial cells of the buds are express high levels of IPF1.* ***C)*** *Adult wt islet stained for IPF1/Pdx1 expression.* ***D,E)*** *Wholemount immuno-histochemistry of e12 Ipf1+/+ and Ipf1-/- embryos using HNF3β antibodies. In Ipf1+/+ embryos, the pancreatic epithelium grows and becomes lobulated (D). In the Ipf1-/- embryos, a bud forms in the dorsal pancreatic epithelium but then becomes growth-arrested (E). Abbreviations; dp, dorsal pancreas; vp, ventral pancreas; dpr, dorsal pancreatic epithelium. Broken line indicates the dorsal pancreatic mesenchyme.*

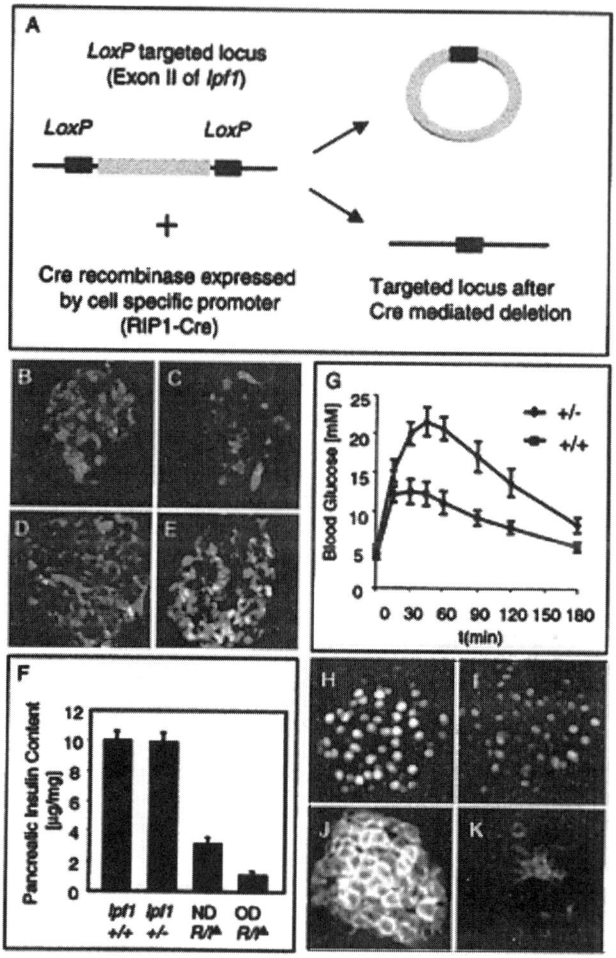

Figure 3. ***A)*** *Strategy for cell type specific knock out of Ipf1 using the Cre-LoxP system for targeted recombination.* ***B-E)*** *Confocal images showing islets from Ipf1 +/+ (B,D) and diabetic Rip1/Ipf1*$^{\blacktriangle}$ *(C,E) in 18 week old mice stained for insulin (B-E, green) and IPF1/Pdx1 (B,C, red) or glucagon (D,E, red). Normally insulin (ins+) cells co-express IPF1/Pdx1 (B) but in the mutant mice, there is a decrease in the number of ins+ cells and only approximately 20% of the ins+ cells still express IPF1/Pdx1 (C). Insulin and glucagon are normally not co-expressed (D) but in the mutants, a significant number of cells co-expressed both hormones (E, yellow). The number of glucagon expressing cells is also markedly increased in the mutant (E).* ***F)*** *Total pancreatic insulin content in 15 weeks old Ipf1 +/+, Ipf1+/-, non-diabetic Rip1/Ipf1*$^{\blacktriangle}$ *and overt diabetic Rip1/Ipf1*$^{\blacktriangle}$ *mice. Insulin is expressed as µ g/mg pancreas protein ± S.E.M in 8 animals in each group.* ***G)*** *Heterozygosity for the Ipf1/Pdx1 null mutation results in impaired glucose tolerance. Glucose challenge of 18 week old Ipf1 +/+ and Ipf1 +/- mice. Diagram showing blood glucose levels at indicated time points after intraperitoneal administration of glucose. Blood glucose levels increase two-fold in the Ipf1 +/- mice as compared to the Ipf1 +/+ mice. Results are mean ± S.E.M. of 8 animals in each group.* ***H-K)*** *Glucose Transporter Type 2 (Glut2) expression is dependent on high level of IPF1/Pdx1 expression. Analysis of Glut2-expression in correlation to IPF1-expression by immunohistochemistry on pancreas from 18-week Ipf1 +/+ (H,J) and Ipf1 +/- mice (I,K). The expression of IPF1/Pdx1 is slightly reduced in islets from Ipf1+/- mice (I) as compared to Ipf1 +/+ mice (H), resulting in dramatically decreased expression of Glut2 in Ipf1 +/- (J) as compared to Ipf1 +/+ mice (K). Abbreviations: OD, Overtly Diabetic; ND, Non Diabetic; R/I*$^{\blacktriangle}$*, Rip1/Ipf1*$^{\blacktriangle}$.

The pancreas of the OD *Rip1/Ipf1*$^{\blacktriangle}$ mutant mice contained about 60% of the normal number of β-cells (45) and ~10% of the normal total pancreatic insulin content (Figure 3F) suggesting a progressive decrease in insulin expression underlies the development of diabetes in these mice. The diabetic mutants responded to insulin administration by transiently reverting to normo-glycaemia (45) excluding insulin resistance as a major cause of diabetes. IPF1/Pdx1 has, however, been suggested to regulate the expression of the *Glut2* and *glucokinase* genes (48,49), two important components of the β-cell glucose sensing system. Glut2-deficient mice show an impaired glucose-induced insulin secretion and develop diabetes (50) and mutation and/or inactivation of the *glucokinase* gene also results in impaired insulin secretion and development of diabetes (51-53) in both mouse and man. Thus, an impaired expression of Glut2 and glucokinase could also contribute to the diabetic phenotype of *Rip1/Ipf1*▲ mutant mice. In the OD *Rip1/Ipf1*▲ mice, Glut2-expression is virtually extinct whereas the expression of glucokinase appears unaffected (25). In non-diabetic (ND) *Rip1/Ipf1*▲ 11-week old mice the pancreatic insulin content is roughly 30% of the normal level (Figure 3F), the number of Glut2-expressing-cells is reduced and the levels of Glut2 expression is highly variable among the cells (45). Thus, excision of the *Ipf1/Pdx1* gene in β-cells leads to an early loss of Glut2 expression that, via impaired glucose stimulated insulin release, probably contributes to the development of hyperglycaemia. The combined, progressive loss of both Glut2 and insulin expression, due to *Ipf1/Pdx1* inactivation leads to the development of overt diabetes in the *Rip1/Ipf1*▲ mice. Interestingly, *Glut2*-deficient mice also show an increased number of α- (glucagon, Glu+) versus β- (insulin, Ins+) cells (50), but, unlike in the *Rip1/Ipf1*▲ mice, the α-cells still remain located at the periphery of the islets (B. Thorens, personal communication). This suggests that the change in the ratio of Glu+- versus Ins+-cells in the *Rip1/Ipf1*▲ mice primarily is mediated by the loss of IPF1/Pdx1 in β-cells resulting in a change in the pattern of hormone production. Early onset type 2 diabetes is associated with heterozygosity for a point mutation in the human *Ipf1* gene, MODY 4 (40,54). Our results raise the possibility that regulation of Glut2 and insulin expression by IPF1/Pdx1 gene dosage is instrumental in the pathogenesis of MODY 4. Mice heterozygous for the original *Ipf1/Pdx1* null mutation are non-diabetic and show blood glucose levels in upper range of normoglycaemia but were found to be glucose intolerant (45). In *Ipf1* +/- mice, intraperitoneal injections of glucose (1g/kg body weight) resulted in dramatically increased blood glucose levels as compared to *Ipf1* +/- littermates (Figure 3F). The glucose intolerance could reflect either impaired insulin or Glut2 expression or both. The *Ipf1/Pdx1* null +/- mice show a normal total pancreatic insulin content and islet architecture (Figures 3F, 3I, and 3K) and the pattern and levels of expression of Isl1, insulin, glucagon, IAPP and Nkx6.1 appear normal (45). In contrast, IPF1/Pdx1 expression is slightly decreased and Glut2 expression is markedly reduced (Figures 3H and 3I). This provides evidence that IPF1/Pdx1 exerts a dosage-dependent regulation of Glut2 expression. Hence, these results offer a plausible explanation for the development of maturity onset diabetes in *Ipf1/Pdx1* haplo-insufficient individuals and identify *Ipf1/Pdx1* null +/- mice as a relevant animal model for studying this disease. These results also strengthen the idea that an early loss of Glut2 expression is involved in the development of hyperglycaemia in the *Ipf1/Pdx1* β-cell specific mutants and that the combined loss of Glut2 and a gradual decrease of insulin expression together lead to the manifestation of diabetes. Intriguingly, four out of five genes presently linked to MODY represent transcription factors; MODY4 as already mentioned to mutations in the Ipf1 gene, MODY1 and -3 to mutations in hepatocyte nuclear factor (HNF)-4α and -1α respectively, MODY 5 to mutations in HNF-1β whereas MODY2 is linked to glucokinase (51,54,55-57). It is thus plausible that mutations in other transcription factors (see introduction to this chapter), regulating the expression of pancreatic β-cell genes will turn out to be linked to other forms of MODY.

ISL1 IN PANCREAS DEVELOPMENT

The LIM homeobox gene *Islet-1 (Isl1)* was defined initially in studies on insulin gene regulation (34). Like other members of the LIM homeodomain family, ISL1 has two copies of a cysteine/histidine rich motif (LIM) believed to mediate protein-protein interactions (33,34). The temporal and spatial expression pattern of ISL1 is well characterized and seems to be more or less conserved between different vertebrate species such as rat, mouse and zebrafish (58-60). During mouse development, Isl1 is expressed in a subset of neurones of the peripheral and central nervous system, diverse groups of mesenchymal cells and a number of endocrine cells types (58,59). Motor neurones are not generated in *Isl1-/-* mice. This prevents the formation of a specific class of ventral interneurones (61). Like other LIM homeodomain proteins, ISL1 thus seem to be an important regulator of cell differentiation (33,62). During pancreas ontogeny Isl1 positive (Isl1+) cells are detected in the dorsal pancreatic epithelium at the 15-16 somite stage, embryonic day 9 i.e. prior to onset of hormone gene expression (63-66). At e9.5 Isl1 is expressed in mesenchymal cells that surround the dorsal but not ventral evagination of the gut endoderm, that together comprise the pancreatic anlagen, thereby patterning the early pancreatic mesenchyme along the dorsal-ventral axis (Figure 4A). Glucagon + cells first appear at the 20-25 somite stage (e9.5) and they all express Isl1 (Figure 4B), whereas insulin, somatostatin and pancreatic polypeptide expressing cells differentiate at later stages (63-65) and also express Isl1 when they first appear (Figure 4B). Mice lacking functional *Isl1* expression are arrested in their development around e9.5 (61). In e9.5 *Isl1 -/-* embryos, the ventral pancreatic epithelium and its associated mesenchyme appear histologically normal (10). In contrast, there is a complete depletion of the mesenchyme flanking the dorsal pancreatic epithelium (compare Figures 4C and 4D). In addition, glucagon+ cells cannot be detected in the dorsal pancreatic anlage of e9.5 *Isl1 -/-* embryos (compare Figures 4C and 4D). These results show that Isl1 is necessary for the formation of the dorsal pancreatic mesenchyme and for the generation of glucagon+ cells as well as for maintaining a high level of Pdx1 expression in the dorsal pancreatic epithelium. To determine whether the absence of hormone-producing cells at e9.5 merely reflects a delayed development rather than a complete block in their differentiation, segments of gut containing the pancreatic anlagen from e9.5 *Isl1 +/-* and *Isl1 -/-* embryos were isolated and cultured *in vitro*. Explants derived from *Isl1+/-* embryos gave rise to glucagon+, insulin+, and somatostatin+ endocrine cells as well as amylase+ exocrine cells (10). In contrast, glucagon+, insulin+, and somatostatin+ cells were not detected in explants derived from *Isl1 -/-* embryos, although, amylase+ exocrine cells were present (10). These results provide evidence that Isl1 expression in pancreatic epithelium is required for the differentiation of pancreatic endocrine, but not exocrine, cells.

The differentiation of pancreatic epithelium is thought to depend on signals provided by the surrounding mesenchyme (1). Since in *Isl1 -/-* embryos, pancreatic mesenchyme surrounds only the ventral pancreatic epithelium it is possible that the amylase+ exocrine cells generated in gut explants from *Isl1-/-* embryos derive solely from the ventral pancreatic epithelium. In support of this observation, amylase + exocrine cells are generated in cultured ventral half-gut explants but not dorsal half gut explants (Figures 4E and 4F). However, dorsal pancreatic mesenchyme derived from wild-type e9.5 embryos can rescue the differentiation of exocrine, but not endocrine, cells in the dorsal epithelium from *Isl1 -/-* embryos (Figure 4G). Both gut explant halves generate amylase+ cells when isolated from *Isl1 +/-* embryos (10). Hence, Isl1 is required at two independent steps during pancreas ontogeny. First,

Isl1 is expressed in and required for the formation of dorsal pancreatic mesenchyme, providing genetic evidence that absence of mesenchyme blocks exocrine cell differentiation. Interestingly, loss of *Isl1* function and thereby dorsal pancreatic mesenchyme is associated with a decreased level of IPF1/Pdx1 expression in the dorsal pancreatic epithelium. The absence of exocrine cells in dorsal *Isl1-/-* pancreas may thus be an indirect consequence of decreased IPF1/Pdx1 expression in the dorsal pancreatic epithelium resulting in an arrested development of the epithelium similar to that seen in *Ipf1/Pdx1-/-* mice (9). Second, Isl1 expression in the pancreatic epithelium is required for the formation of pancreatic endocrine cells. However, the exact role of Isl1 in this process remains unclear. It is possible that Isl1 expressed by the pancreatic epithelium has a cell-autonomous function similar to that reported in motor neuron generation (61). Our results indicate that ISL1 is expressed in the prospective pancreatic endocrine cells after they have passed their final mitotic division. Thus, if islet-cell fate is determined in dividing progenitor cells, ISL1 could play a role in the developmental progression of a previously determined islet cell. In support of this hypothesis, the homeodomain transcription factor Nkx2.2 and the b-HLH gene *NeuroD/BETA2* are still expressed in the dorsal pancreatic epithelium of *Isl1-/-* mice (U. Ahlgren and H. Edlund unpublished results). In *wt* mice both *NeuroD/BETA2* and Nkx2.2 are expressed in the early dorsal pancreatic epithelium as well as in mature islet cells (unpublished results and 67,68) depletion results in arrested islet morphogenesis (17). In *Isl1+/+* mice, initiation of Pax6 expression is restricted to the ISL1 positive cells of the epithelium (unpublished result) and mice carrying a disruption of the Pax6 gene have impaired islet cell differentiation (16,18). Interestingly, expression of the transcription factor Pax6 is absent in *Isl1 -/-* pancreatic epithelium (unpublished result). Together these findings suggest that ISL1 acts upstream of Pax6. Thus, it is likely that endocrine precursor cells are formed in the *Isl1-/-* mice but that in absence of *Isl1* they fail to terminally differentiate.

HB9 FUNCTION IN PANCREATIC DEVELOPMENT

The homeobox gene *HB9* was initially isolated from a human lymphoid B-cell library (69) and has in humans been linked to dominant inherited sacral agenesis (70). In mouse the expression of *HB9* is first evident at the ~8 somites stage (e8) in the notochord, in the entire dorsal gut endoderm and in the ventral endoderm at the prospective pancreatic level (12). The early pancreatic *HB9* expression is however transient and by e9.5 the level of expression of *HB9* is reduced in both the dorsal and ventral pancreatic bud and by e10.5, only very low levels of *HB9* expression remains in the dorsal and ventral pancreatic buds (12). Thus, the early pancreatic expression of *HB9* is down-regulated prior to that of IPF1/Pdx1. However, at late embryonic stages *HB9* expression, alike IPF1/Pdx1, reappears in the insulin producing β-cells, but not in the other endocrine cells of the differentiated pancreas (12). Thus, *HB9* is expressed in two distinct developmental phases, first during the evagination of the pancreatic buds and later in differentiated β-cells (Figure 5).

Mice targeted for mutations in the *HB9* gene have a normal gastrointestinal tract but completely lack the dorsal pancreatic epithelial bud (12). In contrast, the ventral bud, the mesenchyme that normally surrounds the dorsal pancreas and the spleen, are all present and appear to develop normally in these mice (12) (Figure 5). The lack of the dorsal pancreatic bud appears, therefore, to reflect a selective defect in the development of the presumptive dorsal pancreatic epithelium. Analysis of early, e9-e10, *HB9* deficient embryos provides evidence that lack of *HB9* function impairs both the initial stages in dorsal epithelial evagination and the subsequent differentiation of early pancreatic cell types (12). Thus, the arrest in dorsal pancreatic bud development in the *HB9* deficient mice is more severe than that observed in *Ipf1/Pdx1-/-* mice. The selective requirement of *HB9* for specifying the initial stages of dorsal, but not ventral, pancreatic development reveals a molecular distinction between the programs of dorsal and ventral pancreatic development (Figure 5). In addition to the dorsal dependence on *HB9*, the organization and identity of surrounding tissues differs in the dorsal and ventral pancreatic buds (2,10,71). Moreover, pancreatic endocrine cells appear earlier in the dorsal than in the ventral bud and the pancreatic mesenchyme is patterned with respect to Isl1 expression (10) (Figure 4A). The selective dorso-ventral difference in the *HB9* function clearly indicates that the initial programs of dorsal and ventral pancreatic differentiation are different.

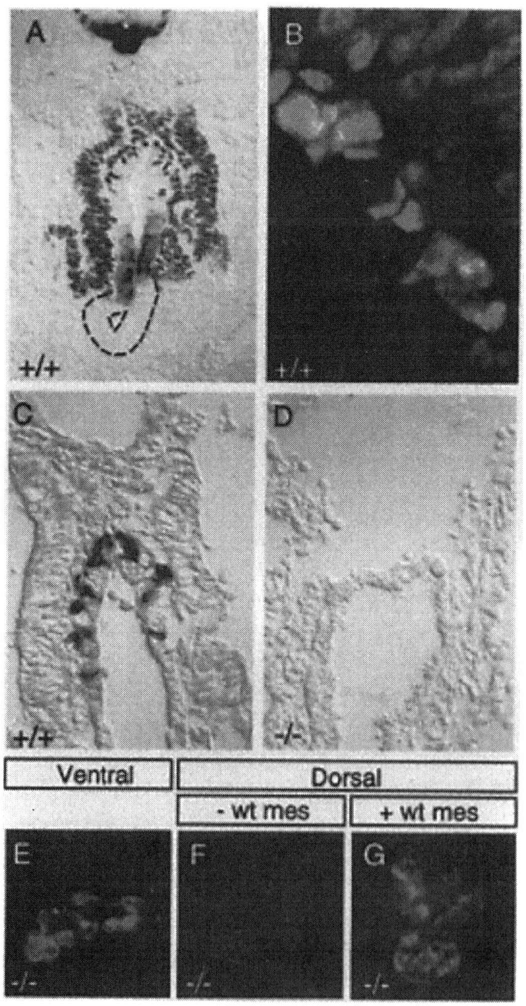

Figure 4. ***A)*** *At e9.5Isl1 (brown) is expressed in a subset of the dorsal epithelial cells and in the dorsal pancreatic mesenchyme. In contrast, Isl1 is not expressed in the ventral pancreatic epithelium (broken line) or in the adjacent mesenchyme. Shh mRNA expression (dark blue) is included to visualise the lateral endoderm.* ***B)*** *Confocal image of the dorsal pancreatic bud of an Isl1+/+ e9.5 embryo showing that all Glu+ cells (green) also are Isl1+ (red).* ***C,D)*** *Transverse sections of Isl1+/+ (C) and Isl1-/- (D) embryos at the level of the pancreas. At e9.5 Glu+ have appeared in the dorsal epithelium in Isl1+/+ embryos (C), whereas in somite matched Isl -/- embryos no Glu+ cells are detected and the dorsal pancreatic mesenchyme is absent (D).* ***E-G)*** *Amylase positive cells are generated in ventral (E) but not in dorsal (F) explants derived from Isl -/- embryos. Recombination of dorsal pancreatic anlagen from Isl -/- embryos with dorsal pancreatic mesenchyme from somite matched Isl1+/+ rescues the differentiation of dorsal exocrine cells (G).*

CONCLUSION

IPF1/Pdx1, ISL1, and *HB9*, all have important instructive roles during pancreatic development albeit at different stages. At first glance the early and late pancreatic expression of IPF1/Pdx1 and *HB9* appear to be almost identical, suggesting a putative coupling between these two genes. However, the normal expression of IPF1/Pdx1 in the ventral bud of *HB9* mutant mice together with the normal expression of *HB9* in the buds of *Ipfl/Pdxl* mutant mice clearly demonstrates that these genes are not genetically linked (12 and our own unpublished observations). Their respective roles during pancreatic development also differ remarkably. *HB9* appears to specify the initial stages of dorsal pancreatic development and thus acts at stages, prior to the function of *Ipfl/Pdxl* (Figure 6). In addition, *HB9* is expendable for ventral pancreatic development, whereas *Ipfl/Pdxl* is required for the development of both pancreatic buds beyond e9.5-e10 (Figure 6).

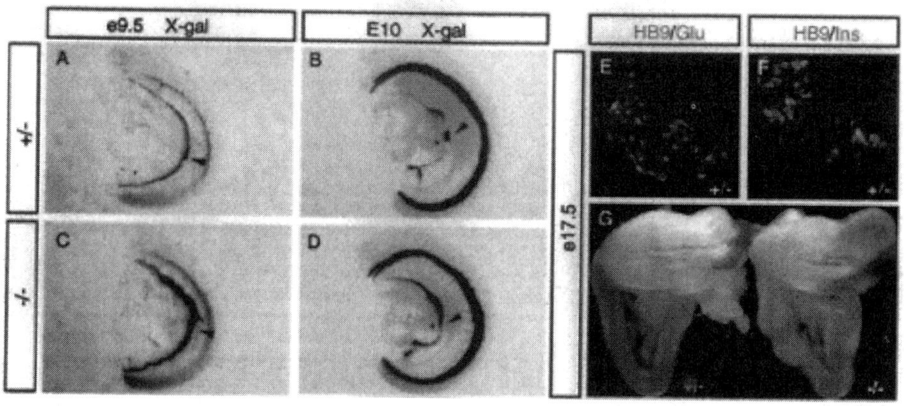

Figure 5. *Selective agenesis of the dorsal pancreas in mice lacking homeobox gene HB9. HB9 is transiently expressed in the early developing pancreatic anlagen but reappears in insulin producing β-cells. The development of the dorsal pancreas is arrested before the stage of epithelial evagination in HB9 mutant embryos.* ***A,C)*** *Whole-mount X-gal staining of e9.5 embryos shows that the protruding, dorsal pancreatic bud can be detected in the heterozygous embryos whereas no equivalent structure is found in the homozygous embryos.* ***B,D)*** *X-gal staining of e10.5 embryos showing that at this stage the ventral bud has formed in both the heterozygous and homozygous embryos whereas there is no evidence of a dorsal pancreatic bud in homozygous embryos.* ***E,F)*** *Double immunohistochemical analysis of e17.5 pancreas using anti-HB9 and anti-glucagon (E), and anti-insulin (F) antibodies. At this stage, HB9 expression is restricted to the insulin producing β-cells.* ***G)*** *Comparison of the gastrointestinal tract derived from e17.5 HB9 heterozygous and homozygous littermates. Note that the dorsal pancreas is completely missing whereas the ventral pancreas is normal in homozygous mutant embryos. (Arrowhead indicates dorsal pancreatic bud.)*

To understand the complete role of these factors during the early stages of development their respective target genes have to be identified. Although the β-cell specific inactivation of *Ipfl/Pdxl* has revealed genes whose expression in adult β-cells is directly or indirectly dependent on *Ipfl/Pdxl*, no such information has yet been obtained regarding genes regulated by *Ipfl/Pdxl* during the first, early phase of expression.

It also remains unclear whether the dependence of dorsal pancreatic differentiation on *HB9* is intrinsic to the gut epithelium or whether the transient expression of *HB9* by notochord cells (12) acts to control dorsal pancreatic specification by regulating the expression of inductive or repressive factors secreted from the notochord (Figure 6). Whether β-cell specific expression of *HB9* correlates with an important function for *HB9* in the adult, differentiated β-cell will also have to be elucidated. The fact that these cells appear to develop normally in the ventral pancreas of *HB9* deficient mice suggests, however, that *HB9* is not required for the differentiation of insulin-producing β-cells.

In contrast to other, hitherto genetically analyzed genes, *Isl1* is the only gene that, when inactivated, leads to a complete loss of all differentiated endocrine cells (12). Nevertheless, the activation of *Isl1* expression around the final mitotis of differentiating endocrine cells together with the appearance of cells expressing early endocrine markers like Nkx2.2 and *NeuroD/BETA2* in the *Isl1* -/- embryos argues against a role for *Isl1* as a pro-endocrine gene. Together these data suggest that *Isl1* is required for the terminal differentiation of endocrine progenitor cells into mature, hormone producing pancreatic endocrine cells. The selective expression of, and requirement for, *Isl1* in the dorsal but not ventral pancreatic mesenchyme also adds to the evidence that the programs of pancreatic differentiation dorsally and ventrally are initially distinct.

Genetic studies in mice have shown that several transcription factors have important roles for pancreatic development and/or glucose homeostasis (72). Many of these transcription factor genes have been linked to human diabetes or dysmorphogenic development of the pancreas in mice, thus demonstrating a conservation in the function of genes that control pancreatic development in mice and humans (72). As described above, in humans as in mice, homozygosity for mutations in the human *Ipf1* gene results in complete pancreas agenesis (8,40). Maturity Onset Diabetes of the Young (MODY) 4 has been linked to heterozygosity for mutations in the human *Ipf1* gene (54) and similarly, mice heterozygous for deletions in the *Ipf1/Pdx1* gene have impaired glucose tolerance (45). The human *HB9* gene, *HLXB9*, has been linked to dominant inherited forms of sacral agenesis (70). No pancreatic or diabetic complications have yet been reported in these patients. However, spontaneous forms of this syndrome have been associated with maternal diabetes (73). Whether mutations in *HLXB9* are also linked to human dorsal pancreatic agenesis syndromes (70) remains to be determined. Lastly, although no linkage has yet been found between *Isl1* and diabetes, a putative linkage has been reported between *Isl1* and morbid obesity (74).

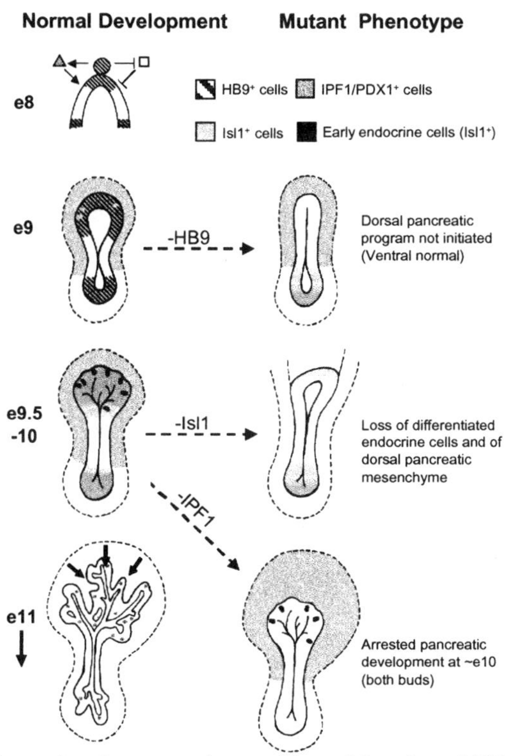

Figure 6. *Model illustrating the expression profile and function of HB9, IPF1/Pdx1 and Isl1 during the development of the pancreas, e8-9; HB9 expressed in the dorsal pancreatic epithelium (dashed lines) may act to provide competence to the epithelium to respond to signals that provoke pancreatic development. HB9 is indispensable for the specification of the dorsal pancreatic program. Thus, when inactivated epithelial evagination, initiation of IPF1/Pdx1 expression and other early pancreatic markers do not occur at the dorsal side. It is possible that in the ventral pancreatic epithelium, the pancreatic program is controlled by a distinct mechanism and other, yet unidentified gene(s) may confer competence to the ventral epithelium to respond to inductive signals resulting in the expression of early pancreatic markers like IPF1/Pdx1. Hence, mice lacking HB9 function have a normally developed ventral pancreas. Alternatively, HB9 through its early expression in the notochord functions to regulate the expression of an inducer (▲) or repressor (■) that in turn may influence the specification of the dorsal pancreatic program. This would suggest that the function of HB9 is not intrinsic to the epithelium but rather that HB9 exert its role by regulating factors provided by the notochord. e9; Isl+ mesenchyme has enveloped the dorsal pancreatic epithelium and a few Isl1+ cells can be detected in the dorsal epithelium (grey dots). e9.5-10; At e9.5, Isl1 is expressed in the dorsal pancreatic mesenchyme and the pancreatic endocrine cells (red dots). IPF1/Pdx1 (green) is expressed in, and acts cell autonomously, within the dorsal and ventral pancreatic epithelium by activating a gene(s) that makes the epithelium competent to grow, branch and differentiate. In the absence of IPF1/Pdx1 the further morphogenesis and differentiation of the epithelium is arrested around e10. e11→ ; Epithelio-mesenchymal interactions (black arrows) lead to morphogenesis of the pancreatic epithelium and is an absolute requirement for exocrine cell differentiation. IPF1/Pdx1 has been downregulated around e10.5 by but later reappears in the differentiating β-cells (green dots), which alike other islet cells also are Isl1+. IPF1/Pdx1 expression in the adult β-cell is required to maintain its hormone producing phenotype by positively regulating insulin and glut 2 and by repressing glucagon expression.*

REFERENCES

1. Golosow N and Grobstein C. Epitheliomesenchymal interaction in pancreatic morphogenesis. Dev Biol 1962;4:242-55.
2. Wessels NK and Cohen JH. Early pancreas organogenesis: morphogenesis, tissue interactions and mass effects. Dev Biol 1967;15:237-70.
3. Fontaine J and Le Douarin NM. Analysis of endoderm formation in the avian blastoderm by the use of quail-chick chimeras. The problem of the neuroectodermal origin of the cells of the APUD series. J Embryol Morphol 1977;41:209-22.
4. Le Douarin NM. On origin of the pancreatic endocrine cells. Cell 1988;53:169-171.
5. Pictet RL, Rall LB, Phelps P, Rutter WJ. The neural crest and the origin of the insulin-producing and other gastrointestinal hormone producing cells. Science 1976;191:191-2.
6. Sander M and German S. The β-cell transcription factors and development of the pancreas. J Mol Med 1997;75:327-40.
7. German M, Ashcroft S, Docherty K et al. The Insulin Promoter. Diabetes 1995;44:1002-4.
8. Jonsson J, Carlsson L, Edlund T, Edlund, H. Insulin-promoter-factor 1 is required for pancreas development in mice. Nature 1994;371:606-9.
9. Ahlgren U, Jonsson J, Edlund, H. The morphogenesis of the pancreatic mesenchyme is uncoupled from that of the pancreatic epithelium in PDX1/IPF1-deficient mice. Development 1996;122:1409-16.
10. Ahlgren U, Pfaff S, Jessel TM, Edlund T, Edlund H. Independent requirement for ISL1 in the formation of the pancreatic mesenchyme and islet cells. Nature 1997;385:257-60.
11. Harrison KA, Druey KM, Deguchi Y, Tuscano JM, Kerhl JH. A novel human homeobox gene distantly related to proboscipedia is expressed in lymphoid and pancreatic tissues. J Biol Chem 1994;269:19968-75.
12. Li H, Arber S, Jessell TM, Edlund H. Selective Agenesis of the Dorsal Pancreas in Mice Lacking Homeobox Gene *HB9*. 1999;Submitted.
13. Sussel L, Kalamaras J, Hartigan-O'Connor DJ, Meneses JJ, Pedersen RA, Rubenstein JLR, German MS. Mice lacking the homeodomain transcription factor Nkx2.2 have diabetes due to arrested differentiation of pancreatic beta cells. Development 1998;125:2213-21.
14. Sander M, Kalamaras J, German MS. The homeobox gene Nkx6.1 is essential for differentiation of insulin-producing β-cells in the mouse pancreas. Abstract from The Keystone Symposium on Vertebrate Development, Steamboat Springs, Colorado, April 3-8, 1998.
15. Sosa-Pineda B, Chowdhury K, Torres M, Oliver G, Gruss P. The Pax4 gene is essential for differentiation of insulin-producing beta cells in the mammalian pancreas. Nature 1997;386:399-402.
16. Sander M et al. Genetic analysis reveals that PAX6 is required for normal transcription of pancreatic hormone genes and islet development. Genes & Dev 1997;11:1662-73.
17. Naya FJ et al. Diabetes, defective pancreatic morphogenesis, and abnormal enteroendocrine differentiation in BETA2/neuroD-deficient mice. Genes & Dev 1997;11:2323-34.
18. St-Onge L, Sosa-Pineda B, Chowdhury K, Mansouri A, Gruss P. Pax6 is required for differentiation of glucagon-producing alpha-cells in mouse pancreas. Nature 1997;387:406-9.
19. Beatson W. Materials for the study of variation. MacMillan & Co 1894.
20. McGinnis W, Garber RL, Wirz J, Kuriowa A, Gehring WJ. A homologous protein-coding sequence in Drosophila homeotic genes and its conservation in other metazoans. Cell 1984;37:403-8.
21. Scott MP and Weiner AJ. Structural relationship between genes that control development: sequence homology between Antennapedia, Ultrabithorax, and fushi tarazu loci of Drosophila. Proc Natl Acad Sci USA 1984;81:4115-9.
22. Manak JR and Scott MP. A class act: conservation of homeodomain protein functions. Development Suppl 1994:61-71
23. McGinnis G and Krumlauf R. Homeobox genes and axial patterning. Cell 1992;63:969-76.
24. Malicki J, Shcugart K, McGinnis W. A human HOX4B regulatory element provides head specific expression in Drosophila embryos. Nature 1990;358:345-7.
25. Rosenfeld MG. POU domain transcription factors: Pou-er-ful developmental regulators. Genes & Dev 1991;5:897-907.
26. Bopp D, Burri M, Baumgartner S, Frigerio G, Noll M. Conservation of a large protein domain in the segmentation gene paired and in functionally related genes of Drosophila. Cell 1986;47:1033-40.
27. Schonemann MD, Ryan AK, Erkman L, McEvilly RJ, Bermingham J, Rosenfeld MG. POU domain factors in neural development. Adv Exp Med Biol 1998;449:39-53.
28. Verrijzer CP, Van OJ, Van der Vliet PC. The Oct-1 POU domain mediates interactions between Oct-1 and other POU proteins. Mol Cell Biol 1992;12:542-51.
29. Ritz-Laser B, Estreicher A, Klages N, Saule S, Philippe J. Pax-6 and Cdx-2/3 interact to activate glucagon gene expression on the G1 control element. J Biol Chem 1999;7:4124-32.
30. Ingraham HA, Flynn SE, Voss JW, Albert VR, Kapiloff MS, Wilson L, Rosenfeld MG. The POU-specific domain of Pit-1 is essential for sequence-specific, high affinity DNA binding and DNA-dependent Pit-1-Pit-1 interactions. Cell 1990;61:1021-33.

31. Chan SK, Mann RS. A structural model for a homeotic protein-extradenticle-DNA complex accounts for the choice of HOX protein in the heterodimer. Proc Natl Acad Sci USA 1996;93:5223-8.
32. Goudet G, Delhalle S, Biemar F, Martial JA, Peers B. Functional and cooperative interactions between the homeodomain PDX1, Pbx, and Prep1 factors on the somatostatin promoter. J Biol Chem 1999;274:4067-73.
33. Freyd G, Kim S, Horowitz R. Novel cysteine-rich motif and homeodomain in the product of the Caenorhabditis elegans cell lineage gene lin-11. Nature 1990;344:876-9.
34. Karlsson O, Thor S, Norberg T, Ohlsson H, Edlund T. Insulin gene enhancer binding protein Isl-1 is a member of a novel class of proteins containing both a homeo- and a Cys-His domain. Nature 1990;344:879-82.
35. Dawid IB, Toyama R, Taira M. LIM domain proteins C R. Acad Sci III 1995;318:295-306.
36. Miller CP, McGehee Jr. RE, Habener JF. IDX-1: a new homeodomain transcription factor expressed in rat pancreatic islets and duodenum that transactivates the somatostatin gene. EMBO J 1994;13:1145-58.
37. Leonard J, Peers B, Johnson T, Ferreri K, Lee S, Montminy MR. Characterization of somatostatin transactivating factor-1, a novel homeobox factor that stimulates somatostatin expression in pancreatic islet cells. Mol Endocrin 1993;7:1275-83.
38. Ohlsson H, Karlsson K, Edlund, T. IPF1, a homeodomain-containing transactivator of the insulin gene. EMBO 1993;12:4251-59.
39. Offield MF, Jetton TL, Labosky PA, Ray M, Stein R, Magnuson MA, Hogan BL M, Wright CVE. PDX-1 is required for pancreatic outgrowth and differentiation of the rostral duodenum. Development 1996;122:983-95.
40. Stoffers DA, Zinkin NT, Stanojevic V, Clarke WL, Habener JF. Pancreatic agenesis attributable to a single nucleotide deletion in the human IPF1 gene coding sequence. Nature Genetics 1997;15:106-10.
41. Guz Y, Montminy MR, Stein R, Leonard J, Gamer LW, Wright, CVE and Teitelman G. Expression of murine STF-1, a putative insulin gene transcription factor, in beta cells of pancreas, duodenal epithelium and pancreatic exocrine and endocrine progenitors during ontogeny. Development 1995;121:11-18.
42. Gu H, Zou Y, and Rajewski K. Independent control of immunoglobulin switch recombination at individual swotch regions evidenced through Cre-loxP-mediated targeting. Cell 1993;73:1155-64.
43. Kilby NJ, Snaith MR and Murray JAH. Site-specific recombinases: tools for genome engineering. TIG 1993;9:413-421.
44. Tsien JZ, Chen DF, Gerber D, Tom C, Mercer EH, Anderson DJ, Mayford M, Kandel ER, and Tonegawa S. Subregion- and cell type-restricted gene knockout in mouse brain. Cell 1997;87:1317-1326.
45. Ahlgren U, Jonsson J, Jonsson L, Simu K, Edlund H. β-cell specific inactivation of the mouse Ipf1/Pdx1 gene results in impaired glucose transporter expression and late onset diabetes. Genes & Dev 1998;12:1763-8.
46. Jensen J, Serup P, Karlsen C, Nielsen TF, Madsen OD. mRNA profiling of rat islet tumors reveals Nkx 6.1 as a beta-cell-specific homeodomain transcription factor. J Biol Chem 1996;271:18749-58.
47. Komuro I, Schalling M, Jahn L, Bodmer R, Jenkins NA, Copeland NG, Izumo S. Gtx: a novel murine homeobox-containing gene, expressed specifically in glial cells of the brain and germ cells of testis, has a transcriptional repressor activity *in vitro* for a serum-inducible promoter. EMBO J 1993;12:1387-401.
48. Waeber G, Thompson N, Nicod P, and Bonny C. Transcriptional activation of the GLUT2 gene by the IPF-1/STF-1/IDX-1 homeobox factor. Mol Endocrinology 1996;10:1327-34.
49. Watada H, Kajimoto Y, Umayahara Y, Matsuoka T, Kaneto H., Fujitani Y, Kamada T, Kawamori R, and Yamasaki Y. The human glucokinase gene β-cell-type promoter: An essential role of insulin promoter factor 1/PDX-1 in its activation in Hit-T15 cells. Diabetes 1996;45:1478-88.
50. Guillam M T, Hümmler E, Schaerer E, Wu J Y, Birnbaum M J, Beermann F, Schmidt A, Dériaz N and Thorens B. Early diabetes and abnormal postnatal pancreatic islet development in mice lacking Glut-2. Nature Genetics 1997;17:327-30.
51. Froguel P, Vaxillaire M, Sun F, Velho G, Zouali H, Butel MO, Lesage S, Vionnet N, Clement K, Fougerousse F, Tanizawa Y, Weissenbach J, Beckmann JS, Lathrop GM, Passa P, Permutt MA, Cohe D. Close linkage of glucokinase locus on chromosome 7p to early-onset non-insulin-dependent diabetes mellitus. Nature 1992;356:162-4.
52. Bali D, Svetlanov A, Lee HW, Fusco-DeMane D, Leiser M, Li B, Barzilai N, Surana M, Hou H, Fleischer N, DePinho R, Rossetti L, Efrat S. Animal model for maturity-onset diabetes of the young generated by disruption of the mouse glucokinase gene. J Biol Chem1995;270:21464-7.
53. Grupe A, Hultgren B, Ryan A, Ma YH, Bauer M, Stewart TA. Transgenic knockouts reveal a critical requirement for pancreatic beta cell glucokinase in maintaining glucose homeostasis. Cell 1995;38:69-7.
54. Stoffers DA, Ferrer J, Clarke WL, Habener JF. Early-onset type-II diabetes mellitus (MODY4) linked to IPF1. Nature Genetics 1997;17:138-9.

55. Yamagata K, Furuta H, Oda N, Kaisaki PJ, Menzel S, Cox NJ, Fajans SS, Signorini S, Stoffel M, Bell GI. Mutations in the hepatocyte nuclear factor-4alpha gene in maturity-onset diabetes of the young. Nature 1996;384:458-60.
56. Yamagata K, Oda N, Kaisaki PJ, Menzel S, Furuta H, Vaxillaire M, Southam L, Cox RD, Lathrop GM, Boriraj VV, Chen X, Cox NJ, Oda Y, Yano H, Le Beau MM, Yamada S, Nishigori H, Takeda J, Fajans SS, Hattersley AT, Iwasaki N, Hansen T, Pedersen O, Polonsky KS, Turner RC, Verlho G, Chevre J-C, Froeguel P, Bell GI. Mutations in the hepatocyte nuclear factor-1alpha gene in maturity-onset diabetes of the young. Nature 1996;384:455-8.
57. Horikawa Y, Iwasaki N, Hara M, Furuta H, Hinokio Y, Cockburn BN, Lindner T, Yamagata K, Ogata M, Tomonaga O, Kuroki H, Kasahara T, Iwamoto Y, Bell GI. Mutation in hepatocyte nuclear factor-1 beta gene (TCF2) associated with MODY. Nat Genet 1997;17:384-385.
58. Thor S, Ericson J, Brannstrom T and Edlund T. The homeodomain LIM protein Isl-1 is expressed in subsets of neurons and endocrine cells in the adult rat. Neuron 1991;7:881-9.
59. Ericson J, Thor S, Edlund T, Jessel TM and Yamada T. Early stages of motor neuron differentiation revealed by expression of homeobox gene Islet-1. Science 1992;256:1555-60.
60. Korzh V, Edlund T and Thor S. Zebrafish primary neurons initiate expression of the LIM homeodomain protein Isl-1 at the end of gastrulation. Development 1993;118:417-25.
61. Pfaff SL, Mendelsohn M, Stewart CL, Edlund T and Jessell TM. Requirement for LIM homeobox gene Isl1 in motor neuron generation reveals a motorneuron-dependent step in interneuron differentiation. Cell 1996;84:309-20.
62. Way JC and Chalfie M. mec-3, a homeobox-containing gene that specifies differentiation of the touch receptor neurons in C. elegans. Cell 1988;54:5-16.
63. Alpert S, Hanahan D, Teitelman G. Hybrid insulin genes reveal a developmental lineage for pancreatic endocrine cells and imply a relationship with neurons. Cell 1988;53:295-308.
64. Herrera PL, Huarte J, Sanvito F, Meda P, Orci L, Vassalli JD. Embryogenesis of the murine endocrine pancreas; early expression of pancreatic polypeptide gene. Development 1991;113:1257-65.
65. Teitelman G, Alpert S, Polak JM, Martinez A, Hanahan D. Precursor cells of mouse endocrine pancreas coexpress insulin, glucagon, and the neuronal proteins tyrosine hydroxylase and neuropeptide Y but not pancreatic polypeptide. Development 1993;118:1031-9.
66. Upchurch BH, Aponte GW, Leiter AB. Expression of peptide YY in all four islet cell types in the developing mouse pancreas suggests a common peptide YY-progenitor. Development 1994;120:245-52.
67. Naya FJ, Stellrecht CM, Tsai MJ. Tissue-specific regulation of the insulin gene by a novel basic helix-loop-helix transcription factor. Genes & Dev 1995;9:1009-19.
68. Lee JE, Hollenberg SM, Snider l, Turner DL, Lipnick N, Weintraub H. Conversion of Xenopus into neurons by NeuroD, a basic helix-loop-helix protein. Science 1995;268:836-44.
69. Harrison, KA, Druey KM, Deguchi Y, Tuscano, JM, Kerhl, JH. A novel human homeobox gene distantly related to proboscipedia is expressed in lymphoid and pancreatic tissues. J Biol Chem 1994;269:19968-75.
70. Ross, AJ Ruiz-Perez V, Wang Y, et al. A homeobox gene, HLXB9, is the major locus for dominantly inherited sacral agenesis. Nature Genet 1998;20:358-61.
71. Slack JMW. Developmental biology of the pancreas. Development 1995;121:1569-80.
72. Edlund H. Transcribing Pancreas. Diabetes 1998;47:1817-23.
73. Wildling, R et al. Agenesis of the dorsal pancreas in a woman with diabetes mellitus and in both her sons. Gastroenterology 1993;104:1182-6.
74. Clement K, Garner C, Hager J, Philippi A, LeDuc C, Carey A, Harris TJ, Jury C, Cardon LR, Basdevant A, Demenais F, Guy-Grand B, North M, Froguel P. Indication for linkage of the human OB gene region with extreme obesity. Diabetes 1996;45:687-90.

12
bHLH Factors and Notch in Pancreatic Development

Jan Jensen, Ph.D., Luis Emilio Flores, Ph.D.,
R. Scott Heller, Ph.D., Palle Serup, Ph.D.,
and Ole D. Madsen, Ph.D.
Hagedorn Research Institute, Niels Steensensvej 6, 2820 Gentofte. Denmark

ABSTRACT

bHLH (basic-Helix-Loop-Helix) transcription factors are essential during the commitment of a multitude of cell fate decisions throughout vertebrate development, most extensively characterized within cells of ectodermal or mesodermal origin. Not surprisingly, members of this protein class are also instrumental in regulating cellular differentiation in the developing endoderm, including the endocrine cells of the lung, pancreas, stomach, and gut (1-4). These observations have begun to unravel an extensive similarity between the developing ectoderm and endoderm - involving not merely the sharing of molecular mechanisms, but include sharing of identical gene networks. These data provide a beginning of understanding the pancreatic precursor cell state and how individual endocrine cells may escape to complete differentiation. This leaves us in possession with an excellent platform from which further insight into endodermal endocrine differentiation may be obtained.

bHLH FACTORS AND CELLULAR DIFFERENTIATION

The bHLH abbreviation is commonly used to group proteins containing a basic-Helix-Loop-Helix domain of approximately 60 amino acids (5). The bHLH domain acts both as a protein dimerization interface and a composite DNA-binding domain upon heterodimerization between different factors (6-8). In certain cases, homodimerization of bHLH factors have been reported, although only in limited circumstances do these seem to play a physiological role (9,10). Members of the bHLH class can be subdivided into seven different classes (11), including ubiquitous activators (Class I, or the A-class, including the E2A, E2-2 and HEB factors); tissue-specific activators (Class II, or the B-class, by far the largest including NeuroD-, ngn-, MATH-, MyoD- and Myogenin-types, as well as many others); tissue specific repressors (class VII, including HES- and Hairy-type factors); non-DNA binding repressors (class V, or the E-class, including the Id-type factors). Yet other families exist including, e.g. the c-myc-type factors, although these will not be discussed here. The possibility of extensive heterodimer formation between members of the different families provides large flexibility in target DNA sequence readout activity and recognition, where the transcriptional activity of bHLH controlled promoters can be regulated either positively or negatively, even from the same site. Apparently, this feature is important, as most of the B-class bHLH components are not only found to control transcription in mature cells, but are pivotal in controlling cellular differentiation events (neural, muscle, hematopoeitic, dermal, skeletal differentiation and more, see((12-18) and references therein), and thus the transcriptional changes associated therewith.

NeuroD

NeuroD (also known as BETA2) was the first tissue-specific bHLH factor identified in pancreatic islets (19). It was identified as a partner for the ubiquitous A-class bHLH factor (E2A), and several studies have shown the importance of this heterodimeric complex in insulin-promoter activation binding directly to the conserved E1-element (20,21). Importantly, mutations either affecting NeuroD DNA binding or transactivation predisposes in the heterozygous state to the development of NIDDM (22). Not restricted to the pancreatic β-cell, NeuroD is also expressed by the remaining islet cells, and is thus apparently not acting in endocrine subtype specification. NeuroD was also identified in the developing nervous system (23), where it is required for the development of post-natally born neurons of the cerebellum and hippocampus (24). Importantly, the initial studies revealed a strong neurogenic activity of NeuroD, where injection of *neuroD* mRNA in Xenopus oocytes lead to an increase in neural differentiation (23). The importance of NeuroD in pancreatic development was revealed by targeted mutation of the *neuroD* gene as mice lacking this gene failed to generate the normal complement of pancreatic islet cells (2). However, few endocrine cells were formed showing that NeuroD is not absolutely required for the differentiation process. Also, studies have shown that those endocrine cells formed, undergo controlled cell death in absence of NeuroD (2). Thus, NeuroD is essential at some still to be determined step for the survival of the differentiated cells. The latter observations may suggest that NeuroD only plays a limited role in the endocrine differentiation process, but the fact that too few endocrine cells at the very initial stages are generated should not be overlooked. It may well be that the position of the *neuroD* gene in the differentiation pathway is late. Alternatively, if NeuroD does play a role in initiating the differentiation program, this particular function may be covered by another redundant component. As we will see, the Ngn3 bHLH factor is an excellent candidate for undertaking such a role.

NGN3 IS A PRO-ENDOCRINE GENE.

Recent data have uncovered how instrumental bHLH components are for the endocrine differentiation choice. Sommer and colleagues were first to discover the expression of another B-class bHLH gene component in the early developing pancreas (25). This gene, *ngn3* (also known as MATH4B, approved gene symbol *Atoh5*), fell within the neurogenin subclass, and is therefore likely to play a role in the initiation of endocrine differentiation in the pancreas. This is due to the fact that other members of the neurogenin subclass are positioned early in the neurogenic program, but not expressed in the mature neuronal types (18,26). In several cases, neurogenin-type factors are found to initiate a neuronal program, and directly activate downstream bHLH components of the NeuroD-subclass (27-29). Also, more recent data have shown that neurogenins are involved in subtype specification of individual neuronal types (14,30-32). The expression pattern of *ngn3* in the developing pancreas has been characterized in more detail by several groups (3,33,34), and several functional investigations have been performed. *ngn3* is expressed in a subset of pancreatic epithelial cells, some of which are still dividing (34). This expression is found at the early budding stages, where glucagon-positive endocrine cells primarily are formed, as well as during the secondary transition, where mature β-cells form. Around the secondary transition, occurring between E13.5-E15.5 in the mouse, *ngn3* expression peaks, coinciding with the largest wave of endocrine differentiation. *ngn3*-expressing cells differ in many respects from mature endocrine cells (34). First, mature endocrine cells prior to E17 in the mouse are mitotically quiescent. Secondly, these endocrine cells have lost their epithelial morphology and start to aggregate via migration. Thirdly, the terminal markers of the endocrine cells, e.g. insulin or glucagon, are never co-expressed with *ngn3*, whereas this is generally the case for *neuroD*. These above observations do not demonstrate that *ngn3* necessarily plays a role in endocrine differentiation, and the gene could serve a role within another lineage in the pancreas. However, both gain-, and loss-of-function studies using *ngn3* proves otherwise. Expression of *ngn3* in the pancreatic epithelial cells using the PDX1-promoter induces widespread endocrine differentiation in most pancreatic cells (33). These develop as the first type of endocrine cells that form during pancreatic development and are glucagon-positive. Conversely, mice lacking *ngn3* completely fail to generate pancreatic endocrine cells, although the expansion and exocrine differentiation of the pancreatic epithelium is normal (3). These results clearly demonstrate that *ngn3* is both necessary and sufficient for pancreatic endocrine differentiation, although it does not provide an explanation for the sub-type specification between α- and β-cells. Also, taking into consideration the temporal expression of *ngn3* preceding *neuroD*, we may convincingly state that this gene serves a pro-endocrine role in the developing pancreas very similar to the pro-neural role of *ngn1* and *ngn2* in the developing nervous system. Finally, the notion that *ngn3* and *neuroD* are positioned in a linear cascade has received further support, as Ngn3 is able to activate the *neuroD* promoter in transfection studies (35).

NOTCH – SETTING A BALANCE

It is often observed that differentiation of tissues relying on B-class bHLH components is also regulated by Notch. Notch is a transmembrane receptor, and an integral part of a functional cassette with the hallmark of controlling bHLH gene activity (36-39). In the following, we will refer to the Notch signalling system, which consists of both upstream and downstream components; together serving to inhibit the cellular differentiation conferred by the various members of the B-class bHLH components. In essence, the Notch signalling system is capable of resolving a binary fate choice between equipotent cells. If these cells are in direct contact, this process may be termed lateral specification, as only one commits itself to differentiation, and the other(s) are assigned an alternative fate or maintained in the undifferentiated state. The Notch signalling system is not necessarily limited to the process of lateral specification. Activity of Notch can well be envisioned to impose a general block on cellular differentiation. This aspect may be important during expansion phases of specific tissues, where proliferation is required. Also, Notch has been shown to be involved in inductive signalling (37), and is also an integrated art of the clock mechanism controlling vertebrate somitogenenesis (40,41). In the process of lateral specification, the cell type undergoing differentiation is always displaying reduced Notch activity. This may be termed the primary (1°) cell fate, whereas in the other, Notch activity is sustained, and this cell is either not allowed to undergo differentiation, or will assume an alternative (2°) fate.

The reason that the Notch system is capable of performing this task is due to feedback regulation between the cells involved. Notch itself acts as receptor for ligands of the Delta and Jagged families. B-class bHLH factors have been shown to directly activate the promoter of the *Delta*-gene (28), whereas it is still unclear if this also is true for the *Jagged*-family. Expression of the ligand at gradually higher level in one cell, will allow increased Notch-activity in neighbours. Within these cells, the intracellular portion of Notch is translocated to the nucleus (Notch itself is proteolytically regulated by several endoproteases, and ligand-induced processing allows release of the intracellular domain (42-46)). The intracellular portion of Notch associates with the RBP-Jκ transcription factor and stimulates target genes. In absence of Notch activation RBP-Jκ serves as a repressor of the same targets (47), and Notch may be viewed as a co-activator converting RBP-Jκ into an activating complex. The main target genes for this complex are members of the *hairy/enhancer-of-split* (HES)-class genes. These are bHLH components acting as dominant repressors, which may directly antagonize both activity and gene expression of the early members of the B-class bHLH components (reviewed in (48,49)).

In sum, the outcome is a sustained expression of B-class bHLH genes in the 1°-fated cell, including increased levels of the Notch ligand, whereas in the 2°-fated cell silencing of both gene types ensues due to the presence of HES-type components.

Such a process is continuously occurring in the vertebrate neural tube, where a constant supply of differentiating neurons is generated. The differentiation of these is also intimately linked to the precursor cell expansion, as their neighbours continue in the precursor pool. However, upon differentiation mature neurons migrate away allowing for a second round of differentiation in those cells initially inhibited.

So does Notch play a role in the developing pancreas, and if so, how does this connect to the morphogenetic program of this organ, that at least superficially shares little resemblance to the nervous system? Recent insight into these questions has been obtained through analysis of phenotypes of mice lacking components of the Notch signalling system.

NOTCH AND THE DEVELOPMENT OF THE PANCREAS

The developing mammalian pancreas offers an impressive array of expression of various members of the Notch signalling system (4,33,34). Of the 4 characterized members of mammalian *notch* genes, *notch-1, 2,* and *3* are expressed throughout pancreagenesis. This is also the case for the mammalian *delta-1* gene (approved gene symbol *dll1*), as well as the two *jagged*-ligands, *jagged-1* and *-2*. With this number of various Notch components present, the inborn complexity does not allow for an easy interpretation of how these factors regulate development. Particularly not so, as specificity between receptors and ligands is far from understood. Furthermore, the expression of these genes is most likely highly dynamic, as this has been observed in most other tissues. Also, it is not yet known what degree of redundancy may be present on either the ligand or the receptor level.

In situ hybridisation analyses have provided some insight as to where and when the Notch receptors and ligands are expressed (4,33,34). The expanding pancreatic epithelium between E10-E14, consisting of primarily undifferentiated PDX1-positive cells express rather uniformly both *notch-1* and *2*, whereas *notch-3* is expressed at much lower levels. At the same time, the neighbouring mesenchymal cells express primarily *notch-2* and *3*, but only minor levels of *notch-1*. Notably, the differentiating endocrine cells do not express either form of Notch, resembling neonatal islets in this respect. *delta-1* is expressed in scattered cells within the pancreatic epithelium at the secondary transition, and is also found in a few cells at the budding stage (E9). Although these cells most likely correspond to the developing endocrine cells this needs to be ascertained using double-labelling techniques. *jagged-1* displays a marked difference to *delta-1*, as this gene is expressed uniformly throughout the pancreatic epithelium. Perhaps Jagged-1 serves a role as a uniform notch agonist, setting a threshold level against differentiation. *jagged-2* is primarily expressed in cells of mesodermal origin, and later in endothelial cells. As the pancreas approaches the onset of terminal differentiation of both the exocrine cells and the β-cells at the secondary transition (E14), a general decline of *notch* expression is observed. In its simplest form this could be interpreted as a possible way of initiating the wave of differentiation events occurring at this time point due to a decrease in threshold. This needs to be experimentally verified. After the secondary transition, at which only few undifferentiated cells are present, *notch-1* and *-2* are primarily expressed within mature exocrine cells. At present, the role of Notch in these cells is not known. However, this is not a unique observation as Notch is, in addition to its role in lateral inhibition in the developing retina, also expressed in certain post-mitotic retinal neurons (50).

The functional importance of the Notch-signalling system in control of pancreatic endocrine differentiation was demonstrated by Apelquist and colleagues analysing pancreatic development in mice lacking various components in the signalling cascade (33). Mice deficient in either *delta-1* or *RBP-Jκ* display increased endocrine differentiation, as would be expected from loss-of-function mutants in the Notch system. As both of these mutants are early embryonic lethal, only the effects on the budding stages of the pancreas could be investigated. However, the "endocrinogenic" phenotype in this endodermal region is rather similar to the "neurogenic" collective group term used to describe the mutant phenotypes observed in the nervous system. The reason for the endocrinogenic effect was hypothesized to be through an increase in *ngn3* expression, and this was indeed found in *delta-1*$^{-/-}$ mice. This result strongly connects the Notch-system to the control of bHLH activity, in particular *ngn3*, which in turn is sufficient to drive the endocrine programme.

HES-1

If the notch-signalling cassette is functionally conserved between the endoderm and the ectoderm, the link between Notch and the bHLH cascade control is presumably via members of the HES-class bHLH repressors. *Hes1*, as well as *Hes5*, are known direct targets of Notch in the nervous system, and are required for the suppressive activity of Notch during neurogenesis (36,51). In the pancreas, and adjacent endoderm, only *Hes1* is expressed at significant levels (4). Therefore, HES-1 appears to be the likely candidate through which Notch would inhibit endocrinogenesis. HES-1 is a bHLH-type DNA-binding active repressor that recruits the co-repressor groucho to target promoters (52-56). In transformed lung cells, HES-1 is capable of repressing the hASH1 (human achaete-scute homologue-1, orthologue to MASH1) promoter (57). As MASH-1 is required for development of the neuroendocrine cells in the lung (1), this suggests that a balance between

MASH1/HES1 is involved in neuroendocrine fate determination in the lung. In the pancreas, one possible target promoter is the insulin promoter. HES-1 is capable of strongly repressing this promoter, and will antagonize the activity of either NeuroD or Ngn3, both of which are capable of transactivation (L. Flores, J. Jensen, unpublished data). Two other likely target promoters are those of *ngn3* and *NeuroD*, but at this time no data regarding HES-1 repression of these promoters are available. Still, we may conclude that HES-1 is capable of functionally antagonizing those B-class members important for the development of the endocrine pancreas. During pancreatic development *Hes1* is expressed in the PDX1-positive precursor cells, but is completely absent in developing endocrine cells (4). Hence, *Notch* and *Hes1* share expression in the pancreatic precursor cells.

Mice lacking *Hes1* display a neurogenic phenotype, where accelerated neuronal differentiation in the CNS results in severe neuronal defects, due to loss of precursor cells at early stages (58). Retinal and thymic development of these mice is also severely affected (59,60). In the endoderm, lack of *Hes1* results in accelerated, and excessive endocrine differentiation along the anterior-posterior length of the stomach-colon axis (4). This includes the pancreas, which is very strongly hypoplasic. Temporally, the pancreas is the first endodermal organ to initiate endocrine development, occurring at the very budding stage (E9). In *Hes1* mutants, most PDX1-positive pancreatic precursor cells differentiate into mitotically silent glucagon-expressing endocrine cells (Figure 1). So similar to that of *RBP-jκ* and *Delta1*, *Hes1* is endocrinogenic in mutant form. Combined with data obtained from the *RBP-jκ* and *Delta1* mutant mice, we can conclude that endocrine fate determination is regulated in a very similar manner as neuronal development. This is schematically shown in Figure 2, which superimposes the classical lateral specification mechanism on the developing pancreatic epithelium.

HES-1 is in addition to the pancreas also expressed in the adjacent endodermal regions at later timepoints. This could imply that *Hes1* also participates in developmental control there. Because these tissues, which include the stomach and intestine, normally commence endocrinogenesis several days later in development, these are less severely affected than the pancreas. However, excessive, and accelerated, endocrine differentiation is also observed in the stomach at E14-E15 and throughout the intestine a day later. This includes the full complement of gastro-intestinal endocrine cell types including CCK, secretin, GIP, glucagon, serotonin, gastrin and somatostatin. Also, in E16 lung, *Hes-/-* mice display increased levels of CGRP-alpha expression (J. Jensen, unpublished), and increased numbers of Goα-positive neuroendocrine cells (61) supporting the balance model of MASH1/HES1 in regulating pulmonary neuroendocrine development. Accordingly, in the stomach and gut, absence of HES-1 is accompanied by transcriptional upregulation of several genes encoding B-class bHLH activators, including *ngn3*, *neuroD*, *math1* and *mash1* as well as the Notch ligands *delta-1* and *–3*. Therefore, HES-1 is a unified general repressor of enteroendocrine differentiation, which in all cases appears to be regulated by positively acting B-class bHLH genes. What's more, these gut endocrine cells are most likely controlled in a similar manner by the Notch-pathway as is observed in the pancreas. This mechanism is apparently operating in the adult intestine as well, as HES-1 is expressed only in the dividing cells in the intestinal crypt (4). Presently, it is unknown if Notch/HES-1 control of Ngn3-NeuroD is also functioning during pancreatic regeneration, where all pancreatic cell types may be formed. This is an important question to verify, as control of pancreatic cell differentiation from adult pancreatic tissue to e.g. β-cells by manipulation of the Notch-system, requires this to be the case.

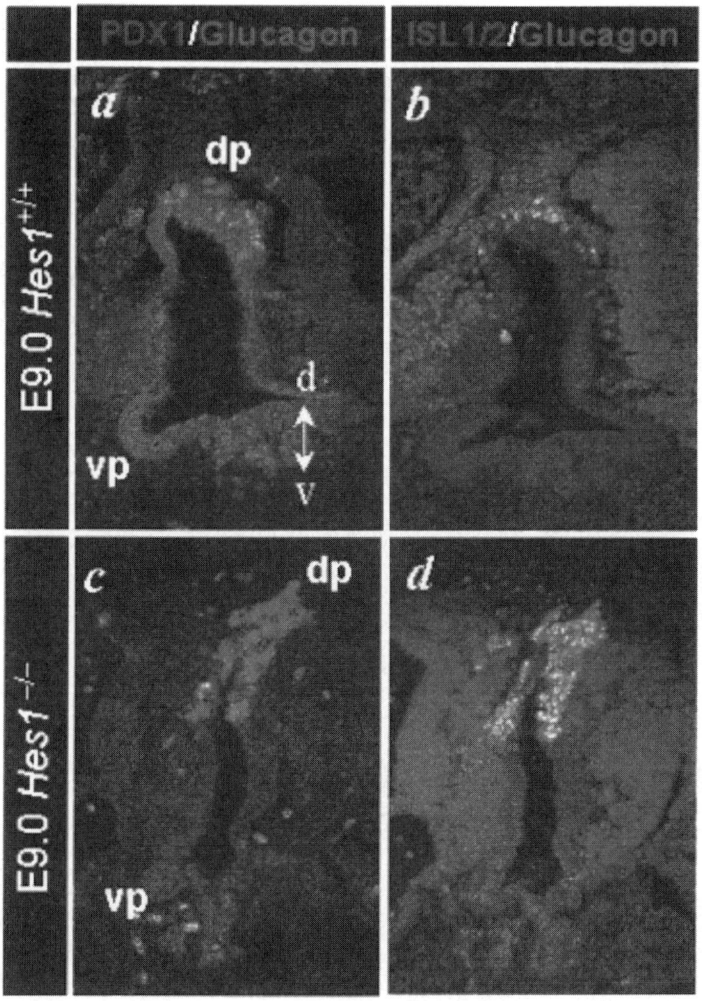

Figure 1. ***Increased endocrine differentiation in absence of Hes1.***
Double-immunofluorescence staining of E9 wildtype **(a,b)** *and* Hes1-/- **(c,d)** *embryos. PDX1 is expressed in the thickened dorsal epithelial bud of the wildtype* **(a)**, *and few PDX1+ cells are also seen in the ventral pancreatic region. Few glucagon-positive cells are observed in the dorsal, but not in the ventral pancreatic bud* **(a)**. *These also express the LIM-homeodomain protein Isl1* **(b)**, *as does the adjacent mesenchymal cells of the dorsal bud. In the dorsal bud of* Hes1 *mutants, only few PDX1+ cells are observed* **(c)**, *whereas increased numbers of glucagon-positive endocrine cells are found. These express Isl1 as well* **(d)**. *The ventral pancreas normally commences endocrine development at E11, but this is initiated at E10 in* Hes1 *mutant pancreas (not shown). The consequence of the loss of PDX1+ precursor cells and the post-mitotic state of the endocrine cells is a strong pancreatic hypoplasia at later stages.*

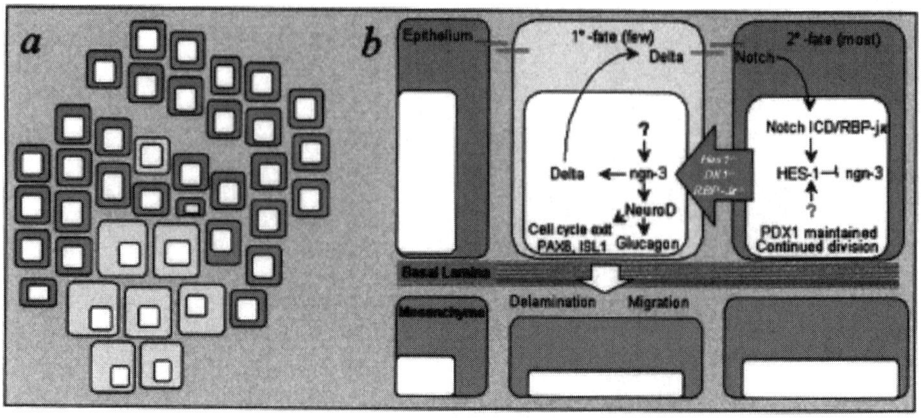

Figure 2. ***Lateral specification in pancreatic endocrine cell development.*** *Schematic drawing of an early pancreatic bud. Endocrine cells (yellow) form as single entities directly from the PDX1-expressing epithelium (green) adjacent to the condensing pancreatic mesenchyme (red). The endocrine cells lose the epithelial morphology, and migrate into clusters consisting only of endocrine cells. During this time, further maturation occurs and the cells increase their cytoplasmatic/nuclear ratio and display specialized functions. At the budding stage, only glucagon-expressing cells form, whereas later, insulin cells may be recruited. Our recent data have indicated that these two cell types develop independently from the precursor epithelium, although sharing a similar molecular mechanism involving Ngn3-NeuroD.* b. *The selection of the endocrine cell is based on a lateral specification mechanism, in which Notch is instrumental. Mutations in the Notch-pathway (*delta-1, RBP-jκ, Hes1*) cause increased endocrine differentiation, increased levels of Ngn3, and loss of precursor cells (red arrow). This model shows* Hes1 *as a downstream target of Notch. One alternative possibility is that the* Hes1 *promoter responds to other activating cues (red question mark), thus pointing to a role of* Hes1 *as a pre-patterning gene. At present, there are no data to discriminate between these possibilities and these are not mutually exclusive. Recent findings have shown that* Hes1 *both plays a pre-patterning, as well as a lateral specification role in development of the olfactory placodes (92).*

HNF6 AND THE INITIATION OF ENDOCRINE DIFFERENTIATION

Although the above observations show that Notch-HES-1 signalling is important in regulating the propensity of a Ngn3-positive cell population to undergo differentiation, they do not explain how this population is established initially. At present it is essentially unknown what signals activate *ngn3* expression at the budding stage. However, recent data have shown that the CUT-homeodomain factor HNF6 (62,63) is important for *ngn3* transcription at the secondary transition. *Hnf6* mutant mice almost completely fail to generate endocrine cells at the secondary transition, whereas the first glucagon cells develop normally (64). In these mice, almost complete absence of *ngn3* expression is observed. Therefore, *Hnf6* is positioned genetically upstream of *ngn3* – a notion supported by the fact that HNF6 is capable of activating the ngn3 promoter (64). In turn, this positions *Hnf6* as an excellent candidate as a target gene for morphogenetic signals needed to establish the *ngn3* expression, although these need to be identified. Interestingly, absence of HNF6 causes massive pancreatic cystic structures to form in late gestational development. These consist of cells mostly resembling those of the undifferentiated epithelium prior to differentiation. This could suggest a general deficiency in accomplishing differentiation, although it must be concluded that exocrine differentiation is less severely affected than endocrine. One additional observation provided by the HNF6 mutant mouse model is far reaching with respect to the importance of lateral specification in relation to the Notch system. Simply speaking, the activity state of Notch could be explained by the presence of differentiating endocrine cells, expressing a Notch ligand. A corollary to this is that in the absence of the endocrine cell, and thus the ligand, Notch activity should decline. However, this is not the case (64). HNF6 mutant embryos display normal levels of *Notch-1*, *2*, and *3* expression, despite the fact that the endocrine cell numbers are severely reduced. Consequently, the major driving force for Notch activation is not lateral specification, but some other, yet to be defined mechanism. A plausible explanation may focus on Jagged-1, but this needs to be verified. However, this possibility deserves attention, as it may be central to the understanding of how the Notch system connects to the epithelial/mesenchymal interaction so important for pancreatic development (65-67).

INDEPENDENT DEVELOPMENT OF THE PANCREATIC α- AND β-CELLS

Primarily due to the finding of double-positive hormone producing cells during pancreas ontogeny, many studies have argued for a direct lineage relationship between the pancreatic α- and β-cells (68-70). Hence, the initially developing glucagon-expressing cells would develop through transient multihormonal stages into all of the mature islet endocrine cells. Several data strongly argues that this is not case. First, the early established glucagon-positive cells are mitotically arrested, and remain so through the secondary transition 4-5 days later (34,71). Thus, they cannot account for the large increase in endocrine cell number observed during pancreas ontogeny. Secondly, the early developing glucagon-positive cells will remain clustered in the period from E10-E14, whereas maturing β-cells, based on high level expression of PDX1 and Nkx6.1, appear as scattered cells in the pancreatic epithelium around E13.5-E14.5 (34). Thirdly, *ngn3* is strongly expressed in the pancreatic epithelium during the secondary transition, arguing that endocrine cell differentiation is occurring at this time point (3,33,34). Fourthly, and of most importance, ablation of the glucagon-expressing cells using the diphteria toxin A-chain only affects the development of the glucagon cell type, whereas insulin producing cells develop normally (72). This argues that insulin-positive cells have not been through a transient glucagon-expressing phase prior to their development. However, as the effectiveness of the DipTox ablation can be discussed, a refined approach was recently carried out (73). Transgenic mice carrying an inactivated loxP-flanked reporter gene (growth hormone) under control of the insulin promoter, were crossed to mice carrying the CRE recombinase controlled by the glucagon promoter. No progeny displayed any insulin-positive cells expressing growth hormone. This would have been expected if these cells had developed through a transient glucagon-expressing stage, during which they would have irreversibly recombined the reporter gene. As the reciprocal experiment also showed that glucagon-cells did not develop through an insulin-expressing stage, it was concluded that these cell types develop independently. However, they develop from PDX1-positive cells, as PDX1-promoter CRE-mice generated an active reporter gene in both α- and β-cells. Using an immunohistochemical approach, our laboratory has reached the same conclusions suggesting a temporal order of gene activation during endocrine development (34). Together with the information obtained from various mouse knock-out studies (71,74-78), we propose a model of endocrine cell development where a dynamic equilibrium between HES-1 and ngn3 is central to initiate endocrine development, whether it be α- , or β-cell development directly from the pancreatic epithelial precursor cell (Figure 3).

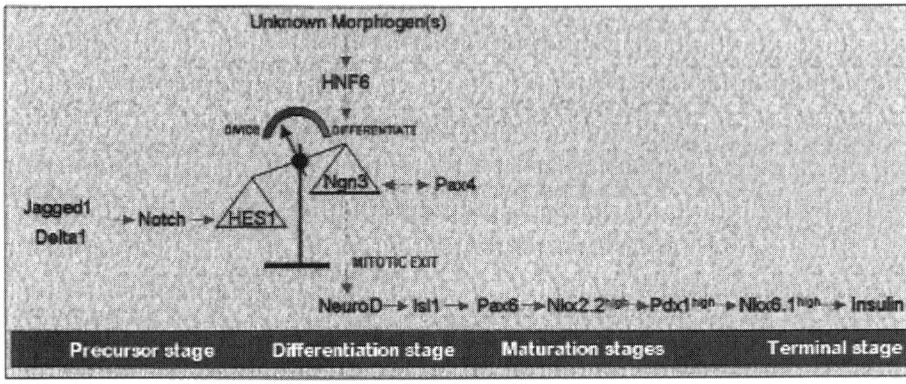

Figure 3. ***A bHLH-balance model of endocrine differentiation.***
With the above schematic model, we have attempted to list a sequential order of gene activation viewed from the perspective of the developing β-cell. This is proposed based on findings from mutant studies, where the epigenetic relationship between genes is determined by the absence of expression of a downstream positioned gene, or, in the case of repressive interactions, by the increase of downstream genes. Several aspects of this model requires further experimental support, and the linear cascade envisioned here of particularly the later transcriptional effectors should be viewed with caution, as the transitional stages ("maturation stages") of the cells may be brief and most genes may act in concert during a short period. However, the essence of the model is the notion of a dynamic equilibrium in cells expressing ngn3 and HES-1. Pancreatic epithelial cells are initially maintained in the precursor stage due to Notch (most likely Notch-1 and 2), activating HES-1. Delta-1 and Jagged-1 are both plausible Notch agonists to accomplish this, although these probably act in different manners. The expression of Jagged-1 within the majority of the precursor cells themselves suggests that this gene may act as a global agonist. It is undetermined whether Jagged-1 is membrane associated, or secreted in a soluble form. Also, production of Notch-ligand by the adjacent mesenchyme may play a role in suppressing differentiation in the endoderm. In contrast to Jagged, Delta-1 is only expressed in scattered cells, and is assumedly involved in fate refinement during lateral specification. Endocrine differentiation commences as cells with certain positional cues start transcribing ngn3. It is undetermined which genes are involved, except that HNF6 is required for ngn3 activation. Also, Pax4 is probably involved at this time point as this gene shares a nearly identical kinetic profile as ngn3. Some, but not all, cells within the ngn3 domain will complete differentiation. This is due to the lateral specification mechanism that allows individual cell selection. The irreversible fate change is instated as NeuroD is activated and the cell cycle arrested. Subsequent changes in gene expression occur as the cell develops to the terminal stage. Most likely, additional morphogenetic signals during this time are interpreted to secure proper specification.

p48 AND THE EXOCRINE FATE CHOICE

Not only endocrine differentiation relies on B-class bHLH components - differentiation of the exocrine pancreas is crucially dependent on p48/PTF1. p48 was identified as a tissue-specific B-class bHLH component of the PTF1 transcription complex (79). This complex activates transcription of a multitude of exocrine gene products, through binding to E-box sites (80). At present, p48 is the most specific exocrine transcriptional regulator known. *p48* mutant mice fail to form an exocrine pancreas (81). Some endocrine development occurs, and the cells generated reside in the spleen. This is less surprising than it sounds, as the splenic stroma condenses from the distal pancreatic mesenchyme between E12-E13. It is thus the tissue in closest connection to the developing pancreas. The involvement of yet another B-class bHLH activator in specification of a pancreatic cell type is fascinating and may lead to the enticing prospect that exocrine development may be regulated by a very similar mechanism as that of the endocrine cells.

NO SURPRISES – AND YET?

The fact that bHLH components are setting the stage for endocrine differentiation can hardly come as a surprise knowing the importance of these in neurogenesis. In many ways, islet cells share remarkable resemblance to neurons, and were once believed to descend from the neural crest. Also, that Notch is central to governing the extent and timing of differentiation in the pancreas is not unexpected, as this is exactly what Notch is capable of in other tissues. Therefore, the scaffold that could be built, even without experimental evidence, using information obtained within other developing systems and organisms, hold true for the pancreas and endoderm in general as well. However, the details of Notch function are still poorly understood. Particularly within the area of ligand/receptor interaction and how this triggers signalling. Presently, it has been observed that Delta itself may be under complex proteolytic control (82,83), and it is still unclear under what circumstances the resulting forms operate as agonists/antagonists of Notch. Also, multiple other signalling systems may feed into the Notch cascade, either extracellularly, or intracellularly. Fringe molecules may modulate ligand availability to Notch (84-86). The Wnt signalling pathway may via Dishevelled act on the intracellular part of Notch (87,88). Numb may control Notch-protein distribution during asymmetrical cell division (89,90). Fringes (all three known members), several Wnt factors, and Numb are all expressed during pancreagenesis (J. Jensen, unpublished). What roles do these factors play in the pancreas? Also, the Notch-system fails to explain how the initial *ngn3* expression is established. Most likely, HNF6 is only part of one of several morphogenetic systems that act on the *ngn3* promoter, allowing endocrinogenesis to proceed correctly in both a temporal and spatially controlled fashion. These signalling molecules and downstream effectors still await identification. Moreover, despite the involvement of bHLH components in neuronal subtype specification, both Ngn3 and NeuroD fail to explain the difference between α- and β-cell development. It is known that the α/β subtype decision is under influence of homeodomain factors including e.g. Pax4 and Brn4 (34,91), but the circumstances under which these factors come into play and how they exert their functions is unresolved. With no doubt, the coming decade will show a strong extension and more rigid wiring of the framework upon which we now base our understanding of pancreatic development. Many of these connections will be based on borrowing concepts from other systems – but who knows? – perhaps the pancreas will, as much due to its simplicity, as to the intensity put into the understanding of its development simply because it generates, and accommodates, the β-cells – lead to a greater understanding of developmental principles applicable to other tissues as well.

ACKNOWLEDGMENTS

The authors would like to thank Jacob Hald, Trine Nørgaard Jørgensen, and Helle V. Petersen for critical reading of the manuscript and Erna E. Pedersen, Tove Funder

Nielsen for expert technical assistance. This work was supported by the JDF (J.J), and the NIH (J.J, P.S, O.D.M). Hagedorn Research Institute is an independent research component of Novo-Nordisk A/S.

REFERENCES

1. Borges M, Linnolia RI, van de Velde HJK, Chen H, Nelkin BD, Mabry M, Baylin SB, Ball DW. An achaete-scute homologue essential for neuroendocrine differentiation in the lung. Nature 1997;386:852-855.
2. Naya FJ, Huang HP, Qiu YH, Mutoh H, Demayo FJ, Leiter AB, and Tsai MJ. Diabetes, defective pancreatic morphogenesis, and abnormal enteroendocrine differentiation in beta2/neurod-deficient mice. Genes Dev 1997;11(18),2323-2334.
3. Gradwohl G, Dierich A, LeMeur M, Guillemot F. neurogenin3 is required for the development of the four endocrine cell lineages of the pancreas. Proc Natl Acad Sci USA 2000;97:1607-1611.
4. Jensen J, Pedersen EE, Galante P, Hald J, Heller RS, Ishibashi M, Kageyama R, Guillemot F, Serup P, Madsen OD. Control of endodermal endocrine development by Hes-1. Nat Genet 20001;24:36-44.
5. Murre C, Schonleber McCaw P, and Baltimore D. A new DNA binding and dimerization motif in immunoglobulin enhancer binding, daughterless, MyoD, and myc proteins. Cell 1989;56(5),777-783.
6. Murre C, Schonleber McCaw P, Vaessin H, Caudy M, Jan LY, Jan YN, Cabrera CV, Buskin JN, Hauschka SD, Lassar AB, Weintraub H, Baltimore D. Interactions between heterologous helix-loop-helix proteins generate complexes that bind specifically to a common DNA sequence. Cell 1989;58:537-544.
7. Ellenberger T, Fass D, Arnaud M, and Harrison SC. Crystal-structure of transcription factor e47 - e-box recognition by a basic region helix-loop-helix dimer. Genes Dev 1994;8(8),970-980.
8. Ma PM, Rould MA, Weintraub H, Pabot CO. Crystal-structure of myod bhlh domain-dna complex - perspectives on dna recognition and implications for transcriptional activation. Cell 1994;77:-451.
9. Shen CP, Kadesch T. β-cell-specific dna-binding by an e47 homodimer. Mol Cell Biol 1995;15:4518-4524.
10. Zhuang Y, Soriano P, and Weintraub H. The helix-loop-helix gene e2a is required for β-cell formation. Cell 1994;79(5),875-884.
11. Massari ME, Murre C. Helix-loop-helix proteins: Regulators of transcription in eucaryotic organisms. Mol Cell Biol 2000;20:429-440.
12. Arnold HH, Braun T. Genetics of muscle determination and development. Curr Top Dev Biol 2000;48:129-164.
13. Weintraub H. The MyoD family and myogenesis: redundancy, networks, and thresholds. Cell 1993;75:1241-1244.
14. Anderson DJ. Lineages and transcription factors in the specification of vertebrate primary sensory neurons. Curr Opin Neurobiol 1999;9:517-524.
15. Brunet JF, Ghysen A. Deconstructing cell determination: proneural genes and neuronal identity. Bioessays 1999;21:313-318.
16. Chan YM, Jan YN. Conservation of neurogenic genes and mechanisms. Curr Opin Neurobiol 1999;9:582-588.
17. Lee JE. Basic helix-loop-helix genes in neural development. Curr Opin Neurobiol 1997;7:13-20.
18. Ma QF, Kintner C, Anderson DJ. Identification of neurogenin, a vertebrate neuronal determination gene. Cell 1996;87:43-52.
19. Naya FJ, Stellrecht CMM, and Tsai MJ. Tissue-specific regulation of the insulin gene by a novel basic helix-loop-helix transcription factor. Genes Dev 1995;9(8),1009-1019.
20. Cordle SR, Henderson E, Masuoka H, Weil PA, Stein R. Pancreatic beta-cell-type-specific transcription of the insulin gene is mediated by basic helix-loop-helix DNA- binding proteins. Mol Cell Biol 1991;11:1734-1738.
21. Peers B, Leonard J, Sharma S, Teitelman G, Montminy MR. Insulin expression in pancreatic-islet cells relies on cooperative interactions between the helix-loop-helix factor e47 and the homeobox factor stf-1. Mol Endocrinol 1994;8:-1798.
22. Malecki MT, Jhala US, Antonellis A, Fields L, Doria A, Orban T, Saad M, Warram JH, Montminy M, Krolewski AS. Mutations in NEUROD1 are associated with the development of type 2 diabetes mellitus. Nat Genet 1999;23:323-328.
23. Lee, J. E., Hollenberg, S. M., Snider, L., Turner, D. L., Lipnick, N., and Weintraub, H. Conversion of xenopus ectoderm into neurons by neurod, a basic helix-loop-helix protein. Science 1995;268(5212),836-844.
24. Miyata T, Maeda T, Lee JE. NeuroD is required for differentiation of the granule cells in the cerebellum and hippocampus. Genes Dev 1999;13:1647-1652.

25. Sommer L, Ma QF, and Anderson DJ. Neurogenins, a novel family of atonal-related bhlh transcription factors, are putative mammalian neuronal determination genes that reveal progenitor-cell heterogeneity in the developing cns and pns. Mol Cell Neurosci 1996;8(4), 221-241.
26. Ma QF, Sommer L, Cserjesi P, and Anderson DJ. Mash1 and neurogenin1 expression patterns define complementary domains of neuroepithelium in the developing cns and are correlated with regions expressing notch ligands. J Neurosci 1997;17(10), 3644-3652.
27. Perez SE, Rebelo S, Anderson DJ. Early specification of sensory neuron fate revealed by expression and function of neurogenins in the chick embryo. Development 1999;126:1715-1728.
28. Ma QF, Chen ZF, Barrantes ID, Delapompa JL, Anderson DJ. Neurogenin1 is essential for the determination of neuronal precursors for proximal cranial sensory ganglia. Neuron 1998;20:469-482.
29. Ma QF, Kintner C, Anderson DJ. Identification of neurogenin, a vertebrate neuronal determination gene. Cell 1996;87:43-52.
30. Fode C, Gradwohl G, Morin X, Dierich A, LeMeur M, Goridis C, Guillemot F. The bHLH protein NEUROGENIN 2 is a determination factor for epibranchial placode-derived sensory neurons. Neuron 1998;20:483-494.
31. Fode C, Ma Q, Casarosa S, Ang SL, Anderson DJ, Guillemot F. A role for neural determination genes in specifying the dorsoventral identity of telencephalic neurons. Genes Dev 2000;14:67-80.
32. Ma Q, Fode C, Guillemot F, Anderson DJ. Neurogenin1 and neurogenin2 control two distinct waves of neurogenesis in developing dorsal root ganglia. Genes Dev 1999;13:1717-1728.
33. Apelqvist A, Li H, Sommer L, Beatus P, Anderson DJ, Honjo T, de Angelis MH, Lendahl U, Edlund H. Notch signalling controls pancreatic cell differentiation. Nature 1999;400:877-881.
34. Jensen J, Heller RS, Funder-Nielsen T, Pedersen EE, Lindsell C, Weinmaster G, Madsen OD, and Serup P. Independent development of pancreatic α- and β-cells from Neurogenin-3 expressing precursors. Diabetes 2000;49,163-176.
35. Huang HP, Liu M, El Hodiri HM, Chu K, Jamrich M, Tsai MJ. Regulation of the pancreatic islet-specific gene BETA2 (neuroD) by neurogenin 3. Mol Cell Biol 2000;20:3292-3307.
36. Jarriault S, Le-Bail O, Hirsinger E, Pourquie O, Logeat F, Strong CF, Brou C, Seidah NG, Israel A. Delta-1 activation of notch-1 signaling results in HES-1 transactivation. Mol Cell Biol 1998;18:7423-7431.
37. Artavanis-Tsakonas S, Rand MD, Lake RJ. Notch signaling: cell fate control and signal integration in development. Science 1999;284:770-776.
38. Kopan, R, Turner, DL. The notch pathway - democracy and aristocracy in the selection of cell fate. Curr Opin Neurobiol 1996;6:594-601.
39. Nye JS, Kopan R. Developmental signaling. Vertebrate ligands for Notch. Curr Biol 1995;5:966-969.
40. Jouve C, Palmeirim I, Henrique D, Beckers J, Gossler A, Ish-Horowicz D, Pourquie O. Notch signalling is required for cyclic expression of the hairy- like gene HES1 in the presomitic mesoderm. Development 2000;127:1421-1429.
41. Dale KJ, Pourquie O. A clock-work somite. Bioessays 2000;22:72-83.
42. Capell A, Steiner H, Romig H, Keck S, Baader M, Grim MG, Baumeister R, Haass C. Presenilin-1 differentially facilitates endoproteolysis of the beta-amyloid precursor protein and Notch. Nat Cell Biol 2000;2:205-211.
43. Brou C, Logeat F, Gupta N, Bessia C, LeBail O, Doedens JR, Cumano A, Roux P, Black RA, Israel A. A novel proteolytic cleavage involved in Notch signaling: The role of the disintegrin-metalloprotease TACE. Mol Cell 2000;5:207-216.
44. Mumm JS, Schroeter EH, Saxena MT, Griesemer A, Tian XL, Pan DJ, Ray WJ, Kopan R. A ligand-induced extracellular cleavage regulates gamma- secretase-like proteolytic activation of Notch1. Mol Cell 2000;5:197-206.
45. De Strooper B, Annaert W, Cupers P, Saftig P, Craessaerts K, Mumm JS, Schroeter EH, Schrijvers V, Wolfe MS, Ray WJ, Goate A, Kopan R. A presenilin-1-dependent gamma-secretase-like protease mediates release of Notch intracellular domain. Nature 1999;398:518-522.
46. Kidd S, Lieber T, Young MW. Ligand-induced cleavage and regulation of nuclear entry of Notch in Drosophila melanogaster embryos. Genes Dev 1998;12:3728-3740.
47. Kao HY, Ordentlich P, Koyanonakagawa N, Tang Z, Downes M, Kintner CR, Evans RM, Kadesch T. A histone deacetylase corepressor complex regulates the notch signal-transduction pathway. Genes Dev 1998;12:2269-2277.
48. Fisher A, Caudy M. The function of hairy-related bhlh repressor proteins in cell fate decisions. Bioessays 1998;20:298-306.
49. Kageyama R, Ohtsuka T. The Notch-Hes pathway in mammalian neural development. Cell Res 1999;9:179-188.
50. Ahmad I, Zaqouras P, Artavanis-Tsakonas S. Involvement of Notch-1 in mammalian retinal neurogenesis: association of Notch-1 activity with both immature and terminally differentiated cells. Mech Dev 1995;53:73-85.
51. Ohtsuka T, Ishibashi M, Gradwohl G, Nakanishi S, Guillemot F, Kageyama R. Hes1 and Hes5 as Notch effectors in mammalian neuronal differentiation. Embo J 1999;18:2196-2207.

52. Grbavec D, Stifani S. Molecular interaction between TLE1 and the carboxyl-terminal domain of HES-1 containing the WRPW motif. Biochem.Biophys.Res.Commun. 1996;223:701-705.
53. Jimenez G, Paroush Z, Ishhorowicz D. Groucho acts as a corepressor for a subset of negative regulators, including hairy and engrailed. Genes Dev 1997;11:-3072.
54. Paroush Z, Finley RL, Kidd T, Wainwright SM, Ingham PW, Brent R, Ishhorowicz D. Groucho is required for drosophila neurogenesis, segmentation, and sex determination and interacts directly with hairy-related bhlh proteins. Cell 1994;79:805-815.
55. Sasai Y, Kageyama R, Tagawa Y, Shigemoto R, and Nakanishi S. 2 mammalian helix loop helix factors structurally related to drosophila hairy and enhancer of split. Genes Dev 1992;6(12B),2620-2634.
56. Fisher AL, Ohsako S, Caudy M. The wrpw motif of the hairy-related basic helix-loop-helix repressor proteins acts as a 4-amino-acid transcription repression and protein-protein interaction domain. Mol Cell Biol 1996;16:2670-2677.
57. Chen H, Thiagalingam A, Chopra H, Borges MW, Feder JN, Nelkin BD, Baylin SB, Ball DW. Conservation of the Drosophila lateral inhibition pathway in human lung cancer: a hairy-related protein (HES-1) directly represses achaete-scute homolog-1 expression. Proc Natl Acad Sci U S A 1997;94:5355-5360.
58. Ishibashi M, Ang SL, Shiota K, Nakanishi S, Kageyama R, and Guillemot F. Targeted disruption of mammalian hairy and enhancer of split homolog-1 (hes-1) leads to up-regulation of neural helix-loop-helix factors, premature neurogenesis, and severe neural-tube defects. Genes Dev 1995;(24),3136-3148.
59. Tomita K, Ishibashi M, Nakahara K, Ang SL, Nakanishi S, Guillemot F, Kageyama R. Mammalian hairy and enhancer of split homolog-1 regulates differentiation of retinal neurons and is essential for eye morphogenesis. Neuron 1996;16:-723.
60. Tomita K, Hattori M, Nakamura E, Nakanishi S, Minato N, Kageyama R. The bHLH gene Hes1 is essential for expansion of early T cell precursors. Genes Dev 1999;13:1203-1210.
61. Ito T. Differentiation and proliferation of pulmonary neuroendocrine cells. Prog Histochem Cytochem 1999;34:247-322.
62. Landry C, Clotman F, Hioki T, Oda H, Picard JJ, LeMaigre FP, Rousseau GG. Hnf-6 is expressed in endoderm derivatives and nervous-system of the mouse embryo and participates to the cross-regulatory network of liver-enriched transcription factors. Dev Biol 1997;192:247-257.
63. Rausa F, Samadani U, Ye HG, Lim L, Fletcher CF, Jenkins NA, Copeland NG, Costa RH. The cut-homeodomain transcriptional activator hnf-6 is coexpressed with its target gene hnf-3-beta in the developing murine liver and pancreas. Dev Biol 1997;192:228-246.
64. Jacquemin P, Durviaux SM, Jensen J, Godfraind G, Gradwohl G, Guillemot F, Madsen OD, Carmeliet P, Deverchin M, Collen D, Rousseau G, and LeMaigre FP. The transcription factor HNF-6 regulates pancreatic endocrine cell differentiation and controls the expression of the pro-endocrine gene ngn3. Mol Cell Biol 2000;In press.
65. Gittes GK, Galante PE, Hanahan D, Rutter WJ, and Debase HT. Lineage-specific morphogenesis in the developing pancreas: role of mesenchymal factors. Development 1996;122(2), 439-447.
66. Golosow N, Grobstein C. Epitheliomesenchymal interaction in pancreatic morphogenesis. Dev Biol 1962;4:242-255.
67. Wessells NK, Cohen JH. Early pancreas morphogenesis: Morphogenesis, tissue interations, and mass effects. Dev Biol 1967;15:237-270.
68. Alpert S, Hanahan D, Teitelman G. Hybrid insulin genes reveal a developmental lineage for pancreatic endocrine cells and imply a relationship with neurons. Cell 1988;53:295-308.
69. Guz Y, Montminy MR, Stein R, Leonard J, Gamer LW, Wright CV, and Teitelman G. Expression of murine STF-1, a putative insulin gene transcription factor, in beta cells of pancreas, duodenal epithelium and pancreatic exocrine and endocrine progenitors during ontogeny. Development 1995;121(1), 11-18.
70. Teitelman G, Alpert S, Polak JM, Martinez A, and Hanahan D. Precursor cells of mouse endocrine pancreas coexpress insulin, glucagon and the neuronal proteins tyrosine hydroxylase and neuropeptide Y, but not pancreatic polypeptide. Development 1993;118(4), 1031-1039.
71. Ahlgren U, Pfaff SL, Jessell TM, Edlund T, and Edlund H. Independent requirement for ISL1 in formation of pancreatic mesenchyme and islet cells. Nature 1997;385(6613),257-260.
72. Herrera PL, Huarte J, Zufferey R, Nichols A, Mermillod B, Philippe J, Muniesa P, Sanvito F, Orci L, Vassalli JD. Ablation of islet endocrine-cells by targeted expression of hormone-promoter-driven toxigenes. Proc Natl Acad Sci U S A 1994;91:12999-13004.
73. Herrera PL. Adult insulin- and glucagon-producing cells differentiate from two independent cell lineages. Development 2000;127, 2317-2322.
74. Jonsson J, Carlsson L, Edlund T, and Edlund H. Insulin-promoter-factor 1 is required for pancreas development in mice. Nature 1994;371(6498),606-609.
75. Offield MF, Jetton TL, Labosky PA, Ray M, Stein RW, Magnuson MA, Hogan BL, and Wright CV. PDX-1 is required for pancreatic outgrowth and differentiation of the rostral duodenum. Development 1996;122(3),983-995.

76. Sander M, Neubuser A, Kalamaras J, Ee HC, Martin GR, and German MS. Genetic analysis reveals that PAX6 is required for normal transcription of pancreatic hormone genes and islet development. Genes and Development 1997;11(13),1662-1673.
77. St-Onge L, Sosa-Pineda B, Chowdhury K, Mansouri A, and Gruss P. Pax6 is required for differentiation of glucagon-producing alpha-cells in mouse pancreas. Nature 1997;387(6631),406-409.
78. Sussel L, Kalamaras J, Hartigan-O'Connor DJ, Meneses JJ, Pedersen RA, Rubenstein JL, German MS. Mice lacking the homeodomain transcription factor Nkx2.2 have diabetes due to arrested differentiation of pancreatic beta cells. Development 1998;125:2213-2221.
79. Krapp A, Knofler M, Frutiger S, Hughes GJ, Hagenbuchle O, and Wellauer PK. The p48 DNA-binding subunit of transcription factor PTF1 is a new exocrine pancreas-specific basic helix-loop-helix protein. Embo Journal 1996;15(16),4317-4329.
80. Petrucco S, Wellauer PK, and Hagenbuchle O. The DNA-binding activity of transcription factor PTF1 parallels the synthesis of pancreas-specific mRNAs during mouse development. Mol Cell Biol 1990;10(1),254-264.
81. Krapp A, Knofler M, Ledermann B, Burki K, Berney C, Zoerkler N, Hagenbuchle O, Wellauer PK. The bHLH protein PTF1-p48 is essential for the formation of the exocrine and the correct spatial organization of the endocrine pancreas. Genes Dev 1998;12:3752-3763.
82. Qi,HL, Rand,MD, Wu,XH, Sestan,N, Wang,WY, Rakic,P, Xu,T, Artavanis-Tsakonas,S: Processing of the Notch ligand delta by the metalloprotease kuzbanian. Science 283:91-94, 1999
83. Klueg KM, Parody TR, Muskavitch MAT. Complex proteolytic processing acts on delta, a transmembrane ligand for notch, during drosophila development. Mol Biol Cell 1998;9:1709-1723,
84. Panin, V. M., Papayannopoulos, V., Wilson, R., and Irvine, K. D. Fringe modulates notch ligand interactions. Nature 387(6636), 908-912. 1997.
85. Rodriguezesteban C, Schwabe JR, Delapena J, Foys B, Eshelman B, Belmonte JI. Radical fringe positions the apical ectodermal ridge at the dorsoventral boundary of the vertebrate limb. Nature 1997;386:-360.
86. Wu JY, Rao Y. Fringe: defining borders by regulating the notch pathway. Curr Opin Neurobiol 1999;9:537-543.
87. Axelrod JD, Matsuno K, Artavanistsakonas S, Perrimon N. Interaction between wingless and notch signaling pathways mediated by dishevelled. Science 1996;271:1826-1832.
88. Uyttendaele H, Soriano JV, Montesano R, Kitajewski J. Notch4 and wnt-1 proteins function to regulate branching morphogenesis of mammary epithelial-cells in an opposing fashion. Dev Biol 1998;196:204-217.
89. Guo M, Jan LY, Jan YN. Control of daughter cell fates during asymmetric division - interaction of numb and notch. Neuron 1996;17:27-41.
90. Zhong WM, Jiang MM, Weinmaster G, Jan LY, Jan YN. Differential expression of mammalian numb, numblike and notch1 suggests distinct roles during mouse cortical neurogenesis. Development 1997;124:-1887.
91. Sosa-Pineda B, Chowdhury K, Torres M, Oliver G, Gruss P. The Pax4 gene is essential for differentiation of insulin- producing beta cells in the mammalian pancreas. Nature 1997;386:399-402.
92. Cau E, Gradwohl G, Casarosa S, Kageyama R, and Guillemot F. Hes genes regulate sequential stages of neurogenesis in the olfactory epithelium. Development 2000;127,2323-2332.

13

IDENTIFICATION, BIOLOGICAL FUNCTIONS, AND CONTRIBUTION TO HUMAN DIABETES OF ISLET-BRAIN 1

Gérard Waeber, M.D. and Christophe Bonny, Ph.D.
Department of Internal Medicine, CHUV, 1011 Lausanne, Switzerland

GLUT2 GENE REGULATION AS A MODEL FOR THE STUDY OF DIABETES

The GLUT2 glucose transporter isoform is important for control of glucose homeostasis in vertebrates (1). GLUT2 facilitates the entry of glucose through the plasma membrane of cells found in liver, kidney, small intestine, some restricted areas of the brain, and in the pancreatic β-cells (1,2). The regulated expression of GLUT2 has been extensively studied *in vitro* and in a number of animal models that have an unbalanced glucose homeostasis. In freshly isolated pancreatic islets or in insulinoma cells, GLUT2 gene expression is positively modulated by glucose (3). In hepatocytes, glucose metabolism upregulates GLUT2 gene expression as assessed by run-on transcription assays (4-6). While glucose increases GLUT2 gene expression *in vitro*, several reports demonstrate that diabetic hyperglycemia is associated with reduced GLUT2 transcripts in β–cells. This has been observed in the neonatal low-dose streptozotocin (STZ)-induced diabetic rat, the GK rat, the *db/db* mouse, the BB/W rat and the Zucker diabetic *fa/fa* rat (7-10). Interestingly, GLUT2 suppression by hyperglycaemia is specific to β-cells, and GLUT2 expression remains unchanged in liver or kidneys of diabetic animals (11-13). Apart from GLUT2, several other β-cell expressed genes were also found to be dysregulated in the pancreatic islets of the diabetic animals (14).

Diabetic hyperglycemia is associated with β-cell dysfunction and we hypothesized that a restricted number of important regulators of β-cell function were direct targets of this diabetic milieu. A restricted set of transcription factors could be modified by the diabetic milieu, and this change may be responsible for disturbed expression of genes in β-cells (15,26). Decreased GLUT2 expression represents a good biochemical marker for β–cell dysfunction associated with diabetes. The characterization of the GLUT2 *cis*-regulatory elements and *trans*-acting factors may therefore provide a valuable insight into the general control of β-cell specific gene expression in diabetes.

β-CELL SPECIFIC TRANSCRIPTIONAL CONTROL OF THE GLUT2 GENE

The human, rat and murine 5' regulatory regions of the GLUT2 gene have been partially characterized (6,16-18). While the nucleic acid sequence of the coding region of GLUT2 is well conserved between the three species, their promoter regions are less conserved. However, some stretches within the 5' untranslated region of the GLUT2 gene are very similar among species. This indicates some functional importance for these putative *cis* regulatory elements (6). A fragment of 1308 bp of the murine GLUT2 promoter confers glucose responsiveness when transfected into an insulin-secreting cell line or into hepatocytes (4-6). The human GLUT2 promoter also responds to changes in extracellular glucose concentrations. Further, a (TAAT) motif is conserved in the human and murine GLUT2 promoters. This site was shown to be one of the preferential binding sites of the homeodomain protein IPF1 (19-21). Mutation of this *cis* element decreases GLUT2 gene transcription, and the GLUT2TAAT element binds IPF1 *in vitro*, as assessed by mobility shift assays (22) (Figure 1). The importance of IPF1 for GLUT2 expression promoter was recently corroborated *in vivo*: β-cell specific inactivation of the mouse IPF1 gene results in the loss of GLUT2 gene expression in β cells and the development of diabetes mellitus (23).

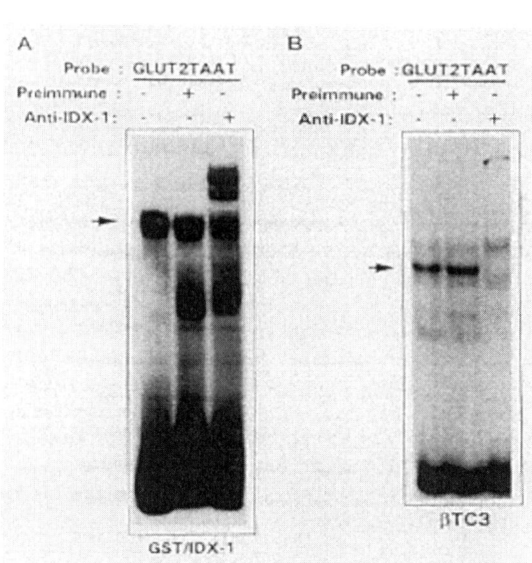

Figure 1. *The IPF1 homeodomain protein interacts with an identified GLUT2TAAT motif of the murine GLUT2 promoter.* ***A)*** *EMSA with bacterially expressed IDX-1 (IPF1) and GLUT2TAAT. The DNA-protein binding complex is disrupted by the addition of the IDX-1 antiserum (+) but not with the preimmune serum (-).* ***B)*** *EMSA with βTC3 nuclear extracts incubated with the GLUT2TAAT motif. The arrow indicates the DNA-protein complex that is selectively supershifted in the presence of the IDX-1 antiserum (reprinted with permission of the Endocrine Society. Molecular Endocrinology, 1996, 10:1327-1334) (22).*

5' deletions of the murine GLUT2 promoter linked to a reporter gene reveal that in transient transfection experiments, the proximal 338 bp of this promoter region directs high reporter gene expression in INS1 and βTC3 cell lines but not in unrelated cell lines (24). This proximal region is also essential for basal transcriptional activity since its deletion from the 1308 bp GLUT2 promoter abolishes reporter gene expression (24). Furthermore, the proximal 338 bp of the GLUT2 promoter also directs reporter gene expression in pancreatic islets of transgenic mice, suggesting that important *cis*-regulatory elements are present within this DNA region (25).

Within the proximal 338 bp of the promoter, three *cis*-elements, GTI, II and III can be identified by DNAse I footprinting, gel retardation and Southwestern experiments in the proximal 338 bp of the promoter (24) (Figure 2). The nucleic acid composition of these *cis*-regulatory elements is well conserved between human and mouse. GTI and GTIII bind distinct but ubiquitously expressed DNA-binding proteins. On the other hand, proteins expressed specifically in pancreatic islets or β-cell lines interact with GTII. Two complexes, GTIIa and GTIIb, are detected in EMSA experiments using GTII labeled oligonucleotides (Figure 3). Interestingly, the GTIIa but not the GTIIb complex is decreased in the pancreatic islets of diabetic animals (26). Therefore, the decreased GLUT2 mRNA expression found in diabetic *db/db* pancreatic islets correlates with a diminution of the β-cell specific complex GTIIa (26). It is not yet clear wheether the loss of GTIIa binding activity found in these diabetic islets is the consequence of the diabetic milieu or a primary event involved in the loss of GLUT2 expression.

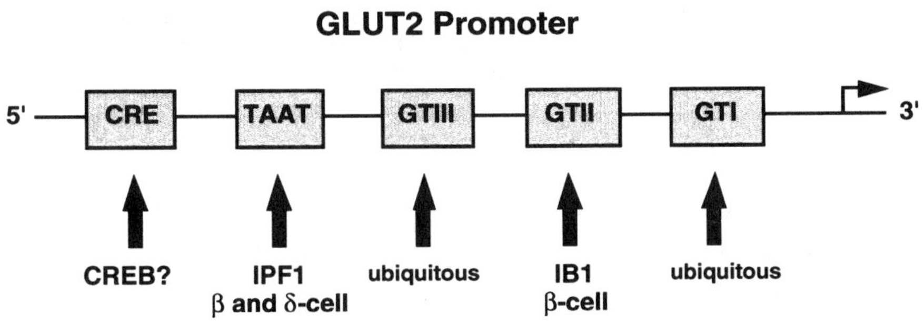

Figure 2. *Schematic representation of the GLUT2 promoter with the localization of the functionally important cis-regulatory elements and trans-acting factors. GTI, GTII, GTIII and TAAT elements are the recognition sites for ubiquitously expressed proteins (GTI and GTIII), for the IPF1 homeodomain (TAAT) and for the β-specific DNA binding protein IB1 (GTII).*

EXPRESSION CLONING OF ISLET-BRAIN 1, AN ISOFORM OF THE C-JUN-N-TERMINAL KINASE INTERACTING PROTEIN JIP-1

An expression cloning strategy was used to identify the GTII binding proteins (27). A differentiated insulinoma (INS1) expression library was constructed and screened by the procedure described by Singh et al. (28) using as probe a radiolabelled concatenated GTII oligonucleotide. A 2953 bp cDNA encoding a 714 amino acid protein was isolated and termed «Islet-Brain 1» (IB1) since its expression was found to be the highest in pancreatic islets and in the brain (27). Northern blot analysis showed that IB1 transcripts are present in all β-cell derived cell lines (INS1, βTC3, MIN6, RIN5F) and in freshly isolated rat pancreatic islets (Figure 4). Varying glucose concentrations in rat pancreatic islets does not regulate IB1 mRNA (Figure 4). In the brain, IB1 mRNA and protein are detected in cortical neurons, in the retina, the hippocampal region and some restricted nuclei in the hypothalamus. IB1 expression is also present, although to a lower extent, in the kidney, the testis and the heart but not in the liver, the lung or the intestine (Figure 4). These data indicate a tissue-specific distribution of IB1, which could be of importance since GLUT2 is dysregulated only in the β-cells of diabetic animals.

IB1 is the rat homologue of a newly identified JIP-1 protein (29). JIP-1 is a cytoplasmic inhibitor of the c-JUN-N-Terminal Kinase activated pathway (JNK) and was cloned from a mouse brain cDNA library using a two-hybrid system with JNK as a bait (29). JIP-1 and IB1 proteins are 97% identical with the exception of a 47 amino-acid insertion present in the carboxyl-terminal part of IB1. Interestingly, this 47 amino acids insertion contains a helix-loop-helix (HLH) and a phosphotyrosine-interaction-domain (PID) absent in JIP-1 (Figure 5). PID domains consist of four conserved block and the first block is contained in the 47 amino acid insertion and therefore absent in JIP-1. JIP-1 is a cytoplasmic protein that binds and retains JNK in the cytoplasm and that inhibits JNK-regulated gene expression. As JNK binds in the nuclei to the transcription factors c-JUN, ATF2 and Elk-1, the sequestration of JNK by JIP-1 in the cytoplasm inhibits the JNK signalling pathway (29). We speculate that in the JIP-1 protein the 47 amino acid that creates a HLH and PID domain allows protein-protein interactions, possibly with other members of the tyrosine kinase signalling pathways or with transcription factors. Computer analysis identifies a putative SH3 domain in the carboxyl-terminal part of the IB1 protein. The functional importance of these domains remains to be established.

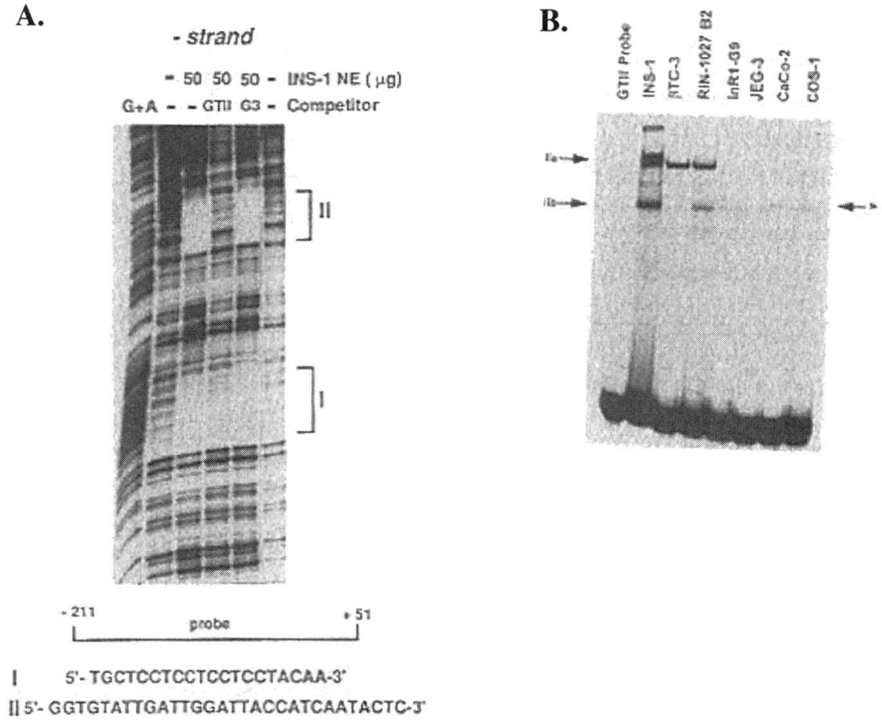

Figure 3. *Identification of the islet-specific GTII binding proteins.* ***A)*** *In vitro DNAse I footprinting competition experiment. The mouse GLUT2 gene 5' sequences from -211 to +51 were used as probe. The GTII double-stranded oligonucleotide prevents formation of the GTII footprint but not GTI or an unrelated G3 oligonucleotide.* ***B)*** *The GTII binding activity is detected only in β cell lines. EMSA with the GTII probe shows the presence of two complexes, IIa and IIb. IIa corresponds to binding factors present only in GLUT2 expressing cell lines (INS1, βTC3 or RIN-1027 B2) and not in glucagon cell line (InR1-G9) or in non-islet derived cell lines (JEG-3, CaCo2 and COS-1). (Reprinted with permission from the Endocrine Society. Molecular Endocrinology, 1995, 9:1413-1426) (24).*

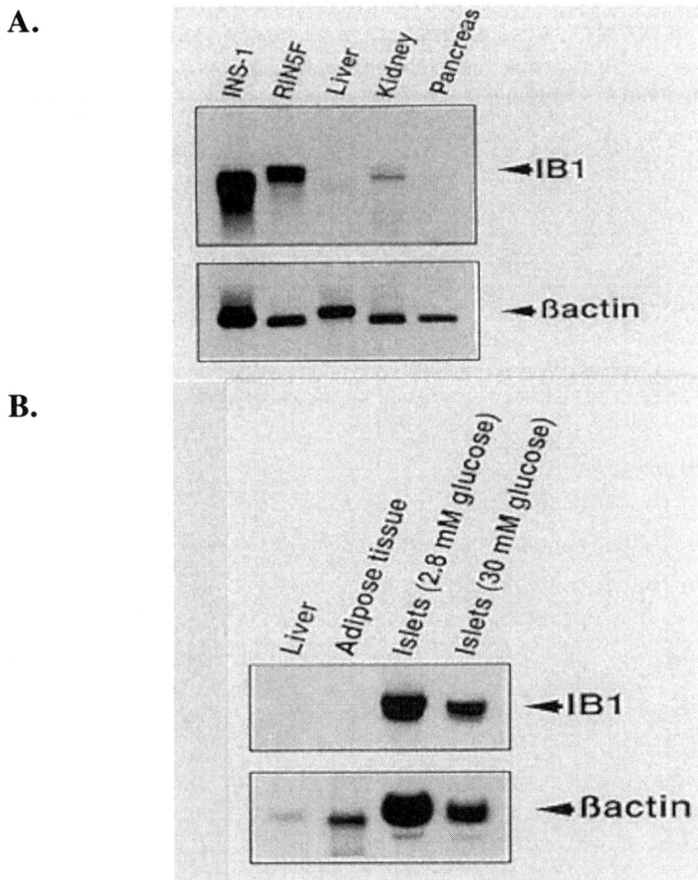

Figure 4. *IB1 mRNA expression is restricted to the insulin-secreting cell lines and to freshly isolated pancreatic islets.* **A)** *Five micrograms of poly(A)$^+$ RNA prepared from two different insulin-secreting cell lines, from rat liver, kidney and whole pancreas were analyzed by Northern blotting for IB1 expression.* **B)** *A total of 5 micrograms of total RNA obtained from isolated rat pancreatic islets incubated in 2.8 or 30 mM glucose for 14 hours were analyzed by Northern blotting, together with rat liver and adipose tissue RNAs (reprinted with permission from the American Society for Biochemistry and Molecular Biology. J Biol Chemistry, 1997, 273:1843-46) (27).*

A.

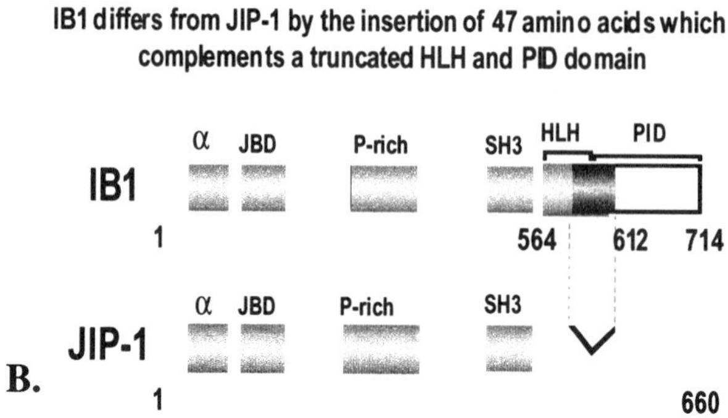

Figure 5. *IB1 differs from JIP-1 by the insertion of 47 amino acids which complement a HLH and PID domain.* ***A)*** *Schematic diagram of IB1 and JIP1 with the putative motifs (HLH= Helix Loop Helix; PID= phophotyrosine interaction domain; SH3= Src homology, P-rich= Proline-rich region; α= a helicoidal acidic stretches)* ***B)*** *amino acid sequence comparison of IB1 with other HLH proteins. Shaded amino acids are conserved in at least five of the sequence presented.* ***C)*** *Sequence alignments of the PID domain of IB1 with several members of PID- containing proteins. (Reprinted with the permission of the American Society for Biochemistry and Molecular Biology. J Biol Chemistry, 1997, 273:1843-46) (27).*

B. **Amino acid sequence comparison of IB1 with other HLH proteins**

```
IB1     RTGARGVFPAYYAIEVTKEPEHMAALAKNS..........KGNDVLCAAMQKLATTR
E47     R-ERRMANNARERLRVRDINEAFRELGRMC..........K-LLILQQAVQVILGLE
MyoD    A-DRRKAATMRERRRLSKVNEAFETLKRCT..........K-VEILRNAIRYIEGLQ
c-myc   N-VKRRTHNVLERQRRNELKRSFFALRDQI..........K-VVILKKATAYILSVQ
E12     K-ERRVANNARERLRVRDINEAFKELGRMC..........K-LLILHQAVSVILNLE
ITF-1   R-ERRMANNARERVRVRDINEAFRELGRMC..........K-LLILQQAVQVILGLE
```

C. **Sequence alignments of the PID domain of IB1 with several members of PID-containing proteins**

```
  consensus  .gdgv.fkvk ..G.vev... .......... ...rd.is.a sea----m.i
jip(mouse)   ..............................................----SVR
  ib1(rat)   SDWIDQFRVK FLGSVQVPY. .......... HKGNDVLCAA MQK----SVR
shc(human)   MGPGVSYLVR YMGCVEVLQS MRALDFNTRT QVTREAISLV CEA----MPI
sck(human)   LGPGVSYVVR YMGCIEVLRS MRSLDFNTRT QVTREAINRL HEA----MSI
 fe65(rat)   DPEAKCFAVR SLGWVEMAE. .......... ...EDLAPGK SSV----GEG
dab(drome)   FGDGVQFKAK LIGILEV... .......... .ARPEVIGCA RRR----AAI
p96(mouse)   KGDGVKYKAK LIGIDDVPD. .......... .ARGDKMSQD SMM----QRI
                                  I

  consensus  t.his..gl. l.d.ktgqii .nhh.q.Isf i.g..dp... nryf.y----
jip(mouse)   GVKIGVKADD ALEAKGNKCS HFFQLKNISF CGY..HPK.N NKYFGF----
  ib1(rat)   GVKIGVKADE AQEAKGNKCS HFFQLKNISF CGY..HPK.N NKYFGF----
shc(human)   TLTVSTSSLN LMAADCKQII ANHHMQSISF ASG.GDPD.T AEYVAY----
sck(human)   SIHISTDGLS LSVPATRQVI ANHHMPSISF ASG.GDTD.M TDYVAY----
 fe65(rat)   KDMYLILEND MLSLVDPMDR SVWHSQPIVS IRVWGVGRDN GRDFAY----
dab(drome)   TIHVTIDGLR LRDEKTGDSL YHHPVHKISF IAQ..DMT.D SRAFGY----
p96(mouse)   WVNISLSGIK IIDEKTGVIE HEHPVNKISF IAR..DVT.D NRAFGY----
                                    II

  consensus  acH.f.ci.. ..lA.a..s. .g.afq..fk q.kke
jip(mouse)   ACHVFVSEDS .TKA..LAES VGRAFQQFYK QFVEY
  ib1(rat)   ACHVFVSEDS .TKA..LAES VGRAFQQFYK QFVEY
shc(human)   ACHILECPEG ..LAQDVIST IGQAFELRFK QYLRN
sck(human)   ACHILECCEG ..LAQSIIST VGQAFELRFK QYLHS
 fe65(rat)   KCHVFRCDT. ..PAKAIATS LHEICSKIMA ERKNA
dab(drome)   SGHRFFGIKT DKAASQVVLA MRDLFQVVFE LKKKE
p96(mouse)   GQHQFFAIKT GQQAEPLVVD LKDLFQVIYN VKKKE
                III              IV
```

Western blot and immunohistochemistry studies reveals that IB1 is present in the cytoplasm and the nuclei of insulin-secreting cells as well as of neurons. IB1 is detected as an approximately 120-kDa protein in both β and non-β cell populations of freshly isolated rat pancreatic islets suggesting that the protein may also be expressed in α or δ cells. The carboxyl-terminal part of the protein (280-714 a.a.) contains the DNA-binding domain of IB1, while the amino-terminal part can act as an activation domain as assessed in a heterologous GAL4 system. Regarding GLUT2 transcriptional activation, IB1 is a weak activator of the GLUT2 promoter. It is not clear whether IB1 functions in the presence of other related HLH proteins and/or whether IB1 functions mainly through the modulation of the JNK-activated pathway.

The role of IB1 in the control of β-cell function was evaluated using a stable insulinoma β-cell line engineered to express IB1 antisense RNA under the control of a doxycycline-dependent transactivator. The conditional expression of the antisense RNA in these cells decreases IB1 protein, which is associated with significantly reduced GLUT2 and insulin expression (30).

IDENTIFICATION AND MAPPING OF THE HUMAN IB1 GENE

The human IB1 cDNA is 94% identical to the rat *IB1* gene and its tissue distribution of expression is similar to that observed in rodents. The human *IB1* structure is very analogous to the murine *IB1* gene. The gene contains 12 exons and maps to chromosome 11p11.2-p12 (31) (Figure 6). Interestingly, the 141-bp sequence present in the IB1 cDNA that is absent in the mouse JIP-1 cDNA is encoded by the 3' portion of exon 8 and the 5' half of exon 9. No GT-AG splice sites flank the 141-bp sequence, suggesting that alternative splicing is not likely to occur within this region of the IB1 gene. The identification of a single *IB1* gene in the human genome and its fine mapping by FISH and radiation hybrid panels argues against the existence of a *JIP-1* gene in human and the mechanism by which JIP-1 may be generated in humans remains to be determined.

Human Genomic Structure of the IB1 gene

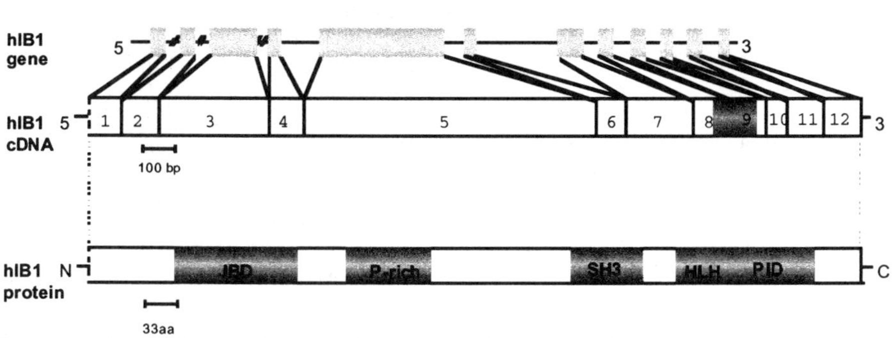

Figure 6. *Genomic organization of the human IB1 gene and schematic representation of the human IB1 cDNA and IB1 protein. The human IB1 gene contains 12 exons and the 141-bp sequence encoding the 47-residue segment that distinguishes IB1 from JIP-1 is indicated as a hatched box (reproduced with permission of Genomics. Genomics 1999, 55:202-8) (31).*

The 11p11.2-p12 region of the human genome has been carefully studied in the case of a rare human syndrome termed DEFECT-11. This syndrome is characterized by **D**eletion of the 11p11.2-p12, **E**nlarged **F**oramina, **E**xostoses, **C**raniofacial dysostosis and mental re**t**ardation. The genes responsible for the exostoses and cranial dysostosis have been mapped to this 11p11.2-p12 region however the neuronal phenotypic manifestation remains unexplained. It is conceivable that the absence of the *IB1* gene in the DEFECT-11 syndrome may underlie the neuronal and metabolic manifestations of the disease.

HUMAN DIABETES ASSOCIATED WITH A MUTATION WITHIN THE IB1 GENE

IB1 was considered as a candidate-gene for human diabetes for several reasons. First, IB1 was identified as a β-cell specific DNA-binding transactivator of the *GLUT2* gene and therefore it may be involved in the dysregulation of GLUT2 in experimental diabetes. Second, the IB1 gene is highly conserved between species including human, rat and mouse. This indicates an important functional role for the protein. Third, IB1 is expressed in human pancreatic islets and in an human insulinoma implying that an altered expression or function of the IB1 gene may have some consequences to the normal function of the islet. Fourth, the IB1 protein is related to JIP-1 and could play some critical role in the control of the activated JNK pathway in β cells. Since this pathway is involved in embryonic development, the immune response, oncogenic transformation and apoptosis, one may speculate that abnormal function of one or several step(s) in this activated pathway may have some important consequences for the normal function of the β-cells (32).

Using polymorphic markers flanking the IB1 gene, 638 individuals collected from 149 French families with Type 2 diabetes were analyzed for possible linkage. Although no evidence of linkage was observed between the IB1 markers and diabetes, an excess in allele sharing was noticed among affected siblings in 23 families. The coding region of the IB1 gene was sequenced in one member of each of these families and a unique missense mutation was identified in one family (Figure 7). The missense mutation results in a serine-to asparagine substitution at codon 59 (S59N), and the mutation was absent in 119 healthy subjects and 436 unrelated subjects with Type 2 diabetes. This mutation segregates with diabetes in all affected members of the family (30). Of interest, some of the diabetic members are also carriers of a second mutation within the IPF1 gene, suggesting a digenic origin of diabetes within this pedigree. The S59N mutation in the IB1 gene is localized close to the JNK domain of the protein. In vitro experiments revealed that the mutated IB1 protein allele increases the susceptibility of the β-cells to apoptosis.

Type 2 diabetes is recognized as a heterogeneous disease of polygenic origin influenced by environmental factors (33-35). Further work will be required to investigate in detail how mutations within the IB1 gene may be responsible for a monogenic non-MODY form of diabetes that seems to enhance the phenotypic expression of a second mutation found in the IPF1 gene in one pedigree. Some of these answers may be resolved by careful transgenesis studies. The selective disruption of the murine IB1 gene is early embryonic lethal (N. Thompson and G. Waeber, manuscript in preparation). It will be of interest to follow the metabolic homeostasis of mice carrying either a functional IB1(+/-) and/or IPF1(+/-) allele. Mutations within the IB1 and IPF1 genes may alter the β–cell function in several ways: they may modify the normal developmental program of the endocrine pancreas and abnormal function of IB1 may decrease the β-cell mass (since the JNK-activated pathway is involved in apoptosis) (32).

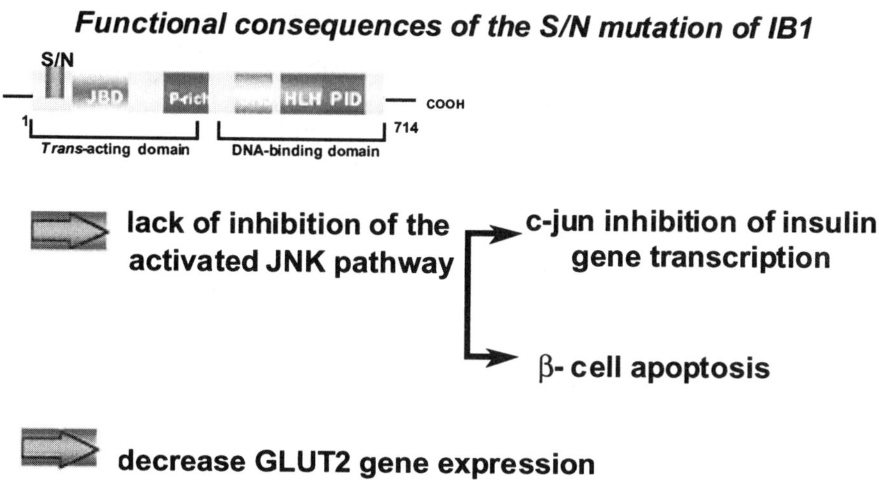

Figure 7. *The S59N mutation in IB1 is localized close to the JNK domain of the protein.*

ACKNOWLEDGEMENTS

This work was supported by the Swiss Foundation for Scientific Research (32-49673.96), the Placide Nicod and Botnar Foundations. The authors are grateful to Vincent Mooser, Nancy Thompson, Myriam Steinmann, Pascal Nicod, and Philippe Froguel for all valuable discussions and excellent technical assistance.

REFERENCES

1. Thorens B. Molecular and cellular physiology of GLUT2, a high Km facilitated diffusion glucose transporter. Int Review of Cytology 1992;137A:209-237.
2. Leloup C, Arluison M, Lepetit N, Cartier N, Marfaing-Jallat P, Ferré P, et al. Glucose transporter 2 (GLUT2): expression in specific brain nuclei. Brain Research 1994;638:221-226.
3. Asano T, Katagiri H, Tsukuda K, Lin JL, Ishihara H, Yazaki Y, et al. Upregulation of GLUT2 mRNA by glucose, mannose, and fructose in isolated rat hepatocytes. Diabetes 1992;41:22-25.
4. Rencurel F, Waeber G, Antoine B, Rocchiccioli F, Maulard P, Girard J. Requirement of glucose metabolism for regulation of glucose transporter type 2 (GLUT2) gene expression in liver. Biochem J 1996;314:903-909.
5. Rencurel F, Waeber G, Bonny C, Antoine B, Maulard P, Girard J, et al. Cyclic adenosine monophosphate prevents the glucose-mediated stimulation of GLUT2 gene transcription in hepatocytes. Biochem J 1997;322:441-448.
6. Waeber G, Thompson N, Haefliger J-A, Nicod P. Characterization of the murine high Km glucose transporter GLUT2 gene and its transcriptional regulation by glucose in a differentiated insulin-secreting cell line. J Biol Chem 1994;269:26912-26919.
7. Orci L, Unger RH, Ravazzola M, Ogawa A, Komiyia I, Baetens D, et al. Reduced B-cell glucose transporter in new onset diabetic BB rats. J Clin Invest 1990;86:1615-1622.
8. Ohneda M, Johnson JH, Inman LR, Chen L, Suzuki KI, Goto Y, et al. GLUT2 expression and function in β-cells of GK rats with NIDDM. Diabetes 1993;42:1065-1072.
9. Johnson JH, Ogawa A, Chen L, Orci L, Newgard CB, Alam T, et al. Underexpression of b-cell high Km glucose transporters in non insulin-dependent diabetes. Science 1990;250:546-548.
10. Thorens B, Wu Y-J, Leahy JL, Weir GC. The loss of GLUT2 expression by glucose-unresponsive

β-cells of db/db mice is reversible and is induced by the diabetic environment. J Clin Invest 1992;90:77-85.
11. Oka Y, Asano T, Shibasaki Y, Lin J-L, Tsukuda T, Akanuma Y, et al. Increased liver glucose-transporter protein and mRNA in streptozocin-induced diabetic rats. Diabetes 1990;39:441-446.
12. Burcelin R, Eddouks M, Kandé J, Assan R, Girard J. Evidence that GLUT2 mRNA and protein concentrations are decreased by hyperinsulinemia and increase by hyperglycemia in liver of diabetic rats. Biochem J 1992;288:675-679.
13. Dominguez JH, Camp K, Maianu L, Feister H, Garvey WT. Am J Physiol 1994;266:F283-290.
14. Tokuyama Y, Sturis J, DePaoli AM, Takeda J, Stoffel M, Tang J, et al. Evolution of β-cell dysfunction in the male Zucker diabetic fatty rat. Diabetes 1995;44:1447-1457.
15. Gremlich S, Bonny C, Waeber G, Thorens B. Fatty acids decrease IDX-1 expression in rat pancreatic islets and reduce GLUT2, glucokinase, insulin and somatostatin levels. J Biol Chem 1997;272:30261-30269.
16. Takeda J, Kayano T, Fukomoto H, Bell GI. Organization of the human GLUT2 (pancreatic β-cell and hepatocyte) glucose transporter gene. Diabetes 1993;42:773-777.
17. Ahn Y-h, Kim J-W, Han G-S, Lee B-G, Kim YS. Cloning and characterization of rat pancreatic β-cell/liver type glucose transporter gene: a unique exon/intron organization. Arch Bioch and Biophysics 1995; 323:387-396.
18. Leibiger B, Leibiger IB. Functional analysis of DNA-elements involved in transcriptional control of the human glucose transporter 2 (GLUT2) gene in the insulin-producing cell line βTC3. Diabetologia 1995;38:112-115.
19. Leonard J, Peers B, Johnson T, Ferreri K, Lee S, Montminy MR. Characterization of somatostatin transactivating factor-1, a novel homeobox factor that stimulates somatostatin expression in pancreatic islet cells. Mol Endo 1993;7:1275-1283.
20. Miller CP, McGehee RE, Jr, Habener JF. IDX-1: a new homeodomain transcription factor expressed in rat pancreatic islets and duodenum that transactivates the somatostatin gene. EMBO J 1994;13:1145-1156.
21. Ohlsson H, Karlsson K, Edlund T. IPF1, a homeodomain-containing transactivator of the insulin gene. EMBO J 1993;12:4251-4259.
22. Waeber G, Thompson N, Nicod P, Bonny C. Transcriptional activation of the GLUT2 gene by the IPF-1/STF-1/IDX-1 homeobox factor. Mol Endo 1996;10:1327-1334.
23. Ahlgren U, Jonsson J, Jonsson L, Simu K, Edlund H. Beta-cell specific inactivation of the mouse IPF1/PDX1 gene results in loss of the beta-cell phenotype and maturity onset diabetes. Genes Dev 1998;15:1763-1768.
24. Bonny C, Thompson N, Nicod P, Waeber G. Pancreatic-specific expression of the glucose transporter type 2 gene: identification of *cis*-elements and islet-specific *trans*-acting factors. Mol Endo 1995;9:1413-1426.
25. Waeber G, Pedrazzini T, Bonny O, Bonny C, Steinmann M, Nicod P, et al. A 338 bp proximal fragment of the glucose transporter type 2 (GLUT2) promoter drives reporter gene expression in the pancreatic islets of transgenic mice. Mol Cell Endocrinol 1995;114:205-215.
26. Bonny C, Roduit R, Gremlich S, Nicod P, Thorens B, Waeber G. The loss of GLUT2 expression in the pancreatic __cells of diabetic db/db mice is associated with an impaired DNA-binding activity of islet-specific trans-acting factors. Mol Cell Endocrinol 1997;135:59-65.
27. Bonny C, Nicod P, Waeber G. IB1, a JIP-1 related nuclear protein present in insulin-secreting cells. J Biol Chem 1998;273:1843-1846.
28. Singh H, LeBowitz JH, Baldwin AS, Sharp PA. Molecular cloning of an enhancer binding protein: isolation by screening of an expression library with a recognition site DNA. Cell 1988;52:415-423.
29. Dickens M, Rogers JS, Cavanagh J, Raitano A, Xia Z, Halpern JR, et al. A cytoplasmic inhibitor of the JNK signal transduction pathway. Science 1997;277:693-696.
30. Waeber G, Delplanque J, Bonny C, Mooser V, Steinmann M, Widman C, et al. The gene MAPK81Pi, encoding islet-Brain1, is a candidate for type 2 diabetes. Nature Genetics 2000;24:291-295.
31. Mooser V, Maillard A, Bonny C, Steinmann M, Shaw P, Yarnall DP, et al. Genomic organization, fine-mapping, and expression of the human islet-brain 1 (IB1)/c-Jun-amino-terminal kinase interacting protein-1 (JIP-1) gene. Genomics 1999;15:202-208.
32. Ip YT, Davis RJ. Signal transduction by the c-Jun N terminal kinase (JNK)-from inflammation to development. Current Opinion in Cell Biology 1998;10:205-219.
33. DeFronzo RA. Pathogenesis of type 2 diabetes: metabolic and molecular implications for identifying diabetes genes. Diabetes Reviews 1997;5:177-269.
34. Kahn BB. Type 2 diabetes: when insulin secretion fails to compensate for insulin resistance. Cell 1998;92:593-596.
35. Polonsky KS, Sturis J, Bell GI. Non-Insulin-Dependent Diabetes Mellitus: a genetically programmed failure of beta cells to compensate for insulin resistance. N Engl J Med 1996;334:777-783.

14

PAX4 AND PAX6 IN ISLET DIFFERENTIATION

Xunlei Zhou, Ph.D. and Peter Gruss, Ph.D.
Max-Planck Institute of Molecular Biology
37077 Göttingen, Germany

INTRODUCTION

After the classical demonstration of the role of the pancreas in diabetes mellitus (1,2), and since the identification of the cellular components of the pancreatic islets and their hormonal products (3-6), the development of the islets of Langerhans of the pancreas has attracted the attention of researchers (7-10). Major progress in the understanding of the cell lineages of the endocrine pancreas has come, among others, from ablation studies (11-13), from analyses of the coexpression of endocrine hormones (14-16) and from transgenic approaches (17,18). In the last five years, however, the primordium of the endocrine pancreas has received special and renewed attention, mainly because advances in the field of molecular biology have brought about new insights into the intricacies of islet differentiation (19-25). Perhaps the most important recent contributions to the field have been a consequence of the study of the pancreatic phenotypes of mouse lines carrying induced mutations of developmental control genes – HNF1-α (26); Isl1 (27); Beta2/NeuroD (28); Nkx2.2 (29); P48 (30); Pax4 (31); Pax6 (32,33); pdx-1 (34-36). A large part of the excitement that surrounds the study of islet development is due to the therapeutic promise harboured by every advance in the understanding of the development and function of the endocrine pancreas.

Cell differentiation, the process by which embryonic cells become different from one another and acquire specialized functions, has been intensively studied in a variety of systems. In every one of the models, one particular differentiation strategy has been found – muscle differentiation is achieved with the help of master genes (37); in the hematopoietic system, pluripotent stem cells and growth factors have a fundamental role (38); in the neural crest, environmental factors found during extensive migrations are probably responsible for the final fate of these multipotent cells (39). Except for the general mechanisms of regulation of gene expression, the details of the differentiation process do not show much similarity between systems – it would seem that, perhaps not surprisingly, cells achieve their differentiated state by different mechanisms – no "model" can possibly be found that applies to the differentiation of every kind of organ or tissue.

Complex combinations of transcription factors control cell differentiation, and although some of them have a very restricted pattern of expression, others are common to many cell types. An emerging concept is that groups of transcription factors perform same or similar work in the differentiation of a variety of tissues or organs (epigenetic code). Perhaps we do not have cellular or organic models of differentiation, but molecular models of co-operation between transcription factors to bring about similar effects in many kinds of cellular systems. One family of transcription factors that is currently under scrutiny from precisely this point of view, and some of whose members have major roles in islet differentiation is formed by the Pax genes.

The Pax gene family
The Pax genes form a family of developmental control genes coding for transcriptional regulator proteins that share a highly conserved 128 amino acid domain or "paired domain" (reviewed in reference 40). Nine mammalian Pax genes have been cloned. Mutations in three of the human Pax genes cause different human developmental phenotypes – a Pax2 mutation causes the renal-coloboma syndrome (41-43), Pax3 mutations cause Waardenburg type I syndrome (44) and mutations of Pax6 have been identified as the cause of aniridia (45). In addition, several human tumors show chromosomal translocations involving Pax genes, or alterations of the regulation of some members of the family (46-53). The implication of Pax genes in carcinogenesis (54-57) and in the development of organs (58,59) has been recently reviewed. Apart from the pancreas, Pax genes have a major involvement in the differentiation of other two organs, the kidney (60-62) and the thyroid gland (63-66).

Vertebrate Pax genes have been classified into four paralogous (related, non-allelic genes within a single species) groups (I-IV) by structural similarities (reviewed in references 58 and 67). The members of each group share a specific assembly of three motifs: the paired box, the homeobox and the octapeptide. Group I is formed by Pax1 and Pax9, Group II by Pax2, 5 and 8, Group III by Pax3 and 7 and Group IV by Pax 4 and 6. Members of a group have very high sequence similarity within the paired domain and show resembling expression patterns during development. In this context, it is also interesting that Pax transcription factors appear in groups of two in a variety of differentiating systems: Pax2 and Pax6 in the eye (68-70), Pax2 and Pax5 in the midbrain and cerebellum (71, 72), Pax2 and Pax8 in the kidney (62,73), Pax3 and Pax7 in the spinal cord (74-76) and of course Pax4 and Pax6 in the pancreas (31,32). In the model of axial mesoderm differentiation, and with respect to the classical homeobox genes, it has been proposed that the identity of a vertebral segment could be determined by the particular combination of Hox genes expressed at a certain time in that particular segment; these significant combinations of transcription factors would form a "Hox code" (77). The paired combinations of Pax transcription factors that cooperate in differentiation processes make it tempting to speculate about the existence of a "Pax code" to cellular identity at work in many tissues or organs.

Pax4 and Pax6
The role of Pax genes in islet development was instantly emphasized in 1997, with the phenotypes of two targeted mutant mouse lines which show major pancreatic differentiation alterations (31,32): Pax4 and Pax6 are essential for the differentiation of the β- and α-cell-lineages, respectively. Analysis of a natural mutant of Pax6 confirmed and extended the data on the involvement of this gene in the differentiation of the α-cells (33). Together, Pax4 and Pax6 form Group IV of the structural classification of vertebrate paired box genes – they have paired box and homeobox, but not the octapeptide (reviewed in reference 58).

Pax6 (78) is widely expressed in the developing nervous system and eye (79) and in the endocrine pancreas (80). The brain phenotype of mice homozygous for the Pax6 mutation Small eye (Sey) (81,82) shows great complexity and is currently the object of intensive studies (69,83-88). There are two known human pathological conditions originated by Pax6 mutations: aniridia (lack of iris (45,82)) and Peter's syndrome (a form of congenital corneal opacity; reviewed in references 89 and 90). As is the case at least for Pax1 (91), Pax2 and Pax3 (92), also Pax6 exhibits haploinsufficiency (their mutations are semidominant, i.e. they have a phenotype in heterozygosis, at least in some of the tissues where they are expressed). Haploinsufficiency is not a common phenomenon (reviewed in reference 93) and reveals the importance that correct protein dosage has for the function of these genes. This importance has been recently confirmed and extended for Pax6 by showing that even overexpression of this gene causes severe ocular developmental alterations (94). Finally, the regulation of the expression of Pax6 is under intensive research (95-100).

Perhaps because of its very restricted territory of expression, together with the fact that no natural mutations of this gene are known in mouse or human, Pax4 (78) had remained a more obscure transcription factor than Pax6. Pax4 has been detected only in a few cells in the ventral spinal cord, and in the endocrine pancreas (101); the only known phenotype of mice deficient in this gene is related to the pancreas (101). Ever since the original description (78), little more had been learned about Pax4 except perhaps its chromosomal localization in human (102). The sudden importance acquired by Pax4 in pancreatic development, however (101), has already spawned several papers reporting the cloning of this gene in human (103) and rat (104), as well as expanding our knowledge about its structure and function (104-106).

The essential role of Pax genes in pancreatic development has been uncovered only recently (31-33,99,100,107,108). Here we will emphasize in the first place the important traits of the mutant phenotypes. Based on these facts, we will see what Pax genes can teach us about the interactions that shape the islet, and which models can account for the observed changes.

PAX4 AND PAX6 IN THE ISLET: EXPRESSION AND PHENOTYPES

What we know about the role of Pax4 and Pax6 in mouse islet differentiation comes fundamentally from studies of null mutation effects on the expression of specific markers. Two studies address the role of Pax6 – one by means of a targeted mutation (32) and the other by analyzing the pancreatic phenotype of Sey^{Neu}/Sey^{Neu} (33) (the Sey^{Neu} allele is an ethylnitrosourea-induced mutation of the Pax6 gene (82)). The role of Pax4 has been analyzed by means of a targeted mutation (31) and also in the double Pax4/6 mutant (32). A description of wild type Pax4 and Pax6 expression can be gleaned from the analyses performed by the groups mentioned (31-33).

Expression of Pax4 and Pax6 in the Wild Type Developing Islet (Table 1)

In the mouse embryo, the pancreatic primordium can be first seen on e9.5, under the appearance of a swelling of the endoderm approximately at the level of the junction of foregut and midgut. Already by this stage, cells containing glucagon can be detected, and one day later insulin-containing cells appear. Exocrine cells become distinguishable from endocrine ones around e14.5. Somatostatin-containing cells appear by e15. Finally, cells producing pancreatic polypeptide (PP) can be detected around the day of birth, on e18.5 (reviewed in references 21 and 33).

On e9, Pax6 protein can be detected in certain cells of the endoderm, at the level where the pancreatic primordium will develop. One half-day later (e9.5), these cells also contain immunoreactive glucagon (33). Pax4 mRNA can be first detected in a few cells in the dorsal primordium of the pancreas on the same day as Pax6 is detected (31,109). By e10.5, insulin can also be detected in the primordium, in some cases colocalized with glucagon (31,33). Essentially the same sequence has been reported by St. Onge and coworkers (32), although their date of colocalization is one day later (e10.5), probably due to genetic background differences or differences in the experimental method. By e13.5, the number of Pax4-expressing cells increases, and they can be found scattered throughout the pancreatic epithelium. Among these Pax4-expressing cells, only a small subpopulation coexpresses insulin (109). As mentioned above, around e14.5 exocrine and endocrine lineages differentiate morphologically and biochemically (reviewed in reference 21). At e15.5, Pax6 mRNA and Pax6 protein can be detected in a large number of pancreatic cells which also contain either glucagon or insulin; from then on, and also in the adult, every hormone-producing pancreatic cell expresses Pax6 (33). On the same day, the number of Pax4-expressing cells in the pancreas reaches its peak. At this age, the cells that coexpress Pax4 and insulin largely outnumber the ones that do not, as opposed to the situation two days earlier (109). By e18.5, the endocrine islets start to be visible (reviewed in reference 21). At the same time, Pax4-expressing cells are reduced in number as compared to e15.5, and their lower immunoreactivity suggests that perhaps they are producing reduced levels of the protein (109). The number of Pax4-expressing cells in the pancreas continues to decrease, until in the adult they are virtually non-existent (109). Based on these data, it seems likely that Pax6 has a role in the development of all the pancreatic endocrine lineages, while Pax4 would be implicated in the development of the β-cell-lineage and δ-cell lineage.

Pax4 Mutant Phenotype

Extensive studies have been possible using the Pax4 knockout model with *e. coli* LacZ replacing the Pax4 coding region. In these animals, cells where Pax4 promoter is active express LacZ and are thus easily identified ("blue cells").

The earliest appearance of the Pax4 mutant pancreas is surprising because of its "normality" – at embryonic day 10.5 (e10.5), no difference in LacZ expression was observed between pancreases from animals heterozygous and homozygous for the Pax4 mutation (31,109). Insulin-containing cells and glucagon-containing cells exist in normal numbers in the mutants at this age. Besides, pdx-1 (a transcription factor with a major involvement in islet development (34,36,111-113)) expression is normal at this stage.

By e15.5, however, expression of LacZ (i.e., Pax4 promoter activity) is diminished in the homozygous pancreas, while it reaches its peak in the heterozygous situation. Almost no insulin can be detected in the mutant, but the distribution of glucagon-containing cells in homozygotes matches that of the wild type pancreas. pdx-1 expression is also altered – while the mutant pancreas shows low levels of pdx-1 in cells all over the pancreatic primordium, the wild type pancreas exhibits pdx-1 that is already sharply restricted to β-cells. Expression of Nkx6.1 (a β-cell-specific homeobox (114-116)) seems unaffected by the mutation at this stage – both in wild type and in mutant pancreatic primordia, Nkx6.1 can be found only in insulin-containing cells (109).

Shortly before birth (e18.5), almost no pdx-1 can be detected in the Pax4 mutant, although the wild type pancreas shows intense expression of this gene (109). Nkx6.1 expression is now severely reduced. Amylin (a β-cell marker (117-121) that starts to appear in β-cells before they are fully mature (122, 123)) can be found in the core of the wild type islet, and is excluded from the peripheral rim (formed by cells that contain either glucagon, somatostatin or PP), while in the Pax4 mutant some of the (very abundant) amylin-containing cells also contain glucagon (109). The most striking histological feature of the Pax4-deficient phenotype is related to the cytoarchitecture of the pancreas, and appears also by this age – while the wild type pancreatic primordium starts showing the characteristic islets of Langerhans for the first time, in the Pax4 mutant there islets do not form, and clusters of glucagon-containing cells are dispersed throughout the primordium.

phase	age	wild type	Pax4 -/-	Pax6 -/-	Pax4/6 -/-
early	e9.0	Pax6		LacZ	
	e9.5	Pax4 Pax6 glu	LacZ	LacZ	
	e10.5	Pax4 Pax6 glu ins	LacZ pdx-1 normal ins normal glu normal	glu reduced	
	e12.5			glu reduced ins reduced	
	e13.5	Pax4$^+$-ins$^+$ Pax4$^+$-ins$^-$	pdx-1 normal ins		
	e14.5				
late	e15.5	Pax4 peaks Pax4$^+$-ins$^+$ increase high pdx-1 in β-cell	glu normal almost no ins low pdx-1		
	e16.5				
	e18.5		pdx-1 very reduced		
	P0	LacZ reduced ins glu	no LacZ expr. no pdx-1 expr. almost no ins, amylin glu increased	LacZ present no islets, almost no glu, ins reduced som reduced PP reduced	no endocrine cells few LacZ cells few pdx-1 cells

Table 1. *Main phenotypical features of the developing pancreas of wild type, Pax4-/- and Pax6-/- mice. See text for details.*

In the newborn Pax4 mutant, LacZ expression is completely absent, few or no insulin-containing cells can be found and both pdx-1 and Nkx6.1 (both β-cell markers in the wild type pancreas at this age) expression are undetectable. Glucagon-containing cells remain abnormally clustered, some of them coexpressing amylin (31,109) – although mature β-cells are absent, some poorly differentiated β-cells seem to exist (31,109). No somatostatin expression is detected, suggesting that the δ-cell-lineage is also affected by the Pax4 mutation. However, expression of somatostatin in the gut seems normal in the mutant (31).

Pax6 Mutant Phenotypes
Sander and her coworkers have analyzed the developmental progression of the phenotype of the Pax6-deficient mice in Sey^{Neu}/Sey^{Neu} (33). At e9.5, the number of glucagon-containing cells is still too small to detect any difference between the wild type pancreas and that of Sey^{Neu}/Sey^{Neu} (33). At e10.5, however, the number of glucagon-containing cells is reduced in the mutant, and by e12.5 it is evident that the number of insulin-containing cells is also reduced in Sey^{Neu}/Sey^{Neu} (33).

By e18.5 all the endocrine cell types of the islet are severely reduced in number, particularly the α-lineage (glucagon). The islets that begin to be visible at this stage, can be found in normal numbers, but the normal distribution of cell types within them is altered – all endocrine cell lineages are mixed throughout the islet. Further, the concentration of the hormones insulin and glucagon in the pancreas of Sey^{Neu}/Sey^{Neu} is extremely reduced.

Analysis of the Pax6 targeted mutation at the newborn stage (32) confirms the total or almost total absence of glucagon-containing cells in the Pax6 deficient pancreas, as well as the cytoarchitectonic alteration in the endocrine cells. The LacZ reporter gene included in the targeting construct of the knockout mice provides additional information – blue cells can be found in the newborn mutant pancreas and they produce either insulin, PP, or somatostatin.

Early phase and late phase?
A common theme seems to emerge from these and other (124,125) studies of the islet differentiation process – there could be an early phase and a late phase in the differentiation of the pancreatic anlage. The transition between both phases would roughly coincide with the separation between endocrine and exocrine (reviewed in reference 21) tissue that takes place at around e14.5.

During the early phase of islet differentiation, hormone expression and pdx-1 expression are independent from Pax4. Pax6, however, seems to have an important role in this phase – at least as early as e10.5, glucagon-containing cells are less numerous in Sey^{Neu}/Sey^{Neu} than in wild type, and by e12.5 it is clear that both insulin-containing and glucagon-containing cells are reduced in number in the mutant. The time of expression of these hormones during development, however, is not delayed.

Expression of the reporter gene β-galactosidase (LacZ) of both targeted mutations (Pax4 and Pax6) shows that both promoters are active during the early phase in the absence of the corresponding proteins – this shows that the promoters of these genes are activated by transcription factors other than the proteins they code for.

In the late phase, the transcription factor requirements for the maintenance of the differentiated state change. Lack of Pax4 in mutant primordium manifests itself through virtually complete absence of insulin- and somatostatin-containing cells and severe cytoarchitectonic alterations. In addition, the absence of β-galactosidase expression at later developmental stages indicates that the Pax4 promoter is not active anymore. In the Pax6 deficient pancreas, glucagon synthesis is extremely reduced or inexistent, but the number of insulin-, somatostatin- and PP-containing cells is also reduced, as well as the amount of the corresponding hormones. The Pax6 promoter, however, is still active, to judge by the presence of "blue cells" in the targeted mutation.

In summary, the early phase of endocrine cell differentiation seems to be independent from Pax4, and dependent on Pax6 only quantitatively (for the right number of cells). In the late phase, the presence of Pax4 determines the existence of mature β-cells and of δ-cells and the correct number of α-cells (in its absence the number of α-cells increases dramatically). Pax6, however, is again in the late phase responsible for the correct number of cells (not of islets) of the four lineages, for the correct amount of the respective hormones and for islet morphology.

PAX4 AND PAX6: STRUCTURE AND REGULATION

Following, we will summarize what is known on the structure and regulation of the Pax4 and Pax6 genes with emphasis on their role in islet differentiation.

Structure and regulation of Pax4

The coding region of the murine Pax4 gene comprises 10 exons and spans 5.5 kb; the full length cDNA is 1.38 kb. It contains an 1047 bp open reading frame encoding 349 amino acids with a predicted molecular weight of 38 kD (126-128). Three isoforms of mouse Pax4 are generated by alternative splicing of its RNA. In the rat, four isoforms have been described (104). Expression data gathered in the Pax4 targeted mutant suggest that pdx-1 and Pax4 could interact with each other, and that correct expression of insulin and Nkx6.1 could be directly and/or indirectly upregulated by both proteins (109). Nkx6.1 might in turn repress glucagon expression in β-cells (36,129).

Structure and regulation of Pax6

Analyses of the primary structure of Pax6 in quail (*Coturnix coturnix*), in the nematode *Caenorhabditis elegans* and in mouse (99,130-133) show that the Pax6 gene contains 10 exons that can give place by alternative transcription initiation to at least three different transcripts, the longest of which has 3 kb (78). These studies also suggest that the expression of Pax6 is under the control of different regulators through alternate promoters. In the human Pax6, multiple cis-regulatory elements with distinct function have been identified (95).

We have found four *cis*-elements in this gene (99). Element A that confers pancreas expression, is a stretch of DNA 1.1 kb long located 4.6 kb upstream of exon 0. Element B, located downstream A (3.6 kb upstream of exon 0), is formed by 107 bp responsible for expression in the lens and cornea. Element C, which is 5 kb long, is found between promoters P0 and P1 and confers expression in the telencephalon. Element D, (530 bp long, located downstream the Pax6 translation start site) that contains all of the 5th exon (exon α), controls expression in the retina. Other two groups have reported essentially similar results about the localization of the pancreatic element (100,107). The results obtained by our group (99) reveal, within the 1100 bp fragment of the pancreas-specific element, a stretch of 120 bp which shares a high degree of sequence identity between the Pax6 control elements of pufferfish, mouse and human.

Which proteins then bind to these *cis*-elements? Among the highly conserved regulatory sequences there are several potential binding sites of transcription factors that could be involved in the regulation of Pax6 expression (99). In particular, the 1.1 kb-long pancreas-specific element contains two motifs for homeodomain binding sites and one reported consensus binding site for PBX1 that may regulate Pax6 expression by direct binding (134).

Which genes are regulated by Pax6 in the pancreas? Pancreas-specific expression of the glucagon gene is conferred by the islet-specific enhancer elements G2, G3 and G4 (135-138) and the α-cell-specific proximal promoter element G1 (136,138-141). Pax6 binds to the islet specific enhancer of the glucagon G3 enhancer element, and Pax6 binds to the glucagon G1 element as a monomer or as a heterodimer with Cdx-2/3 (a homeodomain protein known to regulate glucagon expression (139)). The G1 element of the glucagon promoter confers α-cell-specific expression of the glucagon gene; this suggests that Pax6 could have a role in the restricted cell-type expression of this hormone (143). The islet-specific G3-binding complex has been shown to bind also to the rat insulin I and somatostatin promoters (144), and Pax6 also binds to the promoters of insulin and somatostatin (33). In this way, Pax6 is expressed by the four islet lineages and participates in the regulation of the specific hormone product of at least three of them.

Pax genes in the islet: Masters or team players?
A master gene is one capable of activating the downstream program for terminal differentiation of a cell in a certain direction without the concourse of any other factor. The concept of master gene was coined on the basis of the ability of transcription factor gene MyoD to induce the expression of muscle-specific genes in a variety of already differentiated cells not fated in principle to become muscle fibres (145). The gene eyeless (ey), the Drosophila homolog of Pax6 (146), has been shown to be a master gene for eye differentiation in the fruit-fly (147), and has been suggested to be a universal master gene for the morphogenesis and evolution of the eye (148). In view of the dramatic and specific effects of Pax6 deficiency on the development of the pancreatic α-cell-lineage (32), and of Pax4 deficiency on the β-cell-lineage, the question arises if these genes could be considered master genes for the differentiation of said cell types. However, other factors are involved in the acquisition of pancreatic endocrine phenotypes. In the Pax4 mutant, not only Pax4 is absent, but pdx-1 and Nkx6.1 are also reduced (although present in normal amounts in the earliest stages). This suggests that an interaction between these genes is needed for the terminal differentiation of the β-cell-lineage (109).

HOW DO PAX4 AND PAX6 FIT INTO CURRENT MODELS OF ISLET DIFFERENTIATION? (FIGURE 1)

A generally accepted model of islet differentiation and cell lineage based on the developmental expression of specific markers has been developed and refined in the last decade (14-16,22,150) (reviewed in reference 19). We will base our discussion of the function of Pax genes in islet differentiation on a simplified version of the current model (151) (Figure 1).

Pax genes are not necessary to set up the endocrine lineages of the islet, but to carry out the final differentiation of some of them (Pax4) and to produce the right number of endocrine cells (Pax6). This notion fits well with current models of islet differentiation (Figure 1). In the simplest model, the α-cell fate would be adopted "by default". In this way, β-cell-specific factors like Pax4 or pdx-1 would be able (directly or indirectly) to suppress the glucagon promoter in non-α-islet cells.

Therefore, in the Pax4-/- pancreas, because of the absence of Pax4, cells of the β-cell-lineage choose the α differentiation pathway and express glucagon. The fact that these newly fated α-cells do not express the reporter gene β-galactosidase suggests that repression of the Pax4 promoter is part of the α differentiation pathway. Pax4 would be necessary to activate its own promoter, or other β-cell-specific transcription factors that activate the Pax4 promoter.

The phenotype of the Pax6 mutants is more difficult to assess in terms of cellular models. According to the simplest explanation (152), Pax6 would be necessary for the existence of the α-lineage, much as Pax4 determines the β-cell-lineage. Pax4 and Pax6 would be equivalent and fulfil a similar role, one for the α-cell-lineage and the other for the β-cell-lineage. Cell counting data in the pancreas of mice homozygous for Sey^{Neu} suggests that Pax6 is essential not only for the glucagon-containing cells, but also for the four islet lineages (33).

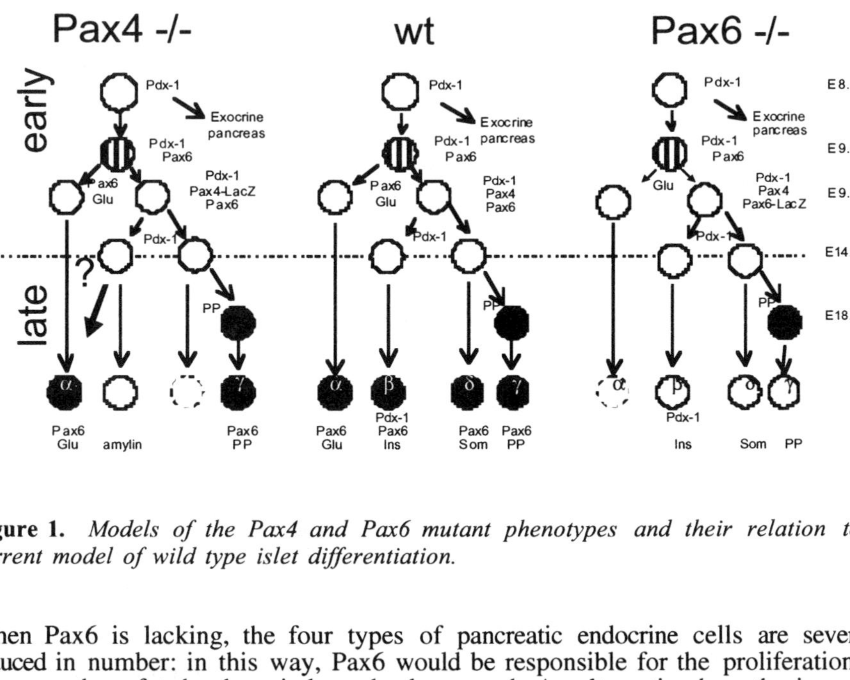

Figure 1. *Models of the Pax4 and Pax6 mutant phenotypes and their relation to a current model of wild type islet differentiation.*

When Pax6 is lacking, the four types of pancreatic endocrine cells are severely reduced in number: in this way, Pax6 would be responsible for the proliferation of lineages whose fate has been independently secured. An alternative hypothesis would make Pax6 necessary for the survival of islet cells – in its absence, large numbers of each of the lineages would die. Data on the incidence of apoptosis and cell proliferation during the normal pancreatic development are currently unavailable to address these questions.

Pax genes have been directly or indirectly implicated in proliferation in different systems, and regulation of cell proliferation has been suggested as a common mechanism used by the genes of this family involved in organogenesis (153). Pax5 plays a role in lymphocyte proliferation (154), Pax3 in the developing muscle of the limbs (155). In particular, Pax6 appears to play a role in cell proliferation in a variety of systems – in the eye primordium (156), in the spinal cord (together with Pax3 (157)), in the diencephalon (158). Finally, in Sey^{Neu}/Sey^{Neu} embryos, some of the precursor cells of the cerebral cortex (the radial glial cells) are decreased in number and suffer also alterations of the cell cycle (84,88).

Do α-cells become β-cells in the absence of Pax6? According to St-Onge and coworkers (159), it is difficult to answer to this question, due to the fact that normally β-cells are already much more numerous than α-cells. The fact that Pax6 is expressed since very early in every pancreatic endocrine cell, and that the four lineages are reduced in number in the Sey^{Neu}/Sey^{Neu} mutant, has prompted the hypothesis that Pax6 could be responsible for adopting the endocrine versus the exocrine fate in the developing pancreas (33).

In the Pax6 mutant mice, the clusters of pancreatic endocrine cells are disorganized. This suggests that Pax6 regulates directly or indirectly the expression of one or several cell adhesion genes or other genes with cytoarchitectonic functions. The role of adhesion molecules in pancreatic development has been recently reviewed (160) – adhesion molecules from both the cadherin and the CAM families have been mapped to the developing pancreas. Evidence linking Pax6 to the regulation of adhesion molecules during development has been obtained by studies of the developing Sey^{Neu}/Sey^{Neu} cerebral cortex (84,88). In this system, Pax6 has been shown to regulate the expression of adhesion molecules R-cadherin (84) and tenascin (88). The promoter of the gene for adhesion molecule L1 (which is not expressed in the pancreas) shows binding sites for Pax6 (161).

FUTURE PERSPECTIVES

The advances in our understanding of cell differentiation in the endocrine pancreas brought about in the last few years by molecular genetics open many possibilities for the therapy of the major conditions related to the physiology of this organ. In the context of the transcription factors, particularly of the Pax genes, some exciting ideas are currently being tested. Specifically, given that the pancreas has a partial regenerative capacity, one might be able to exploit this ability by attempting to trigger specific differentiation processes in the adult pancreas. To this end, obtaining information about the genetic network that leads to β-cell or ultimately islet cell formation is mandatory. Another route that can be used is based on the availability of human embryonic stem cells. The general capacity of pluripotent ES cells to differentiate *in vitro* could be directed in a certain direction, e.g. differentiation into the pancreatic endocrine cells. The general concept of relying on information required for building complex structures during embryonic stages will also undoubtedly be of use in regeneration processes. Consequently, the more we learn about the genetic hierarchies involved in development, the more we can rely on this information for diagnosis and therapy.

ACKNOWLEDGEMENTS

We thank Dr. Sosa-Pineda for sharing unpublished information.

REFERENCES

1. Banting FG, Best CH. Pancreatic extracts. 1922 [classical article]. J Lab Clin Med 1990;115:254-72.

2. Banting FG, Best CH, Collip JB, Campbell WR, Fletcher AA. Pancreatic extracts in the treatment of diabetes mellitus: preliminary report. 1922 [classical article]. Cmaj 1991;145:1281-6.
3. Baum J, Simons BE, Unger RH, Madison LL. Localisation of glucagon in the alpha cells in the pancreatic islet by immunofluorescent technics. Diabetes 1962;11:371-374.
4. Bloom W. New types of granular cell in islets of Langerhans of man. Anat Rec. 1931;49:363-371.
5. Lacy PE, Davies J. Preliminary studies on the demonstration of insulin in the islet by the fluorescent antibody technic. Diabetes 1957;6:354-357.
6. Orci L, Baetens D, Dubois MP, Rufener C. Evidence for the Δ cell of the pancreas secreting somatostatin. Horm Metab Res 1975;7:400-402.
7. Lacy PE, Kostianovsky M. Method for the isolation of intact islets of Langerhans from the rat pancreas. Diabetes 1967;16:35-9.
8. Spooner BS, Walther BT, Rutter WJ. The development of the dorsal and ventral mammalian pancreas in vivo and in vitro. J Cell Biol 1970;47:235-46.
9. Rutter WJ, Kemp JD, Bradshaw WS, Clark WR, Ronzio RA, Sanders TG. Regulation of specific protein synthesis in cytodifferentiation. J Cell Physiol 1968;72:Suppl 1:1-18.
10. Pictet RL, Clark WR, Williams RH, Rutter WJ. An ultrastructural analysis of the developing embryonic pancreas. Dev Biol 1972;29:436-67.
11. Palmiter RD, Behringer RR, Quaife CJ, Maxwell F, Maxwell IH, Brinster RL. Cell lineage ablation in transgenic mice by cell-specific expression of a toxin gene [published erratum appears in Cell 1990 Aug 10;62(3):following 608]. Cell 1987;50:435-43.
12. Evans GA. Dissecting mouse development with toxigenics. Genes Dev 1989;3:259-63.
13. Ohashi PS, Oehen S, Buerki K, et al. Ablation of "tolerance" and induction of diabetes by virus infection in viral antigen transgenic mice. Cell 1991;65:305-17.
14. Teitelman G, Lee JK, Alpert S. Expression of cell type-specific markers during pancreatic development in the mouse: implications for pancreatic cell lineages. Cell Tissue Res 1987;250:435-9.
15. Teitelman G, Lee JK. Cell lineage analysis of pancreatic islet development: glucagon and insulin cells arise from catecholaminergic precursors present in the pancreatic duct. Dev Biol 1987;121:454-66.
16. Teitelman G, Alpert S, Polak JM, Martinez A, Hanahan D. Precursor cells of mouse endocrine pancreas coexpress insulin, glucagon and the neuronal proteins tyrosine hydroxylase and neuropeptide Y, but not pancreatic polypeptide. Development 1993;118:1031-9.
17. Alpert S, Hanahan D, Teitelman G. Hybrid insulin genes reveal a developmental lineage for pancreatic endocrine cells and imply a relationship with neurons. Cell 1988;53:295-308.
18. Upchurch BH, Aponte GW, Leiter AB. Expression of peptide YY in all four islet cell types in the developing mouse pancreas suggests a common peptide YY-producing progenitor. Development 1994;120:245-52.
19. Madsen OD, Jensen J, Blume N, et al. Pancreatic development and maturation of the islet β cell. Studies of pluripotent islet cultures. Eur J Biochem 1996;242:435-45.
20. Habener JF, Stoffers DA. A newly discovered role of transcription factors involved in pancreas development and the pathogenesis of diabetes mellitus. Proc Assoc Am Physicians 1998;110:12-21.
21. Slack JM. Developmental biology of the pancreas. Development 1995;121:1569-80.
22. Teitelman G. Cellular and molecular analysis of pancreatic islet cell lineage and differentiation. Recent Prog Horm Res 1991;47:259-94.
23. Sander M, German MS. The beta cell transcription factors and development of the pancreas. J Mol Med 1997;75:327-40.
24. Rudnick A, Ling TY, Odagiri H, Rutter WJ, German MS. Pancreatic beta cells express a diverse set of homeobox genes. Proc Natl Acad Sci USA 1994;91:12203-7.
25. Yamaoka T, Itakura M. Development of pancreatic islets (Review). Int J Mol Med 1999;3:247-261.
26. Pontoglio M, Sreenan S, Roe M, et al. Defective insulin secretion in hepatocyte nuclear factor 1alpha- deficient mice. J Clin Invest 1998;101:2215-22.
27. Pfaff SL, Mendelsohn M, Stewart CL, Edlund T, Jessell TM. Requirement for LIM homeobox gene Isl1 in motor neuron generation reveals a motor neuron-dependent step in interneuron differentiation. Cell 1996;84:309-20.
28. Naya FJ, Huang HP, Qiu Y, et al. Diabetes, defective pancreatic morphogenesis, and abnormal enteroendocrine differentiation in BETA2/neuroD-deficient mice. Genes Dev 1997;11:2323-34.
29. Sussel L, Kalamaras J, Hartigan-O'Connor DJ, et al. Mice lacking the homeodomain transcription factor Nkx2.2 have diabetes due to arrested differentiation of pancreatic beta cells. Development 1998;125:2213-21.
30. Krapp A, Knofler M, Ledermann B, et al. The bHLH protein PTF1-p48 is essential for the formation of the exocrine and the correct spatial organization of the endocrine pancreas. Genes Dev 1998;12:3752-63.

31. Sosa-Pineda B, Chowdhury K, Torres M, Oliver G, Gruss P. The Pax4 gene is essential for differentiation of insulin-producing beta cells in the mammalian pancreas. Nature 1997;386:399-402.
32. St-Onge L, Sosa-Pineda B, Chowdhury K, Mansouri A, Gruss P. Pax6 is required for differentiation of glucagon-producing alpha-cells in mouse pancreas. Nature 1997;387:406-9.
33. Sander M, Neubuser A, Kalamaras J, Ee HC, Martin GR, German MS. Genetic analysis reveals that PAX6 is required for normal transcription of pancreatic hormone genes and islet development. Genes Dev 1997;11:1662-73.
34. Jonsson J, Carlsson L, Edlund T, Edlund H. Insulin-promoter-factor 1 is required for pancreas development in mice. Nature 1994;371:606-9.
35. Jonsson J, Carlsson L, Edlund T, Edlund H. Insulin-promoter-factor 1 is required for pancreas development in mice. Nature 1994;371:606-9.
36. Ahlgren U, Jonsson J, Jonsson L, Simu K, Edlund H. beta-cell-specific inactivation of the mouse Ipf1/Pdx1 gene results in loss of the beta-cell phenotype and maturity onset diabetes. Genes Dev 1998;12:1763-8.
37. Molkentin JD, Olson EN. Defining the regulatory networks for muscle development. Curr Opin Genet Dev 1996;6:445-53.
38. Morrison SJ, Uchida N, Weissman IL. The biology of hematopoietic stem cells. Annu Rev Cell Dev Biol 1995;11:35-71.
39. Le Douarin NM, Dupin E, Ziller C. Genetic and epigenetic control in neural crest development. Curr Opin Genet Dev 1994;4:685-95.
40. Noll M. Evolution and role of Pax genes. Curr Opin Genet Dev 1993;3:595-605.
41. Sanyanusin P, McNoe LA, Sullivan MJ, Weaver RG, Eccles MR. Mutation of PAX2 in two siblings with renal-coloboma syndrome. Hum Mol Genet 1995;4:2183-4.
42. Schimmenti LA, Pierpont ME, Carpenter BL, Kashtan CE, Johnson MR, Dobyns WB. Autosomal dominant optic nerve colobomas, vesicoureteral reflux, and renal anomalies. Am J Med Genet 1995;59:204-8.
43. Sanyanusin P, Schimmenti LA, McNoe LA, et al. Mutation of the PAX2 gene in a family with optic nerve colobomas, renal anomalies and vesicoureteral reflux [published erratum appears in Nat Genet 1996 May;13(1):129]. Nat Genet 1995;9:358-64.
44. Wilcox ER, Rivolta MN, Ploplis B, Potterf SB, Fex J. The PAX3 gene is mapped to human chromosome 2 together with a highly informative CA dinucleotide repeat. Hum Mol Genet 1992;1:215.
45. Jordan T, Hanson I, Zaletayev D et al. The human PAX6 gene is mutated in two patients with aniridia. Nat Genet 1992;1:328-32.
46. Wang W, Kumar P, Whalley J et al. The mutation status of PAX3 and p53 genes in medulloblastoma. Anticancer Res 1998;18:849-53.
47. Qiu G, Stavnezer J. Overexpression of BSAP/Pax-5 inhibits switching to IgA and enhances switching to IgE in the I.29 mu B cell line. J Immunol 1998;161:2906-18.
48. Morrison AM, Jager U, Chott A, Schebesta M, Haas OA, Busslinger M. Deregulated PAX-5 transcription from a translocated IgH promoter in marginal zone lymphoma. Blood 1998;92:3865-78.
49. Hazen-Martin DJ, Re GG, Garvin AJ, Sens DA. Distinctive properties of an anaplastic Wilms' tumor and its associated epithelial cell line. Am J Pathol 1994; 144:1023-34.
50. Davis RJ, D'Cruz CM, Lovell MA, Biegel JA, Barr FG. Fusion of PAX7 to FKHR by the variant t(1;13)(p36;q14) translocation in alveolar rhabdomyosarcoma. Cancer Res 1994;54:2869-72.
51. Galili N, Davis RJ, Fredericks WJ, et al. Fusion of a fork head domain gene to PAX3 in the solid tumour alveolar rhabdomyosarcoma [published erratum appears in Nat Genet 1994 Feb;6(2):214]. Nat Genet 1993;5:230-5.
52. Shapiro DN, Sublett JE, Li B, Downing JR, Naeve CW. Fusion of PAX3 to a member of the forkhead family of transcription factors in human alveolar rhabdomyosarcoma. Cancer Res 1993;53:5108-12.
53. Dressler GR, Douglass EC. Pax-2 is a DNA-binding protein expressed in embryonic kidney and Wilms tumor. Proc Natl Acad Sci USA 1992;89:1179-83.
54. Schafer BW. Emerging roles for PAX transcription factors in cancer biology. Gen Physiol Biophys 1998; 17:211-24.
55. Mansouri A. The role of Pax3 and Pax7 in development and cancer [In Process Citation]. Crit Rev Oncog 1998;9:141-9.
56. Walker C. Molecular genetics of renal carcinogenesis. Toxicol Pathol 1998;26:113-20.
57. Barr FG. Chromosomal translocations involving paired box transcription factors in human cancer. Int J Biochem Cell Biol 1997;29:1449-61.
58. Dahl E, Koseki H, Balling R. Pax genes and organogenesis. Bioessays 1997;19:755-65.
59. Peters H, Neubuser A, Balling R. Pax genes and organogenesis: Pax9 meets tooth development. Eur J Oral Sci 1998;106 Suppl 1:38-43.
60. Dressler GR. The genetic control of renal development. Curr Opin Nephrol Hypertens 1995;4:253-7.

61. Lipschutz JH. Molecular development of the kidney: a review of the results of gene disruption studies. Am J Kidney Dis 1998;31:383-97.
62. Torban E, Goodyer P. What PAX genes do in the kidney. Exp Nephrol 1998;6:7-11.
63. Mansouri A, Chowdhury K, Gruss P. Follicular cells of the thyroid gland require Pax8 gene function. Nat Genet 1998;19:87-90.
64. Macchia PE, Lapi P, Krude H, et al. PAX8 mutations associated with congenital hypothyroidism caused by thyroid dysgenesis. Nat Genet 1998;19:83-6.
65. Kambe F, Seo H. Thyroid-specific transcription factors. Endocr J 1997;44:775-84.
66. Damante G. Thyroid defects due to Pax8 gene mutations. Eur J Endocrinol 1998;139:563-6.
67. Mansouri A, Hallonet M, Gruss P. Pax genes and their roles in cell differentiation and development. Curr Opin Cell Biol 1996;8:851-7.
68. Torres M, Gomez-Pardo E, Gruss P. Pax2 contributes to inner ear patterning and optic nerve trajectory. Development 1996;122:3381-91.
69. Grindley JC, Davidson DR, Hill RE. The role of Pax-6 in eye and nasal development. Development 1995;121:1433-42.
70. Li HS, Yang JM, Jacobson RD, Pasko D, Sundin O. Pax-6 is first expressed in a region of ectoderm anterior to the early neural plate: implications for stepwise determination of the lens. Dev Biol 1994;162:181-94.
71. Schwarz M, Alvarez-Bolado G, Urbanek P, Busslinger M, Gruss P. Conserved biological function between Pax-2 and Pax-5 in midbrain and cerebellum development: evidence from targeted mutations. Proc Natl Acad Sci U S A 1997;94:14518-23.
72. Urbanek P, Fetka I, Meisler MH, Busslinger M. Cooperation of Pax2 and Pax5 in midbrain and cerebellum development. Proc Natl Acad Sci USA 1997;94:5703-8.
73. Plachov D, Chowdhury K, Walther C, Simon D, Guenet JL, Gruss P. Pax8, a murine paired box gene expressed in the developing excretory system and thyroid gland. Development 1990;110:643-51.
74. Wada H, Holland PW, Sato S, Yamamoto H, Satoh N. Neural tube is partially dorsalized by overexpression of HrPax-37: the ascidian homologue of Pax-3 and Pax-7. Dev Biol 1997;187:240-52.
75. Seo HC, Saetre BO, Havik B, Ellingsen S, Fjose A. The zebrafish Pax3 and Pax7 homologues are highly conserved, encode multiple isoforms and show dynamic segment-like expression in the developing brain. Mech Dev 1998;70:49-63.
76. Mansouri A, Gruss P. Pax3 and Pax7 are expressed in commissural neurons and restrict ventral neuronal identity in the spinal cord. Mech Dev 1998;78:171-8.
77. Kessel M, Gruss P. Homeotic transformations of murine vertebrae and concomitant alteration of Hox codes induced by retinoic acid. Cell 1991;67:89-104.
78. Walther C, Guenet JL, Simon D, et al. Pax: a murine multigene family of paired box-containing genes. Genomics 1991;11:424-34.
79. Walther C, Gruss P. Pax-6, a murine paired box gene, is expressed in the developing CNS. Development 1991;113:1435-49.
80. Turque N, Plaza S, Radvanyi F, Carriere C, Saule S. Pax-QNR/Pax-6, a paired box- and homeobox-containing gene expressed in neurons, is also expressed in pancreatic endocrine cells. Mol Endocrinol 1994;8:929-38.
81. Ton CC, Hirvonen H, Miwa H, et al. Positional cloning and characterization of a paired box- and homeobox- containing gene from the aniridia region. Cell 1991;67:1059-74.
82. Hill RE, Favor J, Hogan BL, et al. Mouse small eye results from mutations in a paired-like homeobox- containing gene [published erratum appears in Nature 1992 Feb 20;355(6362):750]. Nature 1991;354:522-5.
83. Osumi N, Hirota A, Ohuchi H, et al. Pax-6 is involved in the specification of hindbrain motor neuron subtype. Development 1997;124:2961-72.
84. Stoykova A, Gotz M, Gruss P, Price J. Pax6-dependent regulation of adhesive patterning, R-cadherin expression and boundary formation in developing forebrain. Development 1997;124:3765-77.
85. Stoykova A, Fritsch R, Walther C, Gruss P. Forebrain patterning defects in Small eye mutant mice. Development 1996;122:3453-65.
86. Mastick GS, Davis NM, Andrew GL, Easter SS, Jr. Pax-6 functions in boundary formation and axon guidance in the embryonic mouse forebrain. Development 1997;124:1985-97.
87. Grindley JC, Hargett LK, Hill RE, Ross A, Hogan BL. Disruption of PAX6 function in mice homozygous for the Pax6Sey-1Neu mutation produces abnormalities in the early development and regionalization of the diencephalon. Mech Dev 1997;64:111-26.
88. Gotz M, Stoykova A, Gruss P. Pax6 controls radial glia differentiation in the cerebral cortex. Neuron 1998;21:1031-44.
89. Macdonald R, Wilson SW. Pax proteins and eye development. Curr Opin Neurobiol 1996;6:49-56.
90. Graw J. Genetic aspects of embryonic eye development in vertebrates. Dev Genet 1996; 18:181-97.

91. Wilm B, Dahl E, Peters H, Balling R, Imai K. Targeted disruption of Pax1 defines its null phenotype and proves haploinsufficiency. Proc Natl Acad Sci USA 1998;95:8692-7.
92. Chalepakis G, Tremblay P, Gruss P. Pax genes, mutants and molecular function. J Cell Sci Suppl 1992;16:61-7.
93. Engelkamp D, van Heyningen V. Transcription factors in disease. Curr Opin Genet Dev 1996; 6:334-42.
94. Schedl A, Ross A, Lee M et al. Influence of PAX6 gene dosage on development: overexpression causes severe eye abnormalities. Cell 1996;86:71-82.
95. Xu ZP, Saunders GF. Transcriptional regulation of the human PAX6 gene promoter. J Biol Chem 1997;272:3430-6.
96. Plaza S, Turque N, Dozier C, Bailly M, Saule S. C-Myb acts as transcriptional activator of the quail PAX6 (PAX-QNR) promoter through two different mechanisms. Oncogene 1995;10:329-40.
97. Sharon-Friling R, Richardson J, Sperbeck S et al. Lens-specific gene recruitment of zeta-crystallin through Pax6, Nrl- Maf, and brain suppressor sites. Mol Cell Biol 1998;18:2067-76.
98. Xu ZP, Saunders GF. PAX6 intronic sequence targets expression to the spinal cord. Dev Genet 1998;23:259-63.
99. Kammandel B, Chowdhury K, Stoykova A, Aparicio S, Brenner S, Gruss P. Distinct cis-essential modules direct the time-space pattern of the Pax6 gene activity. Dev Biol 1999;205:79-97.
100. Xu PX, Zhang X, Heaney S, Yoon A, Michelson AM, Maas RL. Regulation of Pax6 expression is conserved between mice and flies. Development 1999;126:383-95.
101. Sosa-Pineda B, Chowdhury K, Torres M, Oliver G, Gruss P. The Pax4 gene is essential for differentiation of insulin-producing beta cells in the mammalian pancreas. Nature 1997;386:399-402.
102. Tamura T, Izumikawa Y, Kishino T, Soejima H, Jinno Y, Niikawa N. Assignment of the human PAX4 gene to chromosome band 7q32 by fluorescence in situ hybridization. Cytogenet Cell Genet 1994;66:132-4.
103. Bonthron DT, Dunlop N, Barr DG, El Sanousi AA, Al-Gazali LI. Organisation of the human PAX4 gene and its exclusion as a candidate for the Wolcott-Rallison syndrome. J Med Genet 1998;35:288-92.
104. Tokuyama Y, Yagui K, Sakurai K, Hashimoto N, Saito Y, Kanatsuka A. Molecular cloning of rat Pax4: identification of four isoforms in rat insulinoma cells. Biochem Biophys Res Commun 1998;248:153-6.
105. Tao T, Wasson J, Bernal-Mizrachi E et al. Isolation and characterization of the human PAX4 gene. Diabetes 1998;47:1650-3.
106. Inoue H, Nomiyama J, Nakai K, Matsutani A, Tanizawa Y, Oka Y. Isolation of full-length cDNA of mouse PAX4 gene and identification of its human homologue. Biochem Biophys Res Commun 1998;243:628-33.
107. Williams SC, Altmann CR, Chow RL, Hemmati-Brivanlou A, Lang RA. A highly conserved lens transcriptional control element from the Pax-6 gene. Mech Dev 1998;73:225-9.
108. Tokuyama Y, Yagui K, Sakurai K, Hashimoto N, Saito Y, Kanatsuka A. Molecular cloning of rat Pax4: identification of four isoforms in rat insulinoma cells. Biochem Biophys Res Commun 1998;248:153-6.
109. Sosa-Pineda B, Asano M. personal communication.
110. MacGregor GR, Mogg AE, Burke JF, Caskey CT. Histochemical staining of clonal mammalian cell lines expressing E. coli beta galactosidase indicates heterogeneous expression of the bacterial gene. Somat Cell Mol Genet 1987;13:253-65.
111. Jonsson J, Ahlgren U, Edlund T, Edlund H. IPF1, a homeodomain protein with a dual function in pancreas development. Int J Dev Biol 1995;39:789-98.
112. Ohlsson H, Thor S, Edlund T. Novel insulin promoter- and enhancer-binding proteins that discriminate between pancreatic alpha- and beta-cells. Mol Endocrinol 1991;5:897-904.
113. Ohlsson H, Karlsson K, Edlund T. IPF1, a homeodomain-containing transactivator of the insulin gene. Embo J 1993;12:4251-9.
114. Jensen J, Serup P, Karlsen C, Nielsen TF, Madsen OD. mRNA profiling of rat islet tumors reveals nkx 6.1 as a beta-cell- specific homeodomain transcription factor. J Biol Chem 1996;271:18749-58.
115. Inoue H, Rudnick A, German MS, Veile R, Donis-Keller H, Permutt MA. Isolation, characterization, and chromosomal mapping of the human Nkx6.1 gene (NKX6A), a new pancreatic islet homeobox gene. Genomics 1997;40:367-70.
116. Oster A, Jensen J, Edlund H, Larsson LI. Homeobox gene product Nkx 6.1 immunoreactivity in nuclei of endocrine cells of rat and mouse stomach. J Histochem Cytochem 1998;46:717-21.
117. Nishi M, Sanke T, Seino S, et al. Human islet amyloid polypeptide gene: complete nucleotide sequence, chromosomal localization, and evolutionary history. Mol Endocrinol 1989;3:1775-81.
118. Roberts AN, Leighton B, Todd JA, et al. Molecular and functional characterization of amylin, a peptide associated with type 2 diabetes mellitus. Proc Natl Acad Sci USA 1989;86:9662-6.

119. Cooper GJ, Day AJ, Willis AC, Roberts AN, Reid KB, Leighton B. Amylin and the amylin gene: structure, function and relationship to islet amyloid and to diabetes mellitus. Biochim Biophys Acta 1989;1014:247-58.
120. Westermark P, Wernstedt C, O'Brien TD, Hayden DW, Johnson KH. Islet amyloid in type 2 human diabetes mellitus and adult diabetic cats contains a novel putative polypeptide hormone. Am J Pathol 1987;127:414-7.
121. Cooper GJ, Willis AC, Clark A, Turner RC, Sim RB, Reid KB. Purification and characterization of a peptide from amyloid-rich pancreases of type 2 diabetic patients. Proc Natl Acad Sci USA 1987;84:8628-32.
122. Serup P, Jensen J, Andersen FG, et al. Induction of insulin and islet amyloid polypeptide production in pancreatic islet glucagonoma cells by insulin promoter factor 1. Proc Natl Acad Sci USA 1996;93:9015-20.
123. Sussel L, Kalamaras J, Hartigan-O'Connor DJ et al. Mice lacking the homeodomain transcription factor Nkx2.2 have diabetes due to arrested differentiation of pancreatic beta cells. Development 1998;125:2213-21.
124. Pang K, Mukonoweshuro C, Wong GG. Beta cells arise from glucose transporter type 2 (Glut2)-expressing epithelial cells of the developing rat pancreas. Proc Natl Acad Sci USA 1994;91:9559-63.
125. Ahlgren U, Jonsson J, Edlund H. The morphogenesis of the pancreatic mesenchyme is uncoupled from that of the pancreatic epithelium in IPF1/PDX1-deficient mice. Development 1996;122:1409-16.
126. Tao T, Wasson J, Bernal-Mizrachi E, et al. Isolation and characterization of the human PAX4 gene. Diabetes 1998;47:1650-3.
127. Inoue H, Nomiyama J, Nakai K, Matsutani A, Tanizawa Y, Oka Y. Isolation of full-length cDNA of mouse PAX4 gene and identification of its human homologue. Biochem Biophys Res Commun 1998;243:628-33.
128. Matsushita T, Yamaoka T, Otsuka S, Moritani M, Matsumoto T, Itakura M. Molecular cloning of mouse paired-box-containing gene (Pax)-4 from an islet beta cell line and deduced sequence of human Pax-4. Biochem Biophys Res Commun 1998;242:176-80.
129. Komuro I, Schalling M, Jahn L, et al. Gtx: a novel murine homeobox-containing gene, expressed specifically in glial cells of the brain and germ cells of testis, has a transcriptional repressor activity in vitro for a serum-inducible promoter. Embo J 1993;12:1387-401.
130. Plaza S, Dozier C, Saule S. Quail Pax-6 (Pax-QNR) encodes a transcription factor able to bind and trans-activate its own promoter. Cell Growth Differ 1993;4:1041-50.
131. Plaza S, Dozier C, Turque N, Saule S. Quail Pax-6 (Pax-QNR) mRNAs are expressed from two promoters used differentially during retina development and neuronal differentiation. Mol Cell Biol 1995;15:3344-53.
132. Dozier C, Carriere C, Grevin D, et al. Structure and DNA-binding properties of Pax-QNR, a paired box- and homeobox-containing gene. Cell Growth Differ 1993;4:281-9.
133. Zhang Y, Emmons SW. Specification of sense-organ identity by a Caenorhabditis elegans Pax-6 homologue. Nature 1995;377:55-9.
134. Lu Q, Knoepfler PS, Scheele J, Wright DD, Kamps MP. Both Pbx1 and E2A-Pbx1 bind the DNA motif ATCAATCAA cooperatively with the products of multiple murine Hox genes, some of which are themselves oncogenes. Mol Cell Biol 1995;15:3786-95.
135. Cordier-Bussat M, Morel C, Philippe J. Homologous DNA sequences and cellular factors are implicated in the control of glucagon and insulin gene expression. Mol Cell Biol 1995;15:3904-16.
136. Philippe J, Drucker DJ, Knepel W, Jepeal L, Misulovin Z, Habener JF. Alpha-cell-specific expression of the glucagon gene is conferred to the glucagon promoter element by the interactions of DNA-binding proteins. Mol Cell Biol 1988;8:4877-88.
137. Philippe J, Morel C, Cordier-Bussat M. Islet-specific proteins interact with the insulin-response element of the glucagon gene. J Biol Chem 1995;270:3039-45.
138. Philippe J. Insulin regulation of the glucagon gene is mediated by an insulin- responsive DNA element. Proc Natl Acad Sci U S A 1991;88:7224-7.
139. Laser B, Meda P, Constant I, Philippe J. The caudal-related homeodomain protein Cdx-2/3 regulates glucagon gene expression in islet cells. J Biol Chem 1996;271:28984-94.
140. Morel C, Cordier-Bussat M, Philippe J. The upstream promoter element of the glucagon gene, G1, confers pancreatic alpha cell-specific expression. J Biol Chem 1995;270:3046-55.
141. Philippe J, Morel C, Cordier-Bussat M. Islet-specific proteins interact with the insulin-response element of the glucagon gene. J Biol Chem 1995;270:3039-45.
142. Ritz-Laser B, Estreicher A, Klages N, Saule S, Philippe J. Pax-6 and Cdx-2/3 interact to activate glucagon gene expression on the G1 control element. J Biol Chem 1999;274:4124-32.
143. Ritz-Laser B, Estreicher A, Klages N, Saule S, Philippe J. Pax-6 and Cdx-2/3 interact to activate glucagon gene expression on the G1 control element. J Biol Chem 1999;274:4124-32.
144. Knepel W, Vallejo M, Chafitz JA, Habener JF. The pancreatic islet-specific glucagon G3 transcription factors recognize control elements in the rat somatostatin and insulin-I genes. Mol Endocrinol 1991;5:1457-66.

145. Weintraub H, Tapscott SJ, Davis RL et al. Activation of muscle-specific genes in pigment, nerve, fat, liver, and fibroblast cell lines by forced expression of MyoD. Proc Natl Acad Sci USA 1989;86:5434-8.
146. Quiring R, Walldorf U, Kloter U, Gehring WJ. Homology of the eyeless gene of Drosophila to the Small eye gene in mice and Aniridia in humans [see comments]. Science 1994;265:785-9.
147. Halder G, Callaerts P, Gehring WJ. Induction of ectopic eyes by targeted expression of the eyeless gene in Drosophila [see comments]. Science 1995;267:1788-92.
148. Gehring WJ. The master control gene for morphogenesis and evolution of the eye. Genes Cells 1996;1:11-5.
149. Sander M, Neubuser A, Kalamaras J, Ee HC, Martin GR, German MS. Genetic analysis reveals that PAX6 is required for normal transcription of pancreatic hormone genes and islet development. Genes Dev 1997;11:1662-73.
150. Teitelman G. On the origin of pancreatic endocrine cells, proliferation and neoplastic transformation. Tumour Biol 1993;14:167-73.
151. Guz Y, Montminy MR, Stein R et al. Expression of murine STF-1, a putative insulin gene transcription factor, in beta cells of pancreas, duodenal epithelium and pancreatic exocrine and endocrine progenitors during ontogeny. Development 1995;121:11-8.
152. St-Onge L, Sosa-Pineda B, Chowdhury K, Mansouri A, Gruss P. Pax6 is required for differentiation of glucagon-producing alpha-cells in mouse pancreas. Nature 1997;387:406-9.
153. Dahl E, Koseki H, Balling R. Pax genes and organogenesis. Bioessays 1997;19:755-65.
154. Wakatsuki Y, Neurath MF, Max EE, Strober W. The β cell-specific transcription factor BSAP regulates B cell proliferation. J Exp Med 1994;179:1099-108.
155. Duprez D, Fournier-Thibault C, Le Douarin N. Sonic Hedgehog induces proliferation of committed skeletal muscle cells in the chick limb. Development 1998;125:495-505.
156. Koroma BM, Yang JM, Sundin OH. The Pax-6 homeobox gene is expressed throughout the corneal and conjunctival epithelia. Invest Ophthalmol Vis Sci 1997;38:108-20.
157. Goulding MD, Lumsden A, Gruss P. Signals from the notochord and floor plate regulate the region-specific expression of two Pax genes in the developing spinal cord. Development 1993; 117:1001-16.
158. Warren N, Price DJ. Roles of Pax-6 in murine diencephalic development. Development 1997;124:1573-82.
159. St-Onge L, Sosa-Pineda B, Chowdhury K, Mansouri A, Gruss P. Pax6 is required for differentiation of glucagon-producing alpha-cells in mouse pancreas. Nature 1997;387:406-9.
160. Cirulli V, Hayek A. Developmental roles of cell adhesion molecules: implications for pancreatic islet morphogenesis. In: Sarvetnick N, ed. Pancreatic Growth and Regeneration. Basel: Karger Landes Systems, 1997;154-169.
161. Chalepakis G, Wijnholds J, Giese P, Schachner M, Gruss P. Characterization of Pax-6 and Hoxa-1 binding to the promoter region of the neural cell adhesion molecule L1. DNA Cell Biol 1994;13:891-900.

15

THE ROLE OF THE HEPATOCYTE NUCLEAR FACTOR NETWORK IN GLUCOSE HOMEOSTASIS

Markus Stoffel, M.D., Ph.D.
The Rockefeller University, New York, NY 10021 USA

ROLE OF THE HEPATOCYTE NUCLEAR FACTOR NETWORK IN GLUCOSE HOMEOSTASIS

The Hepatocyte Nuclear Factors

Hepatocyte nuclear factors are a diverse class of transcription factors that were originally identified through their interaction with essential sequences for tissue-specific transcription of liver specific genes. These factors contain DNA-binding domains that have been conserved throughout evolution. Based on the structure of their functional domains, liver-enrichedtranscriptionfactors have been classified into six families. These include HNF-1 [HNF-1α and HNF-1β (vHNF-1)]genes, members of the homeodomain-containing transcription factors; CCAAT/enhancer binding proteins (C/EBPs) that are basic leucine-zipper transcription factors; the winged helix proteins HNF-3 [HNF-3α, HNF-3β and HNF-3γ], members of the HNF-3/forkhead(bZip) transcription factor family; the zinc finger orphan receptor HNF-4 family [HNF-4α and HNF-4β]; D-binding protein [DBP], a member of the proline acid-rich (PAR) subfamily of bZip transcription factors; and HNF-6, which contains two different DNA binding domains, a cut domain and a novel type of homeodomain.

Many studies using biochemical and genetic approaches have demonstrated an important role of HNFs in development, differentiation and metabolism. This chapter will summarize the structure and function of HNF1, 3, 4, and 6 and will discuss their involvement in pancreatic β-cell and liver function and their role in glucose homeostasis and type 2 diabetes (Table 1).

HNF-1

Hepatocyte nuclear factors 1 proteins were first purified from hepatocyte nuclear extracts (1,2). The HNF-1 alpha and -1 beta (HNF-1_ and HNF-1_ (vHNF-1)) proteins are encoded by distinct genes that are localized on human chromosomes 12 and 17, respectively (3). They belong to the large superfamily of homeodomain-containing transcription factors. HNF-1 proteins have a modular structure that is composed of several domains with distinct functions. The DNA-binding activity is localized in the aminoterminal half of the protein and the transcriptional activation domain is localized in the carboxyterminal half. DNA-binding depends on three distinct regions of the proteins, the dimerization domain, the B-domain and the homeo-related domain (4,5). These three domains correspond to the most conserved residues between HNF-1α and HNF-1β. The HNF-1 proteins bind to DNA as homo- and heterodimers (4,6). The DNA consensus is 15 nucleotides long and contains a palindromic structure, which reflects the binding of HNF-1 to DNA as a dimer. The two inverted repeats are often asymmetric (A/GTTAAT), with one half more conserved than the other, and they are separated by one nucleotide. HNF-1 dimers are stabilized by the pterin-4a-carbinolamine dehydratase (PCD), a bifunctional protein also known as DCoH (dimerization co-factor of hepatocyte nuclear factor 1). PCD/DCoH modulates the DNA binding specificity of HNF1, thus acting on its transcriptional activity. In addition, it participates in the recycling of tetra-hydrobiopterin (BH(4)), an essential cofactor of several metabolic reactions (7,8).

Gene Name	Transcription Factor Superfamily	Mutant Mice Phenotype	Molecular Defects	Human Disease
HNF-1α	Homeodomain	Diabetes Fanconi-like Syndrome Laron-type Dwarfism	Glut2, L-PK, HNF-4α, pdx-1, cdx,-2, beta-2, Ins, IGF-2, PAH, others	MODY 3
HNF-1β	Homeodomain	Embryonic lethal (e7.5) Visceral endoderm defect	As above others	MODY 5
HNF-3α	HNF3/forkhead	Persistent hypoglycaemia Pancreatic α- and β-cell defect	Glucagon others	Unknown
HNF-3β	HNF3/forkhead	Embryonic lethal (e7.5) Visceral endoderm defect	HNF-4α, HNF-1α, Pdx-1, serum proteins , apolipoproteins, FABPs, aldoB, L-Pk, others	Unknown
HNF-3δ	HNF3/forkhead	Normal	PEPCK	Unknown
HNF-4α	Steroid Hormone Superfamily (orphan)	Embyonic lethal (e8.5) Visceral endoderm defect	HNF-1α, Pdx-1 Apoplipoproteins, serum proteins, transport proteins AldoB, L-Pk, others	MODY 1
HNF-4γ	Steroid Hormone	Unknown	As above?, others	Unknown
HNF-6	Homeodomain Cut domain	Unknown	HNF-3β, PFK-2 Others	Unknown

Table 1. *HNF transcription factors known to date, their roles in islet-cell and hepatic gene expression and their roles in human disease.*

The HNF-1 genes have an overlapping tissue distribution but the HNF-1α/HNF-1β ratio differs from one organ to another and during different stages of development. HNF-1 proteins are expressed at high levels in liver, intestine kidney and the endocrine pancreas. The expression levels of HNF-1 proteins vary strongly among these organs. HNF-1α protein is predominantly expressed in differentiated hepatocytes, whereas HNF-1β is the major HNF-1 protein in kidney cells. The relative abundance of the proteins within cells determines what protein dimers are present on HNF-1 target sites in promoter elements. In hepatocytes and renal cells, mainly HNF-1α and HNF-1β homodimers exist, respectively. Heterodimers are most frequently found in gut enterocytes.

A role for HNF-1α in controlling development and metabolism in the kidney, liver, and pancreatic islets was suggested by the analysis of mutant mice that lack HNF1α. Two different approaches have been used to inactivate HNF-1α in mice: when HNF-1α was inactivated by a targeted disruption by insertion of a neomycin resistance gene and homologous recombination in ES cells, homozygous HNF-1α deficient animals failed to thrive and usually died before four weeks of age. The mice also exhibited hepatic dysfunction, marked phenylketonuria due to the lack of the enzyme phenylalanine hydroxylase, hyperglycaemia, and a Fanconi-like syndrome including glucosuria (9).

Mutant animals that were generated through the use of Cre-*loxP*-mediated deletion of the first exon and the selectable marker, pgk-neo, developed diabetes two weeks after birth, with no obvious mortality and only minimal renal dysfunction during the first six months of postnatal development. The differences between the mouse models may be explained by strain differences or adverse effects of the selection marker pgk-neo on neighbouring genes surrounding the HNF-1a gene locus. However, mutant mice have in common a marked downregulation of insulin growth factor 2 (IGF2) and phenylalanine hydroxylase (PAH), contributing to a Laron-type dwarfism and elevated serum phenylalanine levels, respectively, in HNF-1α null mice.

Inactivation of the HNF-1β gene in mice results in embryonic lethality by day 7.5 of development. HNF1β-/- embryos display a disorganized visceral endoderm and a significantly reduced size. Studies of ES cell differentiation and aggregation with tetraploid morulae established that HNF1β expression is essential for visceral endoderm differentiation, both *in vitro* and *in vivo* (10, 11).

HNF-3

The hepatocyte nuclear factor 3 (HNF-3)/forkhead (fkh) family of transcription factors in mammals include three distinct genes, designated as HNF-3α, HNF-3β, and HNF-3γ. They all have in common a highly conserved 100 amino acid winged-helix motif that is responsible for monomeric recognition of specific DNA target sites (13). The structure of the highly conserved DNA binding domain of the HNF-3 proteins is similar to that of the linker histones H1 and H5 (13). However, in contrast to linker histones that compact DNA in chromatin and repress gene expression, HNF-3 proteins have been shown to decompact DNA from the nucleosome and are associated with transcriptionally active chromatin (14,15).

HNF-3 proteins were first identified as a binding activity to an enhancer region of the transthyretin (TTR) gene in nuclear liver extracts (16). The HNF-3 genes have overlapping patterns of tissue expression, including gut, central nervous system, neuroendocrine cells, and lung (17-19). During development, HNF-3α and HNF-3β are sequentially expressed in the definite endoderm, notochord, and floorplate of the neural (20,21). Mice with a targeted disruption of the HNF-3α gene develop a complex catabolic phenotype that is characterized by persistent hypoglycaemia, hypotriglyceridaemia, wasting, and neonatal mortality between days 2 and 14 (22,23). Hypoglycaemia in HNF-3α null mice leads to physiological counter-regulatory responses in glucocorticoid and growth hormone production and inhibition of insulin secretion but fails to stimulate glucagon secretion. Glucagon-producing pancreatic α-cells develop normally in HNF-3α mutant mice but proglucagon mRNA levels in pancreatic islets are reduced 50% (22,23). Mice homologous for a null mutation in HNF-3β develop an embryonic lethal phenotype, lack a notochord and exhibit defects in foregut and neural tube development (20,21). HNF-3γ-deficient embryos develop normally with no impairment of glucose homeostasis but exhibit decreased expression levels of the rate-limiting enzyme of gluconeogenesis, phosphoenolpyruvate carboxykinase (PEPCK) (24). Furthermore, biochemical and gene expression studies have shown that HNF-3β is an important regulator of the MODY genes HNF-1α, HNF-4α and IPF-1/PDX-1 (25-27). These studies suggest that normal expression of functional HNF-3 proteins is essential for normal pancreatic α- and β-cell function. However, no sequence variation in the human HNF-3 genes have yet been associated with impaired glucose tolerance or diabetes (28).

HNF-4

Hepatocyte nuclear factor-4α was originally identified as an activity in rat nuclear extracts that bound to a DNA element that is required for transcription of the transthyretin (TTR) as well as to a similar element of the apolipoprotein promoter (apoIII) gene (29). HNF-4α belongs to the steroid hormone receptor superfamily that consists of an increasing number of functionally and structurally related transcription factors (30). HNF-4α binds to the consensus sequence GGGTCAAAGGTCA that consists of two hexamer repeats (underlined). It contains a zinc finger DNA binding domain and binds DNA as a homodimer. Like other steroid hormone receptors, HNF4α contains two transactivation domains: AF1, an N-terminal (acidic) amphipathic α-helical domain spanning the first 24 amino acids and AF2, a complex transactivator domain spanning amino acids 128-366 which also includes the dimerization interface and the ligand binding domains (31). HNF-4α undergoes posttranslational phosphorylation on several consensus sites, however, the functional role of phosphorylation is unknown (32). HNF-4 is highly conserved throughout evolution. The Drosophila homologue (dHNF4) has a 91% identity amino acid sequence in the DNA binding domain compared to the rat HNF-4 (rHNF-4α). Moreover, dHNF-4 and rHNF-4 can heterodimerize, bind to the same sequences and activate gene expression (33). Recently, C14:0 and C16:0 fatty acyl-CoA thioesters have been proposed to act as ligands for the HNF-4 protein (34). We have not been able to reproduce the published data and were unable to show significant activation or inhibition of HNF-4 transcriptional activity by fatty acyl-CoA thioesters (A. Navas and M. Stoffel, unpublished).

In the adult, HNF-4α expression is restricted to liver, kidney, intestine, pancreatic islets (29,37), and the brainstem (M. Stoffel, unpublished). During mouse development, HNF4α is expressed in the primary endoderm at 4.5 days of gestation and is restricted to the visceral endoderm (the progenitor of the yolk sac) from 5.5 to 8.5 days (39). From this stage, HNF4α transcripts are found in the liver diverticulum and hindgut, and at later stages in the mesonephric tubules, stomach, intestine, and pancreas. Disruption of the HNF4α gene in the mouse leads to embryonic death due to a failure of normal gastrulation (39). Mice lacking HNF4α die very early on in embryogenesis: at 7.5 days post coitus the embryos are clearly abnormal and generally by 9.5 days they are reabsorbed (39). The exact cause of death is not known but one explanation might be that HNF4 -/- mice lack the appropriate signals from the visceral endoderm for mesoderm development (40).

Two genes homologous to HNF-4α have recently been identified in Xenopus and human (HNF-4β and HNF-4γ, respectively) (35,36). HNF-4α and HNF-4γ are located on human chromosomes 20 and 8, respectively (37,38). The functional role of HNF-4γ is currently unknown. HNF-4γ is has an overall overlapping expression pattern with HNF-4α, however, mRNAs cannot be detected in the liver (41). Like HNF-4α, HNF-4γ is also expressed in the visceral endoderm. However, although it binds to the same consensus sequences than HNF-4α *in vitro*, it is unable to compensate for the defect in HNF-4α-dependent gene regulation in HNF-4α knockout mice (M. Stoffel, unpublished). In contrast to HNF-4α, no sequence variants have been described in the HNF-4γ gene that are associated with type 2 diabetes (41).

HNF-6

Hepatocyte nuclear factor 6 is a liver-enriched transcription factor that was originally characterized as a transcriptional activator of the liver promoter of the 6-phosphofructo-2-kinase (pfk-2) gene and the HNF-3β gene (42,43). It is expressed in liver, brain, spleen, pancreas, and testis. HNF-6 contains a bipartite DNA-binding domain consisting of a single cut domain and a novel type of homeodomain. Cut homeodomain proteins were originally described as the products of the Drosophila cut gene and of its mammalian homologues, the mclox genes. These proteins contain three cut domains upstream of a homeodomain. Such cut repeats, which are well conserved sequences of 66-88 amino acids, function as DNA-binding domains, alone or in combination with the homeodomain (44). HNF-6 binds to DNA binding sites DHWATTGAYTWWD(where W = A or T, Y = T or C, H is not G, and D is not C) that are found in regulatory sequences of gut epithelium and liver-enriched genes (44). HNF-6 has a similar spatial expression pattern during development than HNF-3β and HNF-4α and it can activate transcription of these genes *in vitro* (45,46). This suggests a role of HNF-6 in several developmental and metabolic pathways. The human HNF-6 gene has been mapped to chromosome band 8 (37). Mutation screening in the coding region of the HNF-6 gene were not associated with type 2 diabetes or with changes in insulin responses to glucose among the Caucasians (47).

THE TRANSCRIPTIONAL NETWORK OF HEPATOCYTE NUCLEAR FACTORS

Several lines of evidence suggest that a transcriptional hierarchy in which HNF4α regulates the expression of HNF-1α is responsible in both the determination and maintenance of the hepatic phenotype. The HNF-1α promoter contains evolutionarily conserved binding sites for transcription factors HNF-4α, AP1 and HNF-3. The presence of the HNF-4 binding site is crucial for HNF-1α activity both *in vivo* and *in vitro* (48-50). Furthermore, stable expression of HNF-4α in a dedifferentiated rat hepatoma cell line has been shown to induce the re-expression of the endogenous HNF-1α gene (51). Analysis of hepatocyte differentiation, using dedifferentiated hepatoma variants and intertypic cell hybrids which show extinction of all or most of the hepatic functions, has revealed that the abolition and re-expression of the hepatic phenotype correlates, respectively, with the disappearance of expression of HNF-4α and HNF-1α and with the re-expression of these two factors (52,53). Evidence that the functional hierarchy may also be important in pancreatic β-cell function comes from human and mouse genetic studies: mutations in the genes encoding the HNF4α and HNF-1α proteins are responsible for two clinically indistinguishable forms of early-onset type 2 diabetes, MODY1 and MODY3 (54,55). Furthermore, a point mutation in the HNF-4 binding site in the HNF-1α promoter leading to loss of HNF-4 binding can also result in the MODY3 phenotype (50). Gene expression studies in islets derived from HNF-1α mutant mice also have reduced steady-state mRNA levels of HNF-4α, cdx-2, pdx-1 and neuroD1/beta2 compared to wildtype littermates, indicating that the expression of these transcription factors is regulated by HNF-4α/HNF-1α. The changes were not only present in adult animals but could be detected shortly after birth, indicating that dysregulation of these genes is caused by HNF-1α insufficiency rather than secondary effect due to impaired glucose tolerance (M. Stoffel, unpublished).

Since HNF-4α and HNF-1α regulate expression of each other and are key regulators of pancreatic islet function, this implies that upstream regulators of HNF-4α/HNF-1α expression may also be critical for controlling similar pathways. The HNF-3 gene family was a good candidate as upstream regulators of HNF-4α/HNF-1α because they both contain evolutionarily conserved HNF-3 binding sites (56). Furthermore, all HNF3 members are expressed in pancreatic islets and the β-cell line MIN6 (37). HNF3-dependent gene expression has been studied *in vivo* and *in vitro*. The expression of HNF-4α and HNF-1α is markedly reduced in the visceral endoderm of HNF-3β-/- embryoid bodies, as are several genes known to be *in vivo* targets of HNF-4α/HNF-1α, including apolipoproteins AI, AII, AIV, B, CII and CIII, transthyretin, aldolase B, and L-pyruvate kinase (25, 57). These results demonstrate that HNF-3β is a major regulator of HNF-4α/HNF-1α gene expression and the master regulator of the hepatocyte nuclear factor transcriptional network (25)(Figure 1).

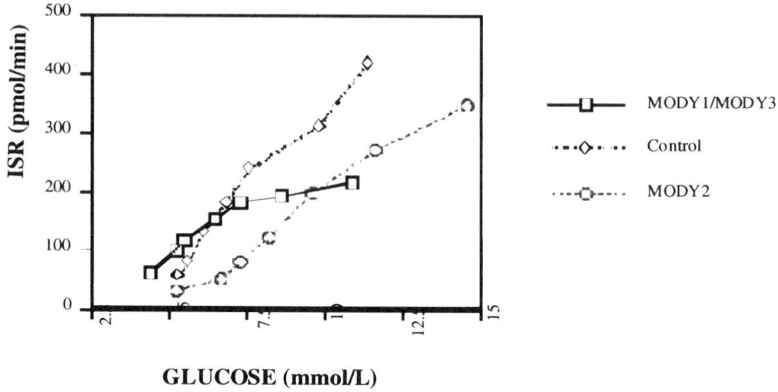

Figure 1. *Insulin secretion rates during a graded intravenous glucose infusion. ISR: Insulin secretion rate, (adapted from ref. 74-76).*

HNF-3β has also been shown to regulate the expression of pdx-1 in pancreatic islet cells (26,27). Furthermore, pdx-1 expression is reduced in embryoid bodies which derived from ES cell in which the HNF-3β gene was inactivated, indicating that HNF-3β is an activator of pdx-1 gene expression (35,36,58). The transcriptional activating properties of HNF-3β on pdx-1 expression are mediated by HNF-3 binding sites in the mouse and human pdx-1 promoters. These sites are evolutionarily conserved and were mapped between -2713 and -1922 bp of the promoter (58). The homeodomain pdx-1 transcription factor plays an essential regulatory role during both early pancreas development and in normal islet β-cell function. Gene disruption studies in which the pdx-1 gene was targeted and inactivated have revealed that this factor serves as an important control switch for expression of both exocrine and endocrine pancreatic programs (59). In early pancreas development, pdx-1 is expressed in both exocrine and endocrine cell types. However, as pancreatic morphogenesis proceeds, pdx-1 expression is eventually restricted to β- and δ-cells of the islets, where it appears to regulate the expression of the insulin, amyloid peptide, and somatostatin genes, respectively (60,61). The pdx-1 gene has also been shown to be essential for pancreatic development and normal pancreatic β-cell function in humans. A subject with complete loss of pdx-1 function due to a homozygous mutation suffers from pancreatic agenesis and individuals with the same heterozygous mutation (P63fsdelC) develop early-onset type 2 diabetes (MODY4)(62,63).

The transcription factor GATA6 has recently been shown to regulate HNF-4α gene expression during embryonic development and to transactivate the HNF-4α promoter *in vitro* (64)(Figure 2). GATA6 belongs to a family of zinc finger transcription factors and is expressed in the extra-embryonic and embryonic endoderm during early development. Later, GATA6, together with GATA4 and GATA5, is expressed in the embryonic heart and gut epithelium. The expression levels of GATA6 in pancreatic islets of adult mice are very low and it is unclear if GATA6 is an important regulator of HNF-4α gene expression in differentiated pancreatic β-cells (M. Stoffel, unpublished) (Figure 2).

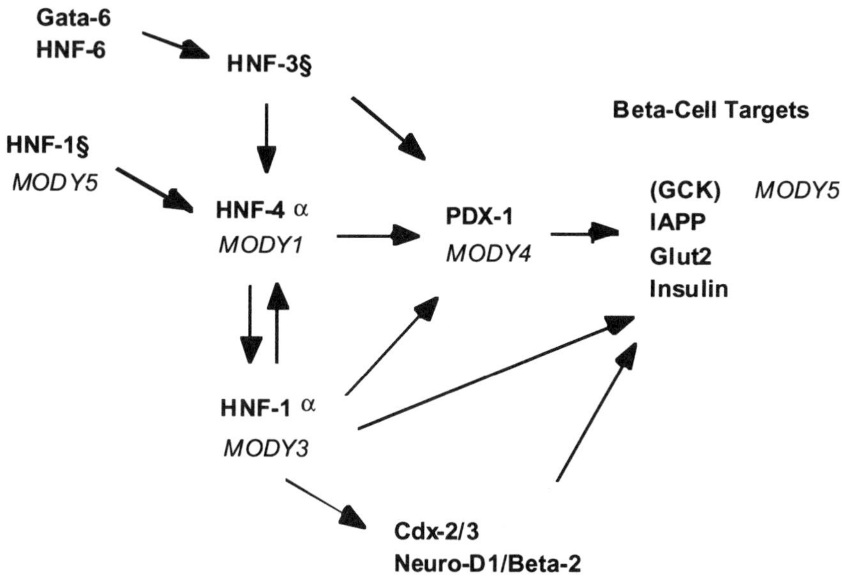

Figure 2. *The Transcriptional HNF-Network and its Regulation of Pancreatic β-Cell Target Genes. Arrows indicate positive transcriptional regulation.*

EARLY-ONSET TYPE 2 DIABETES SUBTYPES ARE CAUSED BY MUTATIONS IN HEPATOCYTE NUCLEAR FACTORS AND DOWNSTREAM TARGET GENES

Maturity-onset diabetes of the young (MODY) is a clinically and genetically heterogenous disease with an autosomal-dominant inheritance and an age of onset of 25 years or younger (65). Using genetic linkage and candidate gene approaches, MODY genes were localized to chromosomes 7, 12, 13, 19 and 20 (66-68) and are believed to be responsible for 1-3% of type 2 diabetes. The gene on chromosome 7 (MODY2) encodes the glycolytic enzyme glucokinase which plays a key role in generating the metabolic signal for insulin secretion and in integrating hepatic glucose uptake (69-71). The genes on chromosomes 20 (MODY1), 12 (MODY3), 19 (MODY5) and 13 (MODY4) are encoded by transcription factors hepatocyte nuclear factor-4α (HNF-4α), -1 alpha (HNF1α), -1β (HNF-1β, vHNF-1)) and homeobox transcription factor-1 (PDX-1, STF-1), respectively (72). Mutations in neuroD1/beta-2 are responsible for an autosomal-dominant form of diabetes with a variable age of onset (17-60 years of age) (73). A significant portion (.20%) of MODY pedigrees do not show linkage to any of the known MODY loci indicating that there is an unknown number of MODY genes that have yet to be identified (Table 2).

Gene mutated	HNF-4α MODY-1	GCK MODY-2	HNF-1α MODY 3	PDX-1 MODY 4	HNF-1β MODY 5	Neuro-D1/ Beta 2
Chromosomal Localization	20	7	12	13	17	2
Frequency	3 –7%	30%	40%	1 –4%	1 –5%	1%
Penetrance	<100%	100%	<100%	<100%	<100%	<100%
Age at diagnosis	Puberty	Childhood	Puberty	(Post)puberty	Puberty	Adulthood
Severity of diabetes	Severe	Mild	Severe	Heterogenous	Severe	Heterogenous
Complications	Frequent	Rare	Frequent	Frequent	Frequent (Kidney)	Heterogenous
Genes abnormally expressed	Glut2, L-Pk, Aldo-B, HNF-1α, PDX-1, CDX-2, Others	GCK	HNF-4α, PDX-1, Glut2, L-Pk, Insulin, Others	Glut-2, GCK Insulin Others	HNF-4α, PDX-1, Glut2, L-Pk, Insulin Others	Insulin Others

Table 2. *MODY genes known to date and characteristics of their phenotypic expression.*

Clinical studies indicate that MODY is associated with reduced and abnormal patterns of glucose-stimulated insulin secretion (74-76). Subjects with glucokinase mutations usually have mild hyperglycaemia that begins in early childhood and, in the absence of other risk factors such as obesity, has little tendency to progress. In contrast, patients with mutations in HNF-1α, HNF-1β and HNF-4α often develop diabetes after puberty. PDX-1 dependent diabetes (MODY4) has a relatively late disease onset (35 years) but pedigrees show autosomal dominant inheritance (63,77,78). MODYs due to defects in the above transcription factors have more severe forms of hyperglycaemia than glucokinase deficient patients and frequently develop complications.

Patients with MODY1 and MODY3 have a clinically indistinguishable form of diabetes. Patients with HNF-1α or HNF-4α mutations have normal insulin sensitivity and normal first phase insulin responses to intravenous glucose. However, they exhibit defects in insulin secretory responses to prolonged glucose infusions, including reduced mean plasma C-peptide levels, decreased insulin secretion rates at blood glucose levels above 7 mmol/l, and a reduced absolute amplitude of ultradian insulin secretory oscillations (75,76). MODY1 patients have also been shown to have decreased ISR to arginine and a decreased suppression of glucagon during a hyperglycaemic clamp, suggesting that mutations in HNF-4α can lead to α-cell as well as β-cell secretory defects (76). In contrast to MODY1/MODY3 patients, subjects with mutations in the glucokinase gene (MODY2) have an earlier time of disease-onset and generally have a milder form of diabetes (70). The fasting and postprandial glucose levels are only moderately elevated in MODY2 patients. First phase insulin secretory responses to intravenous glucose and insulin secretion rates over a 24-hour period on a weight maintenance diet have been found to be similar in subjects with glucokinase mutations and controls (74). However, the dose response curve relating glucose and insulin secretion rates (ISR) insulin secretion rates obtained during a graded intravenous glucose infusion was shifted to the right in the subjects with glucokinase mutations. Average ISRs over a glucose range between 5 and 9 mM were 61% lower than those in controls. In normal subjects, the β-cell is most sensitive to an increase in glucose at concentrations between 5.5 and 6.0 mM, whereas in the patients with glucokinase mutations the point of maximal responsiveness is increased to between 6.5 and 7.5 mM (74) (Figure 2). Patients who have glucokinase mutations that result in a severe impairment of *in vitro* glucokinase enzyme activity may have lower ISRs than subjects with mutations that result only in mild reductions in enzyme activity *in vitro* (74).

Mutations in HNF-1β, the MODY5 gene, are relatively rare and only a few mutations have been described (72,79). Mutations in the HNF-1β gene are associated with a non-insulin dependent subtype of diabetes that often develops early in life (10-25 years) and ultimately requires insulin replacement therapy to control hyperglycaemia. Subjects with HNF-1β haploinsufficiency frequently develop diabetic nephropathy or non-diabetic renal disease (72,79).

MOLECULAR CHARACTERIZATION OF THE HNF-GENE MUTATIONS

The most common forms of MODY result from mutations in the HNF-1α gene (MODY3) More than 50 different mutations have been described in the coding sequence of this gene. They include missense, nonsense, deletion, insertion and frame shift mutations (Figure 3). The molecular mechanism by which mutations in only one allele of the HNF-1α gene impair pancreatic β-cell function is unclear. HNF-1α can form homodimers or heterodimerize with the structurally related protein HNF-1β. Only HNF-1 dimers can bind to promoter elements and activate transcription. HNF-1α is composed of three functional domains: an amino-terminal dimerization domain (amino acids 1-32), a DNA-binding domain with POU-like and homeodomain-like motifs (amino acids 150-280), and a COOH-terminal transactivation domain (amino acids 281-631). Most HNF-1α mutants including defects in the HNF1α promoter or in the dimerization domain can be predicted to result in loss of function. However, mutant HNF-1α proteins with an intact dimerization surface may impair pancreatic β-cell function by forming nonproductive dimers with wild-type protein, hereby inhibiting its activity. This mechanism has been shown for frameshift mutation HNF-1α P291fsinsC, a common mutation in MODY3 patients. P291fsinsC-HNF-1α has lost its transcriptional transactivation activity in HeLa cells, which lack endogenous HNF-1α. Overexpression of HNF-1α (P291fsinsC) in MIN6 cells, a mouse β-cell line, resulted in an approximately 40% inhibition of the endogenous HNF-1α activity in a dosage-dependent manner. Furthermore, heterodimer formation between wildtype and P291fsinsC mutant proteins were observed by electrophoretic mobility shift assay. These data suggest that the HNF-1α (P291fsinsC) mutant protein may have dominant-negative activity (80).

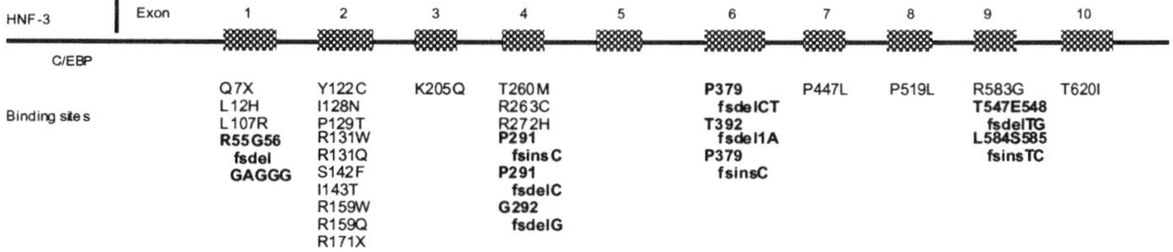

Figure 3. *Mutations in the human HNF-1α gene. Exons of the HNF-1α gene are shown as boxes.*

The first mutation associated with diabetes that was identified in the MODY1 gene HNF-4α was found to be a nonsense mutation in codon 268, Q268X (9) (Figure 4). This mutation generates a truncated protein containing an intact DNA binding domain but lacking part of the AF2 region. The HNF4(Q268X) protein has lost its transcriptional transactivation activity, fails to homo- or heterodimerize and bind to DNA, implying that the MODY1 phenotype is due to a loss of HNF-4α function (81). This also implies that a haploinsufficiency of HNF-4α can lead to the MODY1 phenotype. Additional HNF-4α variants have been associated with type 2 diabetes: K99fsdelAA, R154X , R127W, V255M, E276Q, V393I, and G115S (82-87). Deletion mutant K99fsdelAA leads to a frame shift and truncated protein. Nonsense mutation R154X produces a truncated protein containing only the DNA binding domain and the AF1 transactivation domain. These proteins can be predicted to lack transcriptional transactivation activity. The missense mutation V393I located in the AF2 domain has been shown to lead to a modest decrease in transactivation potential. Three point mutations, R127W, V255M and E276Q, which were identified in Japanese, Danish and UK families, respectively, have also been characterized. Mutation HNF4(E276Q) is a loss of function mutation due to protein instability and loss of DNA binding. Sequence variants HNF4(R127W) and HNF(V255M), located between the DNA binding and AF2 domain and within the AF2 region, respectively, are functionally normal and most likely represent rare polymorphisms. A missense mutation, G115S, located in the DNA binding domain of HNF-4α, leads to an impairment in the ability of the mutant protein to bind to HNF4 consensus binding sites, thereby reducing its transactivation activity. This effect is independent of the type of DNA binding element (DR1 or DR2), suggesting that all target genes are affected similarly. Furthermore, kinetic studies have shown that the dissociation constant (Kd) increases 5- to 6-fold in HNF(G115S), while the maximal binding (Bmax) decreases to a similar extent (88).

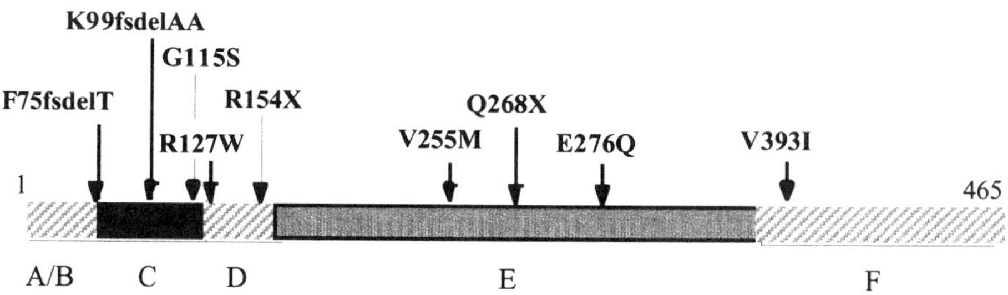

Figure 4. *Mutations in the human HNF-4α protein. A/B: Transactivation domain (ligand-independent), C: DNA binding domain, D: Hinge region, E: Ligand binding domain, Transactivation domain, F: Inhibitory transactivation domain.*

HYPOTHESIS FOR MOLECULAR PATHOMECHANISMS OF MODY-TRANSCRIPTION FACTOR DEFECTS

The finding that mutations in HNF-4α, HNF-1α and HNF-1β can cause early-onset type 2 diabetes suggests that this is a disorder of gene expression and that the HNF-regulatory network plays an important role in pancreatic islet function. Although these factors have been shown to play a significant role in the regulation of many genes expressed in the liver, less information is available on HNF-4α and HNF-1α function in pancreatic β-cells. Based on our emerging knowledge of the role of HNFs in regulating a complex transcription factor network and its downstream target genes, we have hypothesized that an impairment of its pleiotropic actions on gene expression leads to pancreatic β-cell dysfunction through the following mechanism(s):

HNF-transcription factors play a key role in the transcriptional activation of insulin.

HNF1α can bind to the FLAT-F element of the rat insulin I gene promoter and act as a weak activator of insulin transcription (89). Expression studies in pancreatic islets of HNF-1α knockout mice indicate that it may also indirectly control expression of the insulin gene by acting as a positive regulator of the pdx-1, and possibly of cdx-2 and neuroD1/beta-2 genes (M. Stoffel, unpublished). Pdx-1 and neuroD1/beta-2 are both essential transcriptional activators of the insulin gene (90-93). Thus, a decrease in the amount of HNF-4α/1α might have a critical effect on β-cell function by decreasing the expression levels of other transcriptional activators of the insulin gene (Figure 5).

HNF-1α and -4α are important regulators of gene products involved in β-cell glucose sensing and glucose metabolism.

Pancreatic islets and hepatocytes appear to share a glucose sensing mechanism thought to involve glucokinase, a distinct form of hexokinase found in the hepatocyte, pancreatic β-cells and some neuroendocrine cells in the intestinal mucosa, and GLUT2, a member of the glucose transporter family found in the β-cell, liver, kidney and intestine (94-97). The liver-specific glucokinase promoter contains a sequence homologous to the HNF-1 consensus binding site and the GLUT2 promoter appears to contain putative HNF1-binding sites (97). GLUT2 expression is decreased in the visceral endoderm of embryoid bodies of HNF-4α-/- ES-cells compared to HNF-4α+/+ ES-cells (81). Together, this provides evidence that downregulation of key components of the glucose-sensing apparatus of the β-cells may be responsible for impaired insulin secretion and decreased glucose uptake by the liver in MODY1 and/or MODY3 (81). Furthermore, HNF4α regulates three enzymes of glycolysis (L-pyruvate kinase, glyceraldehyde 3-phosphate dehydrogenase and aldolase-B) which could further impair glucose metabolism. The regulation of target gene expression is either direct (HNF-1-independent), mediated through reduced expression of HNF-1α, or more likely is the result of a combination of activating actions of HNF-1α and HNF-4α as well as other transactivating factors. Further support that HNF-1α and HNF-4α regulate glucose metabolism comes from studies in pancreatic islets of HNF-1α knockout mice that showed a lack of GLUT2 expression and reduced pyruvate kinase (liver isoform) protein and mRNA levels (M. Stoffel, unpublished) (Figure 5).

HNF-transcription factors are important regulators of genes involved in detoxification of endogenous and exogenous substances.

HNFs have been shown *in vitro* to play a role in regulating cytochrome P450 genes (cyp2A4 and cyp4A6) (98). Cytochrome P450 are phase I enzymes which are involved in lipid metabolism by oxidizing steroids, fatty acids, prostaglandins and other natural lipophilic compounds as well as drugs, carcinogens and other environmental contaminants. Downregulation of P450 genes might lead to intracellular accumulation of free fatty acids and metabolites that may lead to pancreatic β-cell damage over time. This mechanism may contribute to pancreatic β-cell failure with age. The concept of lipotoxicity has previously been proposed for obesity-associated NIDDM (99), however, this pathway has not yet been studied in pancreatic islets of HNF-dependent diabetes subtypes.

HNF-transcription factors regulate genes responsible for cell lineage proliferation and differentiation.
The strong correlation between extinction and reappearance of HNF-4/HNF-1 binding activities and dedifferentiation and redifferentiation of the hepatic phenotype of hepatoma cell lines strongly imply that HNF-4α and HNF-1α play a crucial role in maintaining hepatocyte specific differentiation (51-53). Pancreatic β-cell lines, like hepatoma cells, can lose their phenotypic characteristics such as glucose-induced insulin secretion. The HNF-transcriptional network regulates the expression of several pancreatic islet-enriched transcription, including pdx-1 and neuroD1/beta-2, that are involved in pancreas development, β-cell differentiation and maintenance or proliferation of islet cells (90,93) (Figure 6).

HNF-REGULATED GENE EXPRESSION IN PANCREATIC β-CELLS AND HEPATOCYTES

Hepatocyte nuclear factors (HNFs) are a diverse class of transcription factors which were initially identified by their binding activity to sites in the regulatory regions of genes that are expressed specifically in the liver. Liver specific transcription depends on the binding of HNFs to distinct cis-acting sequences in gene control regions. The interactions between unique combinations of liver enriched transcription factors and ubiquitous transcription factors regulate and determine maximum transcription of a given target gene. This combinatorial control is an efficient mechanism to generate both diversity and stringency of tissue specific gene expression.

The identification of target genes that are regulated by HNFs and their functional analysis are powerful approaches to study the molecular pathogenesis of MODY. Target genes for different HNFs have mainly been identified based on their ability to bind and activate the promoter of these genes in transient transfection. These target genes that can be classified into the following categories: other transcription factors (see Figure 1), proteins involved in lipid transport, serum proteins, enzymes of lipid and steroid metabolism, amino acid and glucose metabolism (100). Transient transcription assays, have the disadvantage that transcriptional activation is measured in overexpression systems that generate unphysiologically high levels of protein, promoters are not studied in native chromatin and often lack enhancer elements, and that transcriptional activation is measured in transformed cell lines that do not faithfully reflect the biological properties of primary cells. A genetic approach using either genetically manipulated embryonic stem (ES) cells or tissues form mutant mice to study the effect of loss of HNF-function on target gene expression has been shown to be powerful approach to identify HNF-target genes. HNF-1β, HNF-3β and HNF-4α null mice die during development prior to formation of the pancreas and so cannot be used to identify HNF-regulated genes in the pancreatic β-cells. However, the visceral endoderm (VE), which expresses these HNF proteins and its target genes, displays many characteristics of both the liver, gut and endocrine pancreas and has been used as a model to study HNF-regulated gene expression. This system has the advantage that it studies gene regulation of any target gene in a chromosomal context (in native chromatin) and at physiological expression levels of HNF-proteins. Furthermore, the VE is derived from euploid ES-cells which do not have the drawbacks of transformed, genetically abnormal cell lines that are frequently used in *in vitro* studies. ES cells can be grown in suspension in the absence of LIF and can be differentiated to form embryoid bodies (EBs) which contain VE. The VE expresses many genes that regulate glucose metabolism including GLUT2, aldolase B and L-type pyruvate kinase. Inactivation of the HNF- genes by targeted disruption and homologous recombination in ES cells allows to test if loss of function of HNFs leads to an impairment of gene expression of key components of the glucose-stimulated insulin secretion signalling pathway *in vitro*. Gene expression in differentiated wildtype, heterozygous and null HNF (HNF+/+, +/-, -/-) embryoid bodies can be assayed by quantitative RT-PCR. EBs produced from three HNF-4α null ES cell lines, therefore, not expressing HNF-4α mRNA, showed a marked downregulation or lack of four genes involved in glucose transport and metabolism: glucose transporter 2 (GLUT2), aldolase B (aldoB), glyceraldehyde-3-phosphate dehydrogenase (1,3 BGD) and L-pyruvate kinase (L-PK). Furthermore, steady-state mRNA of two transcription factors, HNF-1α and pdx-1, were also reduced. These results also held true *in vivo*, when E.8.5 embryos from crosses of HNF-4+/- mice were studied and VE gene expression in normal or HNF-4α mutant mice were assayed (81). Expression analyses of target genes in embryos of HNF-4α null embryos confirms the results obtained from the ES-cell lines and suggests that downregulation of these genes *in vivo* may be even more dramatic than *in vitro* (81). Similar studies using embryonic bodies that were derived from ES-cell in which HNF-1β or HNF-3β were inactivated showed that HNF-4α expression was absent or reduced, indicating that HNF-4α expression is regulated by these transcription factors. Furthermore, like in mutant HNF-4α EBs, the expression of downstream target genes including glycolytic enzymes, serum factors and apolipoproteins were absent or reduced in null HNF-3β and HNF-1β EBs (11,12,81). The impairment of glucose utilization and mitochondrial oxidation due to reduced gene expression of glucose transporter 2 and several glycolytic enzymes suggest a molecular basis for the diabetic phenotype of MODY1 patients (Figure 2).

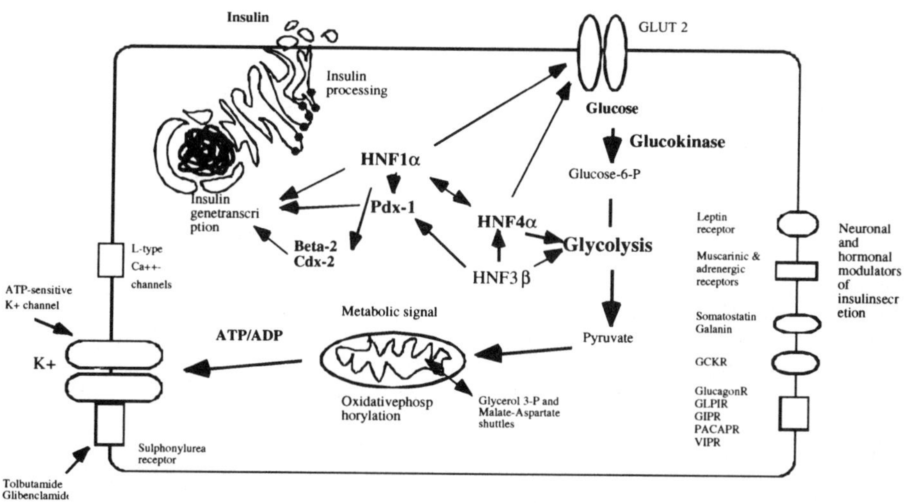

Figure 5. *Glucose stimulated insulin secretion from pancreatic β-cells. Postprandial elevation of blood glucose leads to glucose transport into β-cells via glucose transporter-2 (Glut2), breakdown through the glycolytic pathway and mitochondrial oxidative phosphorylation. As a result, the ATP/ADP ratio increases, leading to an inhibition of ATP-sensitive, transmembrane potassium channels (Kir6.2). The change in membrane potential activates volatage-gated Ca^{++} channels and results in a rise in cytosolic calcium levels that trigger fusion of pre-stored insulin vesicles with the plasma membrane and insulin release. The hepatocyte nuclear transcription factor network regulates the expression of enzymes of glycolysis, Glut-2 and the insulin gene. Abbreviations: SST-R: Somatostatin receptors, GLP1-R: Glucagon-like peptide-1 receptor, GIP-R: Gastric inhibitory protein receptor, VIP-R: Vasoactive inhibitory peptide receptor.*

The target genes of HNF-1α and HNF-4α are believed to be overlapping, since binding elements of both transcription factors are frequently found in close proximity of promoter/enhancer elements and HNF-1α and HNF-4α regulate each others expression. Expression studies in pancreatic islets of HNF-1α mice have shown similar results than in HNF-4α embryoid bodies: glucose transporter 2, L-type pyruvate kinase, pdx-1, HNF-4α and insulin expression was markedly reduced or absent. In addition, the mRNA of cdx-2 and neuroD1/beta-2, two transcriptional activators of the insulin gene, were also reduced. These findings suggested that similar pathomechanism for the development of HNF-4α and HNF-1α-dependent diabetes exist. Other evidence confirming that genes involved in glucose transport, metabolism and insulin transcription are regulated by HNF-1 came from overexpression of wildtype HNF-1α or of a dominant negative form of HNF-1α in INS-1 cells. Graded overexpression of HNF-1α led to an increase, while forced expression of a dominant negative form of this protein was able diminish the expression of the insulin gene, L-pyruvate kinase and glucose transporter 2 genes (101). Physiological evidence for a metabolic defect involving glycolytic flux comes from studies in mice lacking the HNF-1α gene. HNF-1α null mice have impaired insulin secretion and intracellular calcium ($[Ca^{2+}]_i$) responses following stimulation with nutrient secretagogues such as glucose and glyceraldehyde but display normal responses with non-nutrient stimuli such as potassium chloride. Flux of glucose through glycolysis in islets from mutant mice is reduced and results in an impairment of ATP generation in response to glucose. Patch clamp recordings on HNF-1α mutant β-cells show that ATP-sensitive K^+ currents (K_{ATP}) in β-cells are insensitive to suppression by glucose but respond normally to ATP. Furthermore, exposure of HNF-1α null islets to mitochondrial substrates (that bypass glycolysis and enter β-cells independently of Glut-2) suppressed K_{ATP}, elevated $[Ca2+]_i$, and corrected the insulin secretion defect. These results provide strong evidence that hepatocyte nuclear factor-1alpha diabetes also results at least in part from defective β-cell glycolytic signalling (102).

The role of HNF-4α in regulating hepatocyte gene expression in humans has also recently been addressed. HNF-4α target genes that are mainly expressed in the liver including α1-antitrypsin, α1-antichymotrypsin, alpha foetal protein, ceruloplasmin, insulin growth factor binding protein-1, transferrin, and apolipoproteins (apo) AI, AII, B, and CIII were measured in the serum of 24 members of the HNF-4α/MODY1 RW-pedigree (Q268X mutation) including 12 diabetic patients with HNF-4α mutations (D-HNF4+/-), 6 non-diabetic subjects with HNF-4α mutations (N-HNF4+/-), 6 normal relatives (N-HNF-4+/+) as well as 6 unrelated normal matched controls (N-HNF4+/+), and 12 matched diabetic (non-MODY1-5) patients (D-HNF4+/+). Serum levels of apo AII, apo CIII, Lp(a), and triglyceride were significantly reduced in D-HNF4+/- as compared to N-HNF4+/+. This reduction was also found when apoAII, CIII, Lp(a) and triglyceride of N- or D-HNF4+/- individuals were compared to D-HNF4+/+ diabetics, indicating that HNF-4α haploinsufficiency rather than hyperglycaemia is the primary cause of decreased serum protein and triglyceride concentrations (103).

CONCLUSION

Genetic studies in recent years have identified several HNF-proteins to play an essential role in normal pancreatic β-cell function. Haploinsufficiencies in HNF-1α, HNF-1β, and HNF-4α are responsible for early-onset forms of type 2 diabetes (MODY). MODY genes are functionally related and form part of an integral network of transcription factors that regulate gene expression of target genes including insulin, glucose transporter and metabolic enzymes. The molecular and physiological characterization of this network as well as the identification of novel target genes will provide further insights into essential pathways for normal β-cell function as well as pathophysiological mechanisms in type 2 diabetes.

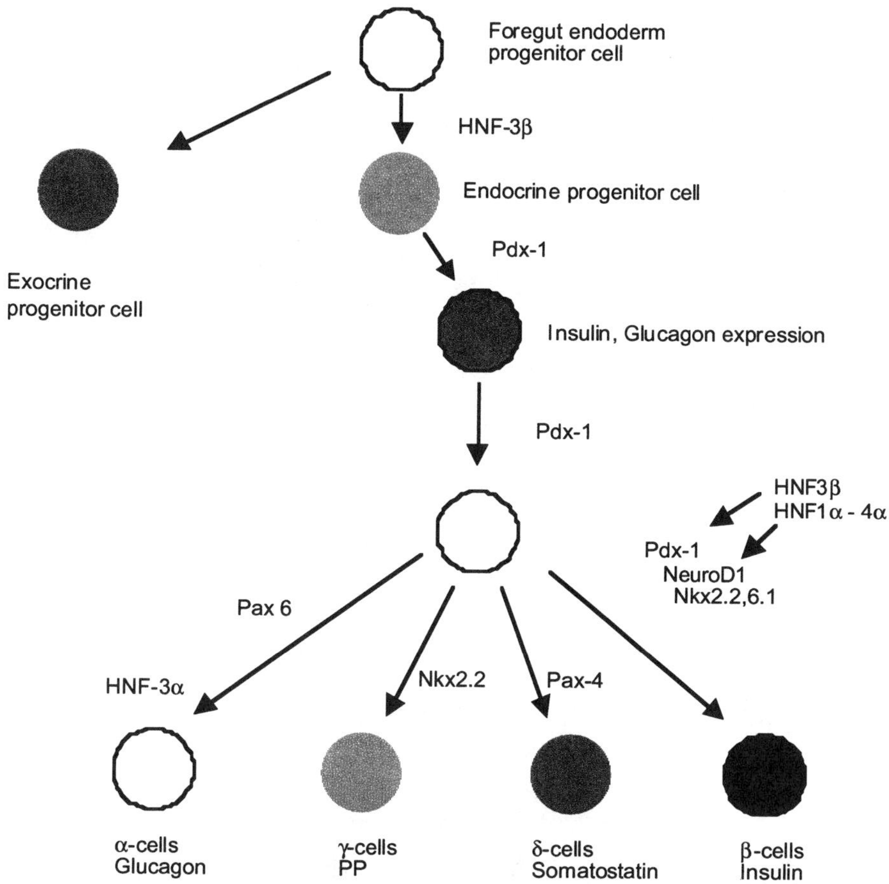

Figure 6. *Involvement of transcription factors in endocrine pancreas development and differentiation.*

REFERENCES:

1. Courtois G, Morgan JG, Campbell LA, Fourel G, Crabtree GR. Interaction of a liver-specific nuclear factor with the fibrinogen and alpha 1-antitrypsin promoters. Science 1987;238:688-92.
2. Courtois G, Baumhueter S, Crabtree GR. Purified hepatocyte nuclear factor 1 interacts with a family of hepatocyte-specificpromoters. Proc Natl Acad Sci USA 1988;85:7937-41.
3. Bach I, Galcheva-Gargova Z, Mattei MG, Simon-Chazottes D, Guenet JL, Cereghini S, Yaniv M. Cloning of human hepatic nuclear factor 1 (HNF1) and chromosomal localization of its gene in man and mouse. Genomics 1990;8:155-64.
4. Nicosia, A, Monaci P, Tomei L, De francesco R, Nuzzo M, Stunnenberg H, Cortese R. A myosin-like dimerization helix and an extra large homeodomainare essential elements of the tripartite DNA binding structure of LFB1. Cell 1990;61:1225.
5. Laughon A. DNA binding specificity of homeodomains. Biochemistry 1991;30:11537.
6. Tomei L, Cortese R, De Francesco R. A POU-A related region dictates DNA binding specificity of

LFB1/HNF1 by orienting the two XL-homeodomains in the dimer. EMBO J 1992;11:4119-29.
7. Mendel DB, Khavari PA, Conley PB, Graves MK, Hansen LP, Admon A, Crabtree GR. Characterization of a cofactor that regulates dimerization of a mammalian homeodomain protein. Science 1991;254:1762-7.
8. Citron BA, Davis MD, Milstien S, Gutierrez J, Mendel DB, Crabtree GR, Kaufman S. Identity of 4a-carbinolamine dehydratase, a component of the phenylalanine hydroxylation system, and DCoH, a transregulator of homeodomain proteins. Proc Natl Acad Sci USA 1992;15;89:11891-4.
9. Pontoglio M, Barra J, Hadchouel M, Doyen A, Kress C, Bach JP, Babinet C, Yaniv M. Hepatocyte nuclear factor 1 inactivation results in hepatic dysfunction, phenylketonuria, and renal Fanconi syndrome. Cell 1996;84:575-585.
10. Lee YH, Sauer B, Gonzalez FJ. Laron dwarfism and non-insulin-dependent diabetes mellitus in the Hnf-1alpha knockout mouse. Mol Cell Biol 1998;18:3059-68.
11. Barbacci E, Reber M, Ott M, Breillat C, Huetz F, Cereghini S. Variant hepatocyte nuclear factor 1 is required for visceral endoderm specification. Development 1999;126:4795-805.
12. Coffinier C, Thepot D, Babinet C, Yaniv M, Barra J. Essential role for the homeoprotein vHNF1/HNF1_ in visceral endoderm differentiation. Development 1999;126:4785-94.
13. Lai E, Clark KL, Burley SK, Darnell JE Jr. Hepatocyte nuclear factor 3/fork head or "winged helix" proteins: a family of transcription factors of diverse biologic function. Proc Natl Acad Sci USA. 1993;90:10421-10423.
14. McPherson CE, Shim EY, Friedman DS, Zaret KS. An active tissue-specific enhancer and bound transcription factors existing in a precisely positioned nucleosomal array. Cell 1993;75:387-398.
15. Shim EY, Woodcock C, Zaret KS. Nucleosome positioning by the winged helix transcription factor HNF3. Genes Dev 1998;12:5-10.
16. Costa RH. Hepatocyte nuclear factor 3/forkhead protein family: mammalian transcription factors that possess divergent cellular expression patterns and binding specificities. In F. Tronche and M. Yaniv (ed), Liver gene expression R.G. Landes Company, Austin, Texas 1994;183-206.
17. Costa RH, Grayson DR, Darnell JE Jr. Multiple hepatocyte-enriched nuclear factors function in the regulation of transthyretin and alpha 1-antitrypsin genes. Mol Cell Biol 1989;9:1415-1425.
18. Lai E, Prezioso VR, Smith E, Litvin O, Costa RH, Darnell JE Jr. HNF-3A, a hepatocyte-enriched transcription factor of novel structure is regulated transcriptionally. Genes Dev 1990;4:1427-1436.
19. Lai E, Prezioso VR, Tao WF, Chen WS, Darnell JE Jr. Hepatocyte nuclear factor 3 alpha belongs to a gene family in mammals that is homologous to the Drosophila homeotic gene fork head. Genes Dev 1991;5:416-427.
20. Weinstein DC, Ruiz i Altaba A, Chen WS, Hoodless P, Prezioso VR, Jessell TM, Darnell JE Jr. The winged-helix transcription factor HNF-3 beta is required for notochord development in the mouse embryo. Cell 1994;78:575-588.
21. Ang SL, Rossant J. HNF-3 beta is essential for node and notochord formation in mouse development. Cell 1994;78:561-574.
22. Kaestner KH, Katz J, Liu Y, Drucker DJ, Schutz G. Inactivation of the winged helix transcription factor HNF3alpha affects glucose homeostasis and islet glucagon gene expression in vivo. Genes Dev 1999;13:495-504.
23. Shih DQ, Navas MA, Kuwajima S, Duncan SA, Stoffel M. Impaired glucose homeostasisand neonatal mortality in hepatocyte nuclear factor 3alpha-deficient mice. Proc Natl Acad Sci USA 1999;96:10152-10157.
24. Kaestner KH, Hiemisch H, Schutz G. Targeted disruption of the gene encoding hepatocyte nuclear factor 3gamma results in reduced transcription of hepatocyte-specific genes. Mol Cell Biol 1998;18:4245-4251.
25. Duncan SA, Navas MA, Dufort D, Rossant J, Stoffel M. Regulation of a transcription factor network required for differentiation and metabolism. Science 1998;281:692-695.
26. Wu KL, Gannon M, Peshavaria M, Offield MF, Henderson E, Ray M, Marks A, Gamer LW, Wright CV, Stein R. Hepatocyte nuclear factor 3beta is involved in pancreatic beta-cell-specific transcription of the pdx-1 gene. Mol Cell Biol 1997;17:6002-6013.
27. Sharma S, Jhala US, Johnson T, Ferreri K, Leonard J, Montminy M. Hormonal regulation of an islet specific enhancer in the pancreatic homeobox gene STF-1. Mol Cell Biol 1997;17:2598-2604.
28. Navas MA, Vaisse C, Boger S, Heimesaat M, Kollee LA, Stoffel M. The Human HNF-3 Genes: Cloning, Partial Sequence and Mutation Screening in Patients with Impaired Glucose Homeostasis. Hum Heredity (in press).
29. Sladek FM, Zhong W, Lai E, Darnell JE Jr. Liver-enriched transcription factor HNF4 is a novel member of the steroid hormone receptor superfamily. Genes Dev 1990;4:2353-2365.
30. Mangelsdorf DJ, Thummel C, Beato M, Herrlich P, Schutz G, Umesono K, Blumberg B, Kastner P, Mark M, Chambon P, et al. The nuclear receptor superfamily: the second decade. Cell 1995;83:835-9.
31. Hadzopoulou-Cladaras M, Kistanova E, Evagelopoulou C, Zeng S, Cladaras C and Ladias JAA. Functional domains of nuclear receptor hepatocyte nuclear factor 4. J Biol Chem 1997;272:539-550.

32. Jiang G, Nepomuceno L, Yang Q, Sladek FM. Serine/threonine phosphorylation of orphan receptor hepatocyte nuclearfactor 4. Arch Biochem Biophys 1997;340:1-9.
33. Zhong W, Sladek FM, Darnell JE Jr. The expression pattern of a Drosophila homolog to the mouse transcription factor HNF-4 suggests a determinative role in gut formation. EMBO J 1993;12:537-44.
34. Hertz R, Magenheim J, Berman I, Bar-Tana J. Fatty acyl-CoA thioesters are ligands of hepatic nuclear factor-4alpha. Nature 1998;392:512-6.
35. Holewa B, Zapp D, Drewes T, Senkel S, Ryffel GU. HNF4beta, a new gene of the HNF4 family with distinct activation and expression profiles in oogenesis and embryogenesis of Xenopus laevis. Mol Cell Biol 1997;17:687-94.
36. Drewes T, Senkel S, Holewa B, Ryffel GU. Human hepatocyte nuclear factor 4 isoforms are encoded by distinct and differentially expressed genes. Mol Cell Biol 1996;16:925-31.
37. Vaisse C, Kim J, Espinosa R 3rd, Le Beau MM, Stoffel M. Pancreatic islet expression studies and polymorphic DNA markers in the genes encoding hepatocyte nuclear factor-3alpha, -3beta, -3gamma, -4gamma, and -6. Diabetes 1997;46:1364-7.
38. Stoffel M, Le Beau MM, Espinosa R 3rd, Bohlander SF, Le Paslier D, Cohen D, Xiang KS, Cox NJ, Fajans SS, Bell CI. A yeast artificial chromosome-based map of the region of chromosome 20 containing the diabetes-susceptibility gene, MODY1, and a myeloid leukemia related gene. Proc Natl Acad Sci USA 1996;93:3937-41.
39. Chen WS, Manova K, Weinstein DC, Duncan SA, Plump AS, Prezioso VR, Bachvarova RF, Darnell JE Jr. Disruptionof the HNF-4 gene, expressed in visceral endoderm, leads to cell death in embryonic ectoderm and impaired gastrulation of mouse embryos. Genes Dev 1994;8:2466-77.
40. Duncan SA, Manova K, Chen WS, Hoodless P, Weinstein DC, Bachvarova RF, Darnell JE Jr. Expression of transcription factor HNF-4 in the extraembryonic endoderm, gut, and nephrogenic tissue of the developing mouse embryo: HNF-4 is a marker for primary endoderm in the implanting blastocyst. Proc Natl Acad Sci USA 1994;91:7598-602.
41. Plengvidhya N, Antonellis A, Wogan LT, Poleev A, Borgschulze M, Warram JH, Ryffel GU, Krolewski AS, Doria A. Hepatocyte nuclear factor-4gamma: cDNA sequence, gene organization, and mutation screening in early-onset autosomal-dominant type 2 diabetes. Diabetes 1999;48:2099-102.
42. Lemaigre FP, Durviaux SM, Truong O, Lannoy VJ, Hsuan JJ, Rousseau GG. Hepatocyte nuclear factor 6, a transcription factor that contains a novel type of homeodomain and a single cut domain. Proc Natl Acad Sci USA 1996;93:9460-4.
43. Samadani U, Costa RH. The transcriptional activator hepatocyte nuclear factor 6 regulates liver gene expression. Mol Cell Biol 1996;16:6273-84.
44. Lannoy VJ, Burglin TR, Rousseau GG, Lemaigre FP. Isoforms of hepatocyte nuclear factor-6 differ in DNA-binding properties, contain a bifunctional homeodomain, and define the new ONECUT class of homeodomain proteins. J Biol Chem 1998;273:13552-62.
45. Landry C, Clotman F, Hioki T, Oda H, Picard JJ, Lemaigre FP, Rousseau GG. HNF-6 is expressed in endoderm derivativesand nervous system of themouse embryo and participatesto the cross-regulatory network of liver-enriched transcription factors. Dev Biol 1997;192:247-57.
46. Rausa F, Samadani U, Ye H, Lim L, Fletcher CF, Jenkins NA, Copeland NG, Costa RH. The cut-homeodomain transcriptional activator HNF-6 is coexpressed with its target gene HNF-3 beta in the developing murine liver and pancreas. Dev Biol 1997;192:228-46.
47. Moller AM, Ek J, Durviaux SM, Urhammer SA, Clausen JO, Eiberg H, Hansen T, Rousseau GG, Lemaigre FP, Pedersen O. Hepatocyte nuclear factor-6: associations between genetic variability and type II diabetes and between genetic variability and estimates of insulin secretion. Diabetologia 1999;42:1011-6.
48. Kuo CJ, Conley PB, Chen L, Sladek FM, Darnell, JE Jr, Crabtree GR. A transcriptional hierarchy involved in mammalian cell type specification. Nature 1992;355:457-461.
49. Sladek, FM. Hepatocyte nuclear factor 4 (HNF4): In Liver gene transcription (Tronche, F, Yaniv, M, eds.) RG Landes Co., Austin, Texas 1994.
50. Gragnoli C, Lindner T, Cockburn BN, Kaisaki PJ, Gragnoli F, Marozzi, G, Bell GI. Maturity-onset diabetes of the young due to a mutation in the hepatocyte nuclear factor-4 alpha binding site in the promoter of the hepatocyte nuclear factor-1 alpha gene. Diabetes 1997;46:1648-51.
51. Bulla, GA, Fournier RE. Genetic analysis of a transcriptional activation pathway by using hepatoma cell variants. Mol Cell Biol 1994;14:7086-7094.
52. Griffo G, Hamon BC, Angrand, PO, Fox M, West L, Lecoq O, Povey S, Cassio D, Weiss M. HNF4 and HNF1 as well as a panel of hepatic functions are extinguished and reexpressed in parallel in chromosomally reduced rat hepatoma-human fibroblast hybrids. J Cell Biol 1993;121:887-898.
53. Cereghini S, Yaniv M, Cortese R. Hepatocyte dedifferentiation and extinction is accompanied by a block in the synthesis of mRNA coding for the transcription factor HNF1/LFB1. EMBO J 1990;9:2257-2263.
54. Yamagata K, Furuta H, Oda N, Kaisaki P, Menzel S, Cox NJ, Fajans SS, Signorini S, Stoffel M and Bell GI. Mutations in hepatic nuclear factor 4 alpha gene in maturity-onset diabetes of the young (MODY1). Nature 1996;384:458-460.
55. Yamagata K, Oda N, Kaisaki PJ, Menzel S, Furuta H, Vaxillaire M, Southam L, Cox RHD, Lathrop

GM, Boriraj VV, Chen X, Cox NJ, Oda Y, Yano H, Le Beau MM, Yamada S, Nishigori H, Takeda J, Fajans SS, Hattersley AT, Iwasaki N, Hansen T, Pederson O, Polonsky KS, Turner RC, Velho G, Chevre J-C, Froguel P, Bell GI. Mutations in the hepatocyte nuclear factor 4 alpha gene in maturity-onset diabetes of the young (MODY3). Nature 1996;384:455-458.

56. Zhang W, Mirkovitch J, Darnell JE. Tissue specific regulation of the mouse HNF-4 expression. Mol Cell Biol 1994;14:7276-7284.
57. Duncan SA, Nagy A, Chan W. Murine gastrulation requires HNF4 regulated gene expression the visceral endoderm: tetraploid rescue of Hnf4 -/- embryos. Development 1997;124:279-287.
58. Stein R, Gerrish K, Gannon M, Shih D, Henderson E, Stoffel M, Wright CVE. Pancreatic beta cell-specific transcription of the pdx-1 gene: The role of conserved upstream control regions and their HNF-3 sites. Mol Cell Biol 1999;in press.
59. Johnsson J, Carlsson L, Edlund T, Edlund H. Insulin promoter factor 1 is required for pancreas development in mice. Nature 1994;371:606-609.
60. Leonard J, Peers B, Johnson T, Ferreri K, Lee S, Montminy M. Characterization of somatostatin transactivating factor-1, a novel homeobox factor which stimulates somatostatin expression in pancreatic islet cells. Mol Endocrinol 1993;7:1275-1283.
61. Serup P, Petersen HV, Pedersen EE, Edlund H, Leonard J, Petersen JS, Larsson LI, Madsen OD. The homeodomain protein IPF-1/STF-1 is expressed in a subset of islet cells and promotes rat insulin 1 gene expression dependent on an intact E1 helix-loop-helix factor binding site. Biochem J 1995;310:997-1003.
62. Stoffers DA, Zinkin NT, Stanojevic V, Clarke WL, Habener JF. Pancreatic agenesis attributable to a single nucleotide deletion in the human IPF1 gene coding sequence. Nature Genetics 1997;15:107-110.
63. Stoffers A, Ferrer J, Clarke WL, Habener JF. Early-onset type-II diabetes mellitus (MODY4) linked to IPF1. Nature Genetics 1997;17:138-139 .
64. Morrisey EE, Tang Z, Sigrist K, Lu MM, Jiang F, Ip HS, Parmacek MS. GATA6 regulates HNF4 and is required for differentiation of visceral endoderm in the mouse embryo. Genes & Dev 1998;12:3579-90.
65. Fajans SS. Maturity-onset diabetes of the young. Diabetes/Metabolism Rev 1989;5:579-606.
66. Bell GI, Xiang KS, Newman MV, Wu S-H, Wright LG, Fajans SS, Spielman RS, Cox, NJ. Gene for non-insulin-dependent diabetes mellitus (maturity-onset diabetes of the young subtype) is linked to DNA polymorphism on human chromosome 20q. Proc Natl Acad Sci USA 1991;88:1484-1488.
67. Froguel P, Vaxillaire M, Velho G, Zouali H, Butel MO, Lesage DS, Vionnet N, Clement, K, Fougerousse F, Tanizawa Y, Weissenbach J, Beckmann,JS, Lathrop JM, Passa P, Permutt, MA, Cohen D. Close linkage of glucokinase locus on chromosome 7p to early-onset non-insulin-dependent diabetes mellitus. Nature 1992;356:162-164.
68. Vaxillaire M, Boccio V, Philippi A, Vigouroux C, Terwilliger J, Passa P, Beckmann JS, Velho G, Lathrop GM, Froguel P. A gene for maturity-onset diabetes of the young (MODY) maps to chromosome 12q. Nature Genetics 1995;9:418-423.
69. Vionnet N, Stoffel M, Takeda J, Yasuda,K, Bell GI, Zouali H, Lesage S, Velho G, Iris F, Passa P, Froguel P, and Cohen D. Nonsense mutation in the glucokinase gene causes early-onset non-insulin-dependent diabetes mellitus. Nature 1992;356:721-722.
70. Froguel P, Zouali H, Vionnet N, Velho G, Vaxillaire M, Sun F, Lesage S, Stoffel M, Takeda J, Passa P, Permutt MA, Beckmann JS, Bell GI and Cohen D. Familial hyperglycemia due to mutations in glucokinase: definition of a subtype of diabetes mellitus. N Engl J Med 1993;328:697-702.
71. Matschinsky FM. Glucokinase as glucose sensor and metabolic signal generator in pancreatic _-cells and hepatocytes. Diabetes 1990;39:647-652.
72. Horikawa Y, Iwasaki N, Furuta H, Hinokio Y, Cockburn BN, Lindner T, Yamagata K, Ogata M, Tomonaga O, Kuroki H, Kasahara T, Iwamoto Y, Bell GI. Mutation in hepatocyte nuclear factor-1 beta gene (TCF2) associated with MODY. Nature Genetics 1997;17:384-5.
73. Malecki MT, Jhala US, Antonellis A, Fields L, Doria A, Orban T, Saad M, Warram JH, Montminy M, Krolewski AS. Mutations in NEUROD1 are associated with the development of type 2 diabetes mellitus. Nat Genet 1999;23:323-8.
74. Byrne MM, Sturis J, Clement K, Vionnet N, Pueyo ME, Stoffel M., Takeda, Passa P, Cohen D, Bell GI, Velho G, Froguel P, and Polonsky KS. Insulin secretion abnormalities in subjects with hyperglycemia due to glucokinase mutations. J Clin Invest 1994;93:1120-1130.
75. Byrne MM, Sturis J, Menzel S, Yamagata Y, Dronsfield MJ, Bain SC, Hattersley AT, Velho G, Froguel P, Bell GI, Polonsky KS. Altered insulin secretory responses to glucose in diabetic and nondiabetic subjects with mutations in the diabetes susceptibility gene MODY3 on chromosome 12. Diabetes 1996;46:1503-1511.
76. Byrne MM, Sturis J, Stoltz A, Oritz FJ, Stoffel M, Smith MJ, Bell GI, Fajans SS, Halter JB and Polonsky KS. Altered insulin secretory responses to glucose in subjects with a mutation in the MODY1 gene on chromosome 20. Diabetes 1994;44:699-705.
77. Macfarlane WM, Frayling TM, Ellard S, Evans JC, Allen LI, Bulman MP, Ayres S, Shepherd M, Clark P, Millward A, Demaine A, Wilkin T, Docherty K, Hattersley AT. Missense mutations in the insulin promoter factor-1 gene predispose to type 2 diabetes. J Clin Invest 1999;104:R33-9.

78. Hani EH, Stoffers DA, Chevre JC, Durand E, Stanojevic V, Dina C, Habener JF, Froguel P. Defective mutations in the insulin promoter factor-1 (IPF-1) gene in late-onset type 2 diabetes mellitus. Clin Invest 1999;104:R41-8.
79. Lindner TH, Njolstad PR, Horikawa Y, Bostad L, Bell GI, Sovik O. A novel syndrome of diabetes mellitus, renal dysfunction and genital malformation associated with a partial deletion of the pseudo-POU domain of hepatocyte nuclear factor-1beta. Hum Mol Genet 1999;8:2001-8.
80. Yamagata K, Yang Q, Yamamoto K, Iwahashi H, Miyagawa J, Okita K, Yoshiuchi I, Miyazaki J, Noguchi T, Nakajima H, Namba M, Hanafusa T, Matsuzawa Y. Mutation P291fsinsC in the transcription factor hepatocyte nuclear factor-1alpha is dominant negative. Diabetes 1998;47:1231-1235.
81. Stoffel M and Duncan SA. The MODY1 transcription factor HNF4a regulates expression of genes required for glucose transport and metabolism. Proc Natl Acad Sci USA 1997;94:13209-13214.
82. Letho M, Bitzen P-O, Isomaa B, Wipemo C, Wesman Y, Forsblom C, Tuomi T, Taskinen M-R, Groop L. Mutations in the HNF4a gene affects insulin secretion and triglyceride metabolism. Diabetes 1999;48:423-425.
83. Lindner T, Gragnoli C, Furuta H, Cockburn BN, Petzold C, Rietzsch H, Weiß U, Schulze J and Bell GI. Hepatic function in a family with a nonsense mutation (R154X) in the hepatocyte nuclear factor4_/MODY1 gene. J Clin Invest 1997;100:1400-1405.
84. Furuta H, Iwasaki N, Oda N, Hinokio Y, Horikawa Y, Yamagata K, Yano N, Sugahiro J, Ogata M, Ohgawara H, Omori Y, Iwamoto Y and Bell GI. Organizationand partial sequence of the hepatocyte nuclear factor-4 alpha/MODY1 gene and identificationof a missense mutation, R127W, in a Japanese family with MODY. Diabetes 1997;46:1652-7.
85. Moller AM, Urhammer SA, Dalgaard LT, Reneland R, Berglund L, Hansen T, Clausen JO, Lithell H, Petersen O. Studies of the genetic variability of the coding region of the hepatocyte nuclear factor-4alpha in Caucasians with maturity onset NIDDM. Diabetologia 1997;40:980-983.
86. Bulman MP, Dronsfield MJ, Frayling T, Appleton M, Bain SC, Ellard S, Hattersley AT. A missense mutation in the hepatocyte nuclear factor 4 alpha gene in a UK pedigree with maturity-onset diabetes of the young. Diabetologia 1997;40:859-862.
87. Malecki MT, Yang Y, Antonellis A, Curtis S, Warram JH and Krolewski AS: Identification of new mutations in the hepatocyte nuclear factor 4alpha gene among families with early onset Type 2 diabetes mellitus. Diabet Med 1999;16:193-200.
88. Navas MA, Breslow B, Krolewski AS, Stoffel M. The MODY1 Gene Mutation HNF4(G115S) Inactivates Hepatocyte Nuclear Factor-4a by Affecting its DNA Binding Activity. (submitted).
89. Emens LA, Landers DW, Moss LG. Hepatocyte nuclear factor 1 alpha is expressed in a hamster insulinoma line and transactivates the rat insulin I gene. Proc Natl Acad Sci USA 1992;89:7300-7304.
90. Ahlgren U, Jonsson J, Jonsson L, Simu K, Edlund H. Beta-cell-specific inactivation of the mouse Ipf1/Pdx1 gene results in loss of the beta-cell phenotype and maturity onset diabetes. Genes Dev 1998;12:1763-8.
91. Dumonteil E, Laser B, Constant I, Philippe J. Differentialregulation of the glucagon and insulin I gene promoters by the basic helix-loop-helix transcription factors E47 and BETA2. J Biol Chem 1998;Aug 7;273(32):19945-54.
92. Naya FJ, Stellrecht CM, Tsai MJ. Tissue-specific regulation of the insulin gene by a novel basic helix-loop-helix transcription factor. Genes Dev 1995;9:1009-19.
93. Naya FJ, Huang HP, Qiu Y, Mutoh H, DeMayo FJ, Leiter AB, Tsai MJ. Diabetes, defective pancreatic morphogenesis, and abnormal enteroendocrine differentiation in BETA2/ neuroD-deficient mice. Genes Dev 1997;11:2323-34.
94. German MS. Glucose sensing in pancreatic _-cells. The key role for glucokinase and glycolytic intermediates. Proc Natl Acad Sci USA 1993;90:1781-1785.
95. Magnuson MA, Andreone TL, Printz RL, Koch S, Granner DK. Rat glucokinase gene: structure and regulation by insulin. Proc Natl Acad Sci USA 1989;86:4838-4842.
96. Thorens B, Sarkar HK, Kaback HR Lodish HF. Cloning and functional expression in bacteria of a novel glucose transporter present in liver, intestine, kidney and _-pancreatic islet cells. Cell 1988;55:281-290.
97. Magnuson MA, Shelton KD. An alternate promoter in the glucokinase gene is active in the pancreatic beta cell. J Biol Chem 1989;164:15936-15942.
98. Nebert DW. Proposed role of drug metabolizing enzymes: regulation of steady state levels of the ligands that effect growth, homeostasis, differentiation, and neuroendocrine functions. Mol Endocrinol 1991;5:1203-1214.
99. Unger RH. Lipotoxicity in the pathogenesis of obesity-dependent NIDDM. Diabetes 1995;44:863-870.
100. Tronche F, Yaniv M, in Liver gene expression, 1994, R.G. Landes Company, Austin.
101. Wang H, Maechler P, Hagenfeldt, KA, Wollheim CB. Dominant negative suppression of HNF-1a function results in defective insulin gene transcription and impaired metabolism-secretion coupling in a pancreatic _-cell line. EMBO J 1998;17:6701-6713.
102. Dukes ID, Sreenan S, Roe MW, Levisetti M, Zhou YP, Ostrega D, Bell GI, Pontoglio M, Yaniv M, Philipson L, Polonsky KS. Defective pancreatic beta-cell glycolytic signaling in hepatocyte nuclear

factor-1alpha-deficient mice. J Biol Chem 1998;273:24457-64.
103. Shih DQ, Dansky HM, Fleisher M, Assmann G, Fajans SS, Stoffel M. Genotype/Phenotype Relationships in Type 2 Diabetes: HNF-4_ haploinsufficiency is Associated with Reduced Apolipoprotein AII, CIII, Lp(a), and Triglyceride Levels (submitted).

16
REGULATION OF *pdx-1* GENE EXPRESSION

Kevin Gerrish, M.S., Susan Samaras, Ph.D.,
Michelle A. Cissell, Ph.D.,
Christopher V.E. Wright, D. Phil.,
and Roland Stein, Ph.D.
Vanderbilt University Medical Center
Nashville, TN 37232, USA

INTRODUCTION

Multiple transcription factors that are enriched within pancreatic islet cells mediate the differentiation of these cells during embryogenesis and the maintenance of their specialized functions in the adult. These proteins are often implicated in diabetes mellitus, a disease caused in part by a failure of β-cells to produce enough insulin to meet the body's needs. One such transcription factor, PDX-1 (pancreatic and duodenal homeobox protein 1) (also known as STF-1, IDX-1, and IPF-1), is integrally involved in both pancreatic physiology and β-cell pathology.

The critical role of PDX-1 in pancreas formation is highlighted by its expression pattern during embryogenesis and by the developmental consequences of inactivating mutations in the *pdx-1* gene. PDX-1 expression is initially observed in the ventral and dorsal walls of the primitive foregut where the pancreatic buds will form (1). Subsequently, PDX-1 is detectable in islet cell precursors and, transiently, in exocrine progenitors (2). A homozygous null mutation within the mouse *pdx-1* locus causes pancreatic agenesis due to a block at a very early developmental stage ((3-5) see chapter by U. Ahlgren and H. Edlund). PDX-1 appears to serve the same essential function in humans, since the pancreas was also not formed in an individual born homozygous for an inactivating mutation in the protein (6).

In the adult pancreas, PDX-1 is selectively expressed in islet β-cells (>90%), and a subset of α- (3%) and δ- (15%) cells (2,7). PDX-1 regulates transcription of several genes associated with β-cell identity and function, including insulin (1,7-9), glucokinase (10), islet amyloid polypeptide (11-14), and glucose transporter type 2 (GLUT2) (15). The importance of PDX-1 in controlling the expression of genes required for the sensing and regulation of blood glucose levels suggested that an inactivating mutation within the protein would result in dysfunctional β-cells. Indeed, mice that are heterozygous mutant carriers of PDX-1 exhibit symptoms of glucose intolerance (16,17), suggesting a dosage effect on insulin expression or β-cell function. More significantly, humans with this condition are susceptible to a form of type 2 (non-insulin dependent) diabetes designated maturity onset diabetes of the young (MODY) (18). In addition, selectively removing PDX-1 from adult islet cells using the *Cre-loxP* system results in the development of diabetes in mice, which appears to be at least partially caused by the reduction in insulin and GLUT2 gene expression levels (17).

Collectively, these data have established a critical role for PDX-1 during both pancreatic differentiation and normal β cell function. However, little is known about what controls *pdx-1* mRNA levels during these processes. In this chapter, our current understanding of *pdx-1* transcriptional regulation will be summarized and experimental strategies that could be used to identify essential *cis*- and *trans*-acting regulatory factors within the transcription control region of the gene will be discussed.

RELEVANCE OF STUDYING *pdx-1* GENE EXPRESSION

Type 1, or insulin-dependent, diabetes is characterized by an irreversible loss of β-cell mass (19). Because of its significant role in islet cell differentiation and β-cell-specific gene transcription, PDX-1 represents a potential target for therapeutic treatments of type 1 diabetes. Moreover, PDX-1 may participate in β-cell neogenesis, a function that would be crucial to successfully engineer transplantable β-cells. The adult β-cell has a lifespan of approximately 30 days after which it undergoes programmed cell death or apoptosis (20). These cells can be replaced in the pancreas through two mechanisms: replication (proliferation) of existing β-cells or neogenesis from progenitor cells in the pancreas (20-22). Significantly, PDX-1 expression is upregulated in models of β-cell neogenesis (21,23,24). Thus, PDX-1 contributes to the maintenance of β-cell numbers necessary for normal islet function and, by extension, to the regulation of glucose homeostasis by supporting the ability of the pancreas to produce sufficient insulin.

In type 2 diabetes, defects in glucose sensing and metabolism result in a hyperlipidemic and hyperglycemic environment that impairs β-cell function (25,26). *pdx-1* mRNA and protein are down-regulated under conditions of chronic hyperglycemia and hyperlipidemia in both *in vitro* and *in vivo* experimental model systems (27-29)(see chapter by R.P. Robertson et al.). Consequently, the β-cells of type 2 diabetics appear to contain reduced levels of factors controlling insulin production and secretion, like PDX-1, and genes that it, in turn, regulates (30,31).

Although the factors responsible for susceptibility to type 2 diabetes are largely unknown, studies suggest a major genetic component to this disease. Susceptibility genes have not yet been identified except in MODY which was found to be caused by single gene deficiencies (32). Four of five known MODY genes encode transcription factors that appear to be necessary for normal β-cell function (MODY1:Hepatic Nuclear Factor 4α (HNF4 α) (33); MODY3:HNF1α (34); MODY4:*pdx-1* (18); MODY5:HNF1β (35)). Glucokinase, an important enzyme for glucose metabolism, is the only non-transcription factor gene (MODY 2) (36). Three MODY factors (HNF1α, HNF1β and HNF4α) interact in a transcription regulatory network required for differentiation and metabolism within both the pancreas and liver (37). Thus, transcription factors involved in β-cell function are also critical determinants of susceptibility to diabetes.

These observations not only highlight the relevance of the *pdx-1* gene to human disease but also illustrate its utility as a prototypical regulatory factor necessary in pancreatic differentiation, β-cell maintenance, and islet-specific gene regulation. As a consequence, identifying the factors involved in regulating *pdx-1* transcription will provide valuable information regarding the biological mechanisms required for these important processes, and conceivably, for those that contribute to β-cell dysfunction in diabetes.

REGULATION OF *pdx-1* TRANSCRIPTION

In all vertebrates examined to date, progenitors of the pancreas and rostral duodenum express the *pdx-1* gene (*Xenopus* (38,39); mouse (1,2,5,40); chicken (41)). In adults, *pdx-1* expression is maintained at high levels in β-cells and the duodenum, and at low levels in pancreatic acinar and islet α- and δ-cells (2,39,42). To understand how *pdx-1* transcription is regulated in these tissues, the essential *cis*- and *trans*-acting factors driving expression during pancreatic development and in β-cells must be identified. Two complementary approaches have been used to broadly define transcription control regions in the *pdx-1* gene. First, mice carrying *pdx-1*-driven transgenes have demonstrated that the *cis*-elements sufficient for expression *in vivo* are located within the region 5' to the transcription start site (42,43). Second, transient transfection analysis of *pdx-1*-driven reporter genes spanning these sequences has begun to identify the regulatory elements critical for β-cell-specific expression of the *pdx-1* gene. Once significant regulatory elements have been defined through detailed mutagenesis analysis, the *trans*-acting factors that mediate activity can be characterized.

The strategy that has been undertaken to identify the proteins regulating *pdx-1* transcription is very similar to that successfully used to characterize the pancreas-enriched hormone and digestive enzyme genes, including insulin (1,7-9) glucagon (44), islet amyloid polypeptide (11-14), and somatostatin (45) of the islet and amylase (46) of the exocrine pancreas. However, little is known about the control mechanisms mediating expression of the *trans*-activators for these genes. Studying these regulators will likely provide additional insight into the processes required in pancreatic function. In this regard, the control region sequences regulating the genes encoding the insulin gene regulator, BETA2/NeuroD1 (47), and the amlyase gene activator, PTF1-p48 (48), have been partially characterized, though the specific elements necessary for selective expression have not been defined. The analysis of the *pdx-1* regulatory sequences is more developed and both published and unpublished data describing their characterization are described below.

IN VIVO ANALYSIS OF THE *pdx-1* TRANSCRIPTION CONTROL REGION

A 14.5 kilobase (kb) fragment of the mouse *pdx-1* gene, which contains 9 kb of 5' flanking sequence, was shown to recapitulate the pancreas and rostral duodenum specific expression of the endogenous *pdx-1* gene by transgenic analysis (42). In addition, PDX-1 protein expression driven by this 14.5 kb fragment as a transgene rescues the pancreatic differentiation deficiency in mice lacking a functional *pdx-1* locus (M. Gannon and C.V.E. Wright, unpublished observations). Progressive 5' deletion analysis has narrowed the important functional sequences required for appropriate developmental- and islet-specific expression to within 4.5 kb of the transcription start site (L. Gamer, M. Offield, and C.V.E. Wright, unpublished observations). A rat *pdx-1*-driven transgene encompassing this region (i.e. -6.5 kb relative to the transcription start site) also directed expression appropriately (43). These transgenic experiments have demonstrated that the regulatory signals required for appropriate *pdx-1* gene transcription *in vivo* are found within sequences from approximately -6.5 (rat) and -4.5 (mouse) kb to the transcription start site.

IN VITRO ANALYSIS OF THE *pdx-1* 5'-FLANKING CONTROL REGION

To identify the specific sequences that mediate transcriptional control, wildtype and mutated experimental gene-driven expression is normally studied with reporter constructs transfected into transformed cell lines, since performing this analysis systematically with transgene constructs *in vivo* is very time-consuming and costly. Unfortunately, a serious limitation of the available pancreatic cell lines is the inability to differentiate them in culture. As a consequence, the signals involved in pancreatic development can not be studied *in vitro*; however, studies conducted with reporter driven constructs in expressing versus non-expressing cell lines can provide insight into the signals involved in cell specific expression. To localize these signals within the rat *pdx-1* gene, a series of 5'-flanking deletion mutants spanning the region from -6.5 kb to the transcription start site were subcloned into a reporter construct and their activity analyzed in transfected *pdx-1*-expressing and non-expressing cell lines. It was interesting that a region from –6200/–5700 bp was shown by this analysis to mediate selective expression in the rat *pdx-1* gene (43), as these sequences reside upstream of those that are sufficient for pancreatic- and duodenal-specific expression in the mouse *pdx-1* transgene (42).

Two distinct experimental approaches were used to localize the 5-flanking control sequences in the mouse *pdx-1* gene: nuclease hypersensitivity and control region-driven transfection analyses (42). The presence of nuclease hypersensitive sites (HSS) within a gene reflects an altered chromatin conformation caused by binding of non-histone proteins (e.g. transcription factors) (see references 49-51 for a discussion of HSS in gene activation). Three nuclease HSS were specifically identified within the endogenous *pdx-1* gene in expressing cells, located between -2560/-1880 bp (HSS1), -1330/-800 bp (HSS2), and -260/+180 bp (HSS3) (42). Pancreatic β-cell-selective expression was analyzed in transfected cells by subcloning mouse *pdx-1* fragments spanning these regions upstream of a herpes virus thymidine kinase (TK) minimal promoter driven reporter. HSS1 was the only region found to selectively direct expression in transfected β-cell lines. The HSS1 region (i.e. -2560/-1880 bp) also directed islet β-cell expression in transgenic mice (42). Interestingly, HSS1 transgene activity was not detected in other *pdx-1* expressing cells, such as those of the exocrine pancreas or duodenum. These results suggest that HSS1 defines an important subdomain of the mouse *pdx-1* gene that is involved in islet-selective transcription.

The ability of the rat -6200/-5700 bp region to direct expression in transgenic mice has not been determined. We have shown by Southern analysis that HSS1 and the -6200/-5700 bp regions are present in similar locations in the rat and mouse *pdx-1* genes. In addition, the rat -6200/-5700 bp sequences selectively stimulated *pdx-1*:TK activity in transfected β cell lines (K. Gerrish, C. Torrez-Sanchez and R. Stein, unpublished observations). These results suggest that both the -6200/-5700 bp and the -2560/-1880 bp regions are involved in appropriate expression of the *pdx-1* gene (Figure 1). Although there is very little sequence identity between the rat -6200/-5700 bp and mouse -2560/-1880 bp regions, a conserved HNF3β binding element is involved in regulation from both regions (42,52) (see below). Collectively, these data suggest that cell specific expression of mammalian *pdx-1* genes is controlled by discrete, but conserved, subdomain sequences found within their 5'-flanking regions.

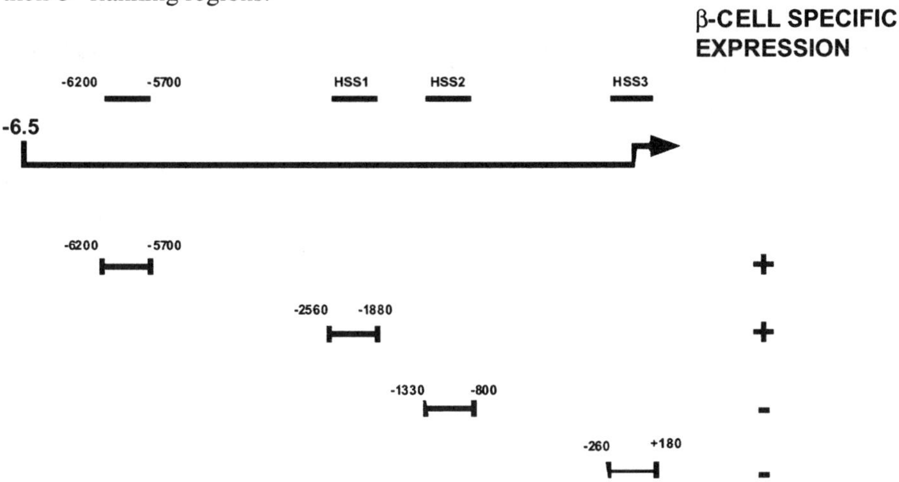

Figure 1. *Transcription control regions of the pdx-1 gene. Schematic of the 5'-flanking region of the vertebrate pdx-1 gene. The location of the rat -6200/-5700 bp region (52) and HSS1 (-2560/-1880 bp), HSS2 (-1330/-800 bp), and HSS3 (-260/+180 bp) are shown. The β-cell selective activity of various pdx-1:pTK transfected constructs in pdx-1:expressing and non-expressing cells is shown; the "+" indicates more activity in β-cells and "-", no detectable difference. The HSS1, HSS2, HSS3-driven reporter results are published (42).*

IDENTIFICATION OF POTENTIAL *PDX-1* GENE ACTIVATORS

Three factors have been identified that can bind and apparently activate *pdx-1* gene transcription: HNF3β (42,52,53), BETA2/NeuroD1 (52), and USF (43). HNF3β, a transcription factor in the fork head family involved in endodermal development (54), binds at elements located within the –6200/–5700 bp (i.e. at -5920/-5910 bp) (52) and HSS1 (i.e. at -2626/-2615 bp (53) and -2007/-1996 bp (42)) regions. In contrast, there is only one characterized site for BETA2/NeuroD1 (-5964/-5968 bp) (52) or USF (-107/-101 bp) (43) within the *pdx-1* transcription control unit. Both BETA2/NeuroD1 and USF are members of the basic helix-loop-helix (bHLH) transcription factor family, with BETA2/NeuroD1 enriched in islet cell types (55) and USF ubiquitously distributed (56). The conservation of the HNF3β and USF binding sites in the human and mouse genes also supports an important function in *pdx-1* transcription (53); conservation of the BETA2/NeuroD1 element has not yet been determined.

Mutation of the HNF3β, BETA2/NeuroD1, or USF binding elements dramatically reduces *pdx-1*-driven reporter gene activity in β-cell lines (42,43,52,53). Does this mean that these factors alone control the selective expression pattern of the *pdx-1* gene? We believe that at least some aspects of *pdx-1* transcription rely on them, as HNF3β (54) and BETA2/NeuroD1 (57) are involved in endodermal development. However, as neither HNF3β nor BETA2/NeuroD1 are restricted to islet β-cells, we expect that selective transcription results from functional cooperation between these factors and others enriched in the β-cell. Support for this proposal is based on several observations. First, HNF3β directs selective expression of genes in hepatocytes (58), yet HSS1-driven constructs are transcriptionally inactive in transfected hepatocyte cell lines (42). Second, mutation in the HNF3β binding site at -2007/-1996 bp affects the level of expression of the -2560/-1880 bp HSS1- driven construct (42), but not the cell specific expression pattern in transfected cells (42) or transgenic mice (M. Gannon and C.V.E. Wright, unpublished observations). Third, mice lacking a functional BETA2/NeuroD1 gene do not exhibit a discernable defect in *pdx-1* expression in the pancreas (57). The role of HNF3β in the expression of *pdx-1 in vivo* cannot be resolved from the phenotype of HNF3β homozygous null mutant mice, since these mice die in early embryogenesis, prior to the differentiation of pancreatic endoderm (59,60).

ANALYSIS OF THE HSS1 REGION

PDX-1 is an essential regulator of the programs leading to the proper development and function of islet β-cells. The important transcriptional regulatory sequences of the *pdx-1* gene appear to be located between -6200/-5700 bp and -2560/-1880 bp (42,43,52). We believe that identifying the essential control factors involved in activation of these regions will provide valuable information regarding the biological mechanisms required for cell type-specific transcription. It is likely that a systematic and detailed analysis of these regions will define target elements for novel, as well as characterized, islet enriched transcription factors (e.g. Brn-4 (61), Hb9 (62), Isl-1 (63), Nkx2.2 (64), Nkx 6.1 (65), PAX-4 (66), PAX-6 (67,68), pdx-1, BETA2/NeuroD1 (55), IB-1 (69)). These studies may also provide insight into how an inactivating mutation within a diabetes susceptibility gene could result in β-cell dysfunction since, strikingly the HSS1 regions contains potential binding site for several MODY genes (i.e. HNF1α, HNF1β, HNF4β) (see below).

The expression pattern and function of pdx-1 appears to be shared amongst vertebrates (frog (38,39,70), chicken (41), rat (8,13,52), and mouse (2,8,70)). Our studies have focused on characterizing HSS1, since the sequences defined by this region (i.e. -2560/-1880 bp) directed pancreatic β-cell-selective reporter activity in transgene and transfection assays (42). Though these experiments unmasked the general location of key elements that were important in selective expression, their precise identification within this ~700 bp region seemed to be a daunting task if an unbiased mutagenesis strategy was utilized. Alternatively, if we assumed that the *cis*-active regulatory sequences required for developmental and adult specific expression from the HSS1 region were maintained amongst vertebrate *pdx-1* genes, then more limited areas of identity should define the sequences essential in transcriptional control.

To test this hypothesis, approximately 4.5 kb of the 5'-flanking region from the chicken and human *pdx-1* genes was sequenced and compared to that of the mouse gene. The HSS1 region contained the only areas of significant identity, which was resolved into three separate conserved subregions, termed Areas I, II, and III (Figure 2). Chicken *pdx-1* does not contain a similarly located region homologous to Area II, although Areas I and III sequences are highly conserved between mouse and chicken. It is presently unclear whether there is a functional consequence to this difference in subdomain organization.

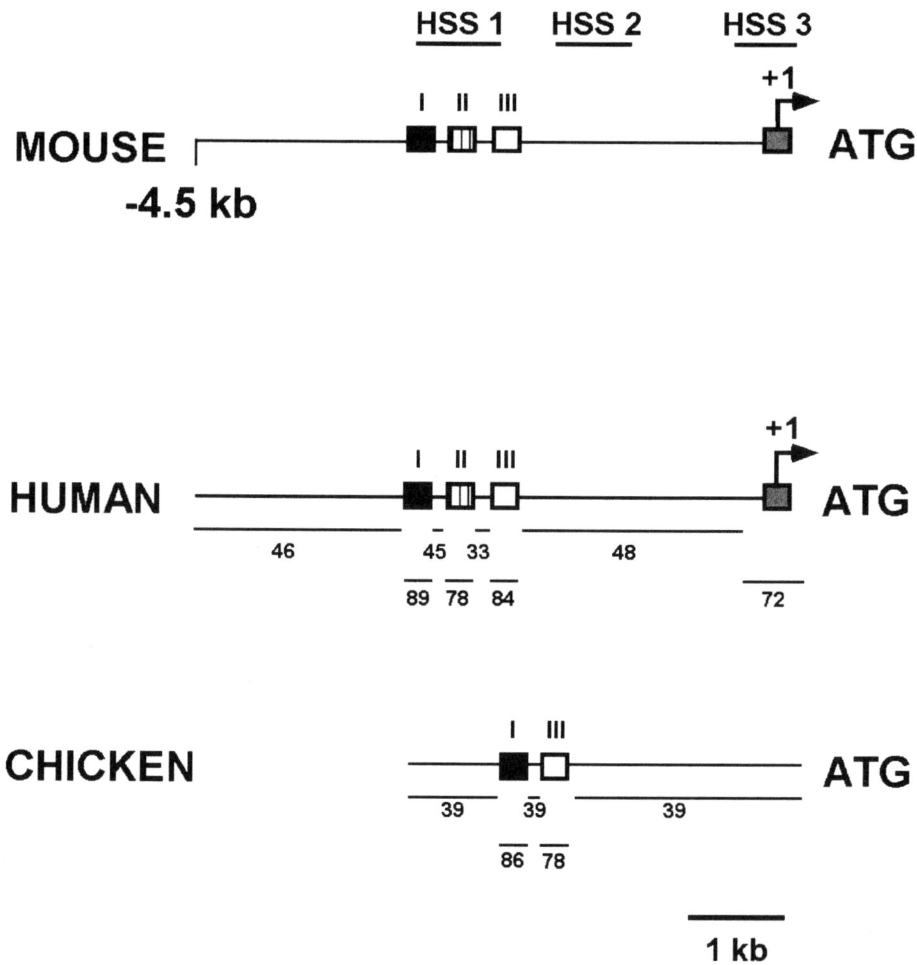

Figure 2. *Sequence similarity within HSS1 in the promoter region of mouse, human, and chicken pdx-1 genes. Diagram of the mouse, human, and chicken promoter region. HSS1, -2560/-1880 bp; HSS2, -1330/-800 bp; HSS3, -260/+180 bp. Area I, -2694/-2561 bp; Area II, -2139/-1958 bp; Area III, -1879/-1799 bp. Because the accuracy in mapping HSS1 was approximately ±150bp (42), all three subdomains were considered to lie within the HSS1 region. The percent identity of the human and chicken sequences to mouse is indicated with bars below the locus diagram. Mouse to human (the numbering is relative to the S1 transcription start site (43)), -4500/-2694, 46%; Area I, 89%; -2435/-2201, 45%; Area II, 78%; -1957/1880, 33%; Area III, 84%; -1799/-364, 48%; HSS3, 72%; mouse to chicken (numbered relative to the chicken protein coding ATG codon), -1731/1265, 39%; Area I, 86%; -1101/-687, 39%; Area III, 78%; -608/+1, 39%.*

Comparison of transfected reporter constructs driven by Areas I, II, and III demonstrated that Area I and Area II could mediate β-cell-selective activation (53). Interestingly, there appear to be few potential binding sites for characterized transcriptional regulators shared between the rat –6200/–5700 bp region or conserved

Area I, Area II, and Area III sequences (Figure 3). Similar to the –6200/–5700 bp region, conserved HNF3β binding sites were also found to be necessary for Area I- and Area II-mediated stimulation (53). These results suggested that HSS1 was regulated by three distinct functional units (i.e. Areas I, II, and III), and furthermore, that conserved sequences within these subdomains define the binding sites for key regulators of *pdx-1* transcription.

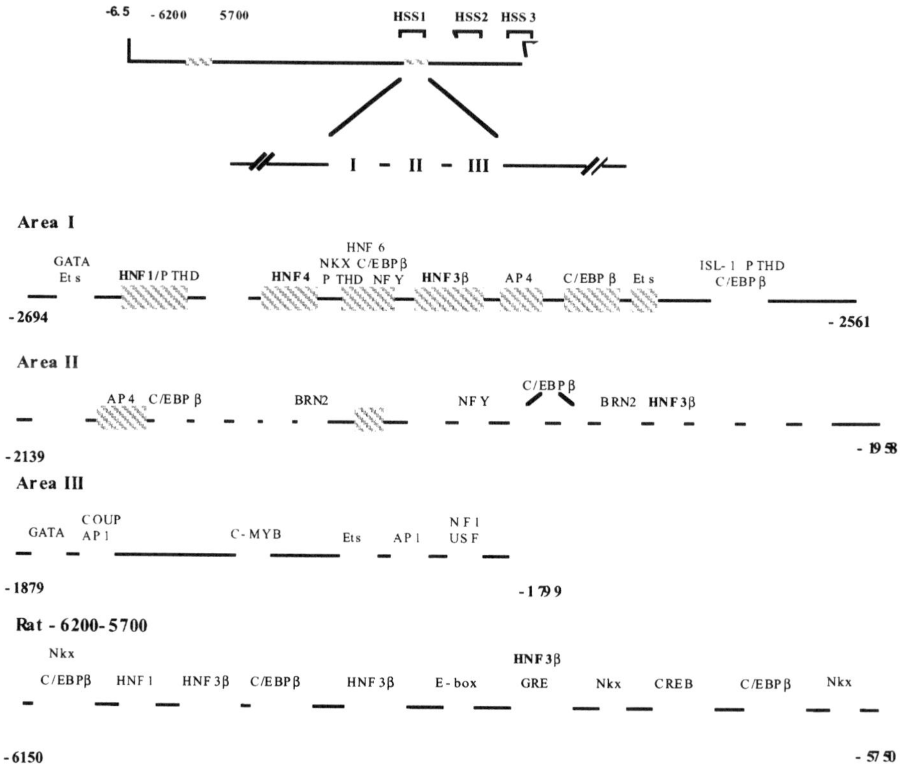

Figure 3. *The potential transcription factor binding sites within the rat –6200/–5700 bp region and conserved Areas I, II, and III sequences. The TRANSFAC database program (79) was used in this analysis of the rat (–6200/–5700 bp) and mouse (Area I, -2694/-2561 bp; Area II, -2139/-1958 bp; Area III, -1879/-1799 bp) sequences. The boxes in Areas I, II, and III represent sequences conserved across species. The potential HNF1α/ HNF1β and HNF4α sites and previously characterized HNF3β binding sites are in bold text. This drawing is not to scale.*

Area I-, Area II-, and Area III-driven β-galactosidase transgenic reporter constructs are presently being analyzed to determine if these distinct sequence domains independently contribute to HSS1 activation during different developmental stages or in particular cell types. In addition, to test if the evolutionarily conserved sequences within Areas I, II, and III are essential for function in β-cells, mutations within these segments will be constructed and their effect on subregion activation analyzed in transfected β-cell lines. Of particular interest are the HNF1α, HNF1β, and HNF4α binding sites within Area I (Figure 3), since these factors are mutated in families with MODY (33,34,35). We and others have proposed that HNF3β may also be a MODY gene, as a result of this factor's ability to regulate many key metabolic processes in β-cells (37,42,53). This raises the possibility that mutations within the HNF1α, HNF1β, HNF3β, and HNF4α genes may compromise insulin synthesis and β-cell function through direct effects on *pdx-1* expression.

The significant sequence identity within HSS1 strongly suggests that valuable information regarding the *cis*-regulatory elements controlling *pdx-1* transcription activation can be obtained by introducing mutations within these segments. These results should provide the framework to define the binding properties and distribution of the activator for a particular control element. If a previously analyzed factor(s) can be identified from these characteristics, then the cognate cDNA, antisera, and activator-null mutant mice can be utilized to determine the precise role the activator plays in pancreatic development and islet function. However, it is also likely that the binding factor for a particular HSS1 region control element will not be a previously characterized activator. Several established protocols can be used to isolate novel DNA binding proteins, including the yeast one hybrid system (71) and λ expression library screening (72,73). In addition, direct biochemical purification of a factor can also be considered from the relatively rare islet β-cell, since the availability of expressed sequence tag information on the majority of the mouse genome means that very little purified protein is required for amino acid sequence and subsequent factor identification. DNA affinity based chromatography strategies have been established and successfully utilized during the isolation of a number of transcription factors (74-76).

PERSPECTIVES

PDX-1 regulates key pathways in pancreatic development and maintenance of the mature β-cell phenotype (1,4-9,11-15,28,77). Upstream regulatory regions of the *pdx-1* gene, conserved through evolution (42,43,52,53), may control many aspects of expression during pancreatic development and in the adult β-cell. Ongoing characterization of the functional elements and their *trans*-acting binding proteins will not only expand the understanding of *pdx-1* gene regulation but will also provide new insights into the mechanisms that confer pancreatic and β-cell identity.

Identification of specific *cis*-elements in the *pdx-1* gene has been facilitated by sequence comparisons across species and subsequent correlation of the conserved regions with *pdx-1*-reporter activity in β-cells. The data obtained from such experiments must also be validated by *in vivo* techniques, such as transgenic analysis, since the degree to which the transformed β-cell lines represent normal islet cells is unclear. In addition, these *in vivo* assays will aid in the dissection of sequences that direct activity in distinct *pdx-1* expressing tissues such as the duodenum and endocrine pancreas. The deletion of critical control regions (or elements), conducted by gene targeting of the endogenous *pdx-1* locus would allow the overall impact of the –6200/–5700 bp and -2560/-1880 bp regions to be broadly assessed. Characterizing the β-cell-enriched factors that mediate selective expression through their elements will be an essential component of this study.

The systematic approach, based on standard molecular biology techniques, outlined in this review provides a template for the study of other transcription factors involved in pancreatic differentiation and function. Many transcription factors that control β-cell specific end-product genes, such as insulin, have subsequently been found to have essential roles in pancreogenesis. For example, "knock-out" of the BETA2/NeuroD1 gene results in a severe loss of islet mass (57). Mice carrying a mutation in the gene for PAX6, another insulin gene regulator (67), display a decrease in all islet α-cells as well as greatly disrupted islet morphology (68). In addition, many transcription factors contribute to pancreatic pathology as evidenced by their identification as MODY genes. Continued efforts to define the transcription regulatory cascades that operate in the β-cell by analyzing the control of the transcription factor genes themselves, is a vital, and attainable, research goal.

Increased understanding of pancreatic development, islet differentiation, and mature β-cell function may eventually lead to the development of new therapeutic treatments for diabetes. For example, β-cell mass is reduced in both type 1 and type 2 diabetes (19,78) due to an imbalance between the rates of β cell neogenesis/proliferation and apoptosis (20). Manipulating the expression of important transcription factors that regulate cellular regeneration may allow the engineering of pancreatic cells *in vitro* for transplantation into patients. Before attempting such therapies, the regulation of these transcription factors under various physiological situations, such as embryonic development, must be understood. Analyzing the impact of removing pancreatic regulatory factors, individually or in combination, from the genome will provide information relevant to the design of such cells. In addition, assessing the role of extracellular influences (e.g. extracellular matrix, cell-cell interactions, hormones) in the function of pancreatic transcription factor networks will be critical for growing transplantable β-cells in culture. Studying the expression of the *pdx-1* gene not only increases our understanding of the role of this critical factor in pancreatic physiology but also advances the discovery of additional transcription factors that coordinately direct β-cell function and identity. Ultimately, the knowledge gained from this research will contribute to the effective management, and possibly to the cure, of a significant human health risk, diabetes mellitus.

ACKNOWLEDGEMENTS

This work was supported by National Institutes of Health grants NIH RO1 DK50203 (to R.S.) and NIH P01 DK42502 (to C.V.E.W.). Partial support was also derived from the Vanderbilt University Diabetes Research and Training Center Molecular Biology Core Laboratory (Public Health Service grant P60 DK20593 from the National Institutes of Health). S.S. is supported by a post-doctoral fellowship from the Juvenile Diabetes Foundation (Number 398212).

REFERENCES

1. Ohlsson H, Karlson K, Edlund T. IPF-1, a homeodomain-containing transactivator of the insulin gene. EMBO J 1993;12:4251-4259.
2. Guz Y, Montminy MR, Stein R, Leonard J, Gamer LW, Wright CVE, Teitelman G. Expression of murine STF-1, a putative insulin gene transcription factor, in β cells of pancreas, duodenal epithelium and pancreatic exocrine and endocrine progenitors during ontogeny. Development 1995;121:11-18.
3. Ahlgren U, Jonsson J, Edlund H. The morphogenesis of the pancreatic mesenchyme is uncoupled from that of the pancreatic epithelium in IPF1/PDX-1 deficient mice. Development 1996;122:1409-1416.
4. Jonsson J, Carlson L, Edlund T, Edlund H. Insulin promoter factor is required for pancreas development in mice. Nature 1994;371:606-609.
5. Offield MF, Jetton TL, Labosky PA, Ray M, Stein R, Magnuson MA, Hogan BLM, Wright CVE. PDX-1 is required for pancreatic outgrowth and differentiation of the rostral duodenum. Development 1996;122:983-995.

6. Stoffers DA, Zinkin NT, Stanojevic V, Clarke WL, Habener JF. Pancreatic agenesis attributable to a single nucleotide deletion in the human IPF1 coding sequence. Nature Genetics 1997;15:106-110.
7. Peshavaria M, Gamer L, Henderson E, Teitelman G, Wright CVE, Stein R. XIHBox8, and endoderm-specific Xenopus homeodomain protein, is closely related to a mammalian insulin gene transcription factor. Mol Endocrinol 1994;8:806-816.
8. Peers B, Leonard J, Sharma S, Teitelman G, Montminy MR. Insulin expression in pancreatic islet cells relies on cooperative interactions between the helix-loop-helix factor E47 and homeobox factor STF-1. Mol Endocrinol 1995;8:1798-1806.
9. Petersen HV, Serup P, Leonard J, Michelsen BK, Madsen OD. Transcriptional regulation of the human insulin gene is dependent on the homeodomain proteins STF1/IPF1 acting through CT boxes. Proc Natl Acad Sci, USA 1994;91:10465-10469.
10. Watada H, Kajimoto Y, Miyagawa J, et al. PDX-1 induces insulin and glucokinase gene expressions in alphaTC1 clone 6 cells in the presence of betacellulin. Diabetes 1996;45:1826-31.
11. Bretherton-Watt D, Gore N, Boam DSW. Insulin upstream factor 1 and a novel ubiquitous factor bind to the human islet amyloid polypeptide/amylin gene promoter. Biochem J 1996;313:495-502.
12. Carty MD, Lilliquist JS, Peshavaria M, Stein R, Soeller WC. Identification of cis and trans-active factors regulating islet amyloid polypeptide expression in pancreatic β cells. J Biol Chem 1997;272:11986-11993.
13. Serup P, Jensen J, Andersen FG, Jorgensen MC, Blume N, Holst JJ, Madsen OD. Induction of insulin and islet amyloid polypeptide production in pancreatic islet glucagonoma cells by insulin promoter factor 1. Proc Natl Acad Sci, USA 1996;93:9015-9020.
14. Watada H, Kajimoto Y, Kaneto H, Matsuoka T, Fujitani Y, Miyazaki J, and Yamasaki Y. Involvement of the homeodomain-containing transcription factor PDX-1 in islet amyloid polypeptide gene transcription. Biochem Biophys Res Commun 1996;229:746-751.
15. Waeber G, Thompson N, Nicod P, Bonny C. Transcriptional activation of the GLUT2 gene by the IPF-1/STF-1/IDX-1 homeobox factor. Mol Endocrinol 1996;10:1327-1334.
16. Dutta S, Bonner-Weir S, Montminy M, Wright CVE. Regulatory factor linked to late-onset diabetes. Nature 1998;392:560.
17. Ahlgren U, Jonsson J, Jonsson L, Simu K, Edlund H. β-cell-specific inactivation of the mouse Ipf-1/Pdx-1 gene results in loss of the β-cell phenotype and maturity onset diabetes. Genes and Dev. 1998;12:1763-1768.
18. Stoffers DA, Ferrer J, Clarke WL, Habener JF. Early-onset type-II diabetes mellitus (MODY4) linked to IPF1. Nature Genetics 1997;17:138-139.
19. Kloppel G, Lohr M, Habich K, Oberholzer M, Heitz PU. Islet pathology and the pathogenesis of type 1 and type 2 diabetes mellitus revisited. Surv Synth Pathol Res 1985;4:110-125.
20. Finegood DT, Scagli L, Bonner-Weir S. Dynamics of β cell mass in the growing rat pancreas; estimation with a simple mathematical model. Diabetes 1995;44:249-256.
21. Fernandes A, King LC, Guz Y, Stein R, Wright CVE, Teitelman G. Differentiation of new insulin-producing cells is induced by injury in adult pancreatic islets. Endocrinology 1997;138:1750-1762.
22. Bonner-Weir S, Baxter LA, Schuppin GT, Smith FE A second pathway for regeneration of adult exocrine and endocrine pancreas: a possible recapitulation of embryonic development. Diabetes 1993;42:1715-1720.
23. Zangen DH, Bonner-Weir S, Lee CH, Latimer JB, Miller CP, Habener JF, Weir G.C. Reduced insulin, GLUT2 and IDX-1 in beta cells after partial pancreatectomy. Diabetes 1997;46:258-264.
24. Sharma A, Zangen DH, Reitz P, Taneja M, Lissauer ME, Miller CP, Weir GC, Habener JF, Bonner-Weir S. The homeodomain protein IDX-1 increases after an early burst of proliferation during pancreatic regeneration. Diabetes 1999;48:507-513.
25. McGarry JD. What if Minkowski had been ageusic? An alternative angle on diabetes. Science 1992;258:766-70.
26. Unger RH. Lipotoxicity in the pathogenesis of obesity-dependent NIDDM. Genetic and clinical implications. Diabetes 1995;44:863-70.
27. Gremlich S, Bonny C, Waeber G, Thorens B. Fatty acids decrease IDX-1 expression in rat pancreatic islets and reduce GLUT2, glucokinase, insulin, and somatostatin levels. J Biol Chem 1997;272:30261-30269.
28. Olson LK, Redmon JB. Towle HC, Robertson R.P. Chronic exposure of HIT cells to high glucose concentrations paradoxically decreases insulin gene transcription and alters binding of insulin gene regulatory protein. J Clin Invest 1993;92:514-519.
29. Tanaka Y, Gleason CE, Tran PO, Harmon JS, Robertson RP. Prevention of glucose toxicity in HIT-T15 cells and Zucker diabetic fatty rats by antioxidants. Proc Natl Acad Sci USA 1999;96:10857-62.
30. Poitout V, Robertson R.P. An integrated view of beta-cell dysfunction in type-II diabetes. Annu Rev Med 1996;47:69-83.
31. Harmon JS, Gleason CE, Tanaka Y, Oseid EA, Hunter-Berger KK, Robertson RP. In vivo prevention of hyperglycemia also prevents glucotoxic effects on PDX-1 and insulin gene expression. Diabetes 1999;48:1995-2000.

32. Hattersley AT. Maturity-onset diabetes of the young: clinical heterogeneity explained by genetic heterogeneity [published erratum appears in Diabet Med 1998 May;15(5):437]. Diabet Med 1998;15:15-24.
33. Yamagata K, Furuta H, Oda N, Kaisaki P, Menzel S, Cox NJ, Fajans SS, Signorini S, Stoffel M, Bell GI. Mutations in hepatic nuclear factor 4 alpha gene in maturity-onset diabetes of the young (MODY1). Nature 1996;384:458-460.
34. Yamagata K, Oda N, Kaisaki PJ, et.al. Mutations in hepatic nuclear factor 1 alpha gene in maturity-onset diabetes of the young (MODY 3). Nature 1996;384:455-458.
35. Horikawa Y, Iwasaki N, Hara M, Furuta H, Hinokio Y, Cockburn BN. Mutation in hepatocyte nuclear factor-1β (TCF2) associated with MODY. Nature Genetics 1997;17:384-385.
36. Tappy L, Dussoix P, Iynedjian P, Henry S, Schneiter P, Zahnd G, Jequier E, Philippe J. Abnormal regulation of hepatic glucose output in maturity-onset diabetes of the young caused by a specific mutation of the glucokinase gene. Diabetes 1997;46:204-208.
37. Duncan SA, Navas MA, Dufort D, Rossant J, Stoffel M. Regulation of a transcription factor network required for differentiation and metabolism. Science 1998;281:692-695.
38. Wright CVE, Schnegelsberg P, DeRobertis EM. XIHBox8: a novel Xenopus homeoprotein restricted to a narrow band of endoderm. Development 1989;105:787-794.
39. Gamer L, Wright CVE. Autonomous endodermal determination on *Xenopus* : Regulation of expression of the pancreatic gene XIHBox8. Dev Biol 1995;171:240-251.
40. Miller CP, McGehee RE, Habener JF. IDX-1: a new homeodomain transcription factor expressed in rat pancreatic islets and duodenum that transactivates the somatostatin gene. EMBO J 1994;13:1145-1156.
41. Kim SK, Hebrok M, Melton DA. Notochord to endoderm signalling is required for pancreas development. Development 1997;124:4243-4252.
42. Wu K-L, Gannon M, Peshavaria M, Offield ME, Henderson EK, Ray M, Marks A, Gamer LW, Wright CVE, Stein R. Hepatocyte nuclear factor 3β is involved in pancreatic β-cell-specific transcription of the pdx-1 gene. Mol Cell Biol 1997;17:6002-6013.
43. Sharma S, Leonard J, Chapman H, Leiter E, Montminy M. Pancreatic islet restricted expression of the homeobox factor STF-1 relies on an E-box motif which binds USF. J Biol Chem 1996;271:2294-2299.
44. Drucker DJ, Philippe J, Jepeal L, Habener JF. Glucagon gene 5'-flanking sequences promote islet cell-specific gene transcription. J Biol Chem. 1987;262:15659-15665.
45. Powers AC, Tedeschi F, Wright KE, Chan JS, Habener JF. Somatostatin gene expression in pancreatic islet cells is directed by cell-specific DNA control elements and DNA-binding proteins. J Biol Chem 1989;264:10048-10056.
46. Cockell M, Stolarczyk D, Frutiger S, Hughes GJ, Hagenbuchle O, Wellauer PK. Binding sites for hepatocyte nuclear factor 3 beta or 3 gamma and pancreas transcription factor 1 are required for efficient expression of the gene encoding pancreatic alpha-amylase. Mol Cell Biol 1995;15:1933-41.
47. Xu W, Murphy LJ. Isolation and characterization of the mouse beta2/neuroD gene promoter. Biochem Biophys Res Commun 1998;247:814-818.
48. Knofler M, Krapp A, Hagenbuchle O, Wellauer PK. Constitutive expression of the gene for the cell-specific p48 DNA-binding subunit of pancreas transcription factor 12 in culture cells is under the control of binding sites for transcription factors Spl and alpha Cbf. J Biol Chem 1996;271:21993-22002.
49. Elgin SCR. The formation and function of DNaseI hypersensitive sites in the process of gene activation. J Biol Chem 1988;263:19259-19262.
50. Felsenfeld G, Boyes J, Chung H, Clark D, Studitsky V. Chromatin structure and gene expression. Proc Natl Acad Sci USA 1996;93:9384-9388.
51. Gross DS, Garrard WT. Nuclease hypersensitive sites in chromatin. Annu Rev Biochem 1988;57:159-197.
52. Sharma S, Jhala US, Johnson T, Fereri K, Leonard J, Montminy MR. Hormonal regulation of an islet-specific enhancer in the pancreatic homeobox gene STF-1. Mol Cell Biol 1997;17:2598-2604.
53. Gerrish K, Gannon M, Shih D, Henderson E, Stoffel M, Wright CVE, Stein R. Pancreatic β cell-specific transcription of the pdx-1 gene: The role of conserved upstream control regions and their HNF3β sites. J boil Chem 2000;275:3485-3492.
54. Zaret KS. Molecular genetics of early liver development. Annu Rev Physiol 1996;58:231-251.
55. Naya FJ, Stellrecht CM, Tsai MJ. Tissue-specific regulation of the insulin gene by a novel basic helix- loop-helix transcription factor. Genes Dev 1995;9:1009-19.
56. Sirito M, Lin Q, Maity T, Sawadogo M. Ubiquitous expression of the 43- and 44-kDa forms of transcription factor USF in mammalian cells. Nucleic Acids Res 1994;22:427-33.
57. Naya FJ, Huang HP, Qiu Y, Mutoh H, DeMaya FJ, Leiter AB, Tsai M-J. Diabetes, defective pancreatic morphogenesis, and abnormal enteroendocrine differentiation in BETA2/NeuroD-deficient mice. Genes Dev. 1997;11:2323-2334.
58. Tronche F, Yaniv M. Liver gene expression. Molecular biology intelligence unit. Austin: CRC Press, 1994:350.

59. Ang S-L, Rossant J. HNF-3β is essential for node and notochord formation in mouse development. Cell 1994;78:561-574.
60. Weinstein DC, Ruiz I, Altaba A, Chen WS, et al. The winged-helix transcription factor HNF-3 beta is required for notochord development in the mouse embryo. Cell 1994;78:575-88.
61. Hussain MA, Lee J, Miller CP, Habener JF. POU domain transcription factor brain 4 confers pancreatic alpha-cell- specific expression of the proglucagon gene through interaction with a novel proximal promoter G1 element. Mol Cell Biol 1997;17:7186-94.
62. Harrison KA, Druey KM, Deguchi Y, Tuscano JM, Kehrl JH. A novel human homeobox gene distantly related to proboscipedia is expressed in lymphoid and pancreatic tissues. J Biol Chem 1994;269:19968-75.
63. Karlsson O, Thor S, Norberg T, Ohlsson H, Edlund T. Insulin gene enhancer binding protein Isl-1 is a member of a novel class of proteins containing both a homeo- and a Cys-His domain. Nature 1990;344:879-82.
64. Sussel L, Kalamaras J, Hartigan-O'Connor DJ, Meneses JJ, Pedeersen RA, Rubenstein JLR German MS. Mice lacking the homeodomain transcription factor Nkx2.2 have diabetes due to arrested differentiation of pancreatic β cells. Development 1998;125:2213-2221.
65. Jensen J, Serup P, Karlsen C, et. al. mRNA profiling of rat islet tumors reveals Nkx 6.1 as a β-cell-specific homeodomain transcription factor. J Biol.Chem 1996;271:18749-18758.
66. Sosa-Pineda B, Chowdhury K, Torres M, Oliver G, Gruss P. The Pax4 gene is essential for differentiation of insulin-producing beta cells in the mammalian pancreas. Nature 1997;386:399-402.
67. Sander M, Neubuser A, Kalamaras J, Ee HC, Martin GR, German MS. Genetic analysis reveals that PAX6 is required for normal transcription of pancreatic hormone genes and islet development. Genes Dev 1997;11:1662-73.
68. St-Onge L, Sosa-Pineda B, Chowdhury K, Mansouri A, Gruss P. Pax6 is required for differentiation of glucagon-producing alpha-cells in mouse pancreas. Nature 1997;387:406-9.
69. Bonny C, Nicod P, Waeber G. IB1, a JIP-1-related nuclear protein present in insulin-secreting cells. J Biol Chem 1998;273:1843-6.
70. Peshavaria M, Henderson E, Sharma A, Wright CVE, Stein R. Functional characterization of the transactivation properties of the PDX-1 homeodomain protein. Mol Cell Biol 1997;17:3987-3996.
71. Li JJ, Herskowitz I. Isolation of ORC6, a component of the yeast origin recognition complex by a one-hybrid system. Science 1993;262:1870-4.
72. Singh H, LeBowitz JH, Baldwin AS, Jr., Sharp PA. Molecular cloning of an enhancer binding protein: isolation by screening of an expression library with a recognition site DNA. Cell 1988;52:415-23.
73. Vinson CR, LaMarco KL, Johnson PF, Landschulz WH, McKnight SL. In situ detection of sequence-specific DNA binding activity specified by a recombinant bacteriophage. Genes Dev 1988;2:801-6.
74. Wang MM, Reed RR. Molecular cloning of the olfactory neuronal transcription factor Olf-1 by genetic selection in yeast. Nature 1993;364:121-126.
75. Cowell IG. Cloning sequence-specific DNA-binding factors from cDNA expression libraries using oligonucleotide binding site probes. Methods Mol Biol 1997;69:161-170.
76. Kadonaga JT. Purification of sequence-specific binding proteins by DNA affinity chromatography. In: Sauer RT, ed. Protein-DNA Interactions. Vol. 208. San Diego: Academic Press, 1991.
77. Watada H, Kajimoto Y, Umayahara Y, Matsuoka T, Kaneto H, Fujitani Y, Kamada T, Kawamori R, Yamasaki Y. The human glucokinase gene β-cell-type promoter: an essential role of IPF-1/PDX-1 in its activation in HIT-T15 cells. Diabetes 1996;45:1478-1488.
78. Clark A, Wells CA, Buley ID, et al. Islet amyloid, increased A-cells, reduced B-cells and exocrine fibrosis: quantitative changes in the pancreas in type 2 diabetes. Diabetes Res 1988;9:151-159.
79. Heinemeyer T, Chen I, Karas H, Kel AE, Kel OV, Leibich I, Meinhardt T, Reuter I, Scherer F, Wingender E. Expanding the TRANSFAC database towards an expert system of regulatory molecular mechanisms. Nucl Acids Res 1999;27:318-322.

17
MECHANISMS OF POSTNATAL β-CELL MASS REGULATION

Susan Bonner-Weir, Ph.D. and Gordon C. Weir, M.D.
Joslin Diabetes Center, Boston, MA 02215, USA

INTRODUCTION

Diabetes results when there is an inadequate functional mass of pancreatic β-cells. In type 1 diabetes immune-mediated destruction of β-cells clearly leaves a markedly reduced β-cell mass, even though as much as 10-20% β-cells can be found in human pancreas after many years of disease (1). In type 2 diabetes, an increased demand for secreted insulin is not met in spite of the presence of β-cell mass that can be near normal. In MODY genetic defects result in impaired β-cell function that appears not to be adequately compensated for by an increase in β-cell mass to maintain glucose homeostasis. Two types of compensation can occur: a functional one in which each β-cell secretes more insulin and a second in which there is change of β-cell mass. Functional adaptations have been shown as changes in threshold for glucose-induced insulin secretion that occurs during pregnancy (2) and glucose-induced increases in glucokinase activity (3). Even so, the major factor in the amount of insulin that can be secreted is the β-cell mass itself. The mass of functional β-cells is dynamic and is regulated to maintain the blood glucose levels in a narrow physiological range. This chapter will describe the mechanisms involved; most of the data have been generated in rodent models but provide insights into what is likely to occur in humans.

PATHWAYS OF FORMATION OF NEW β-CELLS

In embryonic development, β-cells differentiate from pancreatic ducts, a process that is repeated postnatally and is called neogenesis. The cascade of genes expressed during this cell specification process is being defined as described in other chapters of this book. Neogenesis, while clearly the main pathway of β-cell increase during early to mid gestation, still occurs in the normal postnatal animal (4,5) and can be experimentally enhanced (6-11). In the first couple of days after birth, many new islets are formed, and a second wave of neogenesis occurs at about weaning (12). There is evidence that this process continues during adult life, albeit at a slower rate. Numerous experimental models show that neogenesis as well as β-cell replication can be enhanced in the adult rodent. There are no means of determining the rate of neogenesis at present, and even assessment of the presence of neogenesis is difficult. By late fetal stages, replication of the β-cells becomes an important contributor to the expansion of the β-cell mass. Not unexpectedly, both pathways function postnatally even in the adult. The perinatal proliferation rate of β-cells in rodents is high (about 18% at birth) but rapidly drops off during the neonatal period (5,13). Estimates in the 2-4 month old rat suggest a replication rate of just under 3% new β-cells/day.

Further increases in β-cell mass, but without change in cell numbers, occur by increases in cell size, called hypertrophy. This mechanism may have an important role in rapid functional increases. Hypertrophy of β-cells is seen in a variety of rat models: in the last term of pregnancy (12), after 96 hrs of glucose infusion (14); in male ZDF rats (15); in female ZDF rats with impaired GTT (16); in female Zucker lean rats after 48 hrs of dexamethasone (16) and 4 week after partial pancreatectomy (Px) in rats (10,17). This change in cell volume is reversible and may allow a rapid response to changes in insulin demand.

EVIDENCE THAT β-CELL MASS IS DYNAMIC

Lifetime changes in β-cell mass

It is often mentioned that there is a "limited capacity" for β-cell replication after birth. This statement is based on the low replication rate seen in the adult. In fact, in humans the reported replication frequency is extremely low (less than 0.1% labeling for Ki67, a protein expressed through most of the cell cycle, from mid G1 through mitosis) (18-20). However, in rodents, human and cow, the β-cell mass has been shown to increase 12-15 fold from birth to adulthood (5,21,22,24). As seen in rats the β-cell mass is not linear with age but rather has a plateau during the second to third week of life, then linear increase until 10 weeks of age. After the 3-4 month time point, the data have been sparse, but a new longitudinal study (24) shows the addition of new cells account for the increase in β-cell mass through most of the lifespan of rats, but from 15 months onwards hypertrophy of the β-cell was the main mechanism for the expansion of β-cell mass. Analysis of normal mice of the same genetic background found the natural variation in body weight for any age (4 wks to 6 months) and a strong linear correlation of β-cell mass and body weight from 15 to 60 gm (25).

The concept of β-cell turnover

Inherent in the regulation of β-cell mass is the question of β-cell turnover. Apoptosis of β-cells have been shown *in vitro* (26) and *in vivo* during the involution of the β-cell mass in the post partum pancreas (27) and in the normal neonatal rat (13). The normal turnover of β-cells became evident with mathematical modelling of the β-cell mass (5). With almost 3 % per 24 hr (or 0.5% per 6 hrs) replication of β-cells found in the adult rodent pancreas, the β-cell mass could double in about one month. In fact, β-cell mass of Sprague Dawley rats does almost double between 1 to 2, and 2 to 3 months of age, but this monthly doubling does not continue, suggesting a finite lifespan and a normal turnover or loss of β-cells (5). Indeed, in adult (3 month old) rats, the frequency of apoptotic β-cell nuclei was 0.5%. Unfortunately we do not know the <u>rate</u> of apoptosis because there are no data on how long apoptotic β-cell nuclei or bodies are visible *in vivo*; nonetheless visible apoptotic nuclei and bodies are thought to be transient and detectable for less than 4 hrs. If one uses the estimate of 4 hours, then the rate of β-cell apoptosis is nearly equal to that of β-cell replication, resulting in a near steady state of β-cell number. With such a steady state complete replacement of the β-cell population would occur gradually. Thus, the endocrine pancreas should be considered a slowly renewed tissue (5).

Pregnancy

One of the most convincing examples of the dynamic nature of the β-cell mass is the adaptation of β-cells during pregnancy and the subsequent post partum period. During pregnancy there is a 50% increase in β-cell mass, with increased β-cell replication, larger islets and even hypertrophied β-cells (12,28,29). A complex analysis of size and number of islets (using whole mounts) (29) showed a change in size distribution of islets with pregnancy with a shift to larger islets. One of the major stimuli is placental lactogen. With delivery, there are marked changes in the hormonal milieu and decreased demand for insulin. There is a marked involution over the period of lactation that returns the β-cell mass to non-pregnant levels (12,30,31). This involution was achieved by the combination of decreased replication, reduction in cell volume from a hypertrophied state to a transient slightly atrophied one, and an increase of apoptosis of β-cells.

Insulin resistance

Only 20% of those people with severe insulin resistance due to obesity, Cushing's disease, or acromegaly become diabetic, with the other 80% being able to compensate with increased insulin secretion to maintain near normal glycemic levels. While the data for humans is limited, a careful morphometric study of autopsied pancreas from type 2 diabetic and non diabetic patients (24) showed the β-cell mass was about 40% increased in the obese subjects as compared to lean subjects in both the diabetic and non-diabetic, suggesting that there is compensatory growth of β-cell mass with the increasing insulin resistance of obesity. Data supporting the interpretation that insulin resistance drives increased β-cell mass are derived from experiments with mice with a known cause of insulin resistance (32). Mice heterozygous for null deletions of both the insulin receptor and insulin receptor substrate-1 (IRS-1) have marked insulin resistance, but diabetes was not seen until 6 months of age and then only in a portion of the mixed background mice. The mean β-cell mass was 10 fold increased compared to wild type littermates. The β-cell mass increase was selective since that of the non β-endocrine cells of the islets did not differ with wild type littermates. The islets were enlarged and the mantle of non β-cells was disorganized; this phenotype is often seen when there has been increased and sustained replication of β-cells. Some mice that were extremely insulin resistant (plasma insulin levels 26 fold increased over WT) had up to 30 fold increased β-cell mass; paradoxically these were the ones with diabetes. The mixed background of these mice may contribute other genetic factors that modulate the compensatory response.

Challenge with glucose infusions

The glucose-infused rat has served as an important model for understanding β-cell compensation (14,33,34). After 96 hours infusion a 50 % increase in β-cell mass was seen; the β-cell replication was increased 5 fold and cell volume was increased 50% (14). In re-analysis of the data, it would seem that most of the new tissue was from hypertrophy. The cell number as estimated by dividing the β-cell mass by the mean cell volume did not differ between saline- and 50% glucose-infused rats at 96 hr and increased replication was not seen before 72 hr. The involution of β-cell mass after stopping the infusions was slow, β-cell mass had not normalized at 7 days but had by 30 days. More recent studies by Bernard et al. (35) analyzed β-cell compensation in the first 48 hr after glucose infusion. They report a similar increase of β-cell mass by 24 hr as we did at 96 hr. There seemed to be a conservation of cells in that at both 24 and 48 hr the incidence of apoptotic β-cells were decreased (from a basal 0.4% to 0.2%). At 24 hr replication was decreased, which suggests to us that the demand for function with increased insulin secretion occurred at the expense of proliferation. Surprisingly no increase in β-cell size was seen until 48 hr; neogenesis was suggested to be the source of the rapid increase in β-cell mass, but it seems unlikely to us that neogenesis could occur so rapidly. Additionally, if an estimation of β-cell number is made with their data, there was no change of cell number between saline and 48 hr glucose-infused normal rats, but there was a discrepant increase at 24 hr. Further analysis of whether hypertrophy is seen sooner than 48 hr remains to be done.

Zucker Diabetic Fatty rats

Another example of the varied mechanisms of compensation and expansion of the β-cell mass in the adult rodent is the Zucker Diabetic Fatty (ZDF) rat. There is one colony (GMI) of Zucker Fatty (fa/fa) rats in which the male rats become diabetic (at about 9 weeks of age) but the female rats are compensated and have only slightly impaired glucose tolerance. As shown in the prediabetic 6 wk old ZDF male rats, there is an intrinsic defect in the β-cells of this colony as compared to either their lean littermates or the non-diabetic Zucker Fatty rats from other colonies (15). Both male and female ZDF at 12 wks of age (15,16) had increased body weight and increased β-cell mass as compared to the lean littermates (fa^+/fa^- or fa^+/ fa^+). Both the β-cell size and replication were increased compared to the lean animals. In experiments to challenge the compensatory ability of these rats, dexamethasone was given once a day for 2 days (16). Dexamethasone has been shown to increase peripheral insulin resistance and to have direct effects on the β-cell itself. After 48 hrs treatment, lean Zucker females had increased β-cell mass, due to β-cell hypertrophy and increased replication. In contrast, the ZDF females that had been adequately compensated before treatment became frankly diabetic. Their already hypertrophied β-cells did not increase any further in size; their replication was enhanced but due to increased apoptosis, the β-cell mass did not increase. These data suggest that hypertrophy may provide a benefit in terms of increased insulin secretion, but be detrimental in terms of vulnerability to stress such as glucocorticoids. In muscle and renal tissue, hypertrophy has been seen as a rapid response to increased demand, with an arrest in G1 of the cell cycle (36,37). This arrest allows a sustained amplification of gene expression without completing the cell cycle. However, in other tissues hypertrophy has been seen as an early compensatory mechanism that may eventually progress to loss of functioning tissue (38).

REGULATION OF β CELL RENEWAL

β-cell replication has been shown to be stimulated by many factors (growth hormone/prolactin, GLP-1/exendin-4, IGF-I, HGF etc), but glucose is perhaps the best stimulus for β-cell replication *in vitro* and *in vivo* (14,39). In fact, glucose may be the driving force for most β-cell compensation: as glucose uptake by peripheral tissues is diminished by inadequate plasma insulin levels or increased insulin resistance, transient post-prandial hyperglycemic excursions and even modest increases in fasting glucose levels could occur. This mild hyperglycaemia could signal the β-cells that more insulin is needed, leading to compensation with enhanced function as well as increased β-cell replication and cell size. While transient or mild hyperglycaemia may be beneficial to β-cell function, it is clear that chronic or severe hyperglycaemia has a detrimental influence. There are a number of secondary effects of a chronic glycemic environment including the loss of glucose induced insulin secretion (40) and even loss of β-cell differentiation (17). Sometimes even a modest degree of chronic hyperglycaemia can lead to a loss of glucose induced insulin secretion. It must be remembered that a factor does not have to act directly on the β-cell to affect the β-cell mass, an indirect effect that results in transient mild hyperglycaemia can affect the β-cell mass; this should be kept in mind when interpreting the results of transgenic and knock out mice.

β-cell replication

The low proliferation rate of β-cells allows for a slow turnover; the importance of the postnata' proliferation of differentiated β-cells must not be underestimated. It is clear that the replicating cells are truly β-cells: both incorporated bromodeoxyuridine and tritiated thymidine have been localized to cells immunolabelled for insulin, and numerous images of mitotic figures in cells with insulin granules have been published. There still may be differences in function in β-cells that can replicate compared with those that cannot, but such differences have yet to be proven. Such differences may be a matter of differences in pools (replicative versus senescent) or alternatively, those β-cells that replicate may transiently lose function as they replicate.

Neogenesis

Neogenesis of islet tissue originates in mature adult pancreatic ducts. Insulin producing β-cells have been described as comprising only 0.1% of the ductal cells (41). Increased islet budding with some human diseases, such as recent onset of type 1 diabetes and severe liver disease (42) has been reported. In addition, newly formed or budding islets have been found in a number of experimental conditions, including dietary treatment with soybean trypsin inhibitor (6), over-expression of γ-interferon in the β-cells of transgenic mice (7), after partial pancreatectomy (9), after cellophane wrapping of the head of the pancreas (8), after GLP-1/exendin-4 treatment (10) and after ductal ligation (11). A critical question is what induces the differentiation of these cells *in vivo*? When embryonic pancreatic buds are studied *in vitro*, it is found that without mesenchymal tissue, endocrine cells develop in preference to acinar cells; however, with mesenchyme, there was growth of the bud and differentiation of acinar cells (43,44). Thus, islet, in particular β-cell, differentiation has been suggested as the "default pathway" of embryonic pancreatic development (44). An extract from chick embryonic tissue rich in mesenchyme was able to replace the requirement for endogenous mesenchyme for growth and differentiation, but the factors involved have not yet been defined (43). In other systems, the regulation of cellular growth and differentiation has focused on peptide growth factors, their receptors, proto-oncogenes and epithelial-mesenchymal interactions (45,46). An important message from these studies is that the regulation of growth arises from a sequential expression of different growth factors and from differential responses of multiple receptors. Some interactions are dependent on cell-cell contact or cell-extracellular matrix contacts, but there is also considerable evidence for soluble factors.

Neogenesis in adult life: Search for a stem cell

An important question for neogenesis is what cells in the adult have the multipotency to become any or all pancreatic cell types. Our concepts of what is possible have expanded with the demonstration that bone marrow derived stem cells can differentiate into hepatic cells (47). Additionally precursor cells may be the equivalent to the "oval cells" as have been defined in the liver (48,49). Our data suggest that oval or true stem cells are very few, if present at all, in the normal rat pancreas and that neither type of stem cell are not involved in the massive regeneration after partial pancreatectomy (50). The likely source of precursor cells would be the pancreatic ducts since the adult duct epithelium retains the ability to give rise to all the differentiated cell types of the pancreas. In the normal adult pancreas, the ducts are quiescent, being restrained by local factors. If the ducts are isolated from their stroma and put into primary culture, the ducts proliferate extensively showing considerable potential for expansion. Such findings suggest that local effects of matrix components and soluble factors, with TGFβ being a prime candidate, restrict ductal expansion *in vivo*. Separate sets of stimuli lead to expansion of the ductal population by proliferation and to differentiation to the mature phenotypes of endocrine, acinar and duct cells. In the regeneration that occurs after partial pancreatectomy there is a rapid expansion of the duct cells. As they replicate, the duct cells transiently expressed the transcription factor PDX-1/IDX-1 (51). This protein is expressed in the embryonic pancreatic ducts but is repressed in the ducts shortly before birth. We hypothesize that a mature duct cell with rapid replication can transiently regain a less differentiated, and less restricted, phenotype (51). External stimuli, whether soluble factors or matrix components, can then direct differentiation of these multipotent cells to endocrine, acinar or mature duct phenotypes.

Hypertrophy

Hypertrophy has been recognized in many models but the regulation of hypertrophy of β-cells is only now being studied (10,14,17). An increase in cell size without replication could be an efficient and economical mechanism for rapid and transient compensation. After stimulation the earliest that we have seen hypertrophy of β-cells was at 48 hours in the Zucker lean female rats treated with dexamethasone (16), but we have not looked at earlier timepoints. The development of β-cell hypertrophy for increase in β-cell mass in old rats suggests that this mechanism is very important for maintaining glucose homeostasis as these old rats continue to gain weight (24).

Hypertrophy has been well studied in kidney (36-38,52,53), cardiac muscle (54,55) and vascular smooth muscle (56). The mechanisms of hypertrophy seem to differ with tissues but all involve cell cycle kinase inhibitors (cdks) that interfere with the normal progression of the cell cycle from G1 to S. The combination of initiating G1 associated cell growth (protein synthesis) and the prevention of DNA synthesis leads to cellular hypertrophy. In cultured vascular smooth muscle cells angiotensin II can have differential response, resulting in either hyperplasia or hypertrophy (56); in both there was upregulation of cyclin D1, cdk2, and PCNA proteins. In hypertrophy, p27 levels remained high and activation of cdk2 was inhibited, while in hyperplasia the p 27 levels were low, and activation of cdk2 and S phase proceeded. In cardiac muscle hypertrophy, p38 has been implicated (54,55). Since the cells are arrested in G1, hypertrophy can allow a sustained amplification of gene expression (57). However, as a downside of this arrest in G1, the cells may be more vulnerable to apoptosis (58).

Although β-cell hypertrophy in old age and in other situations with increased β-cell demand do not usually lead to decompensation, there are examples where striking rapid failure does occur. The two clear examples of rapid loss of β-cells are the db/db mouse on the C57/Ks background (59) and the desert sand rat (*Psammomys obesus*) (60). However, it is unclear if these rodents have hypertrophied β-cells before their rapid decompensation or involution. We do know that in 4 wk pancreatectomized rats and in ZDF female rats hypertrophy is the response to a sustained hyperglycemic environment; these animals can maintain a stable physiological state with only slightly to moderately impaired glucose tolerance. It may be that they adapted to a gradual exposure of hyperglycaemia. In fact, the 4 wk Px rats have induction of a variety of stress/survival genes (anti-oxidants: heme-oxygenase, Mn-superoxide dismutase, glutathione peroxidase; Fas, A20) possibly allowing the cells to avoid apoptosis (61). It will be important to determine how the β-cells of some animals can successfully adapt to increased demand while those of others rapidly decompensate.

SUMMARY

Experimental paradigms have shown that, *in vivo*, the mass of pancreatic β-cells is dynamic and can be regulated in an effort to maintain euglycaemia. Impressive compensatory growth of the β-cell mass is found in transgenic mice with insulin resistance of defined cause, in Zucker fatty rats and during pregnancy. Inherent in the regulation of β-cell mass is β-cell turnover: the functional mass is maintained by a balance of cell death and cell renewal. The two mechanisms of β-cell renewal, neogenesis (differentiation from ductal precursor cells) and replication of differentiated β-cells, are maintained from the embryo in the postnatal animal. An additional mechanism for increasing β-cell mass is the development of hypertrophy (increase in cell volume). While this mechanism does not change the number of β-cells, it seems to be a common and rapid response to increased demand that leads to increased insulin secretion.

ACKNOWLEDGEMENTS

The authors thank the many scientists who have worked in our laboratory and contributed to the body of work presented here; additionally we thank our collaborators who shared ideas, reagents and precious mice. The research was funded directly by grants from the NIH (DK 35449 and DK 44523).

REFERENCES

1. Pipeleers D and Ling Z. Pancreatic beta cells in insulin-dependent diabetes. Diabetes Metab Rev 1992;8:209-227.
2. Sorenson, RL, Brelje TC, Hegre OD, Marshal S, Anaya P, and Sheridan JD. Prolactin (in vitro) decreases the glucose stimulation, enhances insulin secretion and increases dye coupling among islet β-cells. Endocrinology 1987;121:1447-1453.
3. Chen C, Hosokawa H, Bumbalo LM, and Leahy JL. Regulatory effects of glucose on the catalytic activity and cellular content of glucokinase in the pancreatic β-cell. J Clin Invest 1994;94:1616-1620.
4. Hellerstrom C, Swenne I, and Andersson A. Islet cell replication and diabetes. In The Pathology of the Endocrine Pancreas in Diabetes. P. J. Lefebvre and D. G. Pipeleers, editors. Heidelberg, F.R.G., Springer-Verlag 1988;141-170.
5. Finegood DT, Scaglia L, and Bonner-Weir S. (Perspective) Dynamics of β-cell mass in the growing rat pancreas: estimation with a simple mathematical model. Diabetes 1995;44:249-256.
6. Weaver CV, Sorenson RL, and Kaung HC. Immunocytochemical localization of insulin-immunoreactive cells in the ducts of rats treated with trypsin inhibitor. Diabetologia 1985;28:781-785.
7. Sarvetnick N, Shizuru J, Liggitt D, Martin L, McIntyre B, Gregory A, Parslow T, and Stewart T. Loss of pancreatic islet tolerance induced by beta cell expression of IFN-gamma. Nature 1990;346:844-847.
8. Rosenberg LA, Brown RA, and Duguid WP. A new approach to the induction of duct epithelial hyperplasia and nesidoblastosis by cellophane wrapping of the hamster pancreas. J Surg Res 1983;35:63-72.
9. Bonner-Weir S, Baxter LA, Schuppin GT, and Smith FE. A second pathway for regeneration of the adult exocrine and endocrine pancreas: A possible recapitulation of embryonic development. Diabetes 1993;42:1715-1720.
10. Xu G, Stoffers DA, Habener JF, and Bonner-Weir S. Exendin-4 stimulates both β-cell replication and neogenesis, resulting in increased β-cell mass and improved glucose tolerance in diabetic rats. Diabetes 1999;48:2270-2276.
11. Walker NI, Winterford CM, and Kerr JFR. Ultrastructure of the rat pancreas after experimental duct ligation. II. Duct and stromal cell proliferation, differentiation, and deletion. Pancreas 1992;7:420-434.
12. Scaglia L, Smith FE, and Bonner-Weir S. . Apoptosis contributes to the involution of β-cell mass in the post partum rat pancreas. Endocrinology 1995;136:5461-5468.

13. Scaglia L, Cahill CJ, Finegood DT, and Bonner-Weir S. Apoptosis participates in the remodelling of the endocrine pancreas in the neonatal rat. Endocrinol 1997;138:1736-1741.
14. Bonner-Weir S, Deery D, Leahy JL, and Weir GC. Compensatory growth of pancreatic β-cells in adult rats after short-term glucose infusion. Diabetes 1989;38:49-53.
15. Pick A, Clark J, Kubstrup C, Pugh W, Bonner-Weir S, and Polonsky K. Role of apoptosis in failure of β-cell mass compensation for insulin resistance and β-cell defects in the male Zucker diabetic fatty (ZDF) rat. Diabetes 1998;47:358-364.
16. Pick A, Levisetti M, Baldwin A, and Bonner-Weir S. Failure of β-cell mass compensation for insulin resistance in dexamethasone induced diabetes in female Zucker diabetic fatty (ZDF) rats. *Diabetes* 1998;47 Suppl 1:A258.
17. Jonas J-C, Sharma A, Hasenkamp W, Ilkova H, Patane G, Laybutt R, Bonner-Weir S, and Weir GC. Chronic hyperglycaemia triggers loss of pancreatic β-cell differentiation in an animal model of diabetes. J Biol Chem 1999;274:14112-14121.
18. Wolf G. Molecular mechanisms of renal hypertrophy: role of $p27^{Kip1}$. Kidney Int. 1999;56:1262-1265.
19. Bouwens L, Lu WG, and Krijger RD. Proliferation and differentiation in the human fetal endocrine pancreas. Diabetologia 1997;40:398-404.
20. Bouwens L and Pipeleers DG. Extra-insular beta cells associated with ductules are frequent in adult human pancreas. Diabetologia 1998;41:629-633.
21. Lefebvre V, Otonkoski T, Ustinov J, Huotari M, Pipeleers D, and Bouwens L. Culture of adult human islet preparations with hepatocyte growth factor and 804G matrix is mitogenic for duct cells but not for beta-cells. Diabetes 1998;47:134-137.
22. Kaung H-LC. Growth dynamics of pancreatic islet cell populations during fetal and neonatal development of the rat. Dev Dyn 1994;200:163-175.
23. Kloppel G, Lohr M, Habich K, Oberholzer M, and Heitz PU. Islet pathology and the pathogenesis of type 1 and type 2 diabetes mellitus revisited. Surv Synth Pathol Res 1985;4:110-125.
24. Bonner-Weir S and Like, AA. A dual islet population in bovine pancreas. Cell Tissue Res 1980;206:157-170.
25. Montanya E, Nacher V, Biarnes M, and Soler J. Linear correlation between beta cell mass and body weight throughout life in Lewis rats: role of beta cell hyperplasia and hypertrophy. Diabetes 2000;49:(In Press)
26. Bonner-Weir S. Islet growth and development in the adult. J Mol Endocrinol 2000;24:1-6.
27. Rabinovitch A, Suarez-Pinzon WL, Shi Y, Morgan AR, and Bleackley RC. DNA fragmentation s an early event in cytokine-induced islet beta-cell destruction. Diabetologia 1994;37:733-738.
28. Ledda-Columbano GM, Columbano A, Coni P, Fao G, and Pani P. Cell deletion by apoptosis during regression of renal hyperplasia. Am J Physiol 1989;135:657-662.
29. Parsons JA, Brelje TC, and Sorenson RL. Adaptation of islets to pregnancy: Increased islet cell proliferation and insulin secretion correlates with the onset of placental lactogen secretion. Endocrinology 1992;130:1459-1466.
30. Parsons JA, Bartke A, and Sorenson RL. Number and size of islets of Langerhans in pregnant human growth hormone-expressing transgenic, and pituitary dwarf mice: effect of lactogenic hormones. Endocrinology 1995;136:2013-2021.
31. Marynissen G, Aerts l, and Van Assche FA. The endocrine pancreas during pregnancy and lactation in the rat. J Devel Physiol 1983;5:373-381.
32. Marynissen G, Malaisse WJ, and Van Assche FA. Influence of lactation on morphometric and secretory variables in pancreatic β-cell of mildly diabetic rats. Diabetes 1987;36:883-891.
33. Bruning JC, Winnay J, Bonner-Weir S, Taylor SI, Accili D, and Kahn CR. Development of a novel polygenic model of NIDDM in mice heterozygous for IR and IRS-1 null alleles. Cell 1999;88:561-572.
34. Bonner-Weir S, Leahy JL, and Weir GC. Induced rat models of non-insulin-dependent diabetes mellitus. In Lessons from Animal Diabetes II. E. Shapiro and A. E. Renold, editors. John Libbey, London. 1998;295-300.
35. Leahy JL, Cooper HE, and Weir GC. Impaired insulin secretion associated with near normoglycaemia: study in normal rats with 96-h in in vivo glucose infusions. Diabetes 1987;36:459-464.
36. Bernard C, Berthault M-F, Saulnier C, and Ktorza A. Neogenesis vs. apoptosis as main components of pancreatic β-cell mass changes in glucose-infused normal and mildly diabetic adult rats. FASEB J 1999;13:1195-1205.
37. Preisig P. What makes cells grow larger and how do they do it? Exp Nephrol 1999;7:273-283.
38. Franch HA, Shay JW, Alpern RJ, and Preisig PA. Involvement of pRB family in TGF β-dependent epithelial cell hypertrophy. J Cell Biol 1995;129:245-254.
39. Bonner-Weir S. and Smith FE. Islet cell growth and the growth factors involved. Trends Endocrinol Meta 1994;5:60-64.
40. Leahy JL, Bonner-Weir S, and Weir GC. β-cell dysfunction induced by chronic hyperglycaemia: Current ideas on mechanism of impaired glucose-induced insulin secretion. Diabetes Care 1992;15:442.

41. Madden ME and Sarras, Jr MP. The pancreatic ductal system of the rat: cell diversity, ultrastructure, and innervation. Pancreas 1989;4:472-485.
42. Gepts W. Pathological anatomy of the pancreas in juvenile diabetes. Diabetes 1965;14:619-633.
43. Rutter WJ, Pictet RL, Harding JD, Chirgwin JM, MacDonald RJ, and Przybyla AE. An analysis of pancreatic development: Role of mesenchymal factor and other extracellular factors. Sym Soc Dev Biol 1978;35:205-207.
44. Gittes GK, Galante PE, Hanahan D, Rutter WJ, and Debase HT. Lineage-specific morphogenesis in the developing pancrease: role of mesenchymal factors. Development 1996;122:439-447.
45. Michalopoulos GK. Liver regeneration: molecular mechanisms of growth control. FASEB J 1990;4:176-187.
46. Streuli CH. Extracellular matrix remodelling and cellular differentiation. Current Opin Cell Biol 1999;11:634-640.
47. Petersen BE, Bowen WC, Patrene KD, Mars WM, Sullivan AK, Murase N, Boggs SS, Greenberger JS, and Goff JP. Bone marrow as a potential source of hepatic oval cells. Science 1999;284:1168-1170.
48. Farber E. The multistep nature of cancer development. Cancer Res 1984;44:4217-4223.
49. Evarts RP, Nagy P, Marsden E, and Thorgeirsson SS. A precursor-product relationship exists between oval cells and hepatocytes in rat liver. Carcinogenesis 1987;8:1737-1740.
50. Bonner-Weir S, Stubbs M, Reitz P, Taneja M, and Smith FE. Partial pancreatectomy as a model of pancreatic regeneration. In Pancreatic Growth and Regeneration. N. Sarvetnick, editor. Karger Landes Systems, 1997;138-153.
51. Sharma A, Zangen DH, Reitz P, Taneja M, Lissauer ME, Miller CP, Weir GC, Habener JF, and Bonner-Weir S. The homeodomain protein IDX-1 increases after an early burst of proliferation during pancreatic regeneration. Diabetes 1999;48:507-513.
52. Wolf G, Schroeder R, Ziyadeh FN, Thaiss F, Zahner G, and Stahl RAK. High glucose stimulates expression of $P27^{Kip1}$ in cultured mouse mesangial cells: relationship to hypertrophy. Am J Physiol 1997;42:F348-F356.
53. Preisig P. A cell cycle-dependent mechanism of renal tubule epithelial cell hypertrophy. Kidney Int 1999;56:1193-1198.
54. Wang Y, Huang S, Sah VP, Ross Jr J, Brown JH, Hans J, and Chien KR. Cardiac muscle cellhypertrophy and apoptosis induced by distinct members of the p38 mitogen-activated protein kinase family. J Biol Chem 1998;273:2161-2168.
55. Hunter JJ and Chien KR. Signalling pathways for cardiac hypertrophy and failure. N Engl J Med 1999;341:1276-1283.
56. Braun-Dullaeus RC, Mann MJ, Ziegler A, von der Leyen HE, and Dzau VJ. A novel role for the cyclin-dependent kinase inhibitor p27(kip1) in angiotensin II-stimulated vascular smooth muscle cell hypertrophy. J Clin Invest 1999;104:815-823.
57. Norman JT, Bohman RE, Fischmann G, Bowen JW, McDonough A, Slamon D, and Fine LG. Patterns of mRNA expression during early cell growth differ in kidney epithelial cells destined to undergo compensatory hypertrophy versus regenerative hyperplasia. Proc Natl Acad Sci USA 1998;85:6768-6772.
58. Evan GI, Wyllie AH, Gilbert CS, Littlewood TD, Land H, Brooks M, Waters CM, Penn LZ, and Hancock DC. Induction of apoptosis in fibroblasts by c-myc protein. Cell 1992;69:119-128.
59. Leiter EH, Gapp DA, Eppig JJ, and Coleman DL. Ultrastructural and morphometric studies of delta cells in pancreatic islets from C57BL/Ks diabetes mice. Diabetologia 1979;17:297-309.
60. Gross DJ, Leibowitz G, Cerasi E, and Kaiser N. Increased susceptibility of islets from diabetes-prone psammomys obesus to the delterious effects of chronic glucose exposure. Endocrinol 1996;137:5610-5615.
61. Laybutt DR, Hasenkamp W, Groff A, Jonas J-C, Kaneto H, Grey S, Ferran C, Sharma A, Bonner-Weir S, and Weir GC. Activation of protective and destructive stress genes accompanies beta cell hypertrophy in hyperglycemic rats. Diabetes 2000;49:Suppl 1:(In Press)

18

GENETIC MODELS OF INSULIN RESISTANCE: ALTERATIONS IN β-CELL BIOLOGY

Rohit N. Kulkarni M.D. Ph.D. and C. Ronald Kahn M.D.
Joslin Diabetes Center and Department of Medicine, Harvard Medical School, One Joslin Place, Boston, MA 02215 USA

INTRODUCTION

One of the essential biological actions of insulin in mammals is the maintenance of euglycaemia. This is a complex process and involves the uptake, storage and oxidation of glucose in skeletal muscle and adipose tissues, as well as the suppression of hepatic glucose production. A significant blunting of these actions in spite of the presence of normal or even high circulating levels of insulin indicates the presence of an "insulin resistant" phenotype. A variety of pathological states including type 2 diabetes, obesity, hypertension, atherosclerosis and polycystic ovary disease are characterized by the presence of insulin resistance (1-6). In the case of type 2 diabetes it is generally accepted that insulin resistance must be accompanied by a β-cell defect for the full development of the disease. Although there is some debate as to which of these two defects is primary, longitudinal studies in several populations suggest that insulin resistance may be the first defect to be detected (2,7,8). The early insulin resistance observed in pre-diabetic individuals is initially compensated by an increase in insulin secretion by the islet β-cells that could represent either an enhanced secretory capacity or an increased islet/β-cell mass or a combination of both. Over a period of time, however, the β-cell compensation fails leading to uncontrolled hyperglycaemia and overt diabetes.

The number of functional β-cells is a critical determinant of the insulin secreting capacity of the pancreas. A notable and consistent feature in several rodent models of type 2 diabetes is the presence of islet hyperplasia ranging from mild to massive increases in β-cell mass (9-15). Several nutrient and hormonal factors including glucose, placental lactogen, prolactin and growth hormone have been suggested to contribute to islet growth in different models (for review see (16))(17-23). Recently, overexpression of parathyroid hormone-related protein (24), hepatocyte growth factor (25), cyclin-dependent kinase 4 (26) and IGF-II (27,28) in islets/β-cells have also been shown to cause islet hyperplasia. However, the factors contributing to islet/β-cell hyperplasia in states of insulin resistance are not yet known. Although glucose itself has been shown to stimulate β-cell replication (17,29) the presence of islet hyperplasia even in euglycaemic animal models of type 2 diabetes (12,14,15) strongly predicts the presence of a glucose-independent factor. In humans, very few data exist describing alterations in islet/β-cell mass, however, non-diabetic obese individuals with insulin resistance show a significant increase in β-cell volume (30) and macrosomic infants and foetuses of non-diabetic mothers show islet hyperplasia that correspond to high insulin levels (31). In patients with long-standing type 2 diabetes, on the other hand, the β-cell mass usually shows no change (32) or a mild reduction (33,34). From these observations, it is conceivable that insulin resistance early in the disease is associated with islet growth and a consequent increase in insulin secretion.

GENETIC MODELS OF INSULIN RESISTANCE

Molecular and genetic analysis of complex traits in humans can be limited by the difficulties associated with longitudinal analysis, access to tissues and knowledge of the exact genetic defects. An alternative approach to understanding the pathogenesis of type 2 diabetes has been to create genetically-engineered animal models with specific molecular defects that can be studied longitudinally and at both physiological and molecular levels. To investigate the role of insulin signalling in the pathogenesis of type 2 diabetes, we and others have generated mouse models with global or conditional deletions of one or more proteins in the insulin/IGF-1 signalling pathway (for reviews see (35,36)), (12-14,37-41). In addition, there are several naturally occurring rodent models of insulin resistance, obesity and type 2 diabetes including the *ob/ob* and *db/db* mice and the Zucker *fatty* rat. For the purposes of this review, however, we will focus on some of the recently created genetic models that develop insulin resistance as an approach to understanding islet hyperplasia and effects of insulin resistance on β-cell function.

INSULIN/IGF SIGNALLING PATHWAYS

A schematic overview of the insulin/IGF signalling pathway is shown in Figure 1 and is based on the tyrosine kinase activity of these receptors (for review see (42)). The principal substrates for the insulin and insulin-like growth factor-1 (IGF-1) receptors are a family of cytosolic proteins referred to as insulin receptor substrates -1, -2, -3, and -4. IRS-1 and -2 are expressed in most mammalian tissues (43-45) and tyrosine phosphorylated by the activated insulin receptor, while IRS-3 and -4 have more limited tissue distribution (46,47). In addition to the established role of these substrates and the insulin and IGF signalling pathways in skeletal muscle, liver and adipose tissues, a growing body of evidence suggests that these pathways play an important role in the function and growth of the islet/β-cells. Indeed the insulin and IGF-1 receptors and all four IRS proteins have been detected in islet tissue (15,40,41,48-51), however, the roles of these proteins in islet function has not been fully elucidated.

β-CELL FUNCTION IN THE INSULIN RECEPTOR SUBSTRATE-1 (IRS-1) KNOCKOUT

To evaluate the function of IRS-1, our laboratory and that of Kadowaki have used homologous recombination to create IRS-1 deficient (IRS-$1^{-/-}$) mice (12,13). The IRS-$1^{-/-}$ mice are approximately 50% smaller than wild type controls at birth and throughout life. The IRS-$1^{-/-}$ mice also show mild insulin resistance reflected by elevated plasma insulin levels, a blunted insulin/IGF-1 stimulated glucose uptake, a mildly impaired glucose tolerance in response to intra-peritoneal (IP) injection of glucose, and a ~50% decrease in circulating leptin levels probably secondary to a decrease in fat mass (12,15). Fasting and fed blood glucose levels are similar between control and IRS-1$^{-/-}$ mice, and the knockout animals do not develop overt diabetes even when examined at 12 to 14 months of age. However, fasting insulin and C-peptide levels are ~ 2-fold and 4-fold higher than in wild type controls suggesting an increased basal secretion by islet β-cells.

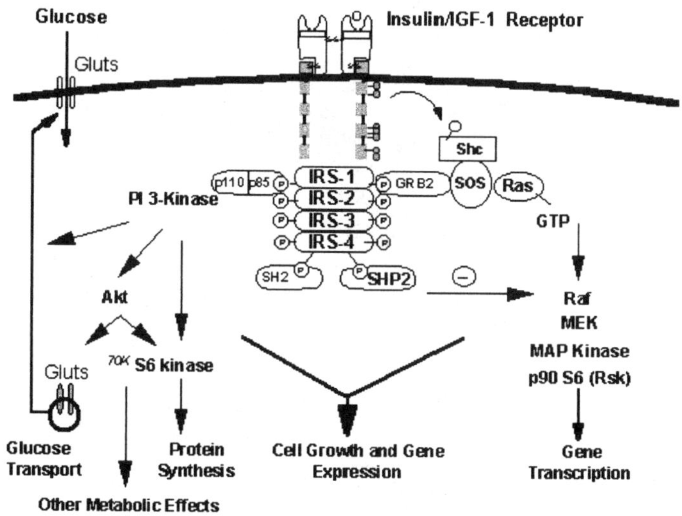

Figure 1. ***The insulin/IGF-1 signalling cascade.*** *A schematic representation at the molecular level showing the current understanding of the cascade of events following insulin/IGF-1 receptor activation and some of the final events associated with insulin/IGF-1 action. Insulin and IGF-1 receptors and their substrates IRS-1,-2,-3 and -4 are present in the pancreatic β-cells. Not shown in the figure is the β-cell transcription factor PDX-1 (pancreatic homeodomain transcription factor) which is localized to the nucleus and may have regulatory interactions with the insulin receptor and/or one or more insulin receptor substrates (see text for discussion).*

Islet Hyperplasia in IRS-1$^{-/-}$ Mice

To evaluate whether IRS-1 contributes to islet/β-cell function we have recently performed a systematic examination of the endocrine pancreas in IRS-1$^{-/-}$ mice. Assessment of islet size in pancreases was carried out by analysis of sections stained with a cocktail of antibodies to the non-β-cells. A minimum of 400 islets were analyzed from multiple sections from each genotype in 4 month-old mice and the mean islet size was measured using a calibrated micrometer. Sections from IRS-1$^{-/-}$ showed three populations of islets. About 54% are "normal-size" islets (118 ± 12 μm) comparable to wild type (112 ± 10 μm), whereas 31% are "large" – i.e., approximately 2-fold greater in size (243 ± 11 μm) than the islets of controls (Figure 2a), reflecting some islet hyperplasia. IRS-1$^{+/-}$ mice also exhibit some "large" islets, however, these are fewer in number (~16%). Interestingly, about 15% of islets in IRS-1$^{-/-}$ pancreas are small (~75 μm), and these are also increased in comparison to <4% of small islets in the wild type mice. Since blood glucose levels are comparable in all three genotypes of mice it is unlikely that glucose alone contributes to the observed islet hyperplasia in the IRS-1$^{-/-}$ animals.

Insulin-staining revealed a spotty distribution of islets throughout the exocrine pancreas of IRS-1$^{-/-}$ mice indicating the presence of insulin-producing cells (Figure 2b). Electron microscopic examination of β-cells in wild type islets shows a electron-dense granulation pattern characteristic of insulin-containing granules. By contrast, the granules in β-cells from IRS-1$^{-/-}$ mice are smaller and distinctly sparse (Figure 2c). Although no differences are observed in the Golgi and endoplasmic reticulum, IRS$^{-/-}$ β-cells display several autophagic vacuoles not evident in wild type β-cells (Figure 2c, arrows).

Reduced insulin secretion and insulin content in IRS-1$^{-/-}$ islets

IRS-1$^{-/-}$ mice show several alterations in insulin secretory patterns *in vivo*. Thus, despite an increase in basal circulating insulin, acute insulin release, as measured by response to intraperitoneal injection of glucose at 2 min, is reduced by 77% in the IRS-1$^{-/-}$ mice when compared to wild type mice (Figure 3a). Furthermore, the acute insulin release in response to IP L-arginine alone and the potentiation of the glucose-stimulated insulin release following IP injection of a mixture of glucose and L-arginine, are both lower in the IRS-1$^{-/-}$ mice (Figures 3b and 3c). These results suggest that a deficiency of IRS-1 results in an altered insulin response when challenged by nutrient secretagogues and indicate a functional insulin signalling pathway in the β-cell.

Insulin content measured in acid-ethanol extracts of size-matched islets is reduced in the heterozygous and homozygous knockout mice by ~34% and ~46%, respectively (Figure 4a). Even the large islets isolated from IRS-1$^{-/-}$ mice have lower (~30%) insulin content than the wild type islets. On the other hand, total pancreatic insulin content (expressed per mg wet weight of pancreas) is similar among the three groups with only a slight trend downwards, suggesting that the insulin content in the pancreas is likely made up by the larger number and size of islets in the IRS-1 deficient mice (Figure 4b).

To assess the glucose-stimulated insulin secretion pattern *in vitro*, islets were cultured for 48 h and then subjected to a glucose dose-response. Blunted insulin secretion is observed in both IRS-1$^{+/-}$ and IRS-1$^{-/-}$ islets when compared to size-matched islets from wild type mice. The reduction is particularly prominent at higher glucose concentrations (8.3 to 22.2 mM) (Figure 5a). Both the normal-size and large islets from the IRS-1$^{-/-}$ mice and the islets from the heterozygous mice show a similarly reduced response (Figure 5a). These responses are evident even when corrected for insulin content indicating alterations at the level of glucose sensitivity in these secretory responses. In time-course experiments, islets from the IRS-1$^{-/-}$ and IRS-1$^{+/-}$ mice show a diminished insulin secretion pattern at all time points from 0 to 60 min. Insulin secretion from the large islets of the IRS-1$^{-/-}$ mice show slightly different kinetics, with reduced insulin secretion early, but a tendency to "catch-up" at the 60 min time-point (Figure 5b). Taken together, these data demonstrate a lower insulin secretory response and altered kinetics to glucose stimulation in the islets isolated from the IRS-1$^{-/-}$ mice.

To evaluate the effect of IRS-1 deficiency on non-β-cell function, glucagon secretion was measured in the culture media in islet incubation experiments. A suppression of glucagon secretion is observed in response to a physiological glucose concentration (8.3 mM) (Figure 5c). An approximately 45% suppression is observed in all three groups and is not significantly different in the IRS-1 deficient islets than wild type islets suggesting a normal α-cell function.

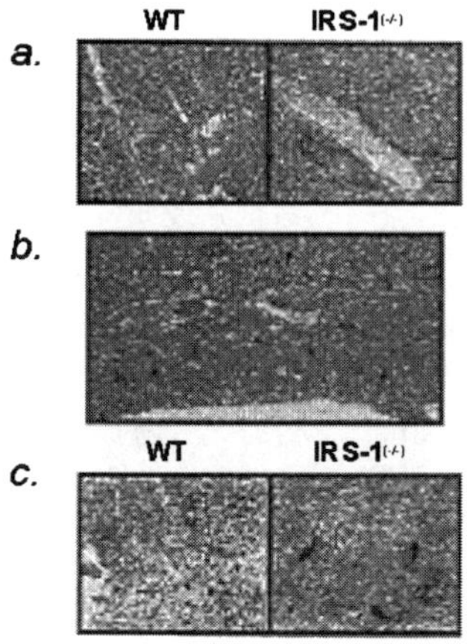

Figure 2. ***Islet morphology and electron microscopy of β-cells in IRS-1$^{-/-}$ mice.*** *(a) Sections of pancreas are stained for non-β-cells using a cocktail antibody against glucagon, somatostatin and pancreatic polypeptide. Representative sections of pancreas from wild type and IRS-1$^{-/-}$ mice show an approximately ~2-fold increase in islet size in the latter. (b) Representative section of pancreas from a IRS-1$^{-/-}$ mouse stained for insulin shows staining of β-cells in the islets. In addition, spotty insulin staining can be observed throughout the exocrine pancreas indicating neogenesis and the presence of differentiated insulin-containing β-cells. (c) Electron microscopic examination of β-cells in islets from IRS-1$^{-/-}$ mice show a scant electron-dense granulation pattern in IRS-1$^{-/-}$ β-cells compared to wild type cells. An increased number of autophagic vacuoles (arrows) are observed in individual IRS-1$^{-/-}$ β-cells. A representative photograph is shown. Magnification x 9690.*

Figure 3. ***Reduced acute phase insulin release in IRS-1$^{-/-}$ mice.*** *Intraperitoneal injection of (a) glucose (3 gm. kg body weight^{-1}), (b) L-arginine (0.3 gm. kg body weight^{-1}) or (c) a mixture of glucose and L-arginine shows a consistent reduced response in IRS-1$^{-/-}$ mice compared with age-matched wild type controls. Whole blood is collected from tail vein samples at the indicated times for insulin measurements. Values are means ± SEM (n=4-6). *, p<0.05 vs WT.*

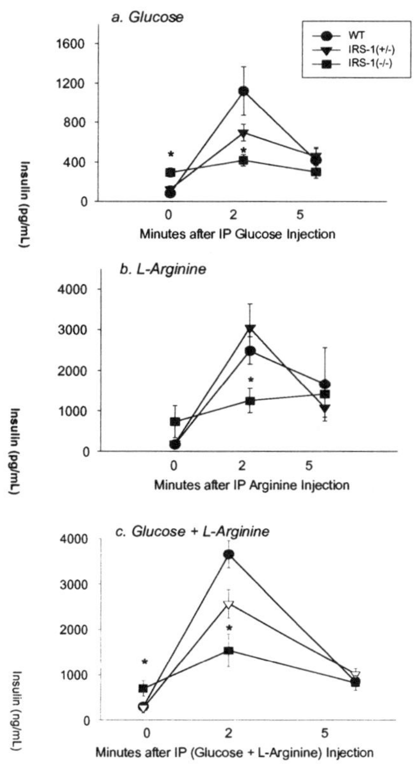

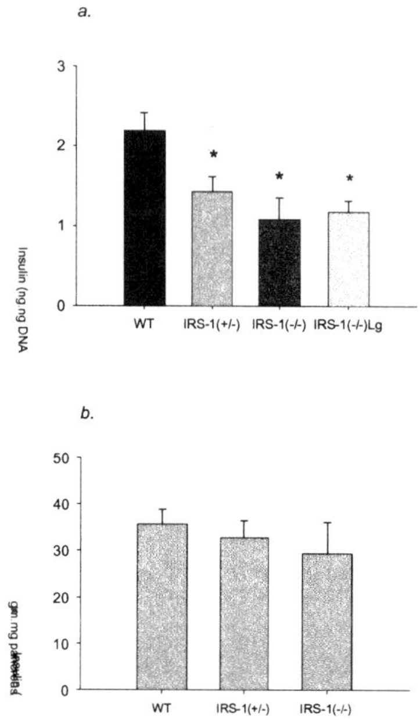

Figure 4. ***Islet and pancreatic insulin content in IRS-1$^{-/-}$ mice.***
*(a) Insulin content is reduced in islets isolated from IRS-1$^{-/-}$ and IRS-1$^{+/-}$ mice. "Large" (Lg) islets show a reduced content compared to wild type islets but are similar to the normal islets isolated from IRS-1$^{-/-}$ mice. Values are means ± SEM (n=35-50 islets each from three mice of each genotype). *, $p<0.05$ vs wild type. (b) Total pancreatic insulin content is similar between the three groups. Pancreases are homogenized in acid ethanol overnight at 4° C and insulin measured by RIA. Values are means ± SEM (n=3).*

Altered Function of IRS-1$^{-/-}$ clonal β-cells

To better assess the influence of IRS-1 deficiency specifically in β-cells, immortalized cell lines were derived by isolating islet tumors from IRS-1$^{-/-}$ and IRS-1$^{+/-}$ mice crossed with mice expressing SV40 T antigen on the rat insulin promoter as described by Hanahan (52,53). As in freshly isolated islets, insulin content is ~34% lower in the IRS-1$^{+/-}$ cells and ~55% lower in the IRS-1 knockout cells compared to wild type cells. Similar results are obtained with cells derived from two different mice of each genotype (data not shown). When the IRS-1$^{-/-}$ cells are transiently transfected with IRS-1 cDNA, the level of expression of IRS-1 protein is restored to 40% of that in wild type cells as assessed by Western blotting. This was accompanied by an increase in insulin content to levels similar to the heterozygote cell line (Figure 6a). The increase in insulin content following re-expression of IRS-1 in IRS-1$^{-/-}$ cells is consistent with a direct role for this protein in maintenance of insulin content.

As in freshly isolated islets, glucose-stimulated insulin secretion is also reduced in the IRS-1$^{-/-}$ and IRS-1$^{+/-}$ β-cell lines. These secretory responses are significantly lower even after correcting for the ~30-50% lower insulin content suggesting a defect in the ability of the β-cells to adequately respond to glucose stimulation (Figure 6b). In addition, these IRS-1 null β-cells show a shift in the glucose sensitivity curve, compared to isolated islets, with higher glucose concentrations being required to produce an increase in insulin secretion. This pattern of lower glucose sensitivity is typical of β-cell lines (54-56) and is similar in IRS-1$^{+/-}$ and IRS-1$^{-/-}$ and wild type cells. A similar blunted secretion pattern is apparent in response to L-arginine mimicking the observations in the islet studies (Figure 6c). Taken together these data indicate a defect in the insulin secretory response to multiple stimuli in β-cells lacking IRS-1.

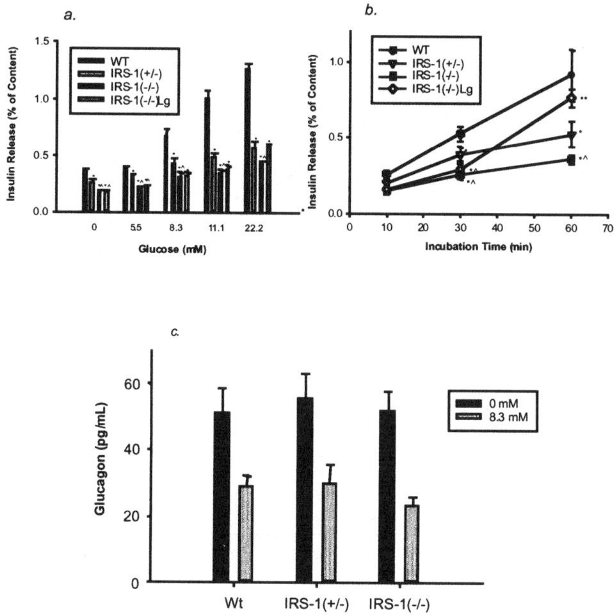

Figure 5. ***Reduced dose- and time-dependent glucose-stimulated insulin secretion in IRS-1 deficient islets.*** *(a) Insulin secretion in response to glucose shows a dose-dependent decrease in insulin secretion in size-matched islets isolated from IRS-1$^{-/-}$ and IRS-1$^{+/-}$ mice compared to wild type controls. Insulin secretion is expressed as a % of the islet insulin content. Values are means ± SEM (n=4-6). *, $p<0.05$ vs wild type; †, $p<0.01$ vs IRS-1$^{+/-}$. (b) Incubation of islets in the presence of 8.3 mM glucose shows a decreased insulin secretion in IRS-1$^{-/-}$ and IRS-1$^{+/-}$ islets compared to wild type islets up to 60 mins. Insulin secretion in IRS-1$^{-/-}$ is lower even when compared to IRS-1$^{+/-}$ islets at 30 and 60 mins. Values are means ± SEM (n=4-6). *, $p<0.05$ vs WT; †, $p<0.02$ vs IRS-1$^{+/-}$; **, $p<0.05$ vs IRS-1$^{+/-}$ or IRS-1$^{-/-}$. (c) Incubation of size-matched islets in a physiological concentration of 8.3 mM glucose shows a suppression of glucagon in all 3 groups. No significant differences are detected between islets isolated from wild type, IRS-1$^{-/-}$ and IRS-1$^{+/-}$ mice. Values are means ± SEM (n=4-6).*

THE IRS-2 KNOCKOUT MOUSE

The observation that IRS-1$^{-/-}$ mice demonstrate residual insulin action even in the presence of significant insulin/IGF-1 resistance led to the isolation of an alternative insulin receptor substrate termed IRS-2 (57). This substrate has since been shown to play a role in signal transduction to proteins mediating several pathways of insulin action such as PI-3 kinase, Grb 2/Sos, NCK and CRK (44;45).

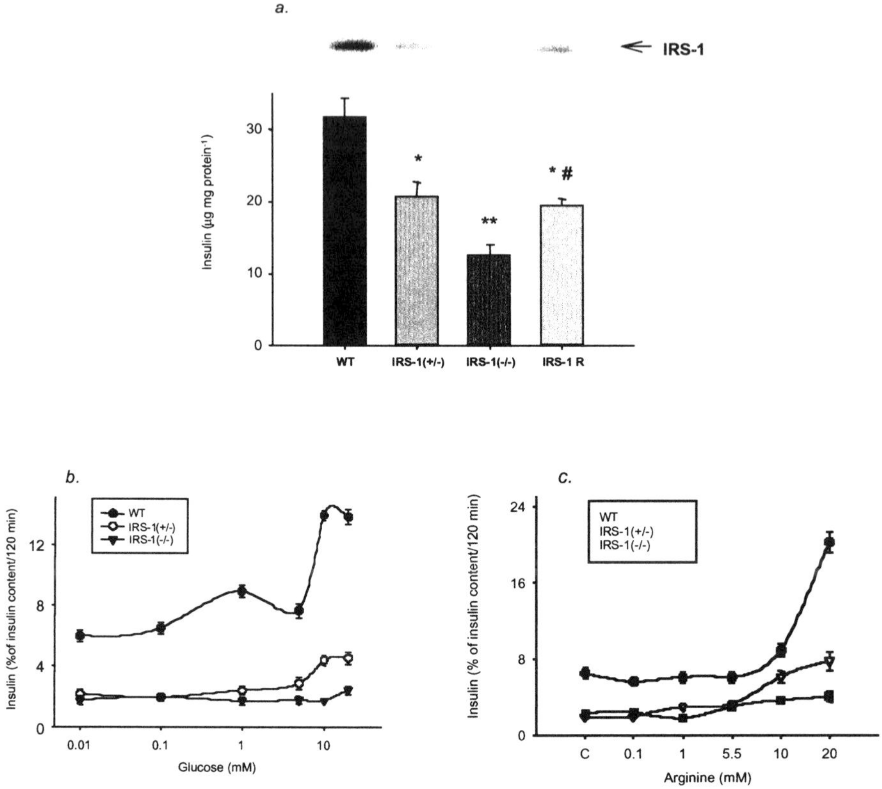

Figure 6. ***Insulin content is partially restored in cultured β-cells re-expressing IRS-1.*** *(a) A reduced insulin content is observed in IRS-1$^{-/-}$ and IRS-1$^{+/-}$ cells compared to WT cells (upper panel). Re-expression of IRS-1 in IRS-1$^{-/-}$ cells shows a partial restoration of insulin content and is significantly higher than IRS-1$^{-/-}$ cells (lower panel). Values are means ± SEM (n=6-7). *, $p<0.05$ vs wild type; **, $p<0.01$ vs wild type; #, $p<0.05$ vs IRS-1$^{-/-}$. Insulin secretion is blunted in response to increasing concentrations of (b) glucose and (c) L-arginine in IRS-1$^{-/-}$ and IRS-1$^{+/-}$ β-cell lines. Results are expressed as a % of the cellular insulin content. Values are means ± SEM (n=6). $p<0.05$ IRS-1$^{+/-}$ or IRS-1$^{-/-}$ vs wild type at all concentrations ; $p<0.05$ IRS-1$^{+/-}$ vs IRS-1$^{-/-}$ at all concentrations except 0.01 and 0.1 mM glucose and 0.1 mM L-arginine.*

To further assess its role in insulin action, Withers et al (40) inactivated the IRS-2 gene by homologous recombination and examined its impact on glucose homeostasis. Breeding the resulting chimeras with C57Bl/6 mice yield IRS-1 heterozygotes which were then intercrossed to produce IRS-2$^{-/-}$ mice. A very early feature (3 weeks) in these mice is the presence of hyperglycaemia in the fasting and fed states that rapidly worsens to severe glucose intolerance by 6 weeks. These mice also develop insulin resistance as shown by elevated fasting serum insulin levels and by the failure of exogenous insulin (2.5 mU.kg/min-1) to increase whole-body glucose disposal and inhibit hepatic glucose production (40).

Alterations in Islet Morphology and Function in IRS-2$^{-/-}$ Mice
As previously discussed early insulin resistance is usually associated with compensation by the β-cell to secrete more insulin to overcome the resistance. The compensatory effect could be due to an increase in secretion and/or an increase in β-cell mass secondary to β-cell neogenesis. Assessment of β-cell mass at 4 weeks of age shows a loss of the increase in β-cell growth normally observed in wild type mice. In fact, the IRS-2$^{-/-}$ mice show hypoplastic islets with a selective loss of β-cell mass and preserved normal non-β-cell mass. The β-cell deficiency is also evident in neonatal pancreas indicating a growth defect secondary to the lack of IRS-2. IRS-2 appears to normally co-localize with insulin in the β-cells and immunofluorescence staining shows the presence of the substrate in ductal epithelium in wild type pancreas. The absence of the protein in ducts isolated from IRS-2$^{-/-}$ mice suggests this protein is associated with β-cell neogenesis (40).

Evaluation of glucose-stimulated insulin secretion in 4-week IRS-2$^{-/-}$ mice, *in vivo*, shows a 2-fold secretory response at 60 minutes which is comparable to that observed in wild type mice (40). However, assessment of insulin release in isolated islets shows either a normal (58) or elevated (59) but not a reduced secretory response, indicating that β-cells lacking IRS-2 are capable of enhanced insulin secretion that may partly contribute to the ambient hyperinsulinemia.

The data from the preceding sections illustrate the contrasting roles of IRS-1 and IRS-2 in islet function and growth. While IRS-1 is involved in the maintenance of islet insulin content and mediates insulin secretory responses, IRS-2 appears to be associated with islet neogenesis. This scenario can be explained at least in part by the fact that these insulin receptor substrates can be phosphorylated by ligands, other than insulin, that can bind to the IGF-1 and cytokine receptors (60-62). In recent studies, intercrossing mice heterozygous for the null alleles of the IGF-1 receptor with mice homozygous for IRS-2 leads to a complete lack of β-cell development in the progeny demonstrating a role for the IGF-1 receptor in IRS-2-mediated β-cell neogenesis (62). Furthermore, prolactin and growth hormone receptors have been shown to activate IRS-1 and IRS-2 (63,64). The presence of receptors for these hormones on insulin-secreting cells (64-66) suggests they may play a potentially crucial role in islet function and/or growth.

In humans, genetic analysis of diabetic populations has shown a two-fold higher incidence of polymorphisms in IRS-1 (67-70) but none to date in IRS-2 (71). Interestingly, patients with the Arg-Gly polymorphism in codon 972 manifest low circulating insulin and C-peptide levels (68). Furthermore, expression of this polymorphism in clonal β-cell lines shows a blunted secretory response to glucose and glibenclamide (72). The impaired insulin secretory response in the IRS-1$^{-/-}$ islets further confirms a role for IRS-1 in β-cell function (15).

In contrast to the significant alterations in growth and glucose homeostasis observed when IRS-1 or IRS-2 are knocked out, global disruption of IRS-3 results in virtually no defects (73), while IRS-4 knockout mice show a ~10% reduction in body mass and very minor alterations in glucose homeostasis manifested by a small decrease in fasting and fed blood glucose concentrations (74). Presently, the precise roles of IRS-3 and IRS-4 in endocrine pancreatic function are still unclear.

INSULIN RECEPTOR KNOCKOUT

The presence and function of the insulin receptor in the β-cells has been a matter of debate for several years. Studies on the β-cell have been limited due to the restricted amount of primary tissue available to perform direct binding assays or autoradiography (75-77) as well as the difficulty in assessing insulin action in a tissue constitutively secreting large quantities of the hormone. Several studies have attempted to address whether insulin regulates its own secretion or synthesis with conflicting results (78-82). Rothenberg *et al* (48) have reported the presence of some components of the insulin signalling pathway by demonstrating the presence of insulin receptor mRNA and IRS-1 in normal islet β-cells and clonal β-cell lines, that has been confirmed by several other laboratories (14,15,49,51,83,84).

WHOLE-BODY DELETION OF THE INSULIN RECEPTOR

Gene-targeting approaches have been used to knockout the insulin receptor either by inserting a stop codon in exon 4 (38) or by deleting part of the insulin receptor gene around exon 2 (39). Mice heterozygous for the insulin receptor null allele develop normally and have relatively normal glucose homeostasis. By contrast $IR^{-/-}$ mice are indistinguishable from the control littermates at birth but develop major metabolic alterations after suckling. Characteristically, these mice manifest hyperglycaemia leading to hyperinsulinemia, and eventually severe diabetes and ketoacidosis. These mice show reduced hepatic glycogen, a decrease in both white and brown fat and marked post-natal growth retardation. All $IR^{-/-}$ mice die within a week after birth precluding a detailed investigation of metabolic and morphological alterations in target tissues. In the limited studies performed, islet size and morphology in the knockout mice are not different compared to controls (Accili D, personal communication).

CONDITIONAL DELETION OF THE INSULIN RECEPTOR IN THE ISLET β-CELL (βIRKO)

In order to study the role of a functional insulin receptor in the islet β-cell we have used the technique of *Cre*-LoxP mediated recombination to inactivate the insulin receptor gene in mice in a tissue-specific manner (14,85,86). To achieve β-cell inactivation we have used a Rip-Cre transgene which is expressed in the islet β-cells 2.5 days after endogenous insulin gene transcription begins at embryonic day 9 (87,88). To generate the βIRKO mice, the IRLox mice (homozygous for the IRlox allele) carrying the *Cre* transgene on the rat insulin promoter, are bred with the IRLox heterozygous mice. This yields the βIRKO mice and several other genotypes among which wild type, Cre and IRLox mice are included as control groups. The efficiency of recombination of the IRLox allele in the islets triggered by *Cre* expression is assessed by a PCR strategy using DNA prepared from islets isolated from βIRKO and IRLox mice. The presence of a single band (300 base pairs) in DNA prepared from the IRLox islets indicates the presence of exon 4 while a smaller band (220 base pairs) in the βIRKO lane indicates the deletion of exon 4 as would occur following *Cre* recombination.

All mice are born at the expected Mendelian frequency and no significant differences are observed in body weights between the different groups up to 6 months. βIRKO mice are fertile and their development is not different from the control littermates.

Fed and fasting serum insulin and blood glucose concentrations are comparable between the different groups up to 6 months of age in the males and a mild degree of hyperinsulinemia can be detected in females at 2 and 6 months (41).

Loss of glucose-stimulated acute phase insulin secretion and mild islet hypoplasia

To further evaluate the effect of loss of the insulin receptor on β-cell function, insulin release is measured in response to stimulation with glucose and L-arginine. While a 3-4-fold stimulation of insulin release is detected in controls, this response is completely absent (males) or blunted (females) in βIRKO mice (Figure 7a). By contrast, the insulin secretory response to L-arginine is intact in all groups examined (Figure 7b), suggesting that a functional insulin receptor is requisite for a normal glucose-stimulated insulin secretory response by the β-cell. To assess the impact of the loss of first-phase insulin secretion on the ability of mice to handle a glucose load, glucose disposal is measured by intraperitoneal (IP) injection of glucose (2 gm/kg body weight) after a 15 hour overnight fast. Both males and females show a significantly impaired glucose tolerance at 2 months that continues to worsen and by 6 months glucose levels are 2-fold higher in the βIRKO mice as controls (Figure 7c).

Analysis of sections of pancreas using a cocktail of antibodies to non-β-cell hormones shows no apparent differences in islet size or in the ratio of β to non-β cells at 2 months (Figure 8a). Measurement of insulin content in the pancreas shows comparable levels at 2 months consistent with the islet morphology. In 4-month-old mice, however, there is a ~ 30% decrease in islet size in the βIRKO mice compared to controls (Figure 8a). While the insulin content in the controls continues to increase in accordance with the growing islet size, this rise is absent in the βIRKO mice resulting in an apparent 35% decrease in insulin content (Figure 8b). Taken together, islet morphology in the whole body insulin receptor knockout and the βIRKO mice suggest it is unlikely that the insulin receptor plays a major role in the regulation of islet development.

Since one of the rate-limiting steps for glucose sensing is its entry into the β-cell, we performed immunofluorescent staining of paraffin sections of pancreas isolated from βIRKO and IRLox controls using Glut2 antibody. The distribution of Glut2 is comparable between the βIRKO and IRLox islets while islets from *ob/ob* mice used as controls show barely detectable Glut2. However, it is possible that the absence of a functional insulin receptor in the βIRKO mice may influence the expression and/or activity of other proteins involved in glucose sensing such as glucokinase. Electron microscopy of β-cells shows no apparent differences in cell membrane, endoplasmic reticulum, Golgi or electron-dense insulin-containing granules within the β-cells in the βIRKO versus IRLox mice indicating an apparently normal secretory machinery (41).

Development of Overt Diabetes in βIRKO Mice

Some of the βIRKO mice that were allowed to age in our animal facility showed signs of diabetes, we therefore studied a large cohort of aged mice maintained on the original mixed genetic background (C57Bl/6 x 129Sv x DBA/2) to evaluate the development of diabetes. Since it is impossible to predict the proportion of each strain in a given mouse, all experiments include littermate controls. Among the 47 male βIRKOs examined at 12 to 14 months, 9 mice tended to be obese and show a greater body weight compared to controls (βIRKO 41 ± 1.1 vs Control 36 ± 1.9 gm, $p<0.01$). Measurement of insulin levels in this obese subgroup show fed hyperglycaemia (βIRKO 197 ± 24 vs Controls 134 ± 22 mg/dL, $p<0.05$, n=9-14), and hyperinsulinemia compared to controls (βIRKO 11.7 ± 2.6 vs Controls 4.7 ± 2.2 ng/ml, p<0.01, n=9-14) as well as severe glucose intolerance. The remainder of the βIRKO mice, however, are lean (38 ± 1.5 gm, p=ns vs Controls) and show no significant elevation in fed glucose or insulin levels (Glucose, 151 ± 28 mg/dL; Insulin, 5.2 ± 1.8 ng/mL, n=38; p=ns vs Controls), but continue to manifest severe glucose intolerance as a consequence of the loss of glucose-stimulated acute phase insulin release.

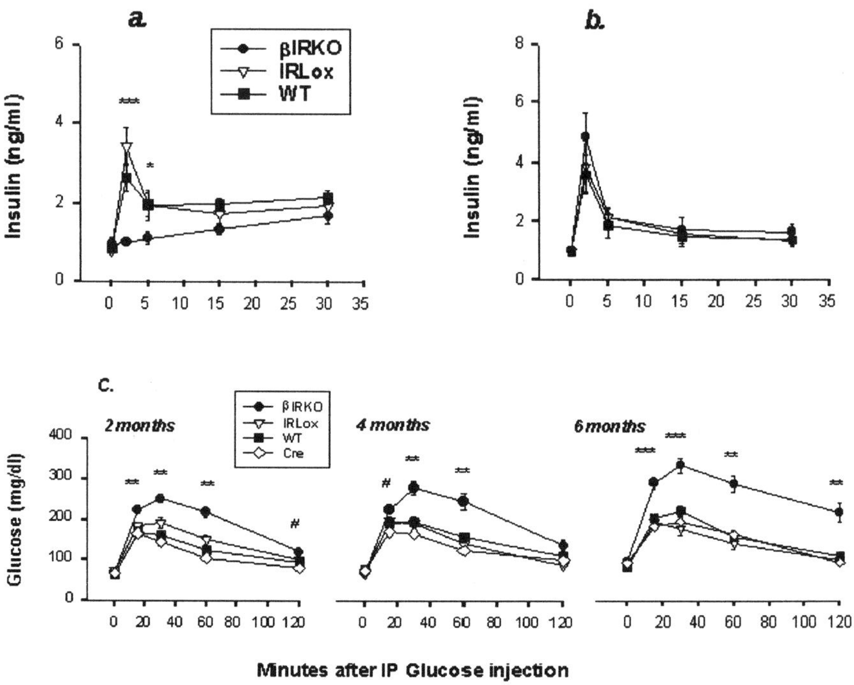

Figure 7. ***βIRKO mice show a selective loss of glucose-stimulated acute phase insulin secretion and a progressive glucose intolerance.*** *A significantly blunted acute insulin secretory response is observed in male βIRKO mice (filled circles) compared with controls (IRLox, inverted triangles; wild type, filled squares), in response to intra-peritoneal injection of (a) glucose (3 g/kg body weight) but not to (b) L-arginine (0.3 g/kg body weight). Similar differences are observed in females (not shown). Values are means ± SEM (n=3-14). *, p<0.05; ***, p<0.001, βIRKO vs wildtype or IRLox or Cre controls. (c) βIRKO mice (filled circles) show an age-dependent progression of glucose intolerance in response to intra-peritoneal injection of glucose compared to controls (wild type, filled squares; IRLox, inverted triangles; Cre, diamonds). Values are means ± SEM. #, p<0.05 βIRKO vs wild type or Cre; **, p<0.01; ***, p<0.001, βIRKO vs wild type, IRLox or Cre.*

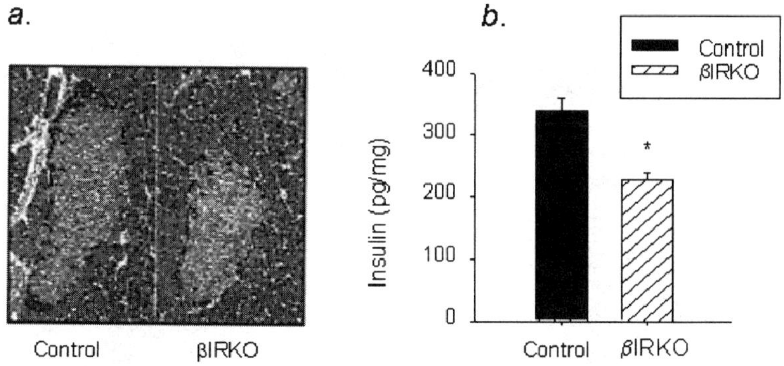

Figure 8. *Mild islet hypoplasia and reduced pancreatic insulin content in normoinsulinemic βIRKO mice. (a) Immunostaining for non-β-cell hormones is performed in pancreatic sections from 4-month-old control and βIRKO mice using a cocktail of antibodies to glucagon, somatostatin and pancreatic polypeptide. Representative sections are shown. (b) Pancreatic insulin content is measured in acid-ethanol extracts from control and βIRKO mice by RIA. Values are means ± SEM (n=3-5). *, $p<0.05$, βIRKO vs Control.*

Similarly, evaluation of islet morphology in the obese βIRKOs shows mild hyperplasia that correlates with the hyperinsulinemia, while the normoinsulinemic lean subgroup from the βIRKOs show islets that are ~ 30 to 40% smaller compared to controls with a corresponding lower islet insulin content similar to the trend observed at 4 months of age (Figures 9a, 9b, and 9c). However, the islet size when expressed as a fraction of the body weight continues to show a slight reduction compared to controls. Recently, Susan Bonner-Weir has reported (112) that islet size appears to be a function of body weight in mice. Although the mechanism underlying the gain in body weight in some βIRKO mice is currently unclear, the reduced islet size in these mice when expressed as a function of body weight supports the notion that the insulin receptor is unlikely to play a primary role in islet growth. Further work is necessary to evaluate whether the insulin receptor contributes in any way to islet hyperplasia in the presence of insulin resistance.

The phenotypes of the βIRKO and the global insulin receptor knockout mice are in some ways different from what is observed in humans with mutations in the insulin receptor. For example, humans with mutations in the insulin receptor (leprechaunism) show severe intrauterine growth retardation and mild hyperglycaemia (89-91), while whole body insulin receptor knockout mice manifest normal birth weights with severe diabetes and ketoacidosis (38,39). Secondly, βIRKO mice manifest impaired insulin secretion (41) whereas humans with insulin receptor mutations display hyperplasia of islets and hypersecretion of insulin (91). Thus, from the data discussed above and from that below (see under Compound Defects - $IR^{+/-}$/$IRS\text{-}1^{+/-}$), it appears that the phenotypes show some variation when a specific mutation is introduced in a different strain even within the same species. This is likely due to heterogeneity in the genetic background and is a feature observed in most knockout mouse models which use 129Sv or FVB embryonic stem cells to generate chimeras and are subsequently bred with C57Bl/6 for germline production. However, there are several advantages in studying mouse models on a mixed genetic background. First, type 2 diabetes in humans is a polygenic disorder with multiple genes contributing to a complex heterogeneous disease, and it is likely that murine models will provide an insight into the mechanisms underlying the pathogenesis of the disease process. Second, the presence of a phenotype on a mixed background will allow mapping and positional cloning in suitable outcrosses to identify modifier alleles that may be causal (or protective) in producing the insulin deficiency or insulin resistance.

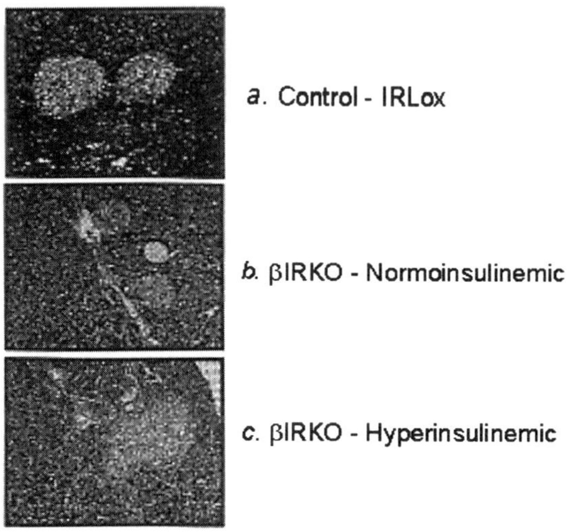

Figure 9. ***Pancreas sections from 12-14 month-old βIRKO mice.*** *Hematoxylin and eosin staining of pancreas sections from (a) control (lox/lox or IRLox), (b) normoinsulinemic βIRKO and (c) hyperinsulinemic βIRKO mice. Representative sections are shown. Magnification 10x.*

MICE WITH COMPOUND DEFECTS $IR^{+/-}$/IRS-$1^{+/-}$

Partial deletion of the insulin receptor in the whole body is not lethal (38,39). $IR^{+/-}$ mice show a small but significant decrease in body weight and mild hyperinsulinemia compared to control littermates (92). IRS-1 heterozygous mice also show a mild reduction in body weight (93) and defects in islet function as discussed above (15). Each of these defects when present separately, however, show minor alterations in glucose homeostasis with only 5% of $IR^{+/-}$ mice becoming diabetic (92). To create a polygenic model that might more closely mimic human disease we generated combined IR/IRS-1 double heterozygous (DH) mice (14).

DH mice are born normally and are fertile, but show a slightly reduced body weight when compared to wild type control littermates. Evaluation of insulin signalling shows additive impairment in several signalling events in the DH mice. Thus, IRS-1 phosphorylation and activation of phosphatidylinositol 3-kinase (PI 3-kinase) are reduced by 50% in either the IRS-$1^{+/-}$ or $IR^{+/-}$ mice and reduced by 75-80% in the double heterozygotes (14).

Physiologically, these defects are synergistic. Thus, mice with simultaneous presence of two partial defects in the insulin signalling pathway show alterations in glucose homeostasis as early as 2 months of age and a 2.6-fold increase in fed insulin levels as compared to wild type controls. By 4 to 6 months, there is a dramatic (~20-fold) elevation in circulating insulin levels and an impaired ability of exogenous insulin to lower glucose indicating severe insulin resistance. Indeed, by this age ~40% of the males progress to overt diabetes (14).

Massive Islet Hyperplasia in IR$^{+/-}$/IRS-1$^{+/-}$ Mice

To evaluate the ability of the β-cell to compensate for the initial insulin resistance in DH animals, maintained on a mixed genetic background (C57Bl X 129Sv), we examined the pancreas histologically after immunostaining for insulin and determined β- and non-β-cell mass by point counting morphometry. At 6 months, although pancreas weights are comparable between the different groups, β-cell mass is increased 2- to 3-fold in IRS-1$^{+/-}$ and IR$^{+/-}$ mice and up to 30-fold in the IR/IRS-1$^{+/-}$ double heterozygous group. The increase in β-cell mass is paralleled by an increase in insulin levels. No differences are observed in non-β-cell mass. The enormous increase in β-cell mass in the DH mice results in distorted islet morphology. In wild type mice the non-β-cells usually form a discontinuous mantle around a core of β-cells, whereas in the DH mice, the non-β-cells are irregularly scattered throughout the islet (14).

Most current models for type 2 diabetes suggest that this decrease is the result of relative failure of β-cells to secrete adequate insulin to compensate for the insulin resistance. Interestingly, in the double heterozygotes the most extensive β-cell hyperplasia is observed in the diabetic mice (fed blood glucose ~300 mg/dL). These animals show a 15-fold increase in β-cell mass and a 21-fold elevated plasma insulin level compared to wild type controls. The euglycaemic DH mice (fed blood glucose ~120 mg/dL) also show a significant increase in β-cell mass and plasma insulin levels but only about 3- to 4-fold (14). These data suggest that diabetes in this model can occur with β-cell failure and that factors other than glucose can significantly contribute to the islet growth in these insulin resistant euglycaemic mice.

To assess the impact of genetic background on glucose homeostasis and islet morphology we have generated DH mice on C57Bl/6, DBA/2 and 129Sv strains to >98% purity. The incidence of diabetes is greatest on the C57Bl/6 background compared to DBA/2 and 129Sv. Evaluation of islet morphology shows marked but uniform hyperplasia on the C57Bl/6 background, while the islet size is less markedly increased in DH mice on the DBA/2 background. Furthermore, islets in pancreas sections from mice in the latter group show disorganized architecture as shown by large vacuoles in the core of the islet which is devoid of β-cells and shows irregularly scattered non-β-cells.

Altered Secretory Function in IR$^{+/-}$/IRS-1$^{+/-}$ Islets

The most striking finding in the severely insulin resistant DH mice is a dramatic increase in insulin content in the hyperplastic islets and in the pancreas compared to single heterozygotes and wild type mice. In spite of the increase in content, assessment of islet function *in vivo* shows a reduced acute insulin secretory response to exogenous administration of glucose and L-arginine. While a 3 to 4-fold increase in insulin secretion is observed at 2 min following glucose injection in wild type mice, a significantly lower (1.7-fold) increase is detectable in DH mice (Figure 10a). A similar pattern is observed in response to L-arginine (Figure 10b) (RN Kulkarni & CR Kahn, unpublished data). Although the absolute levels of insulin are higher in the DH mice, the fold response is consistently lower compared to wild type controls indicating a dysfunctional insulin signalling pathway in the β-cells. Although low insulin content in the β-cells has been shown to influence first and second phase insulin secretion, an impaired secretory response can also occur secondary to perturbations in intracellular Ca^{++} regulation independent of the amount of insulin stores (94). Thus, the presence of more than normal insulin content in the DH islets, indicates that the blunted responses observed in these mice are probably due to a defect in the insulin signalling pathway in the β-cells.

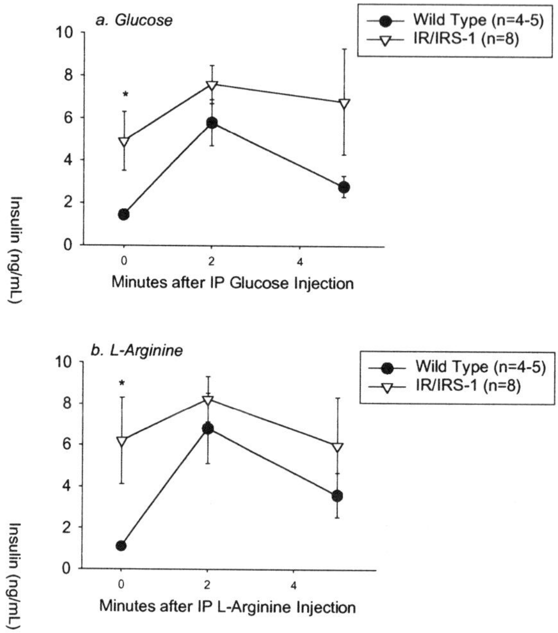

Figure 10. *Reduced acute insulin secretion in IR/IRS-1$^{+/-}$ double heterozygous (DH) mice. Intraperitoneal injection of (a) glucose (3 gm. kg body weight^{-1}), (b) L-arginine (0.3 gm. kg body weight^{-1}) shows a consistent reduced response in the DH mice compared with age-matched wild type controls. Whole blood is collected from tail vein samples at the indicated times for insulin measurements. Values are means ± SEM (n=5). *, p<0.05 vs wild type.*

IRS-1 AND β-CELL GLUCOKINASE

In an attempt to simulate the effects of polygenic defects in type 2 diabetes, Terauchi et al (95) bred IRS-1$^{-/-}$ animals with mice deficient in β-cell glucokinase (GK). The resultant mice with compound defects (IRS-1$^{-/-}$/GK$^{+/-}$) show glucose intolerance at an advanced age (30 to 40 weeks). These mice also show fasting hyperinsulinemia and an impaired insulin tolerance test comparable to IRS-1$^{-/-}$ mice.

Alterations in Islet Morphology and Islet Function

Compared to controls, the IRS-1$^{-/-}$/GK$^{+/-}$ mice demonstrate mild islet hyperplasia. The number of β-cells in the whole pancreas is significantly greater in the IRS-1$^{-/-}$/GK$^{+/-}$ than controls, and is similar to the IRS-1$^{-/-}$ mice. No significant differences are observed in non-β-cell mass indicating a selective β-cell growth effect. Insulin-positive cells are detected in epithelial cells of the pancreatic duct suggesting β-cell differentiation and neogenesis in mice with the compound defects. This mouse model provides another example of islet/β-cell hyperplasia induced by insulin resistance.

IR, IRS-1 AND/OR IRS-2

As noted above, IR and IRS-1 heterozygote knockout mice have enlarged islets, while IRS-2 heterozygotes have decreased β-cell mass. To determine if there might be interactions between insulin receptors and these two substrates, we bred mice heterozygous for IR, IRS-1 and IRS-2 to obtain triple heterozygous animals.
Mice with the IR/IRS-$1^{+/-}$ and IR/IRS-1/IRS-$2^{+/-}$ compound defects show similar growth curves with significantly lower body weights compared to IR/IRS-$2^{+/-}$ mice and wild type controls. At 2 months of age, no significant alterations are observed in blood glucose levels in the various genotypes. However, by 6 months the double and triple heterozygotes show an elevated blood glucose consistent with a progressive deterioration in glucose homeostasis. The number of diabetic mice is highest in the triple heterozygotes (~40%) compared with IR/IRS-$1^{+/-}$ (~20%) and IR/IRS-$2^{+/-}$ (~17%).

Alterations in Islet Morphology

The greatest islet hyperplasia is observed in the IR/IRS-1/IRS-$2^{+/-}$ triple heterozygous mice. The loss of an allele for IRS-2 did not preclude the ambient insulin resistance to induce a robust β-cell hyperplasia in these islets. In fact, the selective β-cell growth is similar to the hyperplasia observed in the IR/IRS-$1^{+/-}$ mice as discussed earlier. The triple heterozygotes and IR/IRS-$1^{+/-}$ mice have significantly elevated plasma insulin levels (~40 to 60 ng/ml) indicating severe insulin resistance. Similarly, IR/IRS-$2^{+/-}$ mice show an increase in islet size and elevated insulin levels comparable to that observed in $IR^{+/-}$ mice alone. The selective increase in β-cell mass in parallel with the increase in plasma insulin levels in all groups indicates an association with insulin resistance. Thus, although IRS-2 deficiency may limit β-cell growth in normal mice, in the context of insulin resistant mice, it does not prevent the development of β-cell hyperplasia.

IR, IRS-1 AND/OR PDX-1

The pancreatic homeodomain transcription factor or PDX-1 (also called STF-1, IPF-1 and IDX-1) has been shown to regulate early pancreatic development and the expression of key endocrine β-cell-specific genes (96-98) Homozygous deletion of PDX-1 results in pancreatic agenesis and early death in mice (98) and humans (99). Heterozygous deletion of PDX-1 in mice results in glucose intolerance and a mild decrease in islet size (100), and β-cell specific inactivation of PDX-1 leads to maturity onset diabetes (101). A relatively new form of early-onset type 2 diabetes in humans has been shown to cosegregate with an inactivation mutation in the PDX-1 gene which has been designated the MODY4 gene (99;101). To evaluate the impact of a β-cell defect on insulin resistance-induced islet hyperplasia, we intercrossed IR/IRS-$1^{+/-}$ mice with PDX-$1^{+/-}$ mice to obtain IR/IRS-$1^{+/-}$, IR/PDX-$1^{+/-}$, IRS-1/PDX-$1^{+/-}$ and IR/IRS-1/PDX-$1^{+/-}$ triple heterozygous mice (102).

Altered Glucose Homeostasis and Islet Morphology in IRS-$1^{+/-}$/PDX-$1^{+/-}$ and $IR^{+/-}$/IRS-$1^{+/-}$/PDX-$1^{+/-}$ Mice

Mice with combined heterozygosities for IR, IRS-1 and PDX-1 are born normally and are fertile but show a significant decrease in growth resulting in reduced body weights compared to the IR/IRS-$1^{+/-}$ and PDX-$1^{+/-}$ mice. By 2 months, fasting and fed blood glucose levels are higher in all groups heterozygous for PDX-1 with the highest levels observed in the triple heterozygotes (Fasting: 101 ± 12 vs 73 ± 5; Fed: 359 ± 45 vs 143 ± 3 mg/dL for triples vs Controls mean ± SEM, both $p<0.05$, n=4-

11). Fasting insulin levels are significantly lower in the $PDX^{+/-}$ (0.4 ± 0.1), $PDX^{+/-}/IR^{+/-}$ (0.3 ± 0.05) and $PDX^{+/-}/IRS\text{-}1^{+/-}$ (0.1 ± 0.01) compared to Controls (0.9 ± 0.1 ng.ml; all $p<0.05$). However, the insulin levels in the triple heterozygotes vary over a wide range. While most mice show barely detectable levels (0.05 ng/ml), insulin concentrations in some animals are comparable to the controls (1.5 ng/ml). By 3 months, an impaired glucose tolerance is evident in PDX-1 heterozygous groups with the highest levels observed in the $IRS\text{-}1^{+/-}/PDX\text{-}1^{+/-}$ and $IR+/-/IRS\text{-}1^{+/-}/PDX\text{-}1^{+/-}$ groups (409 ± 18 and 367 ± 15 vs 184 ± 15 mg/dL for Controls at 60 min; $p<0.05$) (102).

As described previously, $IR/IRS\text{-}1^{+/-}$ mice in this study also show hyperinsulinemia associated with an elevated β-cell mass while $IRS\text{-}1^{+/-}$ mice are mildly insulin resistant and show only a slight increase in islet size. By contrast, $PDX\text{-}1^{+/-}$ mice show low plasma insulin levels and a decrease in islet size due to a defect in islet development. Surprisingly, it is difficult to detect islets in most pancreas sections from $IRS\text{-}1/PDX\text{-}1^{+/-}$ and $IR/IRS\text{-}1/PDX\text{-}1^{+/-}$ mice (Figure 11). However, in some of the sections a few sparsely distributed islets are evident accounting for the barely detectable plasma insulin levels in these mice.

These data indicate the presence of regulatory interactions between the insulin receptor, IRS-1 and the transcription factor PDX-1, and demonstrate how a partial defect in PDX-1 action may limit the ability of the β-cell to functionally compensate in the presence of insulin resistance. Furthermore, this mouse model demonstrates how multiple defects which simultaneously impair insulin action and insulin secretion act synergistically to produce early onset diabetes.

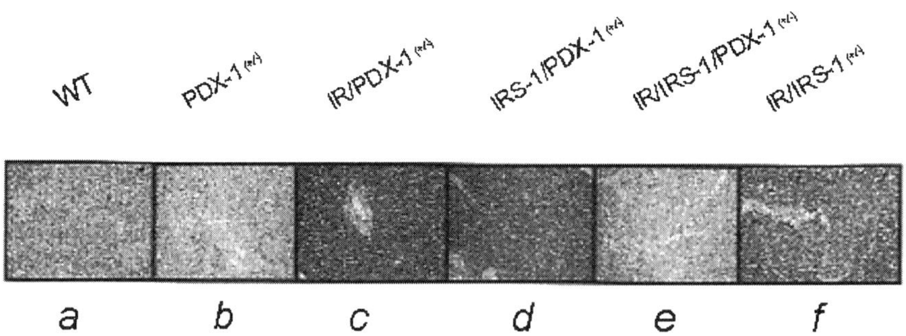

Figure 11. *Reduced islet size in $IRS\text{-}1/PDX\text{-}1^{+/-}$ and $IR/IRS\text{-}1/PDX\text{-}1^{+/-}$ mice*
Examination of islets in pancreas sections shows a mild reduction in size in $PDX\text{-}1^{+/-}$ mice (panel b*) while a greater decrease is observed in $IRS\text{-}1/PDX\text{-}1^{+/-}$ (panel* d*) and $IR/IRS\text{-}1/PDX\text{-}1^{+/-}$ (panel* e*) compared to wild type (panel* a*) mice. Pancreas sections from $IR/IRS\text{-}1^{+/-}$ mice show large islets (panel* f*). Representative sections are shown. Magnification 4x.*

IMPACT OF INSULIN RESISTANCE ON ISLET/β-CELL BIOLOGY

Taken together from the discussion in the preceding sections and reports in the literature, it is becoming increasingly clear that the pancreatic islet is a novel insulin-sensitive tissue and that insulin resistance impacts islet biology in at least two ways. In a regulatory attempt to overcome the early insulin resistance and maintain plasma glucose in the normal range, the organism responds by *islet hyperplasia* leading to a further increase in insulin secretion. As the disease progresses and the insulin levels continue to rise, insulin resistance at the level of the β-cell itself contributes to an *impaired insulin secretion* as part of a unifying hypothesis that ultimately leads to the full blown syndrome of type 2 diabetes. The various roles of the insulin and IGF-1 receptors and the insulin receptor substrates in islet function have been discussed briefly at the end of each section in this chapter.

The factors that promote *islet hyperplasia* during the initial stages of the disease are currently unknown. Some of the animal models of type 2 diabetes manifest hyperglycaemia. Glucose itself may promote islet growth in these animals (17;19;29); however, other models (such as IRS-1$^{-/-}$ and young IR/IRS-1$^{+/-}$ mice) show significant insulin resistance and islet hyperplasia in the presence of normal blood glucose levels. It is likely that the hyperplasia in the latter mice is due to a growth-promoting effect induced by one or more factors in addition to glucose. The presence of islet growth in both males and females suggests that hormones such as prolactin and placental lactogen are unlikely to be major stimuli. It is therefore reasonable to speculate on the presence and source of an insulin resistance-induced factor that can potentially influence islet/β-cell growth. In fact such a factor along with glucose may contribute to islet hyperplasia when hyperglycaemia is part of the insulin resistant phenotype leading to an additive growth effect.

A schematic representation of possible sources of a putative islet growth factor is shown in Figure 12. Insulin secreted by the pancreatic β-cell is normally transported via the portal vein to the liver where ~50% is rapidly metabolized and the remainder enters the systemic circulation. The liver is the first metabolic target for the actions of insulin, which is known to regulate expression of several metabolic enzymes leading to an overall reduction in hepatic glucose output. Furthermore, insulin regulates the hepatic production of IGF-1 and the IGF-binding proteins and hepatocyte growth factor (HGF) (103-105). Both IGF-1 and HGF are involved in islet development and growth (23;25;62). Thus in mice with the insulin resistant phenotype loss of optimal insulin action in the liver leads to altered regulation and production of IGF binding proteins and the growth factors. Whether alterations in these growth-promoting factors or a novel hepatic factor underlie the islet hyperplasia is presently unclear.

Skeletal muscle and adipose tissue constitute two important targets for insulin-mediated glucose disposal. It is conceivable that hyperinsulinemia directly or indirectly induces one or both of these tissues to secrete a circulating factor to communicate with islets to stimulate β-cell proliferation. That such communication between different tissues likely exists is exemplified by our recent experiments on the muscle and β-cell insulin receptor double tissue-specific knockouts (106). Mice lacking functional insulin receptors in both skeletal muscle *and* the β-cell (βIRKO/MIRKO) show a less severe glucose intolerance compared to βIRKO mice alone. One possible explanation for this observation is the presence of a cross talk between the muscle and the β-cell via a circulating factor. In this context it is interesting to note that Heron *et al* (107) recently cloned the cDNA that encodes human α-endosulfine, a 13 kDa peptide that is expressed in skeletal muscle and heart among other tissues. This endogenous ligand for the sulphonylurea receptor has been shown to stimulate insulin secretion, *in vitro*, by activating K_{ATP} channels in islet β-cells and the gene has a locus for susceptibility to type 1 diabetes (108). Another example for tissue-tissue communication is the adipose-tissue hormone leptin. In addition to its appetite regulatory actions it is clear that leptin has significant direct effects on pancreatic β-cells constituting an adipoinsular axis (109;110). Further characterization of this putative growth factor using islet transplantation in suitable insulin resistant models will be useful to evaluate whether local growth factors (25-28;111) and/or islet neuoropeptides play an autocrine role in the observed islet/β-cell growth (Figure 12).

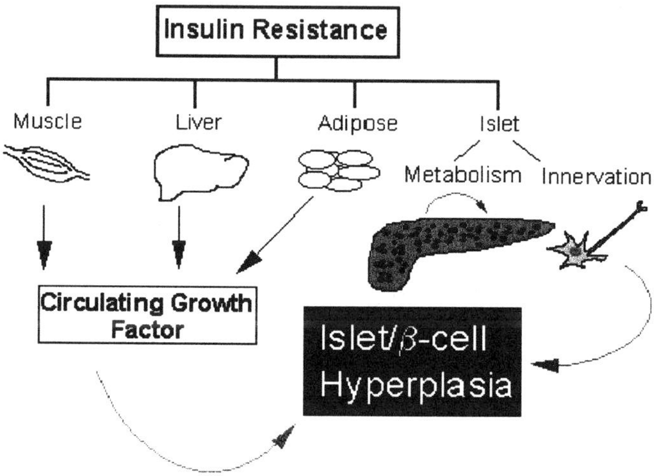

Figure 12. *A hypothetical model depicting the possible sources of a putative insulin-resistance-induced islet growth factor. The presence of insulin resistance in the organism can induce one or more insulin target tissues such as the skeletal muscle, liver and/or adipose to secrete a circulating islet/β-cell-proliferative factor. Alternatively or additively, the high insulin levels can influence islet metabolism and/or islet innervation leading to autocrine or neuronal activation of β-cell growth respectively.*

ACKNOWLEDGEMENTS

Rohit N. Kulkarni was supported by a NIH NRSA Individual Fellowship DK-09825-02. The authors thank Heather L. Brownell for critical reading of the manuscript and Jennifer Konigsberg for excellent secretarial assistance.

REFERENCES

1. Reaven GM. Role of insulin resistance in human disease. Diabetes 1988; 37:1595-1607.
2. Kahn CR. Insulin action, diabetogenes, and the cause of type II diabetes (Banting Lecture). Diabetes 1994; 43(8):1066-1084.
3. Goldberg RB. Cardiovascular disease in diabetic patients. Med Clin North Am 2000; 84(1):81-93.
4. Hansen I, Tsalikian E, Beaufrere B, Gerich JE, Haymond MW, Rizza RA. Insulin resistance in acromegaly: Defects in both hepatic and extrahepatic insulin action. Am J Physiol 1986; 250(3 Pt 1):E269-E273.

5. Weinstein SP, Paquin T, Pritsker A, Haber RS. Glucocorticoid-induced insulin resistance: dexamethasone inhibits the activation of glucose transport in rat skeletal muscle by both insulin- and non-insulin-related stimuli. Diabetes 1995; 44(4):441-445.
6. Franks S, Gilling-Smith C, Watson H, Willis D. Insulin action in the normal and polycystic ovary. Endocrinol Metab Clin North Am 1999; 28(2):361-378.
7. Martin BC, Warram JH, Krolewski AS, Bergman RN, Soeldner JS, Kahn CR. Role of glucose and insulin resistance in development of Type II diabetes mellitus: results of a 25-year follow-up study. Lancet 1992; 340:925-929.
8. Lillioja S, Mott DM, Spraul M, Ferraro R, Foley JE, Ravussin E et al. Insulin resistance and insulin secretory dysfunction as precursors of non-insulin-dependent diabetes mellitus: prospective studies of Pima Indians. N Engl J Med 1993; 329(1988):1992.
9. Gapp DA, Leiter EH, Coleman DL, Schwizer RW. Temporal changes in pancreatic islet composition in C57BL/6J-db/db (diabetes) mice. Diabetologia 1983; 25(5):439-443.
10. Tomita T, Doull V, Pollock HG, Krizsan D. Pancreatic islets of obese hyperglycaemic mice (ob/ob). Pancreas 1992; 7(3):367-375.
11. Tokuyama Y, Sturis J, Depaoli AM, Takeda J, Stoffel M, Tang J et al. Evolution of β-cell dysfunction in the male Zucker diabetic fatty rat. Diabetes 1995; 44(12):1447-1457.
12. Araki E, Lipes MA, Patti ME, Brüning JC, Haag BL, III, Johnson RS et al. Alternative pathway of insulin signalling in mice with targeted disruption of the IRS-1 gene. Nature 1994; 372:186-190.
13. Tamemoto H, Kadowaki T, Tobe K, Yagi T, Sakura H, Hayakawa T et al. Insulin resistance and growth retardation in mice lacking insulin receptor substrate-1. Nature 1994; 372(6502):182-186.
14. Bruning JC, Winnay J, Bonner-Weir S, Taylor SI, Accili D, Kahn CR. Development of a novel polygenic model of NIDDM in mice heterozygous for IR and IRS-1 null alleles. Cell 1997; 88(4):561-572.
15. Kulkarni RN, Winnay JN, Daniels M, Bruning JC, Flier SN, Hanahan D et al. Altered function of insulin receptor substrate-1-deficient mouse islets and cultured β-cell lines. Journal of Clinical Investigation 1999; 104(12):R69-R75.
16. Nielsen JH, Svensson C, Douglas E, Moldrup A, Billestrup N. Beta cell proliferation and growth factors. J Mol Med 1999; 77:62-66.
17. Bonner Weir S, Deery D, Leahy JL, Weir GC. Compensatory growth of pancreatic β-cells in adult rats after short-term glucose infusion. Diabetes 1989; 38(1):49-53.
18. Parsons JA, Brelje TC, Sorenson RL. Adaptation of islets to pregnancy: Increased islet cell proliferation and insulin secretion correlates with the onset of placental lactogen secretion. Endocrinology 1992; 130(3):1459-1466.
19. Hill DJ, Hogg J. Growth factor control of pancreatic β-cell hyperplasia. Baillieres Clin Endocrinol Metab 1991; 5(4):689-698.
20. Sorenson RL, Brelje TC. Adaptation of islets of Langerhans to pregnancy: β-cell growth, enhanced insulin secretion and the role of lactogenic hormones. Horm Metab Res 1997; 29(6):301-307.
21. Nielsen JH, Linde S, Welinder BS, Billestrup N, Madsen OD. Growth hormone is a growth factor for the differentiated pancreatic β-cell. Mol Endocrinol 1989; 3(1):165-173.
22. Swenne I, Heldin CH, Hill DJ, Hellerstrom C. Effects of platelet-derived growth factor and somatomedin- C/insulin-like growth factor I on the deoxyribonucleic acid replication of fetal rat islets of Langerhans in tissue culture. Endocrinology 1988; 122(1):214-218.
23. Otonkoski T, Beattie GM, Rubin JS, Lopez AD, Baird A, Hayek A. Hepatocyte growth factor/scatter factor has insulinotropic activity in human fetal pancreatic cells. Diabetes 1994; 43(7):947-953.
24. Vasavada RC, Cavaliere C, D'Ercole AJ, Dann P, Burtis WJ, Madlener AL et al. Overexpression of parathyroid hormone-related protein in the pancreatic islets of transgenic mice causes islet hyperplasia, hyperinsulinemia, and hypoglycaemia. J Biol Chem 1996; 271(2):1200-1208.
25. Garcia-Ocana A, Takane KK, Syed MA, Philbrick WM, Vasavada RC, Stewart AF. Hepatocyte growth factor overexpression in the islet of transgenic mice increases beta cell proliferation, enhances islet mass, and induces mild hypoglycaemia. J Biol Chem 2000; 275(2):1226-1232.
26. Rane SG, Dubus P, Mettus RV, Galbreath EJ, Boden G, Reddy EP et al. Loss of cyclin-dependent kinase (Cdk4) expression causes insulin-deficient diabetes and cdk4 activation results in β-islet cell hyperplasia. Nat Genet 1999; 22(1):44-52.
27. Petrik J, Pell JM, Arany E, McDonald TJ, Dean WL, Reik W et al. Overexpression of insulin-like growth factor-II in transgenic mice is associated with pancreatic islet cell hyperplasia. Endocrinology 1999; 140(5):2353-2363.
28. Devedjian JC, George M, Casellas A, Pujol A, Visa J, Pelegrin M et al. Transgenic mice overexpressing insulin-like growth factor-II in β-cells develop type 2 diabetes. J Clin Invest 2000; 105(6):731-740.
29. Hugl SR, White MF, Rhodes CJ. IGF-1 stimulated pancreatic β-cell growth is glucose dependent: synergistic activation of IRS-mediated signal transduction pathways by glucose and IGF-1 in INS-1 cells. J Biol Chem 1998; 273(28):17771-17779.
30. Kloppel G, Lohr M, Habich K, Oberholzer M, Heitz PU. Islet pathology and the pathogenesis of type 1 and type 2 diabetes mellitus revisited. Surv Synth Pathol Res 1985; 4(2):110-125.

31. Pinar H, Pinar T, Singer DB. Beta-cell hyperplasia in macrosomic infants and foetuses of nondiabetic mothers. Pediatr Dev Pathol 2000; 3(1):48-52.
32. Stefan Y, Orci L, Malaisse-Lagae F, Perrelet A, Patel Y, Unger RH. Quantitation of endocrine cell content in the pancreas of nondiabetic and diabetic humans. Diabetes 1982; 31(8 Pt 1):694-700.
33. Gepts W, Lecompte PM. The pancreatic islets in diabetes. The American Journal of Medicine 1981; 70:105-115.
34. Westermark P, Wilander E. The influence of amyloid deposits on the islet volume in maturity onset diabetes mellitus. Diabetologia 1978; 15:417-421.
35. Patti ME, Kahn CR. The insulin receptor--a critical link in glucose homeostasis and insulin action. J Basic Clin Physiol Pharmacol 1998; 9(2-4):89-109.
36. Lamothe B, Baudry A, Desbois P, Lamotte L, Bucchini D, De Meyts P et al. Genetic engineering in mice: impact on insulin signalling and action. Biochem J 1998; 335:193-204.
37. Liu JP, Baker J, Perkins JA, Robertson EJ, Efstratiadis A. Mice carrying null mutations of the genes encoding insulin-like growth factor I (Igf-1) and type 1 IGF receptor (Igf1r). Cell 1993; 75:59-72.
38. Accili D, Drago J, Lee EJ, Johnson MD, Cool MH, Salvatore P et al. Early neonatal death in mice homozygous for a null allele of the insulin receptor gene. Nat Genet 1996; 12(1):106-109.
39. Joshi RL, Lamothe B, Cordonnier N, Mesbah K, Monthioux E, Jami J et al. Targeted disruption of the insulin receptor gene in the mouse results in neonatal lethality. EMBO J 1996; 15(7):1542-1547.
40. Withers DJ, Gutierrez JS, Towery H, Burks DJ, Ren JM, Previs S et al. Disruption of IRS-2 causes type 2 diabetes in mice. Nature 1998; 391(6670):900-904.
41. Kulkarni RN, Bruning JC, Winnay JN, Postic C, Magnuson MA, Kahn CR. Tissue-specific knockout of the insulin receptor in pancreatic β cells creates an insulin secretory defect similar to that in Type 2 diabetes. Cell 1999; 96(3):329-339.
42. Cheatham B, Kahn CR. Insulin action and the insulin signalling network. Endocr Rev 1995; 16(2):117-142.
43. White MF, Kahn CR. The insulin signalling system. J Biol Chem 1994; 269(1):1-4.
44. White MF. The IRS-signalling system: a network of docking proteins that mediate insulin and cytokine action. Recent Prog Horm Res 1998; 53:119-138.
45. Virkamaki A, Ueki K, Kahn CR. Protein-protein interaction in insulin signalling and the molecular mechanisms of insulin resistance. J Clin Invest 1999; 103(7):931-943.
46. Anai M, Ono H, Funaki M, Fukushima Y, Inukai K, Ogihara T et al. Different subcellular distribution and regulation of expression of insulin receptor substrate (IRS)-3 from those of IRS-1 and IRS-2. J Biol Chem 1998; 273(45):29686-29692.
47. Fantin VR, Sparling JD, Slot JW, Keller SR, Lienhard GE, Lavan BE. Characterization of insulin receptor substrate 4 in human embryonic kidney 293 cells. J Biol Chem 1998; 273(17):10726-10732.
48. Rothenberg PL, Willison LD, Simon J, Wolf BA. Glucose-induced insulin receptor tyrosine phosphorylation in insulin-secreting β-cells. Diabetes 1995; 44(7):802-809.
49. Leibiger IB, Leibiger B, Moede T, Berggren PO. Exocytosis of insulin promotes insulin gene transcription via the insulin receptor/PI-3 kinase/p70 s6 kinase and CaM kinase. Mol Cell 1998; 1(6):933-938.
50. Xu GG, Rothenberg PL. Insulin receptor signalling in the β-cell influences insulin gene expression and insulin content. Diabetes 1998; 47:1243-1252.
51. Aspinwall CA, Lakey JR, Kennedy RT. Insulin-stimulated insulin secretion in single pancreatic β-cells. J Biol Chem 1999; 274(10):6360-6365.
52. Hanahan D. Heritable formation of pancreatic β-cell tumours in transgenic mice expressing recombinant insulin/simian virus 40 oncogenes. Nature 1985; 315(6015):115-122.
53. Efrat S, Linde S, Kofod H, Spector D, Delannoy M, Grant S et al. Beta-cell lines derived from transgenic mice expressing a hybrid insulin gene-oncogene. Proc Natl Acad Sci U S A 1988; 85(23):9037-9041.
54. Efrat S, Leiser M, Surana M, Tal M, Fusco-DeMane D, Fleischer N. Murine insulinoma cell line with normal glucose-regulated insulin secretion. Diabetes 1993; 42(6):901-907.
55. Knaack DFDM, Surana M, Leiser M, Laurance M, Fusco-DeMane D, Hegre OD et al. Clonal insulinoma cell line that stably maintains correct glucose responsiveness. Diabetes 1994; 43(12):1413-1417.
56. D'Ambra R, Surana M, Efrat S, Starr RG, Fleischer N. Regulation of insulin secretion from beta-cell lines derived from trangenic mice insulinomas resembles that of normal beta-cells. Endocrinology 1990; 126(6):2815-2822.
57. Patti ME, Sun XJ, Bruning JC, Araki E, Lipes MA, White MF et al. 4PS/IRS-2 is the alternative substrate of the insulin receptor in IRS-1 deficient mice. J Biol Chem 1995; 270(42):24670-24673.
58. Bonner-Weir S, Withers DJ, Weir GC, Jonas JC. Impaired survival of differentiating beta cells but no insulin secretory defects result from ablation of IRS-2. Diabetes 48[Suppl.1], A3. 1999. Ref Type: Abstract
59. Kadowaki T, Tobe K, Terauchi Y, Eto K, Yamauchi T, Kubota N. Molecular pathogenesis of type 2 diabetes mellitus and obesity in knockout mice models. Keystone Symposia 2000 , 119. 2000. Ref Type: Abstract

60. Van Schravendijk CF, Foriers A, Van den Brande JL, Pipeleers DG. Evidence for the presence of type I insulin-like growth factor receptors on rat pancreatic A and B cells. Endocrinology 1987; 121(5):1784-1788.
61. Sun XJ, Pons S, Wang LM, Zhang Y, Yenush L, Burks D et al. The IRS-2 gene on murine chromosome 8 encodes a unique signalling adapter for insulin and cytokine action. Mol Endocrinol 1997; 11(2):251-262.
62. Withers DJ, Burks DJ, Towery HH, Altamuro SL, Flint CL, White MF. IRS-2 coordinates IGF-1 receptor-mediated beta cell development and peripheral insulin signalling. Nat Genet 1999; 23(1):32-40.
63. Postel-Vinay MC, Kelly PA. Growth hormone receptor signalling. Baillieres Clin Endocrinol Metab 1996; 10(3):323-336.
64. Bole-Feysot C, Goffin V, Edery M, Binart N, Kelly PA. Prolactin (PRL) and its receptor: actions, signal transduction pathways and phenotypes observed in PRL receptor knockout mice. Endocr Rev 1998; 19(3):225-268.
65. Moldrup A, Billestrup N, Thorn NA, Lernmark A, Nielsen JH. Multiple growth hormone-binding proteins are expressed on insulin-producing cells. Mol Endocrinol 1989; 3(8):1173-1182.
66. Sorenson RL, Stout LE. Prolactin receptors and JAK2 in islets of Langerhans: An immunohistochemical analysis. Endocrinology 1995; 136(9):4092-4098.
67. Laakso M, Malkki M, Kekalainen P, Kuusisto J, Deeb SS. Insulin receptor substrate-1 variants in non-insulin-dependent diabetes. J Clin Invest 1994; 94(3):1141-1146.
68. Almind K, Bjorbaek C, Vestergaard H, Hansen T, Echwald SM, Pedersen O. Amino acid polymorphisms of insulin receptor substrate-1 in non-insulin-dependent diabetes mellitus. Lancet 1993; 342(8875):828-832.
69. Imai Y, Fusco A, Suzuki Y, Lesniak MA, D'Alfonso R, Sesti G et al. Variant sequences of insulin receptor substrate-1 in patients with noninsulin dependent diabetes mellitus. J Clin Endocrinol Metab 1994; 79(6):1655-1658.
70. Zhang Y, Wat N, Stratton IM, Warren-Perry MG, Orho M, Groop L et al. UKPDS 19: Heterogeneity in NIDDM: Separate contributions of IRS-1 and β3-adrenergic-receptor mutations to insulin resistance and obesity respectively with no evidence for glycogen synthase gene mutations. UK Prospective Diabetes Study. Diabetologia 1996; 39(12):1505-1511.
71. Bernal D, Almind K, Yenush L, Ayoub M, Zhang Y, Rosshani L et al. IRS-2 Amino acid polymorphisms are not associated with random type 2 diabetes amoung caucasians. Diabetes 1998; 47:976-979.
72. Porzio O, Federici M, Hribal ML, Lauro D, Accili D, Lauro R et al. The Gly972 to Arg amino acid polymorphism in IRS-1 impairs insulin secretion in pancreatic β cells. J Clin Invest 1999; 104:357-364.
73. Liu SC, Wang Q, Lienhard GE, Keller SR. Insulin receptor substrate 3 is not essential for growth or glucose homeostasis. J Biol Chem 1999; 274(25):18093-18099.
74. Fantin VR, Wang GE, Lienhard GE, Keller SR. Mice lacking insulin receptor substrate 4 exhibit mild defects in growth, reproduction, and homostasis. Am J Physiol 2000; 278:E127-133.
75. Patel YC, Amherdt M, Orci L. Quantitative electron microscopic autoradiography of insulin, glucagon, and somatostatin binding sites on islets. Science 1982; 217(4565):1155-1156.
76. Van Schravendijk CF, Foriers A, Hooghe-Peters EL, Rogiers V, De Meyts P, Sodoyez JC. Pancreatic hormone receptors on islet cells. Endocrinology 1985; 117(3):841-848.
77. Verspohl E, Ammon H. Evidence for the presence of insulin receptors in rat islets of Langerhans. J Clin Invest 1980; 65:1230-1237.
78. Argoud GM, Schade DS, Eaton RP. Insulin suppresses its own secretion *in vivo*. Diabetes 1987; 36(8):959-962.
79. Elahi D, Nagulesparan M, Hershcopf RJ, Muller DC, Tobin JD, Blix PM et al. Feedback inhibition of insulin secretion by insulin: Relation to the hyperinsulinemia of obesity. N Engl J Med 1982; 306(20):1196-1202.
80. Iversen J, Miles DW. Evidence for a feedback inhibition of insulin on insulin secretion in the isolated, perfused canine pancreas. Diabetes 1971; 20(1):1-9.
81. Ammon HP, Reiber C, Verspohl EJ. Indirect evidence for short-loop negative feedback of insulin secretion in the rat. J Endocrinol 1991; 128(1):27-34.
82. Stagner J, Samols E, Polonsky K, Pugh W. Lack of direct inhibition of insulin secretion by exogenous insulin in the canine pancreas. J Clin Invest 1986; 78(5):1193-1198.
83. Velloso LA, Carneiro EM, Crepaldi SC, Boschero AC, Saad MJ. Glucose- and insulin-induced phosphorylation of the insulin receptor and its primary substrates IRS-1 and IRS-2 in rat pancreatic islets. Growth Regul 1995; 377(3):353-357.
84. Harbeck MC, Louie DC, Howland J, Wolf BA, Rothenberg PL. Expression of insulin receptor mRNA and insulin receptor substrate 1 in pancreatic islet β-cells. Diabetes 1996; 45(6):711-717.
85. Gu H, Marth JD, Orban PC, Mossmann H, Rajewsky K. Deletion of a DNA polymerase beta gene segment in T cells using cell type-specific gene targeting. Science 1994; 265(5168):103-106.

86. Metzger D, Clifford J, Chiba H, Chambon P. Conditional site-specific recombination in mammalian cells using a ligand-dependent chimeric Cre recombinase. Proc Natl Acad Sci U S A 1995; 92(15):6991-6995.
87. Pictet R, Rutter WJ. Development of the embryonic endocrine pancreas. In: Steiner DF, Freinkel M, editors. Handbook of Physiology. Washington, D.C.: American Physiological Society, 1972: 25-66.
88. Gannon M, Shiota C, Postic C, Wright CVE, Magnuson M. Analysis of the cre-mediated recombination driven by rat insulin promoter in embryonic and adult mouse pancreas. Genesis 2000; 26(2):139-141.
89. Flier JS, Kahn CR, Roth J, Bar RS. Antibodies that impair insulin receptor binding in an unusual diabetic syndrome with severe insulin resistance. Science 1975; 190:63-65.
90. Taylor SI. Lilly Lecture: Molecular mechanisms of insulin resistance - Lessons from patients with mutations in the insulin receptor gene. Diabetes 1992; 41:1473-1490.
91. Elders MJ, Schedewie HK, Olefsky J, Givens B, Char F, Bier DM et al. Endocrine-metabolic relationships in patients with leprechaunism. J Natl Med Assoc 1982; 74(12):1195-1210.
92. Kido Y, Burks DJ, Withers D, Bruning JC, Kahn CR, White MF et al. Tissue-specific insulin resistance in mice with mjutations in the insulin receptor, IRS-1, and IRS-2. J Clin Invest 2000; 105(2):199-205.
93. Pete G, Fuller CR, Oldham JM, Smith DR, D'Ercole AJ, Kahn CR et al. Postnatal growth responses to insulin-like growth factor I in insulin receptor substrate-1-deficient mice. Endocrinology 1999; 140(12):5478-5487.
94. Anello M, Gilon P, Henquin JC. Alterations of insulin secretion from mouse islets treated with sulphonylureas: perturbations of $Ca2^+$ regulation prevail over changes in insulin content. Br J Pharmacol 1999; 127(8):1883-1891.
95. Terauchi Y, Iwamoto K, Tamemoto H, Komeda K, Ishii C, Kanazawa Y et al. Development of non-insulin-dependent diabetes mellitus in the double knockout mice with disruption of insulin receptor substrate-1 and beta cell glucokinase genes. Genetic reconstitution of diabetes as a polygenic disease. J Clin Invest 1997; 99(5):861-866.
96. Leonard J, Peers B, Johnson T, Ferreri K, Lee S, Montminy MR. Characterization of somatostatin transactivating factor-1, a novel homeobox factor that stimulates somatostatin expression in pancreatic islet cells. Mol Endocrinol 1993; 7(10):1275-1283.
97. Miller CP, McGehee REJ, Habener JF. IDX-1: a new homeodomain transcription factor expressed in rat pancreatic islets and duodenum that transactivates the somatostatin gene. EMBO J 1994; 13(5):1145-1156.
98. Jonsson J, Carlsson L, Edlund T, Edlund H. Insulin-promotor-factor 1 is required for pancreas development in mice. Nature 1994; 371(6498):606-609.
99. Stoffers DA, Zinkin NT, Stanojevic V, Clarke WL, Habener JF. Pancreatic agenesis attributable to a single nucleotide deletion in the human IPF1 gene coding sequence. Nat Genet 1997; 15(1):106-110.
100. Dutta S, Bonner-Weir S, Montminy M, Wright C. Regulatory factor linked to late-onset diabetes? Nature 1998; 392:560.
101. Stoffers DA, Ferrer J, Clarke WL, Habener JF. Early-onset type-II diabetes mellitus (MODY4) linked to IPF1. Nat Genet 1997; 17(2):138-139.
102. Kulkarni RN, Winnay JN, Curtis S, Montminy MR. Creation of a polygenic model of type 2 diabetes: the triple heterozygous knockout. Diabetes 48[Suppl 1], A34. 1999. Ref Type: Abstract
103. Phillips LS, Pao CI, Villafuerte BC. Molecular regulation of insulin-like growth factor-I and its principal binding protein, IGFBP-3. Prog Biophys Mol Biol 1998; 60:195-265.
104. Lawrence JCJ, Fadden P, Haystead TA, Lin TA. PHAS proteins as mediators of the actions of insulin, growth factors and cAMP on protein synthesis and cell proliferation. Adv Enzyme Regul 1997; 37:239-267.
105. Villafuerte BC, Zhang WN, Phillips LS. Insulin and insulin-like growth factor-I regulate hepatic insulin-like growth factor binding protein-3 by different mechanisms. Mol Endocrinology 1996; 10(6):622-630.
106. Mauvais-Jarvis F, Virkamaki A, Michael MD, Kulkarni RN. Double tissue-specific knockout of the insulin receptor in pancreatic beta-cell and in skeletal muscle (BIRKO-MIRKO). Diabetes 48[Suppl. 1], A275. 1999. Ref Type: Abstract
107. Heron L, Virsolvy A, Peyrollier K, Gribble FM, Le Cam A, Ashcroft FM et al. Human alpha-endosulfine, a possible regulator of sulfonylurea-sensitive KATP channel: molecular cloning, expression and biological properties. Proc Natl Acad Sci 1998; 95(14):8387-8391.
108. Heron L, Virsolvy A, Apiou F, Le Cam A, Bataille D. Isolation, characterization, and chromosomal localization of the human ENSA gene that encodes alpha-endosulfine, a regulator of beta-cell K(ATP) channels. Diabetes 1999; 48(9):1873-1876.
109. Kulkarni RN, Wang ZL, Wang RM, Hurley JD, Smith DM, Ghatei MA et al. Leptin rapidly suppresses insulin release from insulinoma cells, rat and human islets and, *in vivo*, in mice. J Clin Invest 1997; 100(11):2729-2736.
110. Kieffer TJ, Habener JF. The adipoinsular axis: effects of leptin on pancreatic beta-cells. Am J Physiol Endocrinol Metab 2000; 278(1):E1-E14.

111. Zarnegar R, Muga S, Rahija R, Michalopoulos G. Tissue distribution of hepatopoietin-A: a heparin-binding polypeptide growth factor for hepatocytes. Proc Natl Acad Sci 1990; 87(3):1252-1256.
112. Bonner-Weir S. Islet growth and development in the adult. J Endocrinology 2000; 24:297-302.

19
CLINICAL CONSEQUENCES OF DEFECTS IN β-CELL GENES

Julie C. Evans, B.Sc., Timothy M. Frayling, Ph.D., and Andrew T. Hattersley, D.M.
Department of Vascular Medicine and Diabetes Research
School of Postgraduate Medicine and Health Sciences
Barrack Road, Exeter, Devon, UK EX2 5AX

INTRODUCTION

Genes critical for β-cell function have been identified by the genetic analysis of families with maturity onset diabetes of the young (MODY). The clinical description of MODY families by Fajans and Tattersall (1,2) and the development of appropriate molecular genetic techniques were both critical in the definition of these genes. In this chapter, we describe the clinical and physiological features of patients with known defects in β-cell genes. This has led to the demonstration of previously un-recognized heterogeneity in clinically defined MODY. In addition, it has given fascinating insights into the role of the genes in the normal β-cell both in post-natal and foetal life.

β-CELL GENE MUTATIONS RESULTING IN MATURITY-ONSET DIABETES OF THE YOUNG

While many genes are important for normal β-cell function, mutations that result in diabetes or hyperglycaemia have been found only in a few of these genes. The majority of these gene mutations result in maturity-onset diabetes of the young (MODY), which is characterized by an autosomal dominant inheritance of early-onset (usually before 25 yr), non-insulin dependent diabetes. MODY is genetically heterogeneous as it can result from mutations in five genes: the pancreatic "glucose-sensing" enzyme glucokinase (MODY2) (3,4), and the transcription factors Hepatocyte Nuclear Factor (HNF)-4α (MODY1) (5), HNF-1α (MODY3) (6), Insulin promoter factor (IPF)-1 (MODY4) (7) and HNF-1β (MODY5) (8). Each genetic sub-group has a distinct phenotype (Table 1).

GLUCOKINASE

Glucokinase as a candidate gene for MODY

The role of glucokinase in insulin secretion made it an ideal candidate gene for MODY. Glucokinase is predominantly expressed in pancreatic β-cells and in hepatocytes where it catalyzes the first step in glucose metabolism, the phosphorylation of glucose to glucose-6-phosphate. In β-cells this step is closely linked with the initiation of insulin secretion (9,10). Unlike other hexokinases, glucokinase has a low affinity for glucose (K_m of 5 mmol/l plasma glucose concentration) and is not inhibited by its product. These features allow β-cells and hepatocytes (the two main organs expressing GLUT2) to be most responsive to changes in glucose concentrations at physiological glucose levels (4-15 mmol/l). Glucokinase has consequently been termed the "pancreatic glucose sensor."

	HNF-4α (MODY 1)	Glucokinase (MODY 2)	HNF-1α (MODY 3)	IPF-1 (MODY 4)	HNF-1β (MODY 5)
Chromosomal location	20q	7p	12q	13q	17q
Frequency in a large UK series	3%	14%	61%	4%	1%
Mutations	No evidence of a common mutation	No evidence of a common mutation	C insertion in the exon 4 C tract (codon 291) in ≅25% of families with mutations	D76N found in many populations	No evidence of a common mutation
Penetrance of mutations at age 40 yrs	>80%	45% (>90% fpg>6 mmol/l)	>95%	>80%	?>95%
Onset of hyperglycaemia	Adolescence Early adulthood	Early childhood (from birth)	Adolesence Early adulthood	?Early adulthood	?Similar to HNF-1α
Severity of hyperglycaemia	Progressive May become severe	Mild with minor deterioration with age	Progressive May be severe	Limited data ? less penetrant than HNF-1α	May be severe
Micro-vascular complications	Frequent	Rare	Frequent	Little data	Frequent
Pathophysiology	β-cell dysfunction	β-cell dysfunction	β-cell dysfunction	?β-cell dysfunction	?β-cell dysfunction
Abnormalityof glucose sensing?	No	Yes	No	?No	?No
Priming with hyperglycaemia	No	Yes	Yes—if normoglycaemic	Not known	Not known
Non-diabetes related features		Reduced birth weight	Low renal threshold and aminoadicuria	Pancreatic agenesis in homozygotes	Renal cysts Proteinuria Renal failure

Table 1. *Comparison of the different sub-types of Maturity-Onset Diabetes of the Young (MODY)*

Glucokinase Mutation Studies

The demonstration of linkage between MODY and the glucokinase gene (3,4) was quickly followed by characterization of the human gene and detection of mutations (11-14). The first mutation was reported in 1992 (11) and over 80 mutations of the glucokinase gene have now been described in many populations although the majority have been found in France (11-13,15-22). These mutations are distributed throughout the gene and no single mutation predominates. All these mutations are associated with hyperglycaemia and reduced enzymatic glucokinase activity *in vitro* (23-25). This subgroup of MODY resulting from glucokinase genes has been designated MODY2.

In a single family, a gain of function mutation has been shown to result in hypoglycaemia (26). This mutation increases the enzyme's affinity for glucose thus glycolysis proceeds faster than normal at relatively low glucose concentrations. Patients heterozygous for the mutation have a lower than normal blood glucose threshold for insulin secretion resulting in mild hypoglycaemia, the opposite situation to MODY2.

Reported glucokinase mutation frequencies in MODY families are very variable. In France, the prevalence of glucokinase mutations is estimated at 56% (18) but in British MODY pedigrees it is approximately 12.5% (4,27-29) and in Japanese less than 1% (30). These differences are likely to be the result of population heterogeneity and the alternative approaches to selecting families used in the separate studies. Screening studies have detected glucokinase mutations in 0.5-2% of type 2 diabetes patients (13,31) and 1-5% of subjects with gestational diabetes (16,31,32).

Glucokinase Phenotype
Different mutations of the glucokinase gene result in a remarkably similar phenotype (33,34). Patients with glucokinase mutations have mild (6-9 mmol/l) fasting hyperglycaemia from early childhood and probably from birth (18). There is a small increment during an oral glucose tolerance test (35); indeed, only 46% of a large French series had diabetes by WHO criteria (18). In keeping with the mild hyperglycaemia found in these patients, diabetic complications, particularly microvascular ones, are rare, and treatment with diet is usually adequate (18,21,36). During pregnancy most patients need, or are given, insulin to attain strict glycaemic control (36). Recently we have shown that glucokinase mutations can be detected in 80% of subjects with gestational diabetes who have a characteristic phenotype (fasting plasma glucose (fpg) > 5.5 mmol/l, 2hr glucose value < 4 mmol/l higher than the fasting value, familial hyperglycaemia and treatment with insulin in pregnancy) (Ellard, S., Beards, F., Hattersley, A.T., personal communication).

β-cell dysfunction has been demonstrated in subjects with a glucokinase mutation using a wide variety of methods of physiological testing (4,36-38). This β-cell defect is an abnormality of glucose sensing as was elegantly demonstrated by Byrne and colleagues, who measured insulin secretion during a slow stepped glucose infusion (38). In glucokinase deficient subjects, the maximum rate of change of insulin secretion was at a glucose value of 7 mmol/l rather than the 5.5 mmol/l seen in controls. This is consistent with the idea of a resetting of the pancreatic glucose sensor as a result of a glucokinase mutation. The increase in the plasma glucose threshold for insulin secretion by the β-cell results in mild hyperglycaemia throughout life. A slight deterioration of β-cell function is seen with age but the rate of decline is similar to that for non-diabetics (36). Glucokinase is also expressed in the liver, and reduced synthesis of glycogen in response to a glucose load has been demonstrated in subjects with glucokinase mutations (39). Insulin resistance has not been demonstrated in MODY2 patients in most studies (4,36). In a large French series there was a slightly increased proportion of MODY2 patients who had frank diabetes rather than just fasting hyperglycaemia or impaired glucose tolerance (40). It is uncertain if this reflects different severity of glucokinase mutations, modifying type 2 diabetes genes or a secondary effect of hyperglycaemia.

HEPATOCYTE NUCLEAR FACTOR-1α

HNF-1α mutations
The transcription factor HNF-1α is a DNA-binding protein that regulates gene expression in many tissues (41-43) and was originally not known to play an important role in β-cells. In contrast to the candidate gene approach to identify glucokinase, HNF-1α was found by linkage analysis. Linkage was first shown to a 10 cM locus on the long-arm of chromosome 12 (MODY3) (44), genetic and clinical

mapping then identified HNF-1α as the MODY3 gene (6). HNF-1α was rapidly shown to be the most common known cause of MODY in UK (45), German (46), French (47), Danish (48), Italian (49) Finnish (50), North American (50) and Japanese (51) pedigrees.

Phenotype of HNF-1α mutations

There are striking differences between the phenotype of patients with HNF-1α and glucokinase mutations. Patients with HNF-1α mutations are usually normoglycaemic in childhood and usually develop diabetes in adolescence or early adulthood. Patients have a progressive deterioration in β-cell function resulting in progressive hyperglycaemia and/or increased treatment requirements with age (29). Patients with a long duration frequently suffer from diabetes complications particularly retinopathy and nephropathy (52,53). As in other types of diabetes, it is important for these patients to aim for tight glycaemic control. Approximately 2/3 of patients will require insulin or oral hypoglycaemic treatment to achieve adequate glucose levels. Caution is needed when first starting HNF-1α patients on sulphonylureas as they can be very sensitive to them and respond with marked hypoglycaemia (54).

The predominant defect is β-cell dysfunction but unlike glucokinase this is not because of a failure of glucose sensing. In contrast to the majority of type 2 diabetes, insulin resistance is not a feature of diabetes in these patients. Non-diabetic subjects with an HNF-1α mutation show normal insulin secretion at normal blood glucose concentrations but once levels exceed 8 mmol/l the insulin secretion response (ISR) is reduced (55). β-cell function progressively deteriorates with age and patients become increasingly hyperglycaemic. This contrasts with subjects with glucokinase mutations who always have a fasting plasma glucose above normal, but the β-cell dysfunction is relatively stable throughout life.

HEPATOCYTE NUCLEAR FACTOR-4α

HNF-4α mutations

The MODY1 gene locus was identified as a 13 cM region on chromosome 20q by linkage analysis in one large North American MODY pedigree (56). Once HNF-1α had been identified as a MODY gene, the functionally similar HNF-4α gene became an obvious candidate for investigation. Sequence analysis of the HNF-4α gene in members of the linked North American family revealed a mutation, Q268X, which results in a truncated HNF-4α protein (5). HNF-4α mutations are relatively rare and have been described in both European and Japanese pedigrees (5,57-61).

Phenotype of HNF-4α mutations

Patients with HNF-4α mutations show a very similar phenotype to those with HNF-1α mutations. This may reflect the similar functions and expression patterns of the two proteins. HNF-4α regulates HNF-1α gene expression, and HNF-4α mutations probably lead to diabetes by reducing the expression of HNF-1α. One clinical difference between MODY 3 and 1 is seen in the responses to a prolonged 18-hour low dose glucose infusion in pre-diabetic subjects. Non-diabetic subjects with HNF-4α mutations show a loss of the priming effect of glucose on the insulin secretion rate (62) whereas subjects with HNF-1α mutations maintain this response until the onset of frank diabetes (55). It has been noted that patients with missense mutations in HNF-4αare often diagnosed later in life than subjects with HNF-1α mutations (57,61).

INSULIN PROMOTER FACTOR-1

IPF-1 as a candidate gene for MODY

Insulin promoter factor (IPF)-1 (also known as IDX-1, STF-1, IUF-1, GSTF, and Pdx1) is a transcription factor that plays an important role in early pancreatic development and regulates several β-cell specific genes, including insulin (63-65). IPF-1 was therefore a good candidate for a role in the pathogenesis of diabetes. Inoue and colleagues reported the cloning of the human form of the gene in 1996 (66).

From mouse knockout to human knockout to MODY4

Targeted disruption of the IPF-1 gene results in pancreatic agenesis (absence of pancreas) in mice (65). When a human subject was identified with this phenotype, the IPF-1 gene was screened and the patient was found to be homozygous for a frameshift mutation, P63fsdelC (67). Further analysis of this patient's extended family shows that this mutation, in heterozygous form, segregates with early onset type 2 diabetes. This led to IPF-1 being designated MODY4 (7). Although this family fits the diagnostic criteria for MODY, only one subject, excluding the homozygous subject with pancreatic agenesis, was diagnosed under 25 years and the average age at diagnosis was 35 years. To date this single family represents the only example of an IPF-1 mutation causing MODY.

IPF-1 mutations may impair the ability of β-cells to compensate for increasing demands as people age (7). A number of mechanisms could explain this, including abnormal β-cell development and decreased expression of β-cell genes such as insulin, GLUT2 and glucokinase (7). Mice with IPF-1 inactivated only in the β-cells develop impaired glucose tolerance and diabetes (68). This suggests that the role of IPF-1 in mature β-cell gene regulation is important in diabetes susceptibility but does not rule out an effect on pancreas development as well in MODY.

HEPATOCYTE NUCLEAR FACTOR-1β

HNF-1β mutations

The identification of HNF-1α as a MODY gene led to the suggestion that mutations in HNF-1β could also result in MODY. Although not previously linked with MODY (as HNF-4α had been) HNF-1β was known to be structurally very similar to HNF-1α, to be expressed in the pancreas and to form heterodimers with HNF-1α (42). Screening of Japanese subjects and of a Norwegian family with MODY revealed three frameshift mutations co-segregating with diabetes in three families (8,69,70).

Phenotype of HNF-1β mutations

Patients with HNF-1β mutations fit the diagnostic criteria for MODY well with all three families showing autosomal dominant inheritance and an average age at diagnosis of 21 years (based on eleven patients). In addition, all eleven patients from these families have renal disease. This varies between renal failure, renal cysts and proteinuria. Renal cysts and impaired kidney function have both been shown to precede the onset of diabetes (69). Hence, mutations in this gene appear to directly cause renal abnormalities rather than renal dysfunction being secondary to diabetes. HNF-1β is expressed very early in renal development. The critical role in nephron development has also been shown in a 17-week foetus with an HNF-1β mutation and no nephrogenesis (Hattersley, A.T. personal communication).

THE POSSIBLE ROLE OF MODY GENES IN TYPE 2 DIABETES MELLITUS

With the exception of MODY, progress in identifying type 2 diabetes genes has been limited and no common predisposing genes have been found. We recently showed that missense mutations in IPF-1 are 3.8 times as common in patients with type 2 diabetes as in the general population (3.8% and 1% respectively (71)). This is the first example of a gene in which a severe mutation (i.e. mutation leading to severely impaired IPF-1 function) causes MODY and a relatively common mild mutation is associated with type 2 diabetes.

Additional studies suggest that there is linkage in type 2 diabetes to the chromosomal regions of MODY genes, but to date no mutations have been shown. A study of 26 families with a high prevalence of type 2 diabetes from the Botnia region of Finland resulted in the identification of the NIDDM2 locus (72). The six families with the lowest insulin secretion response to an oral glucose load demonstrated linkage to the MODY3 region on the long arm of chromosome 12. No variants of the coding region of the HNF-1α gene have been reported. A mutation in an uncharacterized regulatory region of HNF-1αmay be responsible for type 2 diabetes in these families.

Several studies have reported diabetic relatives showing increased allele sharing of chromosome 20 markers close to the HNF-4α gene (73-76). It is uncertain if the diabetes susceptibility gene in this region is HNF-4α or another gene in the vicinity of the HNF-4α locus. HNF-4α may be involved but to date only few mutations have been described. Thus, it is unlikely that HNF-4α mutations contribute in a major way to type 2 diabetes mellitus. In one French family, a later phenotype was observed with a mutation in HNF-4α (61) but this accounted for just one of over 140 French families.

β-CELL GENES AND FOETAL DEVELOPMENT

Insulin as a growth factor

In the foetus, insulin is more important in promoting foetal growth than in regulating foetal blood glucose (which largely depends on the maternal blood glucose) (77-80). In humans, the pancreas forms between the 5th and 8th week of gestation and insulin secretion begins at around the 10th week of gestation. Maternal insulin cannot cross the placenta, and the foetus produces its own insulin in response to hyperglycaemia. Foetal insulin secretion is regulated by maternal glucose concentrations by the beginning of the third trimester. Maternal hyperglycaemia at this time results in increased foetal insulin secretion and in increased size at birth. Mutations that alter β-cell function in the foetus can have profound effects on foetal growth (see Table 2); over-secretion of insulin by the foetus produces a large baby and under-secretion of insulin (or insulin resistance) retards foetal growth. These observations offer potential new insights into the described association between low birth weight and adult onset diabetes (81,82).

Foetal Glucokinase mutations

As described in the previous section, glucokinase is the enzyme important for glucose sensing by the β-cell. A loss of function mutation in glucokinase effectively raises the blood glucose threshold for insulin secretion. Babies who have a glucokinase mutation are born approximately 500g smaller than siblings without the mutation (22). This reflects a reduction in foetal insulin secretion in response to the maternal blood glucose levels as a result of impaired glucose sensing by foetal β-cells. In contrast, babies born to mothers with a glucokinase mutation are approximately 600g heavier than babies born to mothers without the mutation. In this case, the foetus secretes more insulin than normal because of raised maternal blood glucose. When both mother and baby have a glucokinase mutation the two contradictory influences of maternal and foetal mutations cancel each other out and the baby is of normal birth weight (22). No effect on birth weight of the gain of function glucokinase mutation (26) has been reported. It would be expected that increased foetal insulin secretion would mean that babies with the mutation would be heavier than babies without the mutation.

Foetal Sulphonylurea receptor and pancreatic islet potassium inward rectifier mutations.

The sulphonylurea receptor (SUR) and the pancreatic islet potassium inward rectifier, Kir6.2, are subunits of the ATP-sensitive potassium channels that are important in β-cell glucose sensing and insulin secretory response (83). These channels allow small amounts of potassium to leak out of the β-cells and are thus important for maintaining the resting membrane potential. Normally the β-cell potassium channels are closed by an increase in cellular ATP or a decrease in ADP and this triggers insulin release. Mutations in either SUR (84) or Kir6.2 (85) cause Persistent Hyperinsulinaemic Hypoglycaemia of Infancy (PHHI). PHHI is characterized by autosomal recessive inheritance of severe hypoglycaemia. Hypoglycaemia develops soon after birth and often requires removal of most of the pancreas to control it. In PHHI the non-functional potassium channels are in effect always closed such that insulin secretion is constitutive and not regulated by blood glucose levels. In the foetus, this excessive insulin secretion leads to excessive growth so babies born with the disorder are usually large (> 4 kg).

Condition Altered insulin secretion	Genetic defect	Altered physiology	Birth weight
Glucokinase deficiency	Heterozygous mutations in the glucokinase gene (18)	Reduced insulin secretion (to 30% of normal) resulting from reduced glucose sensing by the pancreas (38)	Reduced by 521g compared to unaffected sib (22)
Pancreatic agenesis	Homozygous mutation in IPF-1 gene (67)	No foetal insulin secretion as a result of pancreatic agenesis	Markedly reduced below first centile (90)
Transient neonatal diabetes	Paternal isodisomy or duplication of 6q22-q23 (91,92)	Markedly reduced insulin secretion mechanism uncertain	Markedly reduced most <first centile (93)
Nesideoblastosis	Homozygous mutation in the SUR or Kir6 genes (84,85)	Increased insulin secretion as a result of activation of the SUR receptor	Increased most >90th centile (94)

Table 2: *Monogenic conditions that alter foetal insulin secretion, and insulin resistance and their effect on birth weight.*

Foetal IPF-1 mutations

IPF-1 is expressed very early in the developing pancreas where it promotes proliferation and differentiation of the pancreatic epithelium (86). Mice and humans who are homozygous for inactivating IPF-1 mutations do not develop a pancreas (pancreatic agenesis) (67,65). Babies with pancreatic agenesis cannot produce any insulin and are born small for their gestational age (< 1st centile).

Foetal growth and type 2 diabetes - the foetal insulin hypothesis

The association between low birth weight and the propensity to develop type 2 diabetes (81) has previously been attributed to intrauterine malnutrition with programming of the foetus *in utero* (i.e. the "thrifty" phenotype) (87-89). The effect of β-cell gene defects on birth weight suggest that low birth weight and type 2 diabetes could both be phenotypes of genetic β-cell defects or genetic insulin resistance. This alternative genetic explanation of the association of low birth weight with type 2 diabetes has been termed the "foetal insulin hypothesis" (22,82).

CONCLUSION

Mutations in any of five genes: glucokinase; hepatic nuclear factor 1α (HNF-1α); hepatic nuclear factor 1β (HNF-1β); hepatic nuclear factor 4α (HNF-4α) and insulin promoter factor 1 (IPF-1) can result in diabetes or hyperglycaemia. Mutations in these genes result in discrete clinical and pathophysiological characteristics. New insights into foetal development have come from the observations of foetal growth in the presence of mutations in genes important for β-cell development and/or function.

ACKNOWLEDGEMENTS

The authors are very grateful to the British Diabetic Association, the Medical Research Council, Northcott Devon Medical Foundation, DIRECT, PPP Healthcare Trust, The Darlington Trust, The Royal Devon and Exeter NHS Trust, Perkin Elmer Applied Biosystems and the University of Exeter for supporting the work on MODY in Exeter. Tim Frayling is a career scientist sponsored by the South and West NHS executive. We acknowledge the help of our colleagues, in particular: Sian Ellard, Francis Beards, Mike Bulman, Mark Dronsfield, Lisa Allen, Susan Ayres and Maggie Shepherd.

REFERENCES

1. Tattersall RB. Mild familial diabetes with dominant inheritance. Q J Med 1974;43:339-357.
2. Tattersall RB, Fajans SS. A difference between the inheritance of classical juvenile-onset and maturity-onset type diabetes of young people. Diabetes 1975;24:44-53.
3. Froguel P, Vaxillaire M, Sun F, et al. Close linkage of glucokinase locus on chromosome 7p to early-onset non-insulin-dependent diabetes mellitus. Nature 1992;356:162-4.
4. Hattersley AT, Turner RC, Permutt MA, et al. Linkage of type 2 diabetes to the glucokinase gene. Lancet 1992;339:1307-10.
5. Yamagata K, Furuta H, Oda N, et al. Mutations in the hepatocyte nuclear factor 4 alpha gene in maturity-onset diabetes of the young (MODY1). Nature 1996;384:458-460.
6. Yamagata K, Oda N, Kaisaki PJ, et al. Mutations in the hepatic nuclear factor 1 alpha gene in maturity-onset diabetes of the young (MODY3). Nature 1996;384:455-458.

7. Stoffers DA, Ferrer J, Clarke WL, Habener JF. Early-onset type-II diabetes mellitus (MODY4) linked to IPF1. Nature Genetics 1997;17:138-139.
8. Horikawa Y, Iwasaki N, Hara M, et al. Mutation in hepatocyte nuclear factor-1b gene (TCF2) associated with MODY. Nature Genetics 1997;17:384-5.
9. Meglasson MD, Matschinsky FM. Pancreatic islet glucose metabolism and regulation of insulin secretion. Diabetes/Metabolism Reviews 1986;2:163-214.
10. Matschinsky FM. Glucokinase as glucose sensor and metabolic signal generator in pancreatic β-cell and hepatocytes. Diabetes 1990;30:647-752.
11. Vionnet N, Stoffel M, Takeda J, et al. Nonsense mutation in the glucokinase gene causes early-onset non-insulin-dependent diabetes mellitus. Nature 1992;356:721-2.
12. Stoffel M, Froguel P, Takeda J, et al. Human glucokinase gene: isolation, characterization, and identification of two missense mutations linked to early-onset non-insulin-dependent diabetes. Proc Natl Acad Sci USA 1992;89:7698-702.
13. Stoffel M, Patel P, Lo YM, et al. Missense glucokinase mutation in maturity-onset diabetes of the young and mutation screening in late-onset diabetes. Nature Genetics 1992;2:153-6.
14. Tanizawa Y, Matsutani A, Chiu KC, Permutt MA. Human glucokinase gene: isolation, structural characterization, and identification of a microsatellite repeat polymorphism. Molecular Endocrinology 1992;6:1070-81.
15. Sun F, Knebelmann B, Pueyo ME, et al. Deletion of the donor splice site of intron 4 in the glucokinase gene causes maturity-onset diabetes of the young. J Clin Invest 1993;92:1174-80.
16. Stoffel M, Bell KL, Blackburn CL, et al. Identification of glucokinase mutations in subjects with gestational diabetes mellitus. Diabetes 1993;42:937-940.
17. Shimada F, Makino H, Hashimoto N, et al. Type 2 (non-insulin-dependent) diabetes mellitus associated with a mutation of the glucokinase gene in a Japanese family. Diabetologia 1993;36:433-7.
18. Froguel P, Zouali H, Vionnet N, et al. Familial hyperglycemia due to mutations in glucokinase. Definition of a subtype of diabetes mellitus. N Engl J Med 1993;328:697-702.
19. Hager J, Blanche H, Sun F, et al. Six mutations in the glucokinase gene identified in MODY by using a nonradioactive sensitive screening technique. Diabetes 1994;43:730-3.
20. Eto K, Sakura H, Shimokawa K, et al. Sequence variations of the glucokinase gene in Japanese subjects with NIDDM. Diabetes 1993;42:1133-7.
21. Velho G, Blanche H, Vaxillaire M, et al. Identification of 14 new glucokinase mutations and description of the clinical profile of 42 MODY-2 families. Diabetologia 1997;40:217-224.
22. Hattersley AT, Beards F, Ballantyne E, Appleton M, Harvey R, Ellard S. Mutations in the glucokinase gene of the fetus result in reduced birth weight. Nat Genet 1998;19:268-270.
23. Gidh-Jain M, Takeda J, Xu LZ, et al. Glucokinase mutations associated with non-insulin-dependent (type 2) diabetes mellitus have decreased enzymatic activity: implications for structure/function relationships. Proc Natl Acad Sci USA 1993;90:1932-6.
24. Takeda J, Gidh-Jain M, Zhong Xu L, et al. Structure/Function Studies of Human Beta-cell Glucokinase. J Biol Chem 1993;20:15200-15204.
25. Pilkis SJ, Weber IT, Harrison RW, Bell GI. Glucokinase: structural analysis of a protein involved in susceptibility to diabetes. [Review]. J Biol Chem 1994;269:21925-8.
26. Glaser B, Kesavan P, Heyman M, et al. Familial hyperinsulinism caused by an activating glucokinase mutation. N Engl J Med 1998;338:226-230.
27. Dow E, Gelding SV, Skinner E, et al. Genetic analysis of glucokinase and the chromosome 20 diabetes susceptibility locus in families with type 2 diabetes. Diabetic Medicine 1994;11:856-61.
28. Zhang Y, Warren-Perry MG, Saker PJ, et al. Candidate genes study in pedigrees with maturity-onset diabetes of the young not linked with glucokinase. Diabetologia 1995;38:1055-1060.
29. Hattersley AT. Maturity-onset diabetes of the young: clinical heterogeneity explained by genetic heterogeneity. Diab Med 1998;15:15-24.
30. Katagiri H, Asano T, Ishihara H, et al. Nonsense mutation of glucokinase gene in late-onset non-insulin-dependent diabetes mellitus. Lancet 1992;340:1316-7.
31. Zouali H, Vaxillaire M, Lesage S, et al. Linkage analysis and molecular scanning of glucokinase gene in NIDDM families. Diabetes 1993;42:1238-45.
32. Saker PJ, Hattersley AT, Barrow B, et al. High prevalence of a missense mutation of the glucokinase gene in gestational diabetic patients due to a founder-effect in a local population. Diabetologia 1996;39:1325-1328.
33. Hattersley AT, Turner RC. Mutations of the glucokinase gene and type 2 diabetes. [Review]. Quarterly Journal of Medicine 1993;86:227-32.
34. Hattersley AT. Glucokinase mutations and Type 2 diabetes. In: Lightman S, ed. Horizons in Medicine. Vol. 7. Bristol: Blackwell Science, 1996:440-449.
35. O'Rahilly S, Hattersley A, Vaag A, Gray H. Insulin resistance as the major cause of impaired glucose tolerance: a self-fulfilling prophesy? Lancet 1994;344:585-9.
36. Page RC, Hattersley AT, Levy JC, et al. Clinical characteristics of subjects with a missense mutation in glucokinase. Diab Med 1995;12:209-17.

37. Velho G, Froguel P, Clement K, et al. Primary pancreatic beta-cell secretory defect caused by mutations in glucokinase gene in kindreds of maturity onset diabetes of the young. Lancet 1992;340:444-8.
38. Byrne MM, Sturis J, Clement K, et al. Insulin secretory abnormalities in subjects with hyperglycemia due to glucokinase mutations. J Clin Invest 1994;93:1120-30.
39. Velho G, Hwang J-H, Petersen K, et al. Altered hepatic glycogen synthesis in glucokinase deficient subjects [abstract]. Diabetalogia 1994;37:A131.
40. Clement K, Pueyo ME, Vaxillaire M, et al. Assessment of insulin sensitivity in glucokinase-deficient subjects. Diabetologia 1996;39:82-90.
41. Frain M, Swart G, Monaci P, et al. The liver-specific transcription factor LF-B1 contains a highly diverged homeobox DNA binding domain. Cell 1989;59:145-157.
42. Mendel DB, Hansen LP, Graves MK, Conley PB, Crabtree GR. HNF-1a and HNF-1b (vHNF-1) share dimerisation and homeo domains, but not activation domains, and form heterodimers in vitro. Genes and Development 1991;5:1042-1056.
43. Miquerol L, Lopez S, Cartier N, Tulliez M, Raymondjean M, Kahn A. Expression of the L-type pyruvate kinase gene and the hepatocyte nuclear factor 4 transcription factor in exocrine and endocrine pancreas. J Biol Chem 1994;269:8944-8951.
44. Vaxillaire M, Boccio V, Philippi A, et al. A gene for maturity onset diabetes of the young (MODY) maps to chromosome 12q. Nat Gen 1995;9:418-23.
45. Frayling T, Bulman MP, Ellard S, et al. Mutations in the Hepatocyte Nuclear Factor 1 Alpha gene are a common cause of maturity-onset diabetes of the young in the United Kingdom. Diabetes 1997;46:720-725.
46. Kaisaki PJ, Menzel S, Lindner T, et al. Mutations in the Hepatocyte Nuclear Factor 1 α Gene in MODY and Early-onset NIDDM: Evidence for a Mutational Hotspot in Exon 4. Diabetes 1997;45:528-535.
47. Vaxillaire M, Rouard M, Yamagata K, et al. Identification of nine novel mutations in the hepatocyte nuclear factor 1 alpha gene associated with maturity onset diabetes of the young (MODY3). Human Molecular Genetics 1997;6:583-586.
48. Hansen T, Eiberg H, Rouard M, et al. Novel MODY3 Mutations in the Hepatic Nuclear Factor-1α Gene. Diabetes 1997;46:726-730.
49. Gragnoli C, Lindner T, Marozzi G, Andreani D. Disruption of the HNF-4α promoter in an Italian family with MODY. Diabetologia 1997;40:A7.
50. Glucksmann MA, Lehto M, Tayber O, et al. Novel mutations and a mutational hotspot in the MODY3 gene. Diabetes 1997;46:1081-1086.
51. Iwasaki N, Oda N, Ogata M, et al. Mutations in the Hepatocyte Nuclear Factor-1α/MODY3 gene in Japanese subjects with early- and late-onset NIDDM. Diabetes 1997;46:1504-1508.
52. Velho G, Vaxillaire M, Boccio V, Charpentier G, Froguel P. Diabetes complications in NIDDM kindreds linked to the MODY3 locus on chromosome 12q. Diabetes Care 1996;19:915-919.
53. Isomaa B, Henricsson M, Lehto M, et al. Chronic diabetic complications in patients with MODY3 diabetes. Diabetologia 1998;41:467-473.
54. Sovik O, Njolstad P, Folling I, Sagen J, Cockburn BN, Bell GI. Hyperexcitability to sulphonylurea in MODY3. Diabetologia 1998;41(5):607-8.
55. Byrne MM, Sturis J, Menzel S, et al. Altered insulin secretory responses to glucose in diabetic and nondiabetic subjects with mutations in the diabetes susceptibility gene MODY3 on Chromosome 12. Diabetes 1996;45:1503-1510.
56. Bell GI, Xiang KS, Newman MV, et al. Gene for non-insulin-dependent diabetes mellitus (maturity-onset diabetes of the young subtype) is linked to DNA polymorphism on human chromosome 20q. Proc Natl Acad Sci USA 1991;88:1484-8.
57. Bulman M, Dronsfield MJ, Frayling T, et al. A missense mutation in the hepatocyte nuclear factor 4 alpha gene in a UK pedigree with maturity-onset diabetes of the young. Diabetologia 1997;40:859-863.
58. Lindner T, Gragnoli C, Furuta H, et al. Hepatic function in a family with a nonsense mutation (R154X) in the Hepatocyte Nuclear Factor-4α/MODY1 gene. J Clin Invest 1997;100:1400-1405.
59. Moller AM, Urhammer SA, Dalgaard LT, et al. Studies of the genetic variability of the coding region of the hepatocyte nuclear factor-4α in Caucasians with maturity onset NIDDM. Diabetologia 1997;40:980-983.
60. Furuta H, Iwasaki N, Oda N, et al. Organization and partial sequence of the hepatocyte nuclear factor-4α/MODY1 gene and identification of a missense mutation R127W, in a Japanese family with MODY. Diabetes 1997;46:1652-7.
61. Hani E, Suaud L, Boutin P, et al. A missense mutation in hepatocyte nuclear factor-4 alpha, resulting in a reduced transactivation activity, in human late-onset non- insulin-dependent diabetes mellitus. J Clin Invest 1998;101:521-526.
62. Byrne MM, Sturis J, Fajans SS, et al. Altered insulin secretory responses to glucose in subjects with a mutation in the MODY1 gene on chromosome 20. Diabetes 1995;44:699-704.

63. Marshak S, Totary H, Cerasi E, Melloul D. Purification of the β–cell glucose-sensitive factor that transactivates the insulin gene differentially in normal and transformed islet cells. Proc Natl Acad Sci USA 1996;93:15057-15062.
64. Macfarlane WM, Read ML, Gilligan M, Bujalska I, Docherty K. Glucose modulates the binding activity of the β-cell transcription factor IUF1 in a phosphorylation-dependent manner. Biochem J 1993;303:625-631.
65. Johnsson JL, Carlsson T, Edlund T, Edlund H. Insulin promoter factor 1 is required for pancreas development in mice. Nature 1994;371:606-609.
66. Inoue H, Riggs AC, Tanizawa Y, et al. Isolation, characterization, and chromosomal mapping of the human insulin promoter factor 1 (IPF-1) gene. Diabetes 1996;45:789-794.
67. Stoffers DA, Zinkin NT, Stanojevic V, Clarke WL, Habener JF. Pancreatic agenesis attributable to a single nucleotide deletion in the human IPF1 gene coding sequence. Nat Gen 1997;15:106-110.
68. Ahlgren U, Jonsson J, Jonsson L, Simu K, Edlund H. Beta-cell-specific inactivation of the mouse Ipf1/Pdx1 gene results in loss of the beta-cell phenotype and maturity onset diabetes. Genes Dev 1998;12:1763-8.
69. Nishigori H, Yamada S, Kohama T, et al. Frameshift mutation, A263fsinsGG, in the hepatocyte nuclear factor-1 beta gene associated with diabetes and renal dysfunction. Diabetes 1998;47:1354-1355.
70. Lindner TH, Nj, Horikawa Y, Bostad L, Bell GI, Vik. O. A novel syndrome of diabetes mellitus, renal dysfunction and genital malformation associated with a partial deletion of the pseudo-POU domain of hepatocyte nuclear factor-1beta. Hum Mol Genet 1999;8:2001-2008.
71. Macfarlane W, Frayling T, Ellard S, et al. Missense mutations in the Insulin Promoter Factor 1 (IPF-1) gene predispose to Type 2 diabetes. J Clin Invest 1999;104:R33-R39.
72. Mahtani M, Widen E, Lehto M, et al. Mapping of a gene for type 2 diabetes associated with an insulin secretion defect by a genome scan in Finnish families. Nat Gen 1996;14:90-94.
73. Ji L, Malecki M, Warram HJ, Yang Y, Rich SS, Krolewski AS. New susceptibility locus for NIDDM is localized to human chromosome 20q. Diabetes 1997;46:876-881.
74. Bowden WD, Sale M, Howard TD, et al. Linkage of genetic markers on human chromosomes 20 and 12 to NIDDM in Caucasian sib pairs with a history of diabetic nephropathy. Diabetes 1997;46:882-886.
75. Zouali H, Hani EH, Philippi A, et al. A susceptibility locus for early-onset non-insulin dependent (type 2) diabetes mellitus maps to chromosome 20q, proximal to the phosphoenolpyruvate carboxykinase gene. Human Molecular Genetics 1997;6:1401-1408.
76. Ghosh S, Watanabe RM, Hauser ER, et al. Type 2 diabetes: Evidence for linkage on chromosme 20 in Finnish affected sib pairs. Proc Natl Acad Sci USA 1999;96:2198-2203.
77. Fowden AL. The role of insulin in fetal growth. Early Human Development 1992;29:177-181.
78. Fowden AL. Insulin deficiency: effects on fetal growth and development. Journal of Paediatrics and Child Health 1993;29:6-11.
79. Hill DE. Insulin and fetal growth. Diabetes and Other Endocrine Disorders During Pregnancy and in the Newborn. New York: Alan R Liss Inc., 1976:127-139.
80. Hill DJ, Milner RDG. Insulin as a growth factor. Pediatric Research 1985;19:879-886.
81. Hales CN, Barker DJP, Clark PMS, et al. Fetal and infant growth and impaired glucose tolerance at age 64. BMJ 1991;303:1019-1022.
82. Hattersley AT, Tooke JE. The fetal insulin hypothesis: an alternative explanation of the association of low birth weight with diabetes and vascular disease. Lancet 1999;353:1789-92.
83. Inagaki N, Gonoi T, Clement JP, et al. Reconstitution of I_{KATP}: an inward rectifier subunit plus the sulfonylurea receptor. Science 1995;270:1166-1170.
84. Thomas PM, Cote GJ, Wohllk K, et al. Mutations in the sulfonylurea receptor gene in familial persistent hyperinsulinemic hypoglycemia of infancy. Science 1995;268:426-429.
85. Thomas P, Ye Y, Lightner E. Mutation of the pancreatic islet inward rectifier Kir6.2 also leads to familial persistent hyperinsulinemic hypoglycemia of infancy. Hum Mol Genet 1996;5:1809-1812.
86. Edlund H. Transcribing Pancreas. Diabetes 1998;47:1817-1823.
87. Barker DJ. Intrauterine programming of adult disease. Molecular Medicine Today 1995;1:418-23.
88. Hales CN. The pathogenesis of NIDDM. Diabetologia 1994;37:S162-8.
89. Hales CN, Barker DJP. Type 2 (non-insulin dependent) diabetes mellitus - the thrifty phenotype hypothesis. Diabetologia 1992;35:595-601.
90. Wright NM, Metzger DL, Borowitz SM, Clarke WL. Permanent neonatal diabetes mellitus and pancreatic exocrine insufficiency resulting from congenital pancreatic agenesis. Am J Dis Child 1993;147:607-609.
91. Temple IK, James RS, Crolla JA, et al. An imprinted gene(s) for diabetes? Nat Genet 1995;9:110-112.
92. Temple IK, Gardner RJ, Robinson DO, et al. Further evidence for an imprinted gene for neonatal diabetes localised to chromosome 6q22-q23. Hum Molec Genet 1996;5:1117-1124.
93. Shield JPH. Neonatal diabetes. In: Shield JPH, Baum JD, eds. Childhood Diabetes. Vol. 4. London: Bailliere Tindall, 1996:681-740.

94. Aparicio L, Carpenter MW, Schwartz R, Gruppuso PA. Prenatal diagnosis of familial neonatal hyperinsulinemia. Acta Paediat 1993;82:683-686.

20

PATHOPHYSIOLOGY OF GLUT2 IN DIABETES MELLITUS

Bernard Thorens, Ph.D.
University of Lausanne, 1005, Lausanne, Switzerland

INTRODUCTION

Glucose is a polar molecule and its transport through biological membranes requires the presence of specific transporter proteins. Five structurally related hexose carriers have been described that facilitate the diffusion of glucose and closely related hexoses through the cell membrane. These proteins, referred to as GLUT1 to GLUT5, are the products of different genes located on different chromosomes and are functionally distinguished by their hexose specificity, affinity for glucose, tissue and cellular localization and regulated expression in different metabolic states and in response to different hormones (1,2). GLUT1, GLUT3 and GLUT4, are high affinity glucose transporters (Km for glucose of 1-5 mM), GLUT5 is mostly a fructose transporter and GLUT2 has a uniquely low affinity for glucose (Km for glucose ~17 mM) (3). This transporter is expressed selectively in tissues in which high glucose fluxes are required. In intestine, it is found in the basolateral membrane of epithelial cells and is thought to be responsible for the second step of transepithelial glucose uptake. A similar role for GLUT2 is anticipated in glucose reabsorption in the proximal convoluted tubule where it is located to the basolateral membrane of epithelial cells. GLUT2 is also expressed at a high level in the sinusoidal membrane of hepatocytes where the transporter may function both for glucose uptake and release from the cells. In pancreatic β-cells, GLUT2 may be part of a glucose sensing system-linking variations in plasma glucose to insulin secretion (4).

GLUCOSE-INDUCED INSULIN SECRETION

Glucose is the main physiological stimulus for insulin secretion by pancreatic β-cells. The glucose signalling pathway requires glucose uptake and metabolism. The production of coupling factors, produced most probably at the mitochondrial level upon glucose metabolism, is necessary for the eventual induction of insulin granule exocytosis. An important feature of the pancreatic β-cells is their capability to produce these metabolic coupling factors at a rate proportional to the variations in extracellular glucose concentrations. A rise in the cytoplasmic concentration ratio of ATP to ADP is a consequence of increased glucose metabolism that triggers the closure of a K_{ATP} channel. This leads to plasma membrane depolarization, opening of calcium channels and the resulting influx of calcium eventually stimulates insulin secretion (5-7). Other, as yet less well defined, K_{ATP}-independent, mechanisms also participate in the glucose signalling to insulin secretion in β-cells (8,9).

The unique ability of β-cells to generate a graded insulin exocytosis signal in response to elevations in extracellular glucose over the physiological concentration range is due in great part to specific kinetic properties of the initial steps in glucose metabolism. The phosphorylation of glucose by the high Km (6-8 mM) hexokinase IV isoform, referred to as glucokinase, is the metabolic step with the highest control strength on glycolysis and the subsequent generation of coupling factors (5). This has been demonstrated in early biochemical studies. Recently, transgenic mice with reduced expression of glucokinase have confirmed the role of glucokinase as the rate-limiting step in glucose stimulated insulin secretion (GSIS) (10-12). More striking even, was the discovery that diabetes in MODY-2 patients was caused by mutations in a single allele of the glucokinase gene (13).

GLUT2, because of its high Km for glucose, appears well suited to allow the rate of glucose uptake by β-cells to increase in proportion to the glucose concentrations stimulating insulin secretion. Thus, the presence in β-cells of a high Km transporter together with a high Km phosphorylating enzyme may be required for normal glucose sensing. Numerous studies have however measured the respective rates of glucose uptake and phosphorylation in rodent islets. These studies determined that the uptake rate was approximately 50- to 100-fold in excess over the rate of phosphorylation by glucokinase (14,15). This therefore implies that a low affinity, high capacity transporter may not be needed to permit glucose sensing and that a relatively high expression of, for instance, a low Km transporter may be sufficient to allow an efficient access of glucose to glucokinase and normal sensing.

In human β-cells, GLUT2 expression, although definitively present, is low compared to that found in rodent islets (16). GLUT1 is also expressed in human β-cells (17). From these observations, it can be concluded that GLUT2 is not specifically required for glucose sensing and that GLUT1 or another low Km transporter may replace GLUT2. This is however not really clear since GLUT2 is still present and may be required for a low level of high Km glucose transport. Theoretical considerations on the rates of uptake and phosphorylation also argued against a specific role for GLUT2 (18)

PHENOTYPE OF ISLETS IN THE ABSENCE OF GLUT2

GLUT2 Knockout Mice

Mice with an inactivation of both alleles of GLUT2 by homologous recombination in embryonic stem cells are hyperglycaemic, relatively hypoinsulinemic and have elevated plasma levels of glucagon, free fatty acids and ketone bodies (19). Their glucose tolerance is abnormal. When assessed *in vitro* in islet perifusion experiments, the secretory response to elevations in glucose concentrations from 2.8 to 16.7 mM is suppressed when assessed in the absence of cAMP-elevating agents. When isobutyl-methyl-xanthine is added to the glucose solution, the insulin secretory response is characterized by a lack of first phase but preserved second phase that is of lower magnitude as compared to control islets (Figure 1). This secretory response to glucose can be suppressed by the inhibitor of oxidative phosphorylation, antimycin A1, and by diazoxide and nimodipine that respectively, prevents closure of the K_{ATP} channels and blocks the L-type calcium channels. This indicates that in islets lacking GLUT2 the second phase of insulin secretion requires glucose metabolism and depends on the same membrane depolarization events activated by glucose in normal islets. A remarkable observation is that in the absence of GLUT2, glucose can nevertheless be taken up by β-cells. Glucose uptake probably occurs at a low rate thereby limiting normal access of glucose to glucokinase and thereby suppressing the first phase of secretion. The transporter responsible for the remaining low transport activity is not known. No overexpression of GLUT1 or GLUT3 is observed in the GLUT2 null islets. That the uptake step is limiting for glucose metabolism in GLUT2 null islets has been demonstrated by the fact that 1) glucose consumption increases with elevating external glucose concentrations up to 5 mM but is subsequently blunted at higher concentrations; 2) glucokinase is expressed at normal levels; 3) re-expression of GLUT2 in GLUT2-null islets using a recombinant lentivirus restores normal glucose stimulated insulin secretion (M.-T. Guillam, P. Dupraz, and B.T., submitted). Despite the absence of GLUT2 and impaired secretory response to glucose, insulin secretion is stimulated normally by a combination of leucine and glutamine or by glyceraldehyde. Thus, the lower glycolytic pathway and the mitochondrial metabolism function normally and are still able to couple variations in the extracellular levels of glyceraldehyde and amino acids to insulin granule exocytosis (19).

GLUT2 in foetal and postnatal islet development

GLUT2 is already observed in preimplantation mouse embryos at the morula stage (20). At embryonic day 11 the transporter is detected in the endodermal cells of the intestine at a site where the pancreatic bud will form. GLUT2 is then expressed in the initial pancreatic bud in cells that are distinct from insulin-containing cells. Only at embryonic day 17 does GLUT2 colocalize with insulin positive cells (21,22).

Despite the early appearance of GLUT2 in the developing pancreas, no alteration of the islets of Langerhans can be observed in newborn GLUT2 null mice, either histologically or as evaluated by the pancreatic content of glucagon and insulin (19). GLUT2 is therefore not essential for the formation of the endocrine pancreas. However, within five days after birth, the absence of GLUT2 leads to marked alterations in pancreatic insulin and glucagon content with an absolute increase in glucagon and an absolute decrease in insulin both at the mRNA and peptide levels. This change in hormone expression correlates with a 50 percent increase in α-cell and a 30 percent decrease in β-cell cell islet volume density. We propose that the change in the structure of the endocrine pancreas observed in the absence of GLUT2 may be the consequence of the loss of glucose sensing by β-cells. Indeed, glucose sensing for secretion, but also for proliferation, appears in β-cells approximately at the time of birth (23-25). Only when the normal sensing capability of the β-cells develop will the alteration in endocrine pancreas appear. It may therefore be possible that the lack of glucose uptake coupled to insulin secretion modifies the proliferation of both α- and β-cells. It is known, on the one hand, that insulin has inhibitory effect on α-cells, blocking both glucagon gene expression (26) and secretion (27) and, on the other hand, that insulin has autocrine effects on β-cells, on insulin secretion and transcription, and probably on β-cell development. Insulin action on β-cells leads to increased insulin gene transcription (28). Mouse knockout experiments have shown that selective inactivation of the insulin receptor in pancreatic β-cells leads to a defect in insulin secretion and to the formation of smaller islets (29). Similarly, inactivation of the insulin receptor substrate-2 (IRS-2), but not of IRS-1, leads to profoundly disturbed development of pancreatic islets (30). Loss of glucose sensing is a phenomenon associated with non-insulin-dependent diabetes mellitus. In one study analyzing the structure of the islets of Langerhans of NIDDM patients, an inversion of the α- to β-cell ratio was described (31). Similar to what is found in the GLUT2 null mice, this alteration may be secondary to the loss of glucose sensing by β-cells.

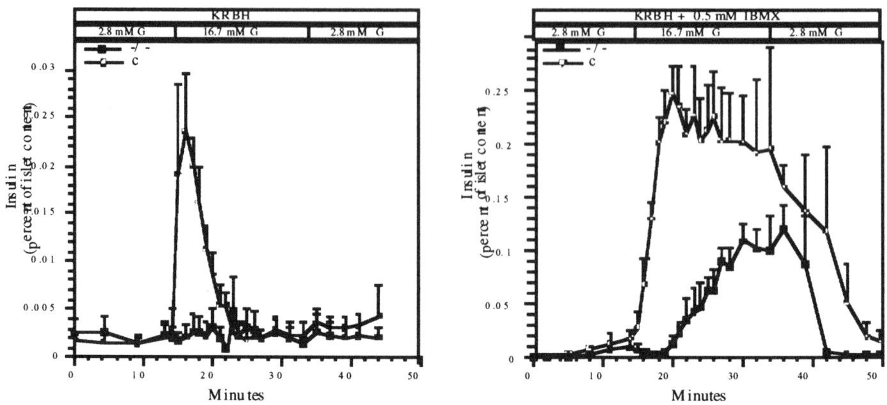

Figure 1. *Glucose-induced insulin secretion by control and GLUT2-deficient islets.* ***A)*** *Islets were perifused with a Krebs buffer solution containing 2.8 to 16.7 mM glucose. Islets from knockout animals do not respond to glucose.* ***B)*** *Glucose-induced insulin secretion by control and GLUT2-deficient islets perifused as in A) but in the continuous presence of 0,5 mM IBMX. There is a robust secretory response in control islets (note that the scale is different from that in panel A) and a qualitatively and quantitatively abnormal secretory response in knockout islets, with a slow onset of secretion but a preserved second phase. (Reprinted from (19) with permission).*

GLUT2 INACTIVATION IN HUMAN: THE FANCONI-BICKEL SYNDROME

The Fanconi-Bickel syndrome is transmitted in an autosomal recessive manner. It is characterized by hepatorenal glycogen accumulation, proximal renal tubular dysfunction and impaired utilization of glucose and galactose (32,33). Fasting is usually accompanied by hypoglycaemia. Recently, Santer et al., (34) described three different homozygous mutations in GLUT2 associated with Fanconi-Bickel syndrome. The parents available for DNA analysis presented the heterozygous mutation. These mutations all led to premature stop within the reading frame of GLUT2. Most, if not all the pathological characteristics of these patients are reproduced in the GLUT2 knockout mouse model. Unfortunately, there is so far no good data on the insulin secretory response in human Fanconi-Bickel patients. Only glucose tolerance tests have been performed and reveal a decreased rate of glucose disappearance (35). As insulin levels were not simultaneously measured, it is not possible to draw any conclusion on the role of GLUT2 for glucose-induced insulin secretion in humans.

REGULATED EXPRESSION OF GLUT2

Fasting, Glucose and Hormonal Regulation

GLUT2 expression in pancreatic β-cells is regulated in several conditions. Fasting leads to decreased GLUT2 expression (36). An important role for glucose in the control of GLUT2 expression in β-cells has also been described. Hypoglycaemia induced by insulin injections decreases GLUT2 expression (37). *In vitro*, the direct effect of glucose on GLUT2 expression is to stimulate its gene transcription rate (38), mRNA and protein level (15,39). The gene promoter region required for this glucose sensitivity appears to lie within the first 338 base pairs upstream of the transcription initiation site as demonstrated by the glucose responsiveness of a luciferase reporter construct expressed transiently in the β INS-1 cell line (40,41). In contrast, no influence of insulin on GLUT2 expression in β-cells has been described so far. Prolactin appears to be a good inducer of GLUT2 expression in β-cells (42).

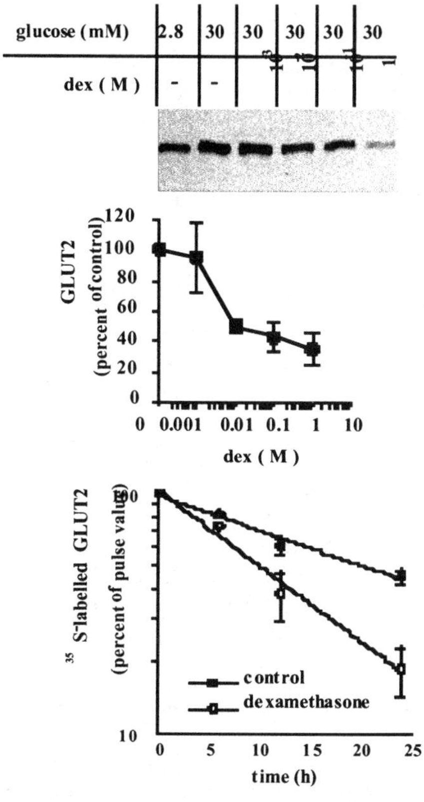

Figure 2. *Dexamethasone decreases GLUT2 expression by a posttranslational mechanism. Top Isolated pancreatic islets were kept in culture for 48 hours in the presence of different concentrations of dexamethasone. After cell lysis, equal amounts of proteins were separated by gel electrophoresis and GLUT2 expression analyzed by Western blotting. Middle. Quantitation of GLUT2 expression relative to control at 30 mM glucose. Lower Pancreatic islets were kept in culture for 48 hours in the presence or absence of dexamethasone. The islets were then pulse-labelled for 5 minutes with ^{35}S-methionine and chased for different periods of time in a fresh medium in the presence of an excess of cold methionine. Following cell lysis GLUT2 was immunoprecipitated, separated by gel electrophoresis and the level of GLUT2 expression was evaluated by scanning densitometry. The graph shows the results expressed as percent of GLUT2 detected at the end of the pulse. The half-life of GLUT2 is decreased from 20 to 10 hours in the presence of glucocorticoid treatment. (Reprinted from (58) with permission).*

Regulated Expression in Diabetes

Because of its possible role in glucose-induced insulin secretion, the expression of GLUT2 has been studied in the pancreatic β-cells of several animal models of diabetes. In every model studied that includes the neonatal streptozocin rat (43), the Zucker diabetic rat (44,45), at the onset of diabetes in the BB/W rat (46) and in db/db mice (47), a strong reduction of GLUT2 expression can be observed. This was measured at the mRNA and protein levels and was correlated with a decrease in the rate of glucose uptake. The reduction of GLUT2 expression in diabetes was correlated with the degree of hyperglycaemia and, in db/ db mice, for instance, the reduction was approximately 90 percent. As mentioned previously, the rate of glucose uptake by β-cells is 50- to 100-fold in excess over the rate of glucose phosphorylation by glucokinase. The observed extent of reduction is therefore unlikely to limit glucose access to glucokinase and cause the reduced glucose responsiveness of the β-cells. The decreased expression of GLUT2 was however a hallmark of glucose unresponsive β-cells from diabetic animals. We have further studied the mechanisms of GLUT2 downregulation with two approaches: islet cross-transplantation and *in vitro* culture of islets that are exposed to putative diabetogenic agents.

Cross-Transplantation Experiments

For transplantation experiments, islets from db/db mice are transplanted under the kidney capsule of control mice or, conversely, islets from control mice are transplanted under the kidney capsule of db/db mice (47). When db/db islets are exposed to a normal environment, GLUT2 expression reappears to normal levels. In contrast, when control islets are exposed to the diabetic environment of db/db mice, GLUT2 expression is lost. This demonstrates that the loss of GLUT2 expression is not due to a β-cell intrinsic defect but is induced by the diabetic environment and, furthermore, that the decrease in GLUT2 expression is fully reversible. Exposure of normal islets to the diabetic environment of streptozocin diabetic mice also led to GLUT2 decreased expression. This indicates that the GLUT2 regulation is found irrespective of the ambient insulin levels: db/db mice are hyperinsulinemic and hyperglycaemic, whereas STZ mice are insulinopenic and hyperglycaemic. As described above, the direct role of glucose on GLUT2 is to stimulate its expression. The diabetic hyperglycaemia could therefore not be the primary cause for decreased expression of GLUT2. In transplantation experiments performed using encapsulated islets transplanted into diabetic rats, correction of hyperglycaemia by phlorizin treatment, which induce renal glycosuria and lowers blood glucose levels, leads to correction of GLUT2 expression (R. Roduit and B.T., unpublished). These data therefore suggest that glucose does not directly down-regulate GLUT2 but allows other factors present in the diabetic milieu to exert their deleterious effects. These observations further suggest that the so-called glucose toxicity may not be a direct effect of glucose on β-cells but may rather be due to other mechanisms which need the presence of high glucose concentrations to be effective and which then become dominant over the effect of glucose.

REGULATION OF GLUT2 EXPRESSION BY DEXAMETHASONE

Dexamethasone administration in humans and in animals as well as hypercortisolism in Cushing's syndrome induce insulin resistance. This is usually accompanied by changes in β-cell functions, in particular by an increase in basal and a decrease in stimulated insulin secretion, an increase in proinsulin mRNA, a decrease in islet insulin stores and hyperplasia and hypertrophy of the β-cells (48-52). Dexamethasone administration to rats does not however induce a decrease in β-cell GLUT2 (53). Only if diabetes is induced, as for example following repeated injections of high doses of dexamethasone to Wistar rats or of relatively lower doses to Zucker fa/fa rats, is a decrease in GLUT2 expression observed (52,54). The exact role of dexamethasone on pancreatic β-cells is however difficult to evaluate when administered to the intact animal. *In vitro*, exposure of RINm5F cells to dexamethasone increases proinsulin mRNA levels but does not alter the insulin secretion rate at any glucose concentration (55,58,59). In HIT cells and isolated β-cells, dexamethasone decreases insulin mRNA and secretion (56). The inhibitory effect on mRNA levels can however be completely prevented by increasing intracellular cAMP (57).

The effect of dexamethasone on GLUT2 expression and insulin secretion was assessed using isolated rat islets maintained in tissue culture (58). Dexamethasone has no effect on GLUT2 mRNA, but decreases GLUT2 protein by about 65 percent (Figure 3). The effect of dexamethasone is more pronounced at high glucose concentrations and is inhibited by the glucocorticoid antagonist RU-486. Biosynthetic labelling experiments reveal that GLUT2 translation rate is only minimally affected by dexamethasone but that the half-life of the protein decreases by 50 percent, indicating that glucocorticoids activates a posttranslational degradation mechanism (Figure 3). This degradation mechanism does not affect all membrane proteins since the expression of the alpha subunit of the $Na^{+}/K^{+}{}_{ATP}$ase remains unchanged under circumstances when GLUT2 is reduced. Because the effect of dexamethasone can be inhibited by the glucocorticoid receptor antagonist RU-486, transcriptional activation of a gene or a set of genes is required to increase the rate of GLUT2 degradation. Furthermore, this transcriptional effect increases in the presence of elevated glucose concentrations. This observation indicates that the deleterious effect of glucocorticoids on β-cell function may increase during the pathogenesis of diabetes as hyperglycaemia progresses.

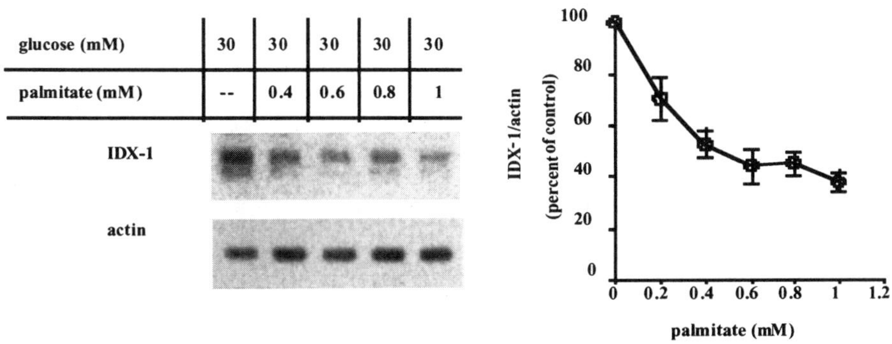

Figure 3. *Palmitic acid regulation of GLUT2 mRNA in isolated pancreatic islets. Top. Northern blot analysis of GLUT2 and actin mRNAs in pancreatic islets incubated for 24 and 48 hours in the presence of 2.8 mM glucose or 30 mM glucose in the presence or absence of 0.6 mM palmitic acid. Bottom. Quantitation of the GLUT2 to actin mRNA ratio in pancreatic islets incubated in the presence of different concentrations of palmitic acid for 48 hours. (Reprinted from (58) with permission).*

REGULATION OF GLUT2 EXPRESSION BY FREE FATTY ACIDS

Elevated circulating free fatty acids and triglycerides are part of the symptoms of both insulin-dependent and non-insulin dependent diabetes mellitus (60,61). Free fatty acids have been shown to induce a state of insulin resistance in peripheral tissues by a glucose/fatty acid cycle that prevents a normal uptake of glucose. The effects of free fatty acids on islet functions have been studied both *in vivo* and *in vitro*. These studies indicated that short-term (1-3 hours) exposure of pancreatic islets to free fatty acids have a stimulatory effect on GSIS (62-64) whereas longer exposure periods tend to suppress insulin secretion (63-65). This inhibitory effect is also accompanied by a decrease in insulin biosynthesis, in glucose oxidation, and a reduction in pyruvate dehydrogenase (PDH) activity with a parallel increase in pyruvate dehydrogenase kinase activity (66,67). A major role for free fatty acids in the development of β-cell glucose-unresponsiveness has thus been proposed. This is further supported by the observation that circulating free fatty acid levels are increased a few weeks before hyperglycaemia develops and GLUT2 expression is lost in male Zucker diabetic rats. Whereas obese female Zucker rats, which do not develop hyperglycaemia and do not lose GLUT2, do not show this increase in free fatty acids even though they develop similar hypertriglyceridaemia (68). Furthermore, incubation of pancreatic islets in the presence of free fatty acids induces an increase in low Km glucose usage (69) and elevates basal insulin secretion rates (65,69). When evaluated in *in vitro* cultures of isolated rat islets, palmitic acid induces a dose-dependent decrease in GLUT2 mRNA levels and a 40 percent decrease in GLUT2 protein. Thus, in contrast to the effect of dexamethasone, free fatty acids regulate GLUT2 expression at a pretranslational level (Figure 4). This is accompanied by a decrease in insulin mRNA and peptide and by a suppression of glucose-stimulated insulin secretion (58).

Free Fatty Acids and the Regulation of pdx-1 Gene Expression
Islet/duodenum homeobox-1 (idx-1 or pdx-1) is a homeobox gene that encodes a 283 amino acid transcription factor. PDX-1 was first described as a transactivator of the insulin (70,71) and somatostatin (72) genes that recognizes a TAATT/G sequence present in their promoters. More recently, it was also shown to transactivate the GLUT2 (73) and glucokinase (74) genes by recognizing similar cis-regulatory elements present in the promoter of these genes. Pdx-1 gene expression is restricted to the duodenum and the pancreatic δ- and β-cells. During embryogenesis, it is expressed starting at e8.5 in the duodenum and pancreatic bud, before the appearance of glucagon or insulin cells (70). PDX-1 importance in pancreas development was further highlighted when pdx-$1^{-/-}$ homozygous knockout mice were shown to fail to develop pancreas, leading to early postnatal death (22,75). More recently, identification of mutations in the human pdx-1 gene was also shown to be responsible for lack of pancreas organogenesis in man (76). It was therefore hypothesized that during development all endocrine and exocrine pancreatic cells originate from pdx-1 expressing cells, and that only β- and δ-cells would retain their expression in mature islets.

To determine whether free fatty acids have a deleterious effect on Pdx-1 mRNA, we exposed isolated rat pancreatic islets to varying concentrations of palmitic acid (Figure 5A) for different time periods (77). Free fatty acids induce a ~70% decrease in Pdx-1 mRNA and protein expression, as well as a 40% and 65% decrease in the binding activity of Pdx-1 to its cognate cis-regulatory elements in the GLUT2 and insulin promoters, respectively (Figure 5B). The inhibitory effect of palmitic acid on Pdx-1 requires its mitochondrial oxidation since the inhibition is prevented by the carnitine palmitoyl transferase I (CPTI) inhibitor bromopalmitic acid. The palmitic acid effect on pdx-1 correlates with a decrease in GLUT2 and glucokinase expression by 40% and 25% respectively, both at the mRNA and protein level. Insulin and somatostatin mRNA expression also decreases by 40% and 60%, whereas glucagon mRNA expression is unchanged. After a 48h exposure to fatty acids, total islet insulin, somatostatin, and glucagon contents are decreased by 85%, 55%, and 65%, respectively.

When the effect of free fatty acids are evaluated on hormone secretion in static culture conditions, secretion of insulin and somatostatin are only marginally stimulated (1.5-fold and 1.7-fold, respectively). In contrast, glucagon secretion is stimulated 13-fold. Because glucagon mRNA levels remain unchanged during the incubation period (24 hours) and the total intracellular and secreted glucagon concentrations increases by more than two-fold, free fatty acids appear not only to stimulate glucagon secretion but also its translation. In summary, fatty acids have pleiotropic diabetogenic effects on pancreatic islet gene expression, some being initiated by a negative control of PDX-1 expression.

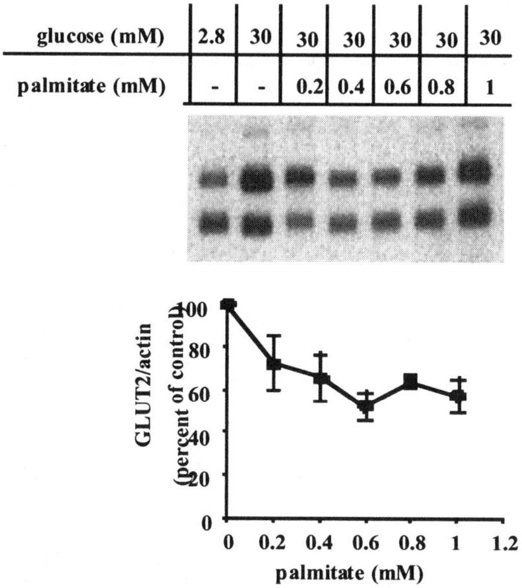

Figure 4. *Palmitic acid induces a reduction in pdx-1 mRNA expression and binding activity to cis-regulatory elements.* ***A)*** *RNA was extracted from islets incubated for 48h in the presence of 30 mM glucose, without or with increasing concentrations of palmitic acid (0.2-1 mM) equilibrated with serum albumin. pdx-1 and actin mRNA levels were evaluated by Northern blot analysis. Quantitation of the pdx-1 to actin ratio is presented in the graph.* ***B)*** *Islets were treated for 48h with 30 mM glucose in the presence or in the absence of 0.6 mM palmitic acid. Nuclear extracts were then prepared and binding activity to the GLUT2-specific pdx-1 cis element and to the GTII and the MLTF binding sequences was analyzed by EMSA. Quantitations of the EMSA analysis is presented in the histogram. There is a marked reduction in pdx-1 binding activity whereas that of GTII or MLTF is unchanged. (Reprinted from (77) with permission).*

The level of PDX-1 expression has an important role on β-cell physiology and whole body glucose homeostasis as is demonstrated by the observation that human individuals with a mutation in one allele of this transcription factor develop diabetes (MODY4) (78). Further, mice in which the pdx-1 gene was progressively deleted in the postnatal period specifically in the pancreatic β-cells develop diabetes between three to five months of age accompanied by a strong decrease in both insulin and GLUT2 expression (79). A similar inverse correlation between hyperglycaemia, on one hand, and reduced GLUT2, insulin and PDX-1 levels, on the other, is found in the partially pancreatectomized rat model (80). Therefore, both genetic and metabolic alterations leading to decreased expression of PDX-1 may lead to the same β-cell dysfunction that ultimately induces diabetes.

Not all forms of diabetes show a decrease in PDX-1 expression. Islets from db/db mice that are severely obese and diabetic, present a very strong reduction of GLUT2 expression and loss of glucose-stimulated insulin secretion in face of increased pdx-1 expression (47). However, the binding activity of GTIIa is decreased (81). GTIIa has been defined as a nuclear binding activity that recognizes the GLUT2 proximal promoter sequence and that is specifically present in β-cells and brain (40). GLUT2 down-regulation in db/db islets is thus not correlated with PDX-1 expression but rather with GTIIa activity. Further, the lack of decreased PDX-1 expression in the islets of these mice that are diabetic due to the absence of a functional leptin receptor suggests that PDX-1 expression may be under the control of this hormone. In ZDF rats that also have a nonfunctional leptin receptor (82), impaired glucose-induced insulin secretion is corrected by reexpression of this receptor using recombinant adenoviruses (83). This impairment is correlated with a decrease in triglyceride stocks, an increase in lipid catabolizing enzymes (carnitine palmitoyl transferase, acyl-CoA oxidase), a decrease in lipid biosynthetic activity (acyl-CoA carboxylase, glycerol phosphate acetyl transferase) (84), a return to normal expression of GLUT2 and glucokinase (83). Although our studies have been limited to PDX-1, it would be interesting to evaluate the regulation of these other transcription factors in similar conditions.

CONCLUSIONS

The role of the GLUT2 transporter isoform as an obligatory component of pancreatic β-cell glucose sensing system has not yet been established. The formal proof that this transporter plays a specific role in β-cell physiology will only be tested when GLUT2 null mice will be rescued by reexpression by transgenesis of GLUT1 or GLUT2 in β-cells followed by a careful comparison of the glucose signalling pathway. Although glucose is the major regulator of insulin secretion by β-cells, its role in these cells is, however, much more complex. Indeed, glucose is also a strong inducer of gene transcription of translation of several pre-existing mRNA's, including that of insulin and of β-cell proliferation. Whether GLUT2 may have some specific signalling function in addition to its role in glucose uptake has been suggested but not yet proven (85,86).

The absence of GLUT2 expression in knockout mice reveals that this transporter is essential for first phase insulin secretion. Glucose can, however, still enter the cells and induce a second phase of secretion. The uptake is, by far, a so far unknown mechanism which does not involve increased expression of GLUT1 or GLUT3. It may thus be through an, as yet, unknown member of the glucose transporter family or through other related transporter molecules which show some transport capacity for glucose. In human Fanconi-Bickel patients, the consequence of the absence of GLUT2 has not yet been evaluated on insulin secretion. Less than forty patients have been described since the original description of the syndrome in 1949 (87). It would, however, be very interesting to get a better assessment of their β-cell secretory capacity. These measurements may, however, be complicated by the general metabolic abnormalities that these patients display which may adversely affect their endocrine pancreas.

The down-expression of GLUT2 in diabetes which is specifically observed in β-cells and not in other tissues, provides an important starting point to understanding some of the pathophysiological mechanisms inducing β-cell dysfunctions in diabetes. Following the decreased expression of these markers, which always correlated with a decreased glucose stimulated insulin secretory capability, we demonstrated that the initial defects were not in the β-cells themselves. Instead, the β-cell dysfunctions appeared secondary to other metabolic alterations. These included a possible role of glucocorticoids. Dexamethasone was indeed demonstrated to regulate GLUT2 expression through the glucose-dependent induction of a degradation system which showed specificity for the transporter. Although this degradative system has not been characterized, it may well be similar to the ubiquitin/proteasome-dependent degradation system induced in muscle by glucocorticoids (88). Free fatty acids have been demonstrated by many groups to have deleterious effects on β-cell function. We demonstrated that one of their mechanisms of action was to decrease GLUT2 expression in isolated islets and that this effect may be secondary to an initial down-expression of the transcription factor PDX-1. These studies supported the essential role that a subset of transcription factors may play in the pathogenesis of diabetes and demonstrated that circulating nutrients or other circulating substances may regulate their expression. Many studies, by others, have demonstrated that mutations in PDX-1, HNF-1α, HNF-1β and HNF4 may cause diabetes. Although our studies have been limited to PDX-1, it would be interesting to evaluate the regulation of these other transcription factors in similar conditions.

ACKNOWLEDGEMENTS

The work performed in my laboratory has been supported by grants from the Swiss National Science Foundation and the Juvenile Diabetes Foundation International.

REFERENCES

1. Gould GW, Holman GD. The glucose transporter family: structure, function and tissue-specific expression. Biochem J 1993;295:329-341.
2. Mueckler M. Facilitative glucose transporters. Eur J Biochem 1994;219:713-725.
3. Thorens B. Glucose transporters in the regulation of intestinal, renal and liver glucose fluxes. Am J Physiol 1996;270:G541-G553.
4. Thorens B. Molecular and cellular physiology of GLUT2, a high-Km facilitated diffusion glucose transporter. Int Rev Cytol 1992;137A:209-238.
5. Matschinsky FM. A lesson in metabolic regulation inspired by the glucokinase sensor paradigm. Diabetes 1996;45:223-241.
6. Prentki M, Glennon MC, Geschwing J-F, Matschinski FM, Corkey BE. Cyclic AMP raises cytosolic Ca2+ and promotes Ca2+ influx in a clonal pancreatic b-cell line (HIT T-15). FEBS l 1987;220:103-107.
7. Henquin JC, Debuyser A, Drews G, Plant TD. Regulation of K+ permeability and membrane potential in insulin-secreting cells. In: Flatt PR, ed. Nutrient Regulation of Insulin Secretion. London, Chapel Hill: Portland Press, 1992:173-191.
8. Gembal M, Gilon P, Henquin J-C. Evidence that glucose can control insulin release independently from its action on ATP-sensitive K+ channels in mouse B cells. J Clin Invest 1992;89:1288-1295.
9. Gembal M, Detimary P, Gilon P, Gao Z-Y, Henquin J-C. Mechanisms by which glucose can control insulin release independently from its action on adenosine triphosphate-sensitive K+ channels in mouse β-cells. J Clin Invest 1993;91:871-880.
10. Efrat S, Leiser M, Wu Y-J, et al. Ribozyme-mediated attenuation of pancreatic β-cell glucokinase expression in transgenic mice results in impaired insulin secretion. Proc Natl Acad Sci USA 1994;91:2051-2055.
11. Grupe A, Hultgren B, Ryan A, Ma YH, Bauer M, Stewart TA. Transgenic knockouts reveal a critical requirement for pancreatic β-cell glucokinase in maintaining glucose homeostasis. Cell 1995;83:69-78.
12. Piston DW, Knobel SM, Postic C, Shelton KD, Magnuson MA. Adenovirus-mediated knockout of a conditional glucokinase gene in isolated pancreatic islets reveals an essential role for proximal metabolic coupling events in glucose-stimulated insulin secretion. J Biol Chem 1999;274:1000-1004.
13. Froguel P, Vaxillaire M, Sun F, et al. Close linkage of glucokinase locus on chromosomes 7p to early-onset non-insulin-dependent diabetes mellitus. Nature 1992;356:162-164.
14. Heimberg H, De Vos A, Vandercammen A, Van Schaftingen E, Pipeleers D, Schuit F. Heterogeneity in glucose sensitivity among pancreatic β-cells is correlated to differences in glucose phosphorylation rather than glucose transport. EMBO J 1993;12:2873-2879.
15. Tal M, Liang Y, Najafi H, Lodish HF, Matschinsky FM. Expression and function of GLUT-1 and GLUT-2 glucose transporter isoforms in cells of cultured rat pancreatic islets. J Biol Chem 1992;267:17241-17247.
16. Ferrer J, Benito C, Gomis R. Pancreatic islet GLUT2 glucose transporter mRNA and protein expression in humans with and without NIDDM. Diabetes 1995;44:1369-1374.
17. De Vos A, Heimberg H, Quartier E, et al. Human and rat beta cells differ in glucose transporter but not in glucokinase gene expression. J Clin Invest 1995;96:2489-2495.
18. Sweet IR, Matschinsky FM. Are there kinetic advantages of GLUT2 in pancreatic glucose sensing? Diabetologia 1997;40:112-119.
19. Guillam M-T, Hümmler E, Schaerer E, et al. Early diabetes and abnormal postnatal pancreatic islet development in mice lacking GLUT2. Nature Gen 1997;17:327-330.
20. Hogan A, Heyner S, Charron MJ, et al. Glucose transporter gene expression in early mouse embryos. Development 1991;113:363-372.

21. Pang K, Mukonoweshuro C, Wong GC. Beta cells arise from glucose transporter type 2 (Glut2)-expressing epithelial cells of the developing rat pancreas. Proc Natl Acad Sci USA 1994;91:9559-9563.
22. Offield MF, Jetton TL, Labosky PA, et al. PDX-1 is required for pancreatic outgrowth and differentiation of the rostral duodenum. Development 1996;122:983-995.
23. Hole RL, Pian-Smith MCM, Sharp GWG. Development of the biphasic response to glucose in fetal and neonatal rat pancreas. Am J Physiol 1988;254:E167-E174.
24. Kervran A, Randon J. Development of insulin release by fetal rat pancreas in vitro. Effects of glucose, amino acids, and theophylline. Diabetes 1980;29:673-678.
25. Swenne I. Glucose-stimulated DNA replication of the pancreatic islets during the development of the rat fetus. Effects of nutrients, growth hormone, and triiodothyronine. Diabetes 1985;34:803-807.
26. Philippe J. Glucagon gene transcription is negatively regulated by insulin in a hamster islet cell line. J Clin Invest 1989;84:672-677.
27. Samols E, Stagner JI. Intraislet and islet-acinar portal systems and their significance. In: Samols E, ed. The Endocrine Pancreas. New York: Raven Press, 1991:93-124.
28. Leibiger IB, Leibiger B, Moede T, Berggren P-O. Exocytosis of insulin promotes insulin gene transcription via the insulin receptor/PI-3 kinase/p70 s6 kinase and CaM kinase pathways. Mol Cell 1998;1:933-938.
29. Kulkarni RN, Brüning JC, Winnay JN, Postic C, Magnuson MA, Kahn CR. Tissue-specific knockout of the insulin receptor in pancreatic β-cells creates an insulin secretory defect similar to that in type 2 diabetes. Cell 1999;96:329-339.
30. Withers DJ, Sanchez Gutierrez J, Towery H, et al. Disruption of IRS-2 causes type 2 diabetes in mice. Nature 1998;391:900-904.
31. Rahier J, Goebbels RM, Henquin JC. Cellular composition of the human diabetic pancreas. Diabetologia 1983;24:366-371.
32. Odièvre M. Glycogénose hépato-rénale avec tubulopathie complexe. Deux observations d'une entité nouvelle. Rev Inst Hépatol 1966;16:1-70.
33. Brivet M, Moatti N, Corriat A, Lemonnier A, Odièvre M. Defective galactose oxidation in a patient with glycogen storage disease and Fanconi syndrome. Pediat Res 1983;17:157-161.
34. Santer R, Schneppenheim R, Dombrowski A, Götze H, Steinmann B, Schaub J. Mutations in GLUT2, the gene for the liver-type glucose transporter, in patients with Fanconi-Bickel syndrome. Nature Gen 1997;17:324-326.
35. Manz F, Bickel H, Brodehl J, et al. Fanconi-Bickel syndrome. Ped Nephr 1987;1:509-518.
36. Tiedge M, Lenzen S. Effects of glucose refeeding and glibenclamide treatment on glucokinase and GLUT2 gene expression in pancreatic β-cells and liver from rats. Biochem J 1995; 308:139-144.
37. Chen L, Alam T, Johnson JH, Hughes S, Newgard CB, Unger RH. Regulation of β cell glucose transporter gene expression. Proc Natl Acad Sci USA 1990;87:4088-4092.
38. Waeber G, Thompson N, Haefliger J-A, Nicod P. Characterization of the murine high Km glucose transporter GLUT2 and its transcriptional regulation by glucose in a differentiated insulin-secreting cell line. J Biol Chem 1994;269:26912-26919.
39. Ferrer J, Gomis R, Fernadez-Alvarez J, Casamitjna R, Vilardell E. Signals derived from glucose metabolism are required for glucose regulation of pancreatic islet GLUT2 mRNA and protein. Diabetes 1993;42:1273-1280.
40. Bonny C, Thompson N, Nicod P, Waeber G. Pancreatic-specific expression of the glucose transporter type 2 gene: identification of cis-elements and islet-specific trans-acting factors. Mol Endo 1995;9:1413-1426.
41. Waeber G, Pedrazzini T, Bonny O, et al. A 338 bp proximal fragment of the glucose transporter type 2 (GLUT2) promoter drives reporter gene expression in the pancreatic islets of transgenic mice. Mol Cell Endocrinol 1995;9:1413-1426.
42. Weinhaus AJ, Stout LE, Sorensen RL. Glucokinase, hexokinase, glucose transporter 2, and glucose metabolism in islets during pregnancy and prolactin-treated islets in vitro: mechanisms for long term up-regulation of islets. Endocrinol 1996;137:1640-1649.
43. Thorens B, Weir GC, Leahy JL, Lodish HF, Bonner-Weir S. Reduced expression of the liver/beta-cell glucose transporter isoform in glucose-insensitive pancreatic beta cells of diabetic rats. Proc Natl Acad Sci USA 1990;87:6492-6406.
44. Johnson JH, Ogawa A, Chen L, et al. Underexpression of β-cell high Km glucose transporters in noninsulin-dependent diabetes. Science 1990;250:546-549.
45. Orci L, Ravazzola M, Baetens D, et al. Evidence that down-regulation of β–cell glucose transporters in non-insulin-dependent diabetes may be the cause of diabetic hyperglycemia. Proc Natl Acad Sci U S A 1990; 87:9953-9957.
46. Orci L, Unger RH, Ravazzola M, et al. Reduced β-cell glucose transporter in new onset diabetic BB rats. J Clin Invest 1990; 86:1615-1622.

47. Thorens B, Wu Y-J, Leahy JL, Weir GC. The loss of GLUT2 expression by glucose-unresponsive β-cells of db/db mice is reversible and is induced by the diabetic environment. J Clin Invest 1992;90:77-85.
48. O'Brien TD, Westermark P, Johnson KH. Islet amyloid polypeptide and insulin secretion from isolated perfused pancreas of fed, fasted, glucose-treated, and dexamethasone-treated rats. Diabetes 1991;40:1701-1706.
49. Orland MJ, Permutt MA. Comparative modulation of insulin secretion, pancreatic insulin content, and proinsulin mRNA in rats. Effects of 50% pancreatectomy and dexamethasone administration. Diabetes 1991;40:181-189.
50. Mulder H, Ahren B, Stridsberg M, Sundler F. Non-parallelism of islet amyloid polypeptide (amylin) and insulin gene expression in rat islets following dexamethasone treatment. Diabetologia 1995;38:395-402.
51. Lenzen S, Bailey CJ. Thyroid hormones, gonadal and adrenocortical steroids and the function of the islets of Langerhans. Endocrine Rev 1984;5:411-434.
52. Ogawa A, Johnson JH, Ohneda M, et al. Roles of insulin resistance and β-cell dysfunction in dexamethasone-induced diabetes. J Clin Invest 1992;90:497-504.
53. Koranyi L, Bourey R, Turk J, Mueckler M, Permutt MA. Differential expression of rat pancreatic islet beta-cell glucose transporter (GLUT2), proinsulin and islet amyloid polypeptide genes after prolonged fasting, insulin-induced hypoglycaemia and dexamethasone treatment. Diabetologia 1992;35:1125-1132.
54. Ohneda M, Johnson JH, Inman LR, et al. GLUT2 expression and function in β-cells of GK rats with NIDDM. Dissociation between reduction in glucose transport and glucose-stimulated insulin secretion. Diabetes 1993;42:1065-1072.
55. Fernandez-Mejia C, Davidson MB. Regulation of glucokinase and proinsulin gene expression and insulin secretion in RINm5F cells by dexamethasone, retinoic acid, and thyroid hormone. Endocrinol 1992;130:1660-1668.
56. Philippe J, Missotten M. Dexamethasone inhibits insulin biosynthesis by destabilizing insulin messenger ribonucleic acid in hamster insulinoma cells. Endocrinol 1990;127:1640-1645.
57. Philippe J, Giordano E, Gjinovci A, Meda P. Cyclic adenosine monophosphate prevents the glucocorticoid-mediated inhibition of insulin gene expression in rodent islet cells. J Clin Invest 1992;90:2228-2233.
58. Gremlich S, Roduit R, Thorens B. Dexamethasone,induces posttranslational degradation of GLUT2 and inhibition of insulin secretion in isolated pancreatic β-cells. Comparison with the effects fo fatty acids. J Biol Chem 1997;272:3216-3222.
59. Lambillotte C, Gilon P, Henquin JC. Direct glucocorticoid inhibition of insulin secretion. An in vitro study of dexamethasone effects in mouse islets. J Clin Invest 1997;93:414-423.
60. McGarry JD. What if Minkovski had been ageusic? An alternative angle on diabetes. Science 1992;258:766-770.
61. Unger RH. Lipotoxicity in the pathogenesis of obesity-dependent NIDDM: genetic and clinical implications. Diabetes 1996;44:863-870.
62. Crespin SR, Greenough WBIII, Steinberg D. Stimulation of insulin secretion by long-chain free fatty acids. A direct pancreatic effect. J Clin Invest 1973;52:1979-1984.
63. Sako Y, Grill VE. A 48-hour lipid infusion in the rat time-dependently inhibits glucose-induced insulin secretion and β-cell oxidation through a process likely coupled to fatty acid oxidation. Endocrinol 1990;127:1580-1589.
64. Elks ML. Chronic perifusion of rat islets with palmitate suppresses glucose-stimulated insulin release. Endocrinol 1993;133:208-214.
65. Zhou Y-P, Grill VE. Long-term exposure of rat pancreatic islets to fatty acids inhibits glucose-induced insulin secretion and biosynthesis through a glucose fatty acid cycle. J Clin Invest 1994;93:870-876.
66. Zhou Y-P, Grill VE. Palmitate-induced β-cell insensitivity to glucose is coupled to decreased pyruvate dehydrogenase activity and enhanced kinase activity in rat pancreatic islets. Diabetes 1995;44:394-399.
67. Zhou Y-P, Grill VE. Long term exposure to fatty acids and ketones inhibits β-cell functions in human pancreatic islets of Langerhans. J Clin End Metab 1995;80:1584-1590.
68. Lee Y, Hirose H, Ohneda M, Johnson JH, McGarry JD, Unger RH. β-cell lipotoxicity in the pathogenesis of non-insulin-dependent diabetes mellitus of obese rats: impairment in adipocytes β-cell relationship. Proc Natl Acad Sci USA 1994;91:10878-10882.
69. Hirose H, Lee YH, Inman LR, Nagasawa Y, Johnson JH, Unger RH. Defective fatty acid-mediated β-cell compensation in Zucker diabetic fatty rats. Pathogenic implications for obesity-dependent diabetes. J Biol Chem 1996;271:5633-5637.
70. Ohlsson H, Karlsson K, Edlund T. IPF1, a homeodomain-containing transactivator of the insulin gene. EMBO J 1993;12:4251-4259.
71. Petersen HV, Serup P, Leonard J, Michelsen BK, Madsen OD. Transcriptional regulation of the human insulin gene is dependent on the homeodomain protein STF1/IPF1 acting through the CT boxes. Proc Natl Acad Sci USA 1994;91:10465-10469.

72. Leonard J, Peesrs B, Johnson t, Ferreri K, Lee S, Montminy MR. Characterization of somatostatin transactivating factor-1, a novel homeobox factor that stimulates somatostatin expression in pancreatic islet cells. Mol Endo 1993;7:1275-1283.
73. Waeber G, Thompson N, Nicod P, Bonny C. Transcriptional activation of the GLUT2 gene by the IPF-1/STF-1/IDX-1 homeodomain factor. Mol Endo 1996;10:1327-1334.
74. Watada H, Kashimoto Y, Miyagawa J-I, et al. PDX-1 induces insulin and glucokinase gene expression in aTC1 clone 6 cells in the presence of betacellulin. Diabetes 1996;45:1826-1831.
75. Jonsson J, Carlsson L, Edlund T, Edlund E. Insulin-promoter-factor 1 is required for pancreas development in mice. Nature 1994;371:606-609.
76. Stoffers DA, Zinkin NT, Stanojevic V, Clarke WL, Habener JF. Pancreatic agenesis attributable to a single nucleotide deletion in the human IPF1 gene coding sequence. Nature Gen 1997;15:106-110.
77. Gremlich S, Bonny C, Waeber G, Thorens B. Fatty acids decrease IDX-1 expression in rat pancreatic islets and reduce GLUT2, glucokinase, insulin, and somatostatin levels. J Biol Chem 1997;272:30261-30269.
78. Stoffers DA, Ferrer J, Clarke WL, Habener JF. Early-onset type II diabetes mellitus (MODY4) linked to IPF1. Nature Gen 1997;17:138-139.
79. Ahlgren U, Jonsson J, Jonsson L, Simu K, Edlund H. β-cell-specific inactivation of the mouse Ipf1/Pdx1 gene results in loss of the β-cell phenotype and maturity onset diabetes. Genes Dev 1998;12:1763-1768.
80. Zangen DH, Bonner-Weir S, Lee CH, et al. Reduced insulin, GLUT2, and IDX-1 in _ cells after partial pancreatectomy. Diabetes 1997;46:258-264.
81. Bonny C, Roduit R, Gremlich S, Thorens B, Nicod P, Waeber G. The loss of GLUT2 expression in the pancreatic β cells of diabetic db/db mice is associated with a decrease in binding DNA-binding activity of islet-specific trans-acting factors. Mol Cell Endocrinol 1997;135:59-65.
82. Chua SC, Chung WK, Wu-Peng S, et al. Phenotypes of mouse *diabetes* and rat *fatty* due to mutations in the OB (leptin) receptor. Science 1996;271:994-996.
83. Wang M-A, Koyama k, Shimabukuro M, Mangelsdorf D, Newgard CB, Unger RH. Overexpression of leptin receptors in pancreatic islets of Zucker diabetic fatty rats restores GLUT2, glucokinase, and glucose-stimulated insulin secretion. Proc Natl Acad Sci USA 1998; 95:11921-11926.
84. Wang M-Y, Koyama k, Shimabukuro M, Newgard CB, Unger RH. OB-Rb gene transfer to leptin-resistant islets reverses diabetogenic phenotype. Proc Natl Acad Sci USA 1998;95:714-718.
85. Hughes SD, Quaade C, Johnson JH, Ferber S, Newgard CB. Transfection of AtT-20ins cells with GLUT-2 but not GLUT-1 confers glucose-stimulated insulin secretion. Relationship to glucose metabolism. J Biol Chem 1993;268:15205-15212.
86. Antoine B, Lefrançois-Martinez A-M, Le Guillou G, Leturque A, Vandewalle A, Kahn A. Role of the GLUT2 glucose transporter in the response of the L-type pyruvate kinase gene to glucose in liver-derived cells. J Biol Chem 1997;272:17937-17943.
87. Fanconi G, Bickel H. Die chronische Aminoacidurie (Aminosäurediabetes oder nephrotisch-glucokisurischer Zwergwuchs) bei der Glycogenose und Cystinkrankheit. Helv Ped Acta 1949;4:359-396.
88. Tiao G, Fagan J, Roegner V, et al. Energy-ubiquitin-dependent muscle proteolysis during sepsis in rats is regulated by glucocorticoids. J Clin Invest 1996;97:339-348.

21

USE OF A CRE/LOXP STRATEGY IN MICE TO DETERMINE THE CELL-SPECIFIC ROLES OF GLUCOKINASE IN MODY-2

Catherine Postic, Ph.D. and Mark A. Magnuson, M.D.
Vanderbilt University, Nashville, TN 37232, USA

INTRODUCTION

Mutations of glucokinase (GK) cause maturity-onset diabetes of the young type 2 (MODY-2), a monogenic form of diabetes that is characterized by an early age of onset and autosomal dominant inheritance. We have used a Cre/*loxP* strategy to generate pancreatic β-cell and hepatocyte-specific knockouts of GK in mice and have studied glucose homeostasis in these mice. The studies clearly demonstrate that diminished pancreatic β-cell GK accounts for most of the hyperglycaemia in MODY-2. Mice deficient in hepatic GK are only moderately hyperglycaemic and have impaired insulin secretion. The mechanism by which the loss of hepatic GK impairs insulin secretion by the β-cell is not understood and requires further study.

Glucokinase, by virtue of kinetic characteristics that distinguish it from other hexokinases, has long been recognized to play an essential role in glucose homeostasis. The discovery in 1992 that GK gene mutations cause MODY-2, propelled GK into a position of being one of only a few molecules in which genetic haploinsufficiency causes diabetes (1). This finding led us to pursue detailed studies in mice, making use of both transgenic and gene targeting strategies, to learn more about the relationship between GK gene expression and glycaemia. Initially, these studies examined the effect of increased GK on blood glucose homeostasis (2-4). More recently, we have studied how diminished GK activity actually causes hyperglycaemia, as occurs when one of the two genes that encode this enzyme is mutated.

GK is expressed in several neural and neuroendocrine cell types, most importantly the pancreatic β-cell as well as in hepatocytes (5). The cell-specific expression of GK is regulated by two widely separated promoters (6). The upstream promoter drives expression in neural and neuroendocrine cell types whereas the downstream promoter confers expression in hepatocytes. GK function has been most extensively studied in β-cells where the enzyme has long been proposed to be an important component of the glucose sensing machinery (7). Phosphorylation of glucose in the β-cell is tightly coupled to insulin secretion, and GK accounts for the majority of the hexokinase activity in this cell. Mathematical modelling of glucose flux in the β-cell indicates that GK has a control strength of close to 1, which means that the enzyme essentially determines the rate at which glucose entering the cell is phosphorylated, and consequently, how much insulin is secreted (8). Indeed, discovery of a novel GK gene mutation that lowers the $K_{cat}S_{0.5}$ of the enzyme in a pedigree with persistent hyperinsulinemic hypoglycaemia of infancy (PHHI) (9) supports the importance of the enzyme kinetics of GK. Thus, for these and a variety of additional reasons, GK is an important part of the enzymatic machinery that enables the β-cell to sense and respond to fluctuations of the plasma glucose concentration.

In contrast, the role of GK in the liver is less firmly established, even though the enzyme was first discovered in this tissue nearly fifty years ago (10). GK is been thought to play a role in determining rates of both glucose uptake and glycogen synthesis. In transgenic mice, increased hepatic GK causes hypoglycaemia (3,4) whereas in primary hepatocytes GK over-expression increases both glycolysis and glycogen synthesis (11,12). Increased GK expression in liver modulates the expression of several glycolytic (13,14), gluconeogenic (15,16) and lipogenic (17,18) genes. The expression levels of these genes are also regulated by glucose. The mechanism whereby glucose regulates these genes is not fully understood, although GK is considered to play an essential role in mediating the effects of glucose on gene expression (13).

In addition to the β-cell and hepatocytes, GK has been identified in pancreatic α-cells (19), in the hypothalamus and in certain enteroendocrine cells of the gut (5). The precise function of GK in each of these locations has not yet been determined. Since the hypothalamus contains glucose responsive neurones, and the gut contains cells that – in response to meal intake - secrete incretins that stimulate insulin secretion (20,21), it is likely that GK functions in these cells, much like it does in the pancreatic β-cell, as a central constituent of the glucose sensing machinery.

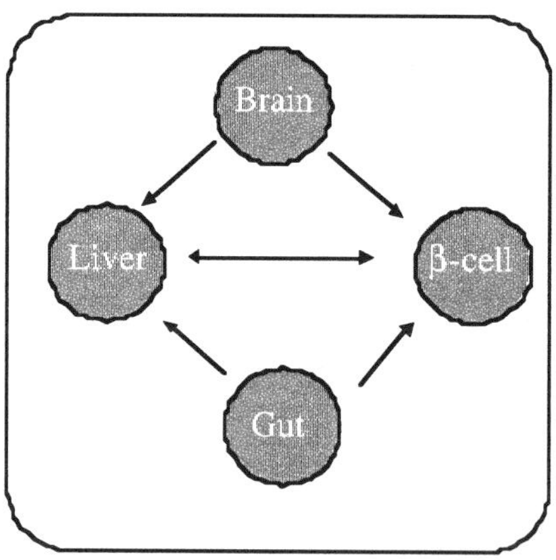

Figure 1. *Multiple sites of GK expression and function. The four tissues shown, all of which express GK, play major roles in glucose homeostasis, and interact with each other in complex ways. Thus, conventional gene knockouts of GK are of only limited value in studying the pathophysiology of MODY-2.*

Studies of MODY-2 patients suggest that impaired insulin secretion is largely responsible for the persistent hyperglycaemia that occurs in this disease. To further understand how this occurs, a variety of mouse models have been generated in which the expression of GK is either increased or decreased (22-24). In all cases, heterozygous GK knockout mice are hyperglycaemic and have defective insulin secretion in response to glucose (22-24). While this indicates that the mouse is a relevant experimental model for MODY-2, these studies have fallen short of clearly explaining the pathophysiology of MODY-2. Indeed, given that GK is expressed in multiple tissues that play important roles in glucose homeostasis, and that the interactions between these different tissues is complex (Figure 1), further knowledge of the cell-specific functions of GK is necessary to fully understand how mutations in this gene cause hyperglycaemia. Therefore, to clearly determine the cell-specific roles of GK in glucose homeostasis, we have used a Cre/*loxP* strategy to begin to precisely define the pathophysiological basis of this disease. Our initial studies focused on the roles of GK in the liver and β-cell.

GENERAL FEATURES OF CRE/LOXP STRATEGY AND APPLICATION TO GK

Conventional gene targeting techniques that typically result in mice that lack a gene in all cell types, often lead to severe developmental defects or embryonic lethality that may preclude or confuse analysis of post-developmental gene functions. Indeed, mice that either globally lack GK (22,23), or even just the islet isoform (24), do not survive more than a few days after birth. Thus, while conventional knockout studies clearly validate the physiological importance of GK, detailed physiological studies in adult animals can only be performed in mice that are heterozygous for the null allele. To overcome these difficulties, we have made use of a conditional targeting strategy that use Cre, a site-specific DNA recombinase, to excise any DNA fragment flanked by two 34 bp DNA sequences termed *loxP* sites (25,26). Gene targeting strategies that use the Cre/*loxP* technology can overcome many of the limitations of conventional gene targeting approaches. Cre is expressed in defined cells of a transgenic mouse under control of a tissue-specific promoter (i.e. insulin promoter). This mouse line is then bred with a mouse line carrying the gene of interest (i.e. GK) flanked by LoxP sites. In the new litter the gene of interest is ablated only in cells that express the Cre recombinase.

We first created a triple-loxed *gk* allele in mice by gene targeting ($gk^{lox+neo}$). As shown in Figure 2, two of the *loxP* sites in this allele flank a neomycin resistance (neo^R) cassette that lies downstream of exon 10. A third *loxP* site is located between exons 8 and 9. This triple-loxed allele was converted to *gk* alleles containing either dual or single *loxP* sites by exposure to Cre. The conversion from 3 to 2 *loxP* sites was achieved in two different ways. The first was by transfection of ES cells with a Cre expression plasmid. The second method was to microinject the same Cre expression plasmid into single cell mouse embryos that were heterozygous for the $gk^{lox+neo}$ allele. Both methods resulted in removal of neo^R, thereby creating a *gk* allele (gk^{lox}) that was identical to the wild type allele, except for the presence of the *loxP* sites. The second method had the advantage that animals containing alleles with either 3, 2 or 1 *loxP* sites can all be derived from a single ES cell clone and provided experimental flexibility.

The microinjection method has two main advantages over the transfection method. First, several variant alleles can be created from a single gene-targeting event after germline transmission has been achieved. Second, since variable amounts of the Cre expression plasmid can be microinjected, some control over the efficiency of the recombination can be achieved. Microinjection of low concentrations of Cre result in more partial recombination events whereas higher concentrations result in complete recombination events, as shown in Table 1.

For generating β-cell and hepatocyte-specific GK gene knockout mice, first transgenic mouse lines that expressed Cre in a large fraction of the desired cell type were established. Cre expression in pancreatic β-cells was achieved using a transgene that contains a fragment of the rat insulin II promoter region whereas expression of Cre in hepatocytes was obtained using albumin promoter/enhancer sequences (Figure 3).

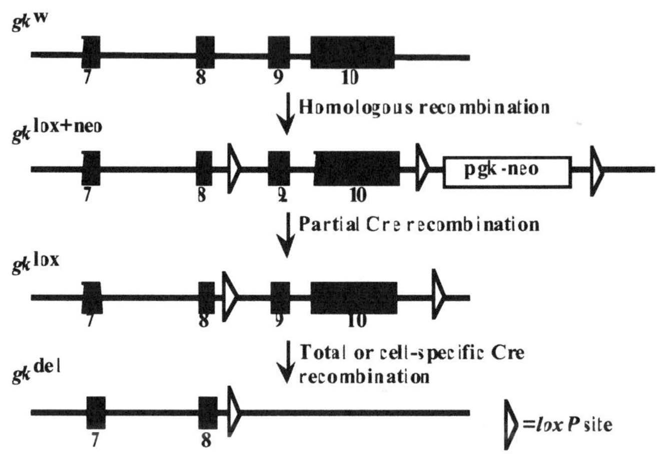

Figure 2. *Generation of mice with conditional gk gene alleles. Exons are indicated as solid rectangles. A partial map of the wild type allele (gk^{w}) is shown. Conditional gk^{lox} and $gk^{lox+neo}$ alleles were obtained by homologous recombination in ES cells and partial cre recombination, respectively (27). The deleted allele (gk^{del}) lacks exons 9 and 10 and was obtained by microinjection of a Cre expression plasmid into single cell mouse embryos (see Table 1) or by cell-specific expression of Cre in transgenic mice (see Figure 3).*

Several features pertaining to the design of these transgenes merit comment. First, human growth hormone gene (hGH) sequences were placed downstream of Cre. Intronic sequences of the hGH gene are thought to be important in determining nucleosome spacing (29,30), which may facilitate expression of upstream coding sequences. We found that inclusion of the hGH sequences is required for high expression of Cre. An earlier version of each of these transgenes that contained metallothionein sequences downstream of Cre did not express the transgene efficiently in the target tissues. Second, the transgenes contained Cre coding sequences that had been modified by insertion of both a nuclear localization sequence and a Kozac consensus sequence, the latter for proper translation initiation.

PHENOTYPE OF MICE THAT HAVE A GLOBAL DEFECT IN GK

Generation of mice with a null GK allele (gk^{del}) by microinjections of a Cre-expression plasmid allowed us first to confirm the effects of either a reduction or total absence of GK on glucose homeostasis. Heterozygous GK null mice ($gk^{del/w}$) were viable, but had both fed (+75%) and fasting hyperglycaemia (+40%) compared to controls. Physiological studies were then performed using chronically catheterized mice. This approach, in which two catheters are implanted prior to performing the physiological studies, allows for determination of rates of hepatic glucose utilization, and rates of insulin secretion under both basal and hyperglycaemic conditions.

During the hyperglycaemic clamp study, a variable infusion of glucose is used to raise blood glucose levels at ~300 mg/dl. Glucose turnover and glucose clearance rates as well as net hepatic and muscle glycogen synthesis are determined by use of [3-^{3}H] glucose as a metabolic tracer in the infusion solution. The glucose infusion rate required to maintain the plasma glucose at this level provides an index of glucose tolerance. During a hyperglycaemic clamp the $gk^{del/w}$ mice had a ~50% reduction in basal glucose turnover rates, as well as marked glucose intolerance as reflected by a ~70% reduction in glucose turnover rates and a ~60% decrease in the peak of insulin secretion (27).

DNA concentration (ng/µl)	1	0.1	0.01	0.001
Embryos injected	74	119	123	82
Embryos survival (%)	66	53	58	63
Pups	21	10	16	9
Total deletion (%)	29	40	0	0
Partial deletion (%)	0	30	20	22

Table 1. *Results of Cre expression plasmid microinjections into single cell $gk^{lox+neo}$ mouse embryos. Different concentrations of supercoiled CMV-Cre plasmid DNA (pBS185) were microinjected into single cell $gk^{lox+neo}$ heterozygous mouse embryos (28) and the recombination events in each surviving animal was determined by southern blot and PCR analysis. A total recombination event eliminates the DNA between the two outer most loxP sites, thereby removing exons 9 and 10, as well as neo^R, whereas a partial recombination event removed either neo^R or exons 9 and 10, but not both. A total of 398 embryos were microinjected and 56 pups were born.*

Interbreeding of $gk^{del/w}$ mice resulted in animals that totally lacked GK ($gk^{del/del}$). All of these mice died within the first few days of life. At 2 days of age they were markedly hyperglycaemic and had low plasma insulin concentrations. In fact, all of the metabolic alterations observed in mice that totally lack GK (e.g. hepatic steatosis, elevated FFAs, and glycogen depletion) are consistent with low plasma insulin concentrations. Overall, the phenotype of GK null mice closely matched that previously reported by Grupe et al. (23), but differed from that of Bali et al. (22) who observed embryonic lethality at ~E9.5. This difference is likely due to the random insertion of a second copy of the targeting vector in the genome of the Bali et al. mice that may have led to the inadvertent knockout of a gene that is essential during early embryogenesis.

ROLE OF β-CELL GK IN GLUCOSE SENSING AND GLUCOSE HOMEOSTASIS

To unambiguously determine the role of GK in pancreatic β-cells, mice with two conditional alleles ($gk^{lox/lox}$) were bred with animals that express Cre under the control of the rat insulin promoter (Figure 4). In this manner, β-cell-specific GK knockout mice (e.g. $gk^{lox/lox}$+*Rip-cre)* were obtained. These mice exhibited a phenotype nearly identical to that of global GK knockout animals. Most died within a few days of birth as a result of severe diabetes, and two day-old pups exhibited identical metabolic and biochemical alterations that were observed in GK null neonates, namely steatosis and depletion of hepatic glycogen content due to ~70% decrease in plasma insulin concentrations. Thus, mice that lack GK only in β-cells are phenotypically similar to animals with a global GK knockout, as well as animals that lack only the islet isoform of GK (24). While they do not exhibit as strikingly high blood glucose concentrations as the global GK null animals do, the glycaemia is high enough to kill most animals. The lack of 100% mortality is probably because the Rip-Cre transgene is expressed in only about 85% of pancreatic β-cells, presumably due to variegated expression of Cre. Thus, the lack of total lethality is probably a reflection of the incomplete conversion of the gk^{lox} allele to the gk^{del} allele in β-cells, which allows a few animals to survive.

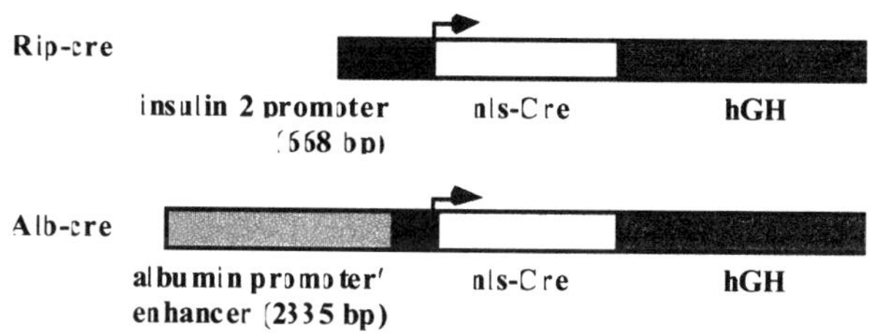

Figure 3. *Design of Cre transgenes. Cre expression in pancreatic β-cells was achieved using a transgene containing a fragment of the rat insulin II promoter region whereas expression in hepatocytes was obtained using albumin promoter/enhancer sequences. To increase the fidelity of expression of the Cre transgenes human growth hormone gene (hGH) sequences were placed downstream of the Cre coding sequences. In addition, the Cre sequences contained both a nuclear localization signal (nls) sequences and an optimized translation start site.*

As for the heterozygous GK global knockout mice, physiological indices of glucose turnover and insulin secretion were determined for the heterozygous β-cell-specific GK knockout mice by chronic catheterization. Heterozygous β-cell-specific GK knockout mice had fasting hyperglycaemia (+25%) without measurable difference in basal insulin levels. During the hyperglycaemic clamp, glucose turnover rates and insulin secretion were reduced by ~70%. As a consequence of diminished insulin secretion, net glycogen synthesis in liver was also reduced by ~50%.

Results from the β-cell-specific GK knockout mice further strengthen the notion that GK plays an essential role in the function of the β-cell glucose sensor, as has been proposed by Matschinsky et al. (8). In addition, they suggested that extrapancreatic glucose sensing might only play a minor role in whole-body glucose homeostasis. Terauchi et al. (24) eliminated the islet isoform of GK in all tissues of the organism with the exception of hepatocytes. However, in these animals, the deficiency of GK in either, the brain or in enteroendocrine cells, might have contributed to the hyperglycaemia of MODY-2. It remained unclear how important the GK defect in β-cells was for the MODY-2 phenotype to develop. Given that our β-cell-specific GK gene knockout mice have a phenotype very similar to the mice made by Terauchi et al., which totally lack the islet GK isoform, it is clear that the haploinsufficiency of GK in the β-cell is the main reason for hyperglycaemia in MODY-2. Extrapancreatic sites of the islet GK isoform (e.g., the brain and gut) cannot compensate for the absence of GK in the β-cell.

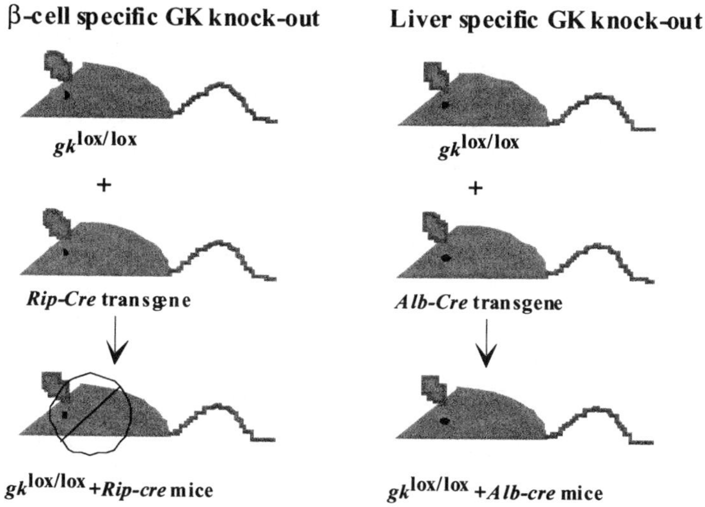

Figure 4. *Strategy for β-cell and liver-specific deletion of the gk^{lox} allele in mice. Intercrossing of either Rip-cre or Alb-cre transgenic mice with mice bearing the gk^{lox} allele resulted in mice with either a β-cell- or liver-specific knockout of GK. The β-cell-specific knockout mice die within a few days of birth whereas the liver-specific knockout mice are viable.*

While our data indicate that, in the pancreatic β-cell, GK is an essential component of the glucose sensing machinery, it is not the only component. Evidence obtained from studies of cultured $gk^{lox/lox}$ islets in which GK was partially knocked-out using a recombinant adenovirus that expresses Cre (31) suggests that a second hexokinase with a lower K_m is present in islet cells. However, whether this second hexokinase plays any role in glucose sensing in the presence of GK is questionable since GK activity yields higher concentrations of glucose-6-phosphate that would suppress the lower K_m hexokinase activity under most physiological conditions.

ROLE OF HEPATIC GK IN GLUCOSE HOMEOSTASIS

In liver, GK has been thought to participate in a substrate cycle that determines whether glucose is either utilized or produced by the liver (32). Metabolic flux in the liver reflects the net activities of several major enzymes that are regulated at the transcriptional level by the metabolism of glucose itself, perhaps involving glucose-6-phosphate as a mediator (13). Hepatic GK gene transcription is increased by insulin and inhibited by glucagon (33,34). In addition, GK activity in liver is acutely regulated by interactions with a GK regulatory protein (GKRP) (35). While it has been difficult to directly assess the role that a deficiency of hepatic GK plays in the pathogenesis of MODY-2, there has been a large amount of indirect information suggesting a major role for this enzyme in regulating hepatic glucose fluxes. For instance, the selective inhibition of hepatic GK activity in the rat by the infusion of glucosamine impairs the ability of hyperglycaemia to suppress endogenous glucose production (36). Moreover, hyperglycaemia fails to fully suppress hepatic glucose production in heterozygous null global GK knockout mice (37). These findings suggest that the haploinsufficiency of GK in MODY-2 disturbs hepatic glucose metabolism, and limits the ability of the liver to normally suppress glucose production rates in response to hyperglycaemia.

To directly determine the role of hepatic GK in glucose homeostasis, liver-specific GK knockout mice (e.g. $gk^{lox/lox}$+*Alb-Cre*) were made by breeding albumin-Cre transgenic mice with animals bearing the loxed GK allele (Figure 4). In contrast to the perinatal death in β–cell GK knockout mice, the total loss of hepatic GK was not associated with mortality. Instead, mice totally lacking hepatic GK showed fed blood glucose values that were only ~10% higher that their $gk^{lox/lox}$ littermates (27). To explore the consequences of the total loss of hepatic GK on both insulin secretion and hepatic fluxes, basal and hyperglycaemic clamp studies were performed. After an 8-hour fast, no differences were detected in either plasma insulin concentration or glucose turnover rate, even though the blood glucose concentrations were 40% higher than the controls. The fact that basal glucose turnover rates in mice totally lacking GK is similar to control animals suggests that normal or near normal hepatic glucose flux rates are maintained by one or another of the low K_m hexokinases in the basal state. The absence of hepatic GK only becomes apparent under hyperglycaemic conditions. In this situation, glucose turnover, glucose clearance, hepatic glycogen synthesis and insulin secretion rates (as shown in Figure 5) are all markedly decreased.

A blunted insulin secretory response to the hyperglycaemic clamp was an unexpected result, particularly since these mice have only slightly elevated basal plasma glucose concentrations. The cause of the impaired insulin secretion in a situation of unimpaired β-cell GK remains unexplained. Sustained mild hyperglycaemia has been shown to cause β-cells to become unresponsive to glucose, and to show impaired glucose-induced insulin-secretion (38,39). However, this circumstance seems unlikely in light of a very slight elevation of basal glucose levels in these animals. Alternatively, the lack of hepatic GK may impair the ability of the liver to sense and respond to hyperglycaemia. Indeed, GK might be considered part of the glucose sensing machinery in hepatocytes. In the absence of hepatic GK, the liver may fail to respond in a variety of ways to hyperglycaemia. For instance, it is conceivable that glucose stimulates the secretion of one or more undefined factors whose function is to modulate insulin secretion. Another possibility is that the lack of hepatic GK affects the function of a neural regulatory loop. In any case, these results clearly demonstrate a role for hepatic GK in glucose homeostasis, by both a direct effect on hepatic glucose utilization and an indirect effect on insulin secretion.

IMPLICATIONS OF THESE FINDINGS FOR THE PATHOGENESIS OF OTHER TYPES OF MODY

The data obtained from cell-specific knockouts of both pancreatic β-cell and hepatic GK clearly show that the hyperglycaemia that occurs in MODY-2 is largely due to diminished β-cell GK. However, diminished hepatic GK is likely to exacerbate the deficiency of GK in the β-cell, even though mice that completely lack hepatic GK have only a small increase in their basal blood glucose concentration. The information from these studies, while primarily related to the pathogenesis of the hyperglycaemia in MODY-2, may also be relevant to understanding the origin of the hyperglycaemia in other types of MODY and in Type 2 diabetes. For instance, other types of MODY are caused by mutations in HNF-1α (40), HNF-4α (41), HNF3-β (42), and Pdx1 (43,44). All of these genes, with the exception of Pdx1, are expressed in both the liver and pancreatic islet cells. Whereas studies of patients with these different MODY syndromes have revealed deficits in insulin secretion, thereby implicating impaired β-cell function; it remains possible that mutations in one or another of the HNFs might also lead to defects in hepatic glucose metabolism. Thus, impaired liver glucose metabolism in individuals with defects in their HNF-1α, HNF-4α or HNF-3β genes might also contribute to the insulin secretory defect observed in these individuals.

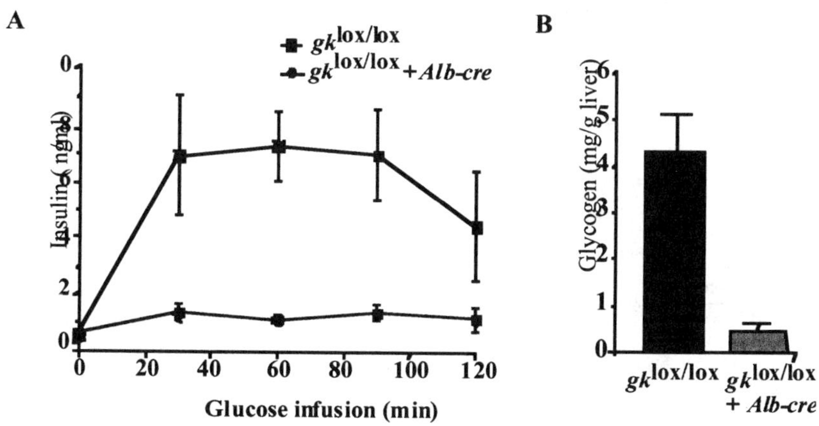

Figure 5. *Impaired insulin secretion and reduced glycogen content in liver of gk$^{lox/lox}$+Alb-cre mice. **A)** gk$^{lox/lox}$+Alb-cre mice secreted 70% less insulin in response to the glucose stimulus compared to controls **B)** Net hepatic glycogen synthesis, measured at the end of the 2-hour hyperglycaemic clamp, was reduced by ~90% in liver of gk$^{lox/lox}$+Alb-cre mice compared to their controls.*

Type 2 diabetes is a complex metabolic disorder characterized by peripheral insulin resistance and impaired β-cell function. Recently, Cre/*loxP* methodology has also been used to dissect the physiological effects of impaired insulin function separately in various tissues. Elegant studies of mice with a muscle-specific insulin receptor knock-out (MIRKO) (45) and a β-cell-specific insulin receptor knock-out (BIRKO) (46) have yielded novel insights into the implication of these two tissues in the development of insulin resistance and Type 2 diabetes (47). Surprisingly, although skeletal muscle is the primary site of glucose disposal *in vivo*, MIRKO mice have normal fasting glucose levels and normal glucose tolerance. Normal glucose clearance in response to insulin was observed in these mice because insulin action in liver was not impaired (45). BIRKO mice are model for insulin resistance in pancreatic β-cells, exhibiting a defect in glucose-stimulated insulin secretion, leading to progressive impairment in glucose tolerance (46). These studies provide evidence that a specific genetic defect in β-cells may not only cause the peripheral tissues to become insulin resistant, but also cause a direct failure of the β-cell function leading to insulin deficiency.

FUTURE USE OF CRE/LOXP STRATEGIES

The unambiguous information that can be obtained by cell-specific knockout models will lead to a more widespread use the Cre/*loxP* methodology. Indeed, a large number of cell-specific gene knockouts are likely to prove necessary to sort out the physiological roles of the many different molecules that are involved in glucose homeostasis. Use of Cre/*loxP* should also be useful in determining the role of GK in other sites of expression, such as the brain (5). Neurones in certain brain nuclei respond to changes in glucose concentration and are thought to mediate counterregulatory responses to hypoglycaemia or affect feeding behaviour (48). However, to perform studies like those described here, a greater collection of Cre-expressing mice needs to be developed and characterized. Alternatively, and at least in the case of the brain, it may be possible to perform intracranial injections of recombinant adenoviruses that express Cre to perform gene deletions in specific nuclei. In any case, it is likely that new physiological interactions pertinent to glucose homeostasis will be discovered with the ability to introduce precise biochemical mutations within specific cell types.

ACKNOWLEDGMENTS

These studies were supported by grants from the NIH (DK42612 and DK42502). We thank M. Shiota, K.D. Niswender, Y. Chen, J.M. Moates, K.D. Shelton, J. Lindner, S. Knobel, D. Piston and A.D. Cherrington for their participation in the primary studies that are summarized here.

REFERENCES

1. Froguel P, Vaxillaire M, Sun F, et al. Close linkage of glucokinase locus on chromosome 7p to early-onset non-insulin-dependent diabetes mellitus. Nature 1992;356:162-164.
2. Ferre T, Riu E, Bosch F, Valera A. Evidence from transgenic mice that glucokinase is rate limiting for glucose utilization in the liver. FASEB J 1996;10:1213-1218.
3. Hariharan N, Farrelly D, Hagan D, et al. Expression of human hepatic glucokinase in transgenic mice liver results in decreased glucose levels and reduced body weight. Diabetes 1997;46:11-16.
4. Niswender KD, Shiota M, Postic C, Cherrington AD, Magnuson MA. Effects of increased glucokinase gene copy number on blood glucose homeostasis and hepatic glucose metabolism. J Biol Chem 1997;272:22570-22572.
5. Jetton T, Liang Y, Petterpher CC, et al. Analysis of upstream glucokinase promoter activity in transgenic mice and identification of glucokinase in rare neuroendocrine cells in the brain and gut. J Biol Chem 1994;269:3641-3654.
6. Magnuson MA. Glucokinase gene structure: Functional implications of molecular genetic studies. Diabetes 1990;39:523-527.
7. Matschinsky FM. Glucokinase as glucose sensor and metabolic signal generator in pancreatic beta-cells and hepatocytes. Diabetes 1990;39:647-652.
8. Matschinsky FM, Glaser B, Magnuson MA. Pancreatic β-cell glucokinase. Closing the gap between theoretical concepts and experimental realities. Diabetes 1998;47:307-315.
9. Glaser B, Kesavan P, Heyman M, et al. Familial hyperinsulinism caused by an activating glucokinase mutation. N Engl J Med 1998;338:226-230.
10. Grossman SH, Potter VR. Identification of rat hepatic glucokinase after polyacrylamide disc electrophoresis. Anal Biochem 1974;59:54-62.
11. Agius L, Peak M, Newgard CB, Gomez-Foix AM, Guinovart JJ. Evidence for a role of glucose-induced translocation of glucokinase in the control of hepatic glycogen synthesis. J Biol Chem 1996;271:30479-30486.

12. O'Doherty RM, Lehman DL, Seoane J, Gomez-Foix AM, Guinovart JJ, Newgard CB. Differential metabolic effects of adenovirus-mediated glucokinase and hexokinase I overexpression in rat primary hepatocytes. J Biol Chem. 1996;271:20524-20530.
13. Girard J. Mechanisms by which carbohydrates regulate expression of genes for glycolytic and lipogenic enzymes. Annu Rev Nutr 1997;17:325-352.
14. Vaulont S, Kahn A. Transcriptional control of metabolic regulation genes by carbohydrates. FASEB J 1994;8:28-35.
15. Scott DK, O'Doherty RM, Stafford JM, Newgard CB, Granner DK. The repression of hormone-activated PEPCK gene expression by glucose is insulin-independent but requires glucose metabolism. J Biol Chem 1998;273:24145-24151.
16. Massillon D, Chen W, Barzilai N, et al. Carbon flux via the pentose phosphate pathway regulates the hepatic expression of the glucose-6-phophatase and phophoenolpyruvate carboxykinase genes in conscious rats. J Biol Chem 1998;273:228-234.
17. Foufelle F, Girard J, Ferre P. Regulation of lipogenic enzyme expression by glucose in liver and adipose tissue: a review of the potential cellular and molecular mechanisms. Adv Enzyme Regul 1996;36:199-226.
18. Prip-Buus C, Perdereau D, Foufelle F, Maury J, Ferre P, Girard J. Induction of fatty-acid-synthase gene expression by glucose in primary culture of rat hepatocytes. Dependency upon glucokinase activity. Eur J Biochem 1995;230:309-315.
19. Heimberg H, De Vos A, Moens K, et al. The glucose sensor protein glucokinase is expressed in glucagon-producing alpha-cells. Proc Natl Acad Sci USA 1996;93:7036-7041.
20. Mojsov S, Weir GC, Habener JF. Insulinotropin: glucagon-like peptide I (7-37) co-encoded in the glucagon gene is a potent stimulator of insulin release in the perfused rat pancreas. J Clin Invest 1987;79:616-619.
21. Thorens B, Waeber G. Glucagon-like peptide-I and the control of insulin secretion in the normal state and in NIDDM. Diabetes 1993;42:121-125.
22. Bali D, Svetlanov A, Lee H-W, et al. Animal model for maturity onset diabetes of the young generated by disruption of the mouse glucokinase gene. J Biol Chem 1995;270:21464-21467.
23. Grupe A, Hultgren B, Ryan S, Ma YH, Bauer M, Stewart TA. Transgenic knockouts reveal a critical requirement for pancreatic β-cell glucokinase in maintaining glucose homeostasis. Cell 1995;83:69-78.
24. Terauchi Y, Sakura H, Yasuda K, et al. Pancreatic β-cell specific targeted disruption of glucokinase gene. J Biol Chem 1995;270:30253-30256.
25. Rajewsky K, Gu H, Kuhn R, et al. Conditional gene targeting. J Clin Invest 1996;98:600-603.
26. Sauer B. Inducible gene targeting in mice using the Cre-loxP system. Methods 1998;14:381-392.
27. Postic C, Shiota M, Niswender KD, et al. Dual roles for glucokinase in glucose homeostasis as determined by liver and pancreatic β cell specific gene knock-outs using cre recombinase. J Biol Chem 1999;274:305-315.
28. Araki K, Araki M, Miyazaki J, Vassalli P. Site-specific recombination of a transgene in fertilized eggs by transient expression of Cre recombinase. Proc Natl Acad Sci USA 1995;92:160-164.
29. Liu K, Sandgren EP, Palmiter RD, Stein A. Rat growth hormone gene introns stimulate nucleosome alignment in vitro and in transgenic mice. Proc Natl Acad Sci USA 1995;92:7724-7728.
30. Palmiter RD, Sandgren EP, Avarbock MR, Allen DD, Brinster RL. Heterologous introns can enhance expression of transgenes in mice. Proc Natl Acad Sci USA 1991;88:478-482.
31. Piston DW, Knobel SM, Postic C, Shelton KD, Magnuson MA. Adenovirus-mediated knockout of a conditional glucokinase gene in isolated pancreatic islets reveals an essential role for proximal metabolic coupling events in glucose-stimulated insulin secretion. J Biol Chem 1999;274:1000-4.
32. Pilkis SJ, Granner DK. Molecular physiology of the regulation of hepatic gluconeogenesis and glycolysis. Annu Rev Phys 1992;54:885-909.
33. Iynedjian PB, Jotterand D, Nouspikel T, Asfari M, Pilot PR. Transcriptional induction of glucokinase gene by insulin in cultured liver cells and its repression by the glucagon c-AMP system. J Biol Chem 1989;264:21824-29.
34. Magnuson MA, Andreone TL, Printz RL, Koch S, Granner DK. Rat glucokinase gene: structure and regulation by insulin. Proc Natl Acad Sci USA 1989;86:4838-4842.
35. Van Schaftingen E, Vandercammen A, Detheux M, Davies DR. The regulatory protein of liver glucokinase. Adv Enzyme Regul 1992;32:133-48.
36. Barzilai N, Hawkins M, Angelov I, Hu M, Rossetti L. Glucosamine-induced inhibition of liver glucokinase impairs the ability of hyperglycaemia to suppress endogenous glucose production. Diabetes 1996;45:1329-1335.
37. Rossetti L, Chen W, Hu MZ, Hawkins M, Barzilai N, Efrat S. Abnormal regulation of HGP by hyperglycaemia in mice with a disrupted glucokinase allele. Am J Physiol 1997;36:E743-E750.
38. Leahy JL, Bonner-Weir S, Weir GC. β-cell dysfunction induced by chronic hyperglycaemia. Diabetes care 1992;15:442-455.
39. Rossetti L, Giaccari A, Defronzo RA. Glucose toxicity. Diabetes care 1990;13:610-630.
40. Yamagata K, Oda N, Kaisaki PJ, et al. Mutations in the hepatocyte nuclear factor-1alpha gene in maturity-onset diabetes of the young (MODY3). Nature 1996;384:455-458.

41. Yamagata K, Furuta H, Oda N, et al. Mutations in the hepatocyte nuclear factor-4alpha gene in maturity-onset diabetes of the young (MODY1). Nature 1996;384:458-460.
42. Horikawa Y, Iwasaki N, Hara M, et al. Mutation in hepatocyte nuclear factor-1 beta gene (TCF2) associated with MODY. Nat Genet 1997;17:384-355.
43. Stoffers DA, Zinkin NT, Stanojevic V, Clarke WL, Habener JF. Pancreatic agenesis attributable to a single nucleotide deletion in the human IPF1 gene coding sequence. Nat Genet 1997;15:106-110.
44. Stoffers DA, Ferrer J, Clarke WL, Habener JF. Early-onset type-II diabetes mellitus (MODY4) linked to IPF1. Nat Genet 1997;17:138-139.
45. Bruning JC, Michael M, Winney J, et al. A muscle-specific insulin receptor knockout exhibits features of the metabolic syndrome of NIDDM without altering glucose tolerance. Mol Cell 1998;2:559-569.
46. Kulkarni RN, Bruning JC, Winnay JN, Postic C, Magnuson MA, Kahn CR. Tissue-specific knockout of the insulin receptor in pancreatic beta cells creates an insulin secretory defect similar to that in type 2 diabetes. Cell 1999;96:329-339.
47. Taylor SI. Deconstructing Type 2 Diabetes. Cell 1999;97:9-12.
48. Navarro M, Rodriquez de Fonseca F, Alvarez E, et al. Colocalization of glucagon-like peptide-1 (GLP-1) receptors, glucose transporter GLUT-2, and glucokinase mRNAs in rat hypothalamic cells: evidence for a role of GLP-1 receptor agonists as an inhibitory signal for food and water intake. J. Neurochem 1996;67:1982-1991.

22

DEVELOPMENT OF β-CELL LINES FOR TRANSPLANTATION IN TYPE 1 DIABETES MELLITUS

Shimon Efrat, Ph.D.
*Department of Human Genetics and Molecular Medicine
Sackler School of Medicine, Tel Aviv University,
Ramat Aviv, Tel Aviv 69978, Israel*

INTRODUCTION

For the better part of the 20th century, people with insulin-dependent (type 1) diabetes mellitus (IDDM) have relied on insulin administration as a life-saving treatment. However, periodical insulin injections are a crude substitute for the fine-tuned regulation of insulin release from the pancreatic islet β-cells, which is continuously and accurately adjusted to changing physiological conditions. As a result, most IDDM patients are exposed to episodes of hyperglycaemia and hypoglycaemia, leading to the development of severe complications. Modern diabetes research has two major goals: the first is to understand the aetiology of the disease sufficiently to be able to identify individuals at risk for developing IDDM and to intervene to prevent it. The second goal is to replace β-cell function in people who already have developed the disease with a safe, efficient, and convenient treatment that will prevent the complications of IDDM. This chapter summarizes the state of the art in the development of new approaches for β-cell replacement and evaluates the potential of cell therapy for treatment of IDDM.

ECTOPIC INSULIN PRODUCTION

An obvious solution for substitution of insulin production by the islet β-cells is the engineering of ectopic insulin biosynthesis and secretion in autologous non-β-cells. This could be achieved by transfer of the preproinsulin gene to various tissues *in vivo* or by engineering of cells explanted from the patient and subsequently reintroduced into their tissue of origin. The greatest advantage of this approach is the likelihood that the engineered autologous cells will be protected from graft rejection and from recurring autoimmunity to β-cells. Proinsulin synthesis and processing has been achieved in a variety of heterologous cell types in experimental animals (1-4) and in cultured cell lines (5-7). It may also become possible to activate insulin expression in non-β-cells from the endogenous insulin gene, as demonstrated by introduction of the gene encoding the transcription factor Pdx1 into a glucagonoma cell line, which resulted in activation of the insulin gene, as well as other β-cell genes (8). Correct proinsulin processing has been obtained in non-β-cells, by replacing the cleavage sites in proinsulin, which are recognized by the PC2 and PC3 prohormone convertases expressed in β-cells, with sites that can be cleaved by ubiquitously expressed endoproteases, such as furin (9). Alternatively, expression of PC2 and PC3 in non-β-cells has allowed correct processing of native proinsulin (10,11). In addition, a number of neuroendocrine cell types considered for ectopic insulin production naturally express these enzymes.

Ectopic insulin expression, however, has two major drawbacks. The first is the difficulty to reproduce in non-β-cells the highly regulated insulin secretion of the normal β-cell. The mechanisms within the β-cell that couple insulin secretion in response to changes in extracellular levels of glucose and other secretagogues are poorly understood. A large number of β-cell specific proteins, including the glucose transporter isotype GLUT2, the glucose phosphorylating enzyme glucokinase, the ATP-sensitive potassium channel, specialized calcium-binding proteins and Ca^{2+}-channels, and poorly characterized secretory vesicle and plasma membrane components have been identified as components of the β-cell sensing and secretory machinery (12). A second-best alternative to glucose-regulated insulin release could be glucose-regulated insulin gene transcription, by driving ectopic insulin gene expression with regulatory regions of genes that include glucose-response elements (13). However, this regulation is likely to be rather coarse, as the kinetics of feedback loops based on transcriptional changes is much slower than that of the secretory response. Thus, the best that ectopic insulin biosynthesis could hope to achieve is a low, steady state supply of insulin, that will have to be supplemented by exogenous insulin.

The second limit to this approach is the current state of the gene targeting technology *in vivo* (14,15). New and improved viral vectors are being developed, however at present there are no efficient ways for cell-specific gene delivery *in vivo* that will result in lasting gene expression. It is easier to perform the genetic manipulations *in vitro*, on cells explanted from the patient, however this approach is limited to those few cell types that can be expanded in culture and used to repopulate their organs of origin. In addition, the cell numbers required to deliver sufficient amounts of insulin may be relatively large, which could create an imbalance of the natural products of the non-β-cells that are utilized. Genetic modification of autologous cells carries risks of introducing potentially neoplastic mutations into cells that cannot be destroyed by the immune system. These risks can be reduced by using insulin-producing allogeneic non-β-cell lines, in which case cell encapsulation is required to protect the transplanted cells from immune rejection. However, in this scenario β-cell lines are a far superior choice, since their insulin release can be tightly regulated, as described below.

β-CELL TRANSPLANTATION

Given the shortcomings of non-β-cells to provide regulated insulin secretion, the optimal replacement for the endogenous β-cells would consist of an alternative source of β-cells. However, allogeneic pancreas or islet tissue is in short supply. Recent progress in islet encapsulation (16) has facilitated transplantation of xenogeneic islets in animal experimental systems (17-19). Nevertheless, islet xenotransplantation remains immunologically difficult and controversial, mainly because of the risk of introduction of animal pathogens into the human population (20).

An alternative to isolated islets is the development of β-cell lines. Cell lines offer the advantage of an abundant and reproducible cell source, which can be modified by gene transfer *in vitro* to optimize its properties. The use of rodent β-cell lines in diabetic animals has shown that pure β-cells can effectively replace the function of intact islets for long periods of time (21). The hormones produced by islet non-β-cells are also important for glucose homeostasis. However, the pancreas of IDDM patients contains sufficient numbers of α-, δ-, and PP cells to meet the physiological requirements for non-β-cell hormones. Functional regulation among the different islet cell types through cell-to-cell contacts and paracrine effects is apparently less crucial than the endocrine feedback loops for most aspects of glucose homeostasis. Pure β-cells may also prove to be less immunogenic than intact islets, since the latter may contain antigen-presenting cells, such as dendritic cells. This chapter will consider a number of approaches for developing animal and human β-cell lines. An equally challenging aspect of β-cell transplantation is the protection of the transplanted cells from allograft rejection and recurring autoimmunity. Potential approaches to cell engineering with genes that increase cell resistance to immune effector molecules are discussed below.

DEVELOPMENT OF β-CELL LINES

Propagation of mature islet β–cells in culture is difficult. Most of the adult islet cells are post-mitotic. They do not divide either *in vivo* or in culture, and, when explanted from their tissue context, are stressed and tend to senesce and die. Although some growth factors can induce limited replication of foetal or neonatal rodent islets (22), the natural growth and survival factors of β-cells that could enable significant cell mass expansion in culture remain largely unknown. Recent findings on the ability of telomerase overexpression to immortalize human fibroblasts (23) have raised hopes for immortalization of other human cell types. However, the data indicates that fibroblasts may be a special case, and that other human cell types, particularly epithelial cells, may require changes in expression of additional genes to remain in cycle and avoid senescence (24).

Given the low replicative potential of adult islets, research efforts have focused on propagation of islet precursor cells. Recent reports on the propagation of human embryonic stem cell lines (25) may open the way for the generation in tissue culture of various differentiated human cell types for transplantation. The emerging understanding of genes involved in early pancreas development from the gut endoderm in the mouse (26) and chick (27) embryo may provide tools for expansion of cells committed to pancreas or islet development from animal or human foetuses. Foetal islets have been used in attempts to develop human β-cell lines (28,29). The ability of pancreatic duct cells to regenerate islets in the adult pancreas in rodents (30-32) has provoked interest in deriving human ductal cell lines that could potentially be induced to differentiate in culture into β-cells. The major hurdle in these efforts is likely to be the induction and maintenance of β-cell differentiation, as characterized by the amounts of insulin produced and stored in the cells, and its regulated secretion in response to physiological secretagogues. At the present state of our knowledge it appears more feasible, to induce replication in differentiated human or animal β-cells than to induce complete differentiation in β-cell precursors.

To circumvent the difficulty of propagating differentiated β-cells, several groups have employed oncogenes, in particular the SV40 large T antigen (Tag), to derive β-cell lines from transformed adult or foetal islets (21,28,29,33-40). Expression of the

Tag oncoprotein in β-cells bypasses senescence and inactivates the gate-keepers to the entrance into the cell cycle and DNA replication, p53 and the retinoblastoma (Rb) proteins, which act at the checkpoint between the G1 and S phases. Rodent β-cell lines transformed by Tag maintain low levels of insulin production and secretion. However, their secretory response to glucose is often abnormal, and they tend to lose their limited differentiation during propagation in culture (38,39). Apparently, cell transformation interferes with the differentiated functions of β-cells. In addition, the transformed cells replicate without control and are thus not suitable for transplantation. In contrast to the success in deriving rodent β-cell lines, β-cell transformation has been less successful in human islets (28,29). Introduction of the Tag and H-ras oncogenes into foetal human islets resulted in cell growth, however insulin expression was essentially lost.

It is conceivable that β-cell dedifferentiation resulting from cell transformation reflects a mutually exclusive relationship between cell replication and differentiation, as observed in many cell types. Most highly specialized cells must withdraw from the cell cycle to fully manifest their differentiated phenotype. Conversely, when induced to resume replication, the cells must turn off genes related to differentiation to allow expression of the genetic program required for cell replication. Thus, the dedifferentiation observed in replicating β-cells might be reversible upon growth arrest. To test this concept, we have used a conditional gene expression system to reversibly turn on and off Tag expression and cell replication in β-cells in transgenic mice (21). This system is based on the bacterial tetracycline (tet) operon elements, as adapted by Gossen and Bujard for use in mammalian cells (tet-off) (41). Using this system, we were able to tightly and reversibly regulate Tag expression in β-cells by exposing the cells both *in vivo* and *in vitro* to tet and its derivatives. The transformed β-cells were completely dependent on the continuous expression of Tag for their proliferation, and suppression of Tag expression induced growth arrest. This finding is key to the approach, since one can expect cell transformation to activate endogenous genes that could allow cell replication independent of Tag expression (42).

The effects of growth arrest on the transformed β-cell viability and function were studied in detail in one cell line, denoted βTC-tet (21,43). Both proliferating and growth-arrested cells produced high amounts of insulin and secreted it in response to physiological glucose concentrations. However, the insulin content of growth arrested cells was three- to five-fold higher, compared with proliferating cells. The phenotype of the proliferating cells was stable for over 60 passages in culture. Eventually, the cells developed an abnormal secretory response to subphysiological glucose levels that was associated with upregulation of hexokinase expression, as has been observed in other β-cell lines. This phenomenon may be related to the increased energy consumption of transformed cells, for which the higher metabolic capacity of hexokinase at low glucose levels may provide a selective advantage. Abnormal overexpression of hexokinase represents a significant impediment to the use of transformed β-cell lines in cell therapy. However, unlike other β-cell lines, in βTC-tet cells this abnormality can essentially be corrected by growth arrest, which induces a downregulation of the elevated hexokinase activity close to the normal range, supporting the correlation between elevated hexokinase activity and β-cell proliferation. The major advantage of this system is the ability to control cell number following transplantation. The βTC-tet cells were able to restore euglycaemia in syngeneic streptozotocin (STZ)-diabetic mice (21). Treatment of the mice with tet prevented abnormal cell expansion, and the cells remained fully functional *in vivo* for months in the growth-arrested state. They were capable of resuming replication if the tet block was removed. Insulin secretion *in vivo* was regulated by hyperglycaemia in hyperglycaemic clamp studies (43).

These results demonstrate that reversible transformation is a promising approach for growing large numbers of β-cells in culture, while providing a tight control of cell replication and improved cell function following transplantation *in vivo*. Conditional transformation of cultured human islets, with the hope that these cells, unlike constitutively transformed human β-cells may manifest enhanced differentiation when induced to undergo growth arrest, is a next step in β-cell engineering. Recent development of lentivirus vectors allows infection of non-replicating cells with high efficiency, and stable integration of the introduced genes into the infected cells (44). Other approaches for regulation of oncogene expression, such as the tet-on system (45), may be required, to avoid the need for continuous ligand administration *in vivo* to maintain growth arrest. Nonetheless, the road is open for the development of conditionally transformed human β-cell lines. The concerns about using transformed cells in humans may be addressed by cell encapsulation, by designing ways to eliminate the oncogenes from the cells using the Cre-loxP DNA recombination approach (46), and by introduction of suicide mechanisms into the engineered cells, such as the herpes simplex thymidine kinase gene, which will allow cell elimination in case of escape from the encapsulation device.

ENGINEERING β-CELLS FOR PROTECTION FROM IMMUNE DESTRUCTION

The development of immunoisolation techniques allows transplantation of allograft and xenograft cells without immunosuppression (16-18). Encapsulation devices can protect the cells from damaging cell-to-cell contacts with immune effector cells and from large proteins such as antibodies and complement. However, encapsulated β-cells may be exposed to recurring autoimmunity mediated by agents that can pass through the pores of encapsulation device membranes. These pores, that should be large enough to allow the passage of nutrients and insulin, cannot exclude small immune effector molecules released by inflammatory cells outside the encapsulation device. These may include cytokines and free radicals, which could compromise the long-term survival of encapsulated β-cells by induction of apoptotic β-cell death. Engineering β-cell lines with genes that will increase the resistance of the encapsulated cells to apoptosis is likely to improve their function and survival within the capsule. In addition, encapsulated cells could be engineered to release small immunosuppressive molecules that will pass through the membrane pores and inhibit immune effector cells in the vicinity of the encapsulation device.

Cytokine-induced β-cell apoptosis is mediated through elevated expression of nitric oxide synthase (iNOS) and an intracellular increase in nitric oxide (NO) free radicals (47-49). β-cells express normally very low levels of enzymes capable of inactivating free radicals, which renders them highly susceptible to their damage (50). By increasing the activity of such enzymes in β-cells, cell survival may be improved. Overexpression of the radical scavenging enzyme copper/zinc superoxide dismutase (SOD) in β-cells in transgenic mice enhanced their resistance to oxidative stress induced by administration of alloxan and STZ (51). In a more recent study, overexpression of the manganese SOD (MnSOD) gene in INS-1 cells resulted in reduction in IL-1β-induced iNOS and NO levels and provided protection against cell death induced by the cytokine (52). It remains to be shown whether SOD overexpression in β-cells has any deleterious effects on insulin production and regulated secretion. In a similar study using catalase, overexpression of this enzyme in islets and in a β-cell line conferred resistance to oxidative agents (53). Catalase overexpression in human islets preserved the normal insulin secretion in the presence of the oxidative stress. Another antioxidative protein, thioredoxin, has been overexpressed in β-cells of non-obese diabetic (NOD) mice, a well-studied animal model of autoimmune diabetes. Thioredoxin expression lead to a significant reduction in the incidence of diabetes, without affecting the development of insulitis, and without altering the normal insulin secretion of the transgenic islets (54). The transgenic mice were also resistant to the oxidative effects of STZ.

Oxidative agents induce apoptosis in β-cells. This cascade of biochemical events results in the activation of proteases and nucleases that cause DNA fragmentation and organelle condensation (55,56). A major role in both the initiator and effector stages of this process is played by a family of cysteine proteases termed caspases. Activation of some of the caspases is modulated by the bcl-2 family of proteins, which in mammals includes over 15 members. Bcl-2 and bcl-X_L are suppressors of apoptosis, while Bax, Bad, and Bid promote it (57). Overexpression of bcl-2 in mouse insulinoma cell lines (βTC) has been shown to confer partial resistance to cytokine-induced apoptosis in tissue culture (58,59). Bcl-2 overexpression does not seem to affect β-cell function.

Another group of antiapoptotic genes that showed promise in prevention of autoimmune diabetes is the adenovirus early 3 (E3) genes. These genes encode several proteins that downregulate class I MHC-mediated antigen presentation on cell surface and provide protection from apoptosis (60). Induction of apoptosis is an antiviral strategy of the infected organism. The E3 genes, like other viral immunomodulatory and antiapoptotic genes, evolved to protect virus-infected cells and permit virus propagation. Expression of the E3 genes in β-cells in transgenic mice, denoted RIP-E3, allowed transplantation of islets from these mice into allogeneic strains without significant rejection (61). By crossing the RIP-E3 mice into a mouse model of autoimmune diabetes, the RIP-LCMV mice, the E3 genes were shown to provide protection from the autoimmune destruction of β-cells (62). The RIP-LCMV mice express antigens of the lymphocytic choriomeningitis virus (LCMV) in β-cells. Following infection with LCMV they develop autoimmunity to their β-cells, resulting in islet destruction similar to that of IDDM (63). Expression of the E3 genes in the double transgenic mice effectively prevented the islet damage.

Encapsulated β-cells that are exposed to cytokines may fight back with the same weapon, by secreting cytokines that can inhibit the inflammatory reactions. The balance between effector and suppressor T cells is thought to be modulated by a complex array of cytokines in a way that remains poorly understood. Expression of certain cytokines in β-cells may shift the local balance between these subsets of T lymphocytes towards a suppressive phenotype. The candidate molecules that can be considered should be small enough to pass through the pores of encapsulation membranes, such as interleukin (IL)-4, IL-10, and transforming growth factor β1 (TGF-β1). In naked islet transplants, larger secreted molecules with immunosuppressive potential, such as CTLA4-Ig (a fusion protein between cytotoxic T lymphocyte-associated antigen 4 with the immunoglobulin Fc region, which can block co-stimulation of T cells), can be used (64,65).

Expression of IL-4 in β-cells of NOD mice prevented autoimmune diabetes (66). More recently, islets from NOD/severe-combined immunodeficiency (SCID) mice were transduced with lentivirus vector encoding IL-4 (67). When transplanted into syngeneic hosts together with NOD splenocytes, both the transplant and endogenous islets were protected from immune destruction.

Paracrine protection of β-cells was obtained by expression of TGF-β1 in islet α-cells in NOD mice, which prevented the development of spontaneous and cyclophosphamide-induced diabetes (68). In contrast, expression of TGF-β1 in β-cells failed to inhibit autoimmunity in the RIP-LCMV model (69). Expression of another cytokine, IL-10, also lead to conflicting results (70), causing both a delay in the onset and a reduction in the incidence of diabetes when administered into adult NOD mice, and an accelerated disease when transgenically expressed in β-cells, reflecting perhaps differences between local and systemic effects. Mammalian IL-10 has apparently both immunosuppressive and immunostimulatory properties. A viral homologue of IL-10 (vIL- 10) encoded by the Epstein-Barr virus (71) lacks the immunostimulatory capacity and may be more promising in induction of T-cell suppression (72). Nonetheless, these results suggest that more work is needed to elucidate the complex cytokine effects, before they can be safely and effectively manipulated to achieve local immunosuppression.

CONCLUSION

Conditional transformation of murine β-cells has provided an abundant supply of highly differentiated cells with tightly regulated growth properties. Immunoisolation, combined with cell engineering with immunomodulatory genes and with genes that provide resistance to cytokine-induced damage, may allow transplantation of such cells into IDDM patients. Efforts to apply similar approaches to the generation of a human β-cell line have been unsuccessful so far, however this remains a desirable goal in the development of cell therapy for IDDM. At present, many parameters of β-cell xenotransplantation remain to be investigated. In general, xenografts are rejected much more vigorously than allografts, however in a host primed to destroy human β-cells, xenogeneic β-cells could be less susceptible to recurring autoimmunity. In addition, transformed xenogeneic β-cells transplanted in immunoisolation devices should be more readily destroyed by the immune system in case of cell escape from a failing device, compared with allogeneic cells. On the other hand, human β-cells are likely to be more compatible with the human physiological environment, compared with most animal β-cells, and human insulin may be more effective in humans and perhaps less immunogenic than most animal insulins. Nonetheless, non-human insulins, such as porcine, have been successfully used in humans. In addition, IDDM patients often develop antibodies to human insulin; therefore, a non-human insulin should not be necessarily more immunogenic. If needed, xenogeneic β-cells can be engineered to produce human insulin. Beyond these considerations of immunogenicity and efficacy, xenografts have raised safety concerns, chief among which is the introduction of unknown animal pathogens into the human population. Another concern is that immunogenic peptides shed by xenografts may elicit immune responses, which could result in cross-reactivity to host proteins. Despite these reservations, in the absence of human β-cell lines, the potential of xenograft β-cell lines in IDDM therapy is worth pursuing.

Some of the immunomodulatory and antiapoptotic genes used to engineer β-cells for transplantation may also be useful in prevention of IDDM, if targeted by viral vectors to islets in people at risk of developing the disease. This prospect will require further advancements in genetic and serological screening for pre-diabetes, as well as the development of safe and efficient ways for gene targeting and sustained expression in islets *in vivo*.

ACKNOWLEDGEMENTS

My work has been supported by the Juvenile Diabetes Foundation International, the National Institute for Diabetes and Digestive and Kidney Diseases, by a Career Scientist Award from the Irma T. Hirschl Foundation, and by the Israel Science Foundation.

REFERENCES

1. Valera A, Fillat C, Costa C et al. Regulated expression of human insulin in the liver of transgenic mice corrects diabetic alterations. FASEB J 1994;8:440-447.
2. Kolodka TM, Finegold M, Moss L, Woo SL. Gene therapy for diabetes mellitus in rats by hepatic expression of insulin. Proc Natl Acad Sci USA 1995;92:3293-3297.
3. Lipes MA, Cooper EM, Skelly R et al. Insulin-secreting non-islet cells are resistant to autoimmune destruction. Proc Natl Acad Sci USA 1996;93:8595-8600.
4. Goldfine ID, German MS, Tseng HC et al. The endocrine secretion of human insulin and growth hormone by exocrine glands of the gastrointestinal tract. Nat Biotechnol 1997;15:1378-1382.
5. Moore H-P, Walker MD, Lee F, Kelly RB. Expressing a human insulin cDNA in a mouse ACTH-secreting cell: intracellular storage, proteolytic processing, and secretionon stimulation. Cell 1983;35:531-538.
6. Vollenweider F, Irminger JC, Gross DJ, Villa-Komaroff L, Halban PA. Processing of proinsulin by transfected hepatoma (FAO) cells. J Biol Chem 1992;267:14629-14636.
7. Simpson AM, Tuch BE, Swan MA, Tu J, Marshall GM. Functional expression of the human insulin gene in a human hepatoma cell line (HEP G2). Gene Therapy 1995;2:223-231.
8. Serup P, Jensen J, Andersen FG et al. Induction of insulin and IAPP production in pancreatic islet glucagonoma cells by insulin promoter factor 1. Proc Natl Acad Sci USA 1996;93:9015-9020.
9. Groskreutz DJ, Sliwkowski MX, Gorman CM. Genetically engineered proinsulin constitutively processed and secreted as mature, active insulin. J Biol Chem 1994;269:6241-6245.
10. Vollenweider F, Kaufmann J, Irminger J-C, Halban PA. Processing of proinsulin by furin, PC2, and PC3 in (co)transfected COS (monkey kidney) cells. Diabetes 1995;44:1075-1080.
11. Kaufmann JE, Irminger J-C, Mungall J, Halban PA. Proinsulin conversion in GH3 cells after coexpression of human proinsulin with the endoproteases PC2 and/or PC3. Diabetes 1997;46:978-982.
12. Efrat S, Tal M, Lodish HF. The pancreatic β-cell glucose sensor. Trends in Biochem Sci 1994;19:535-538.
13. Vaulont S, Kahn A. Transcriptional control of metabolic regulation genes by carbohydrates. FASEB J 1994;8:28-35.
14. Crystal RG. Transfer of genes to humans: Early lessons and obstacles to success. Science 1995;270:404-410.
15. Anderson WF. Human gene therapy. Nature 1998;392 (6679 suppl.):25-30.
16. Lanza RP, Chick WL. Transplantation of pancreatic islets. Ann NY Acad Sci 1997;831:321-331.
17. Sullivan SJ, Maki T, Borland KM et al. Biohybrid artificial pancreas: long-term implantation studies in diabetic, pancreatectomized dogs. Science 1991;252:718-721.
18. Lacy PE, Hegre OD, Gerasimidi-Vazeou A, Gentile FT, Dionne KE. Maintenance of normoglycaemia in diabetic mice by subcutaneous xenografts of encapsulated islets. Science 1991;254:1782-1784.
19. Sun Y, Ma MX, Zhou D, Vacek I, Sun AM. Normalization of diabetes in spontaneously diabetic cynomolgus monkeys by xenografts of microencapsulated porcine islets without immunosuppression. J Clin Invest 1996;98:1417-1422.
20. Bach FH, Fishman JA, Daniels N et al. Uncertainty in xenotransplantation: individual benefit versus collective risk. Nature Med 1998;4:141-144.
21. Efrat S, Fusco-DeMane D, Lemberg H, Emran OA, Wang S. Conditional transformation of a pancreatic β-cell line derived from transgenic mice expressing a tetracycline-regulated oncogene. Proc Natl Acad Sci USA 1995;92:3576-3580.
22. Hellerstrom C, Swenne I. Functional maturation and proliferation of foetal pancreatic β-cells. Diabetes 1991;40 (Suppl.2):89-93.
23. Bodnar AG, Ouellette M, Frolkis M et al. Extension of life-span by introduction of telomerase into normal human cells. Science 1998;279:349-352.

24. Kiyono T, Foster SA, Koop JI, McDougall JK, Galloway DA, Klingelhutz AJ. Both Rb/p16INK4a inactivation and telomerase activity are required to immortalize human epithelial cells. Nature 1998;396:84-88.
25. Thomson JA, Itskovitz-Eldor J, Shapiro SS et al. Embryonic stem cell lines derived from human blastocysts. Science 1998;282:1145-1147.
26. Edlund H. Transcribing pancreas. Diabetes 1998;47:1817-1823.
27. Kim SK, Melton DA. Pancreas development is promoted by cyclopamine, a Hedgehog signaling inhibitor. Proc Natl Acad Sci USA 1998;95:13036-13041.
28. Levine F, Wang S, Beattie G et al. Development of a cell line from the human foetal pancreas. Transplant Proc 1995;27:3410.
29. Wang S, Beattie G, Mally M et al. Isolation and characterization of a cell line from the epithelial cells of the human foetal pancreas. Cell Transplant 1997;6:59-67.
30. Bonner-Weir S, Baxter LA, Schuppin GT, Smith FE. A second pathway for regeneration of adult exocrine and endocrine pancreas: a possible recapitulation of embryonic development. Diabetes 1993;42:1717-1720.
31. Wang RN, Kloppel G, Bouwens L. Duct-to islet-cell differentiation and islet growth in the pancreas of duct-ligated adult rats. Diabetologia 1995;38:1405-1411.
32. Gu D, Sarvetnick N. Epithelial cell proliferation and islet neogenesis in IFN-α transgenic mice. Development 1993;118:33-46.
33. Santerre RF, Cook RA, Crisel RMD et al. Insulin synthesis in a clonal cell line of simian virus 40-transformed hamster pancreatic beta cells. Proc Natl Acad Sci USA 1981;78:4339-4342.
34. Efrat S, Linde S, Kofod H et al. β-cell lines derived from transgenic mice expressing hybrid insulin-oncogenes. Proc Natl Acad Sci USA 1988;85:9037-9041.
35. Miyazaki J-I, Araki K, Yamato E et al. Establishment of a pancreatic β–cell line that retains glucose-inducible insulin secretion: special reference to expression of glucose transporter isoforms. Endocrinology 1990;127:126-132.
36. Hamaguchi K, Gaskins HR, Leiter EH. NIT-1, a pancreatic β-cell line established from a transgenic NOD/Lt mouse. Diabetes 1991;40:842-849.
37. Radvanyi F, Christgau S, Baekkeskov S, Jolicoeur C, Hanahan D. Pancreatic β–cells cultured from individual preneoplastic foci in a multistage tumorigenesis pathway: a potentially general technique for isolating physiologically representative cell lines. Mol Cell Biol 1993;13:4223-4232.
38. Efrat S, Leiser M, Surana M et al. Murine insulinoma cell line with normal glucose-regulated insulin secretion. Diabetes 1993;42:901-907.
39. Knaack D, Fiore DM, Surana M et al. Clonal insulinoma cell line which stably maintains correct glucose responsiveness. Diabetes 1994;43:1413-1417.
40. Soldevila G, Buscema M, Marini V et al. Transfection with SV40 gene of human pancreatic endocrine cells. J Autoimmun 1991;4:381-396.
41. Gossen M, Bujard H. Tight control of gene expression in mammalian cells by tetracycline-responsive promoters. Proc Natl Acad Sci USA 1992;89:5547-5551.
42. Ewald D, Li M, Efrat S et al. Time-sensitive reversal of hyperplasia in transgenic mice expressing SV40 T antigen. Science 1996;273:1384-1386.
43. Fleischer N, Chen C, Surana M et al. Functional analysis of a conditionally-transformed pancreatic β-cell line. Diabetes 1998;47:1419-1425.
44. Naldini L, Blomer U, Gage FH, Trono D, Verma IM. Efficient transfer, integration, and sustained long-term expression of the transgene in adult rat brains injected with a lentivirus vector. Proc Natl Acad Sci USA 1996;93:11382-11388.
45. Gossen M, Freundlieb S, Bender G, Muller G, Hillen W, Bujard H. Transcriptional activation by tetracyclines in mammalian cells. Science 1995;268:1766-1769.
46. Sauer B, Henderson N. Cre-stimulated recombination at loxP-containing DNA sequences placed into the mammalian genome. Nuc Acids Res 1989;17:147-161.
47. Welsh N, Eizirik DL, Bendtzen K, Sandler S. Interleukin-1β-induced nitric oxide production in isolated rat pancreatic islets requires gene transcription and may lead to inhibition of the Krebs cycle enzyme aconitase. Endocrinology 1991;129:3167-3173.
48. Eizirik DL, Cagliero E, Bjorklund A, Welsh N. Interleukin-1β induces the expression of an isoform of nitric oxide synthase in insulin-producing cells, which is similar to that observed in activated macrophages. FEBS Lett 1992;308:249-252.
49. Mauricio D, Mandrup-Poulsen T. Apoptosis and the pathogenesis of IDDM. A question of life and death. Diabetes 1998;47:1537-1543.
50. Lenzen S, Drinkgern J, Tiedge M. Low antioxidant enzyme gene expression in pancreatic islets compared with various other mouse tissues. Free Radical Biol Med 1995;20:463-466.
51. Kubisch HM, Wang J, Luche R et al. Transgenic copper/zinc superoxide dismutase modulates susceptibility to type I diabetes. Proc Natl Acad Sci USA 1994;91:9956-9959.
52. Hohmeier HE, Thigpen A, Tran VV, Davis R, Newgard CB. Stable expression of manganese superoxide dismutase (MnSOD) in insulinoma cells prevents IL-1 beta-induced cytotoxicity and reduces nitric oxide production. J Clin Invest 1998;101:1811-1820.

53. Benhamou PY, Moriscot C, Richard MJ et al. Adenovirus-mediated catalase gene transfer reduces oxidant stress in human, porcine, and rat pancreatic islets. Diabetologia 1998;41:1093-1100.
54. Hotta M, Tashiro F, Ikegami H et al. Pancreatic β–cell-specific expression of thioredoxin, an antioxidative and antiapoptotic protein, prevents autoimmune and streptozotocin-induced diabetes. J Exp Med 1998;188:1445-1451.
55. Vaux DL, Strasser A. The molecular biology of apoptosis. Proc Natl Acad Sci USA 1996;93:2239-2244.
56. Raff M. Cell suicide for beginners. Nature 1998;396:119-122.
57. Adams JM, Cory S. The Bcl-2 protein family: arbiters of cell survival. Science 1998;281:1322-1326.
58. Iwahashi H, Hanafusa T, Eguchi Y et al. Cytokine-induced apoptotic cell death in a mouse pancreatic β-cell line: inhibition by bcl-2. Diabetologia 1996;39:530-536.
59. Liu Y, Rabinovitch A, Suarez-Pinzon W et al. Expression of the bcl-2 gene from a defective HSV-1 amplicon vector protects pancreatic β-cells from apoptosis. Human Gene Therapy 1996;7:1719-1726.
60. Wold WSM, Gooding LR. Region E3 of adenovirus: a cassette of genes involved in host immunosurveillance and virus-cell interactions. Virology 1991;184:1-8.
61. Efrat S, Fejer G, Brownlee M, Horwitz MS. Prolonged survival of murine pancreatic islet allografts mediated by adenovirus early region 3 immunoregulatory transgenes. Proc Natl Acad Sci USA 1995;92:6947-6951.
62. von Herrath MG, Efrat S, Oldstone MBA, Horwitz MS. Expression of adenoviral E3 transgenes in β-cells prevents autoimmune diabetes. Proc Natl Acad Sci USA 1997;94:9808-9813.
63. Oldstone MBA, Nerenberg M, Southern P, Price J, Lewicki H. Virus infection triggers insulin-dependent diabetes mellitus in a transgenic model: Role of anti-self (virus) immune response. Cell 1991;65:319-331.
64. Lenschow DJ, Zeng Y, Thistlethwaite JR et al. Long-term survival of xenogeneic pancreatic islet grafts induced by CTLA4Ig. Science 1992;257:789-792.
65. Weber CJ, Hagler MK, Chryssochoos JT et al. CTLA4-Ig prolongs survival of microencapsulated neonatal porcine islet xenografts in diabetic NOD mice. Cell Transplant 1997;6:505-508.
66. Mueller R, Krahl R, Sarvetnick N. Pancreatic expression of interleukin-4 abrogates insulitis and autoimmune diabetes in nonobese diabetic (NOD) mice. J Exp Med 1996;184:1093-1099.
67. Gallichman WS, Kafri T, Krahl T, Verma IM, Sarvetnick N. Lentivirus-mediated transduction of islet grafts with interleukin 4 results in sustained gene expression and protection from insulitis. Hum Gene Ther 1998;9:2717-2726.
68. Moritani M, Yoshimoto K, Wong SF et al. Abrogation of autoimmune diabetes in nonobese diabetic mice and protection against effector lymphocytes by transgenic TGF-β. J Clin Invest 1998;102:499-506.
69. Lee M-S, Stephen S, Arnush M et al. Transforming growth factor-β fails to inhibit allograft rejection or virus-induced autoimmune diabetes in transgenic mice. Transplantation 1996;61:1112-1113.
70. Balasa B, Sarvetnick N. The paradoxical effects of interleukin 10 in the immunoregulation of autoimmune diabetes. J Autoimmun 1996;9:283-286.
71. Moore KW, Vieira P, Fiorentino DF, Trounstine ML, Khan TQ, Mosmann TR. Homology of cytokine synthesis inhibitory factor (IL-10) tto the Epstein-Barr virus gen BCRFI. Science 1990;248:1230-1234.
72. Suzuki T, Tahara H, Narula S, Moore KW, Robbins PD, Lotze MT. Viral interleukin 10 (IL-10), the human herpes virus 4 cellular IL-10 homologue, induces local anergy to allogeneic and syngeneic tumors. J Exp Med 1995;182:477-486.

23

GENE THERAPEUTIC APPROACHES FOR β-CELL REPLACEMENT

Alberto Hayek, M.D., Gillian M. Beattie, Ph.D., and Fred Levine, M.D.

University of California at San Diego School of Medicine, La Jolla, CA 92037 USA

INTRODUCTION

In this chapter, special emphasis is placed on human cells as potential cell-based insulin delivery systems in type 1 diabetes. At this time, the only viable alternative for cell therapy in diabetes is the use of isolated human islets, either fresh or cryopreserved, as is utilized in clinical transplantation protocols. A recent review of islet transplantation for patients with type 1 diabetes concluded that although there are some important reasons for optimism, the treatment remains experimental (1) and the current outcome of the procedure is quite negative. Of a total of 305 patients receiving islet transplants between 1974 and 1996, only 10% of recipients were insulin-free at one year and of those, only one patient remained insulin-independent for more than five years. Of the many obstacles to successful islet transplantation, two remain of paramount importance: islet destruction by immune processes (either allo- or autoimmune), and the shortage of tissue for islet isolation. As more islet transplantation centers are being developed, the scarcity of tissue will become more acute, and the need for innovative methods to increase existing cell supplies will become more relevant. Thus, in this chapter we will focus on efforts to develop cell-based strategies to obtain physiologic insulin replacement.

CELL-BASED DIABETES THERAPY

Many different cell types have been studied for possible use in cell-based diabetes therapy including β-cells, non-β-cells, and primary cells versus cell lines. The cells could potentially come from the diabetic patient (which for type 1 diabetics would require the use of autologous non-β-cells), allografted cells from other human beings, or xenogeneic cells from a different species such as pigs. The use of β-cells from humans requires the ability to expand the limited amount of available tissue *in vitro* in sufficient quantities for treatment of a large number of patients.

Cell candidates for transplantation therapies for diabetes

β-cells are the only cell type in the body able to sense glucose within a limited threshold and to respond with a well-defined insulin release mechanism. Therefore, β-cells represent a first-line choice for cell transplantation in diabetes.

Human islets

The use of primary human islets is a logical approach to cell transplantation therapies for diabetes. Recurrent immune response towards β-cells may be more of a problem with allografted β-cells than with allografted non-β-cells or with xenografts (2). Additionally, like xenografts, successful allografts require long-term immunosuppression. Thus, islet and pancreas transplants are most often performed in the context of simultaneous kidney transplants, i.e. in patients who will be immunosuppressed anyway (10). To reduce or eliminate the need for systemic immunosuppression, much effort has been devoted to developing immunoisolation devices that separate the transplanted allogeneic and xenogeneic cells from the graft recipient's immune response (3,11-13,16,17). Apart from the problem of allograft rejection, the major problem with the use of human β-cells for diabetes treatment is the insufficient supply of primary human islets. This problem could potentially be overcome with strategies to expand the number of primary cells *in vitro*.

Xenogeneic islets

The species that has been most studied as a replacement for human β-cells is the pig (3-5). Porcine β-cells function in a manner very similar to those of humans and are available in potentially unlimited quantities. A major problem with the use of porcine islets for cell transplantation therapies is the need to overcome the xenograft immune barrier. Concerns have been raised about the potential risk of infection with previously unrecognized viruses following transplantation of xenogeneic cells into humans (6). Although most of the debate has revolved around previously unrecognized exogenous viruses, endogenous viruses such as the porcine retrovirus that can infect human cells may also be a significant problem (7). Even human cell lines might carry some risk in this regard since endogenous retroviruses and retrotransposons exist in humans (8) and retrotransposition events have been shown in some cases (9).

EXPANSION OF PRIMARY HUMAN β-CELLS

Pancreatic endocrine cells have a low mitotic index compared to endocrine precursors that divide actively. This characteristic has been one of the driving forces behind the use of foetal tissue for islet transplantation. In mature animals, islet cell regeneration can be induced by disruption of the pancreas by inflammation involving cytokine production (18), mechanical damage (19), or growth factors (20). However, actively dividing primary cells have not been shown to function as mature endocrine cells. A number of growth factors are present in the human pancreas, including TGF-α and IGF-II (21). Moreover, a substantial number of protein tyrosine kinase growth factor receptors have been found to be expressed in pancreatic endocrine cells (22). Unfortunately, it is difficult to determine which of the many growth factors and growth factor receptors that are found in the endocrine pancreas are active *in vivo* as β-cell growth factors.

Prolactin stimulates cell division in the endocrine pancreas (23,24). Reg protein, also known as pancreatic stone protein, is expressed at high levels in regenerating islets and induces replication in rat and hamster β-cells (25,26) but this has not yet been shown with human islets (27). Betacellulin is a member of the EGF family of growth factors that was isolated from a rodent insulinoma cell line (28). In some systems, it plays a role in endocrine cell development, but this remains controversial

(28,29). Perhaps the best candidate for a physiologic regulator of pancreatic β-cell growth is hepatocyte growth factor/scatter factor (HGF/SF). The HGF/SF receptor, c-met, is present on the surface of human pancreatic epithelial cells, and is more highly expressed on developing and mature β-cells (30). It is possible that once the factors that govern β-cell growth and regeneration from the ductal epithelium are understood, β-cell expansion could be induced by expression of the appropriate growth and differentiation factors.

SOURCES OF HUMAN CELLS FOR EXPANSION

Stem Cells

Two recent independent reports have recently described methods to isolate pluripotent stem cells from cultured human primordial germs cells (31) or from human blastocysts (32). The isolated cells contained markers of stem cells such as alkaline phosphatase, and several immunological markers characteristic of embryonic stem cells. The cells are able to continually proliferate with a stable and normal karyotype. Stem cells have already been shown to generate differentiated cells such as neurones, skeletal muscle and vascular endothelial cells *in vitro*. It is conceivable that β-cells could also be created from stem cells, providing that the appropriate combination of growth and differentiating factors is provided.

Foetal pancreatic cells

The regulation of proliferation and differentiation in foetal pancreatic islets is dependent on interactions between cell-cell and cell-matrix contacts and specific growth factors. However, the nature of these interactions is not fully understood, and the relative effects of matrix and growth factors on growth versus differentiation remain unclear. The extracellular matrix (ECM) is a complex of glycoproteins including fibronectin, laminin, heparan, and dermatan sulfate proteoglycans and collagens (33), serving as the scaffolding in tissue organization and migration especially of embryonic cells during development (34). More recently, it has been shown that components of ECM play an important role in tissue-specific gene expression (35). Complex matrices are preferable to simple matrices such as collagen and matrigel (36), and the matrix generated by the rat bladder carcinoma line 804G is preferable to that made by bovine corneal endothelial cells (37). Growth of cells on 804G results in a ten-fold increase in cell number (37) when the foetal cells were expanded in monolayers, but proliferation is associated with marked downregulation of islet-specific gene expression. Cell transplantation experiments performed with this expanded cell mass failed to produce mature endocrine cells, in contrast to the transplantation of unexpanded islet-like cell clusters into nude mice (38). However, following reaggregation of the cell suspension in the presence of nicotinamide (37) new islet formation was documented in all the nude mice receiving the grafts.

In order to determine the relationship between matrix and growth factor effects on growth versus differentiation we have addressed the question of whether it is possible to expand foetal endocrine cells in culture while minimizing the loss of hormone production. Extracellular matrices tested for effects on growth and differentiation are shown in Table 1.

After five days in culture, proliferation was highest in foetal cell monolayers growing on the matrices made by the bladder carcinoma cell lines, 804G, NBT-11 and HTB-9. Addition of HGF/SF augmented the proliferative responses observed on these matrices. However, the thymidine incorporation was significantly higher in cells growing on the matrix made by the human cell line HTB-9 both with and without HGF/SF. Maximal expansion using the same matrix in the presence of HGF/SF reached a 200-fold increase but simultaneous with undetectable levels of cellular insulin.

Cell line	Species	Tumour	Growth stimulation
804G	rat	Bladder carcinoma	+++
NBT-11	rat	Bladder carcinoma	+++
HTB-9	human	Bladder carcinoma	++++
SCC-25	human	Squamous carcinoma	+++
HaCaT	human	Keratinocyte	-
UCLA	human	Lung carcinoma	++
TRM-1	human	Foetal pancreas	-

Table 1. *Source of extracellular matrices*

Bladder carcinomas were chosen because we had previously shown that ICCs grow well as monolayers on the matrix from 804G (37), which is rich in laminin 5 (39). SSC-25 and HACAT have also been shown to secrete laminin or laminin 5 (40,41). UCLA was chosen as an epithelial cell line of human origin and TRM-1 since it comes from the same tissue as the ICCs.

Growth factors secreted by bladder carcinoma cells *in vitro* include ECGF (42), TGF-1 (43), and under certain conditions HGF/SF (44). The lack of effects of neutralizing antibodies to HGF/SF suggest that the proliferative effect of HTB-9 matrix is not because of secretion and storage of HGF/SF in matrix by HTB-9 cells.

Adult islets

Cells of the adult brain and pancreas are terminally differentiated and have been thought not to be able to replicate. We recently reported that adult islets cells, like human foetal pancreatic cells, could be induced to undergo cell division under the combined influence of extracellular matrix and HGF/SF (45). Also, it has been reported that terminally differentiated human brain cells can proliferate. This indicates that other differentiated tissues have the potential to proliferate as well (46).

Culture of human adult islets on HTB-9 matrix without HGF/SF produces a three-fold increase in DNA content with no loss of insulin expression or response to glucose, and a five-fold increase in DNA content with only a 25% loss of insulin expression. Thus, matrices derived from bladder carcinoma cell lines, and especially of human origin, significantly stimulate the proliferation of pancreatic endocrine cells. However, the combined synergistic effects of the matrix and the growth factor on proliferation is counterbalanced by the diminished expression of islet-specific genes (37) and the loss of function as measured in the decreased insulin content and release.

Isolated Adult β-cells

The downregulation of insulin expression upon growth stimulation (37) makes it difficult to definitively identify replicating cells. In addition, further cell expansion is limited because the cultures are invariably overgrown by fibroblasts. Because fibroblasts have a higher replication rate than epithelial cells, they eventually overtake the epithelial cells in long-term cultures. To overcome the problem of fibroblast contamination and resolve the question of whether human β-cells divide *in vitro*, we used two methods of β-cell enrichment: fluorescent activated cell sorting (FACS) and partial dissociation of intact islets to select for the inner cell core that consists primarily of β-cells. Using these techniques, we have been able to determine whether β-cell DNA synthesis that we observed previously could be translated into significant expansion in the number of β-cells.

Although FACS is highly effective in eliminating fibroblast contamination and enriching for β-cells, it has the disadvantage of a low yield and poor viability of sorted cells. To retain the advantages of fibroblast elimination and β-cell enrichment while improving the cell yield, a technique based on partial dissociation of the islets to generate populations of "outer" and "inner" cells was pursued. Using this approach, the "outer" cell population contained 15±5% insulin positive and 68±11% non-β-cells, whereas the "inner" cell population comprised 76±3% insulin positive cells and 22±3% non-β-cells as determined by immunohistochemical analysis. In contrast whole islets contained 56±3% insulin positive cells (Figure 1). These data were validated by comparing insulin contents of the different cell populations by RIA.

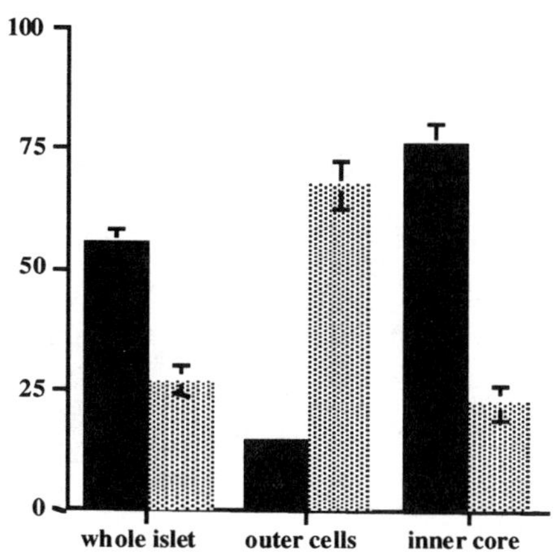

Figure 1. *Immunohistochemical analysis of cells from whole islets, outer cells and inner core. Immunostaining for insulin (solid bars) or for a combination of glucagon, somatostatin and pancreatic polypeptide (open bars) was scored in >300 cells per sample (n=4;*P<0.005). Reprinted with permission from Diabetes, 1999;48:1014.*

Using the replication marker Ki-67, little if any proliferation of these enriched β-cells is detectable before day 5. Immunohistochemical analysis reveals that the majority of the cells contain insulin and Pdx1 (Figure 2A). Glucagon or somatostatin positive cells are rarely observed. There are only isolated CK-19-positive cells, some of which are also positive for insulin. CK-19 positive cells that do not co-express insulin do not stain for Pdx1 either. By day 7 there are modest numbers of proliferating cells, both positive (Figure 2B) and negative for insulin. By day 12 there is a marked increase in proliferating cells. Although there is much heterogeneity between islet cell preparations, in all instances the majority of the proliferating cells contain neither insulin nor CK-19. The cells co-expressing insulin and Ki-67 invariably stain less intensely for insulin than the surrounding non-proliferating β-cells, consistent with previous data showing that insulin is lost in dividing β-cells (37,47). The proliferating cells continue to divide *in vitro* with a doubling time of 24.5 hours (Figure 3). Cells are subcultured approximately weekly at 1:8 dilution through 4-5 passages at which time they experienced growth arrest, becoming large and vacuolated. Thus, allowing for cell loss through passaging, a roughly three-fold doubling in cell number per passage could theoretically result in a 30,000-fold increase in total cell number over five passages or fifteen doublings

Insulin, glucagon and somatostatin transcripts are present as detected by RNase protection assay in the enriched population before culture. Somatostatin disappears after the first passage, and insulin and glucagon message decrease gradually over three passages.

Because insulin is rapidly lost from the expanded cells, it was important to determine whether these cells retain any other β-cell markers. By RT-PCR, the expanded cells at passage 5 expressed a level of Pdx1 that is intermediate between two independent adult preparations of human islets.

Immunohistochemical analysis of replicating cells from passage 3 show that all the cells are epithelial. They are negative for pancreatic hormones, as expected, but stain for Pdx1 (Figure 2C). Parallel staining of expanded ductal cell monolayers derived from isolated ducts are CK-19 positive and Pdx1 negative.

Thus, it is possible to expand human islet cells by 30,000 fold in response to HTB-9 ECM and HGF/SF. In the normal human pancreas, the HGF/SF receptor, c-met, is expressed at high levels only on β-cells (30). Therefore, these are the cells that are most responsive to HGF/SF treatment. Accordingly, the phenotype of the predominant cell type in the expanded cell populations is consistent with an origin from β-cells.

It this is unlikely that these proliferating cells are non-β-cells because the cultures were initiated with cells that had been enriched for β-cells as opposed to duct or other islet cells. Also, the presence of Pdx1 in the expanded cells and its absence in expanded ductal cells makes it unlikely that they are of ductal cell origin.

PANCREATIC ENDOCRINE CELL LINES

Although it is now possible to expand human β-cells 30,000-fold, the lack of sufficient amounts of starting tissue provides a rationale for using transformed β-cell lines as a source of cells for cell transplantation therapies (48-51). Additionally, pancreatic endocrine cell lines have been of critical importance for elucidating the mechanisms that are important for controlling glucose-responsiveness, as well as serving as a source of material for the isolation of pancreas-specific genes (48,52,53).

However, formidable technical problems remain to be overcome before β-cell lines can be used for therapeutic purposes.

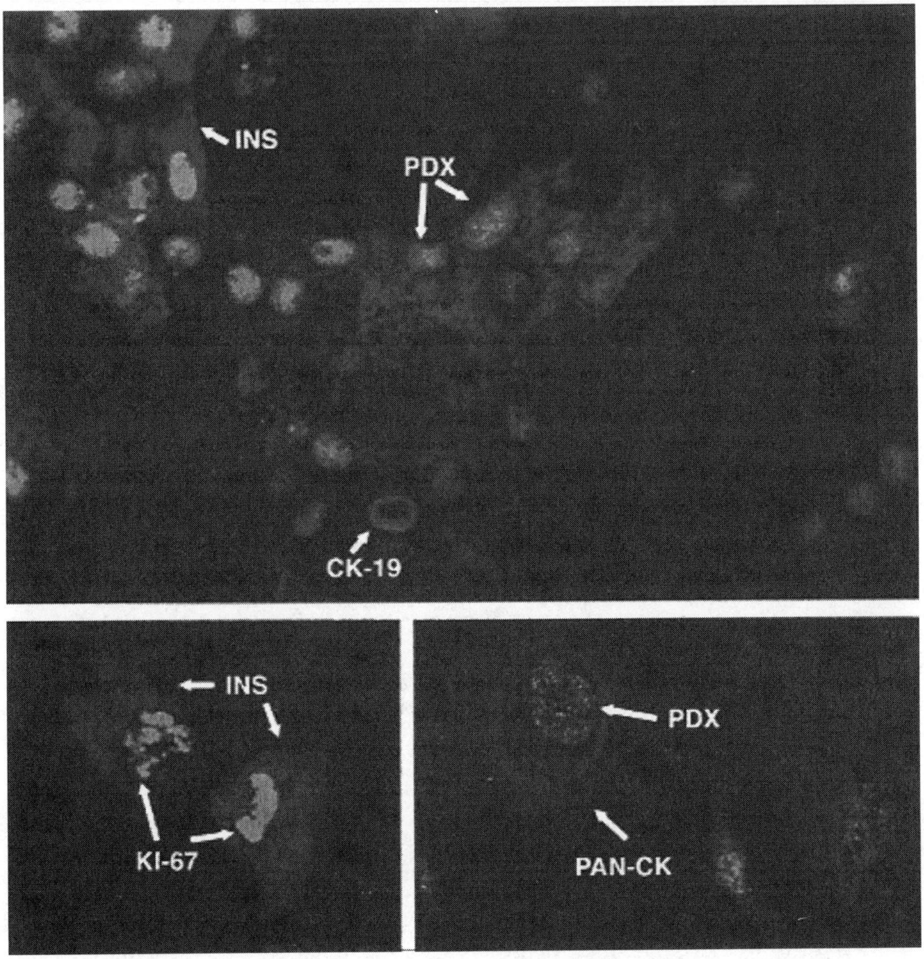

Figure 2. *Confocal microscopic analysis of proliferating islet cells after culture of five days (A), seven days (B) and three passages (C). Cells were triple immunostained for insulin (red A-C), Pdx1 (green A,C), Ki-67 (green B), CK-19 (blue A,B) and Pan-CK (blue C). Reprinted with permission from Diabetes, 1999; 48:1015.*

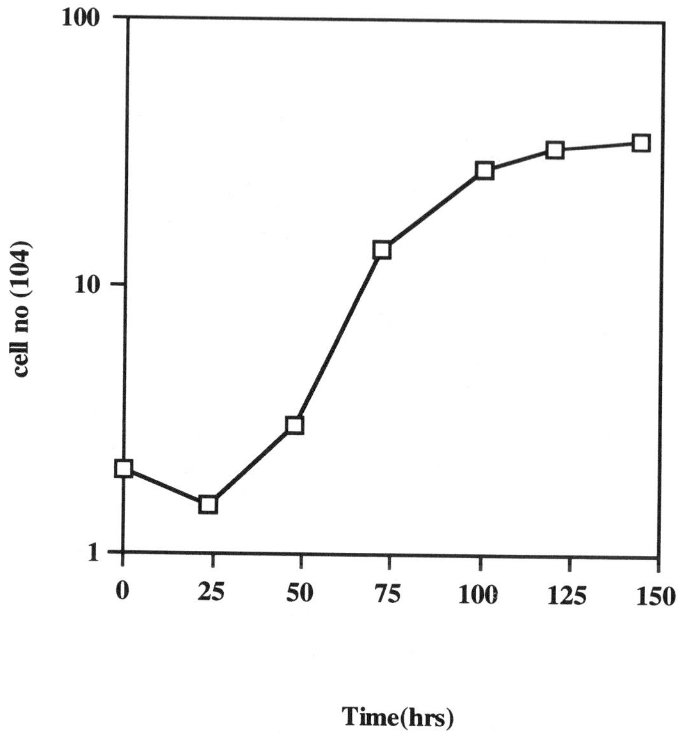

Figure 3. *Replication curve of passage 3 enriched human β-cells. Cell population doubling time was 24.5 hr. during exponential growth phase. Reprinted with permission from Diabetes, 1999; 48:1016.*

Rodent cell lines

Most β-cell lines have been derived from rodents (54). The cell lines have come from a variety of sources: spontaneous insulinomas (55), insulinomas induced by carcinogens (56), insulinomas induced by oncogenic viruses (57), insulinomas induced by a combination of carcinogen treatment and oncogenic viruses (57) and insulinomas from transgenic mice expressing dominant oncogenes, particularly SV40 T antigen under the control of the insulin promoter (58-60). A common feature of all β-cell lines is that formation of the cell line requires multiple genetic events in addition to the initiating event. For example, in the case of rodent β-cell lines expressing SV40 T antigen under the control of the insulin promoter, activation of IGF-II occurs after SV40 T antigen expression (61). Thus, formation of β-cell lines is a multistep process, requiring a substantial (as yet undefined) number of genetic events. These genetic events, while vital for the ability of the cell line to grow *in vivo* and *in vitro*, are largely unknown, and likely contribute to the aberrant regulation of hormone production and secretion that is a feature of all of the cell lines that have been developed to date.

Human cell lines

It is exceedingly difficult to develop human pancreatic endocrine cell lines from spontaneous tumours. With few exceptions (62,63) cell lines from the human pancreas have a pancreatic ductal phenotype (62,64). However, it is not known whether the tumours actually arise from ductal cells or whether malignant transformation of other pancreatic epithelial cell types leads to dedifferentiation to a ductal phenotype. Tumours of human pancreatic endocrine cells are rare, and it is difficult to adapt primary human pancreatic endocrine tumours to *in vitro* culture (65). There is a single report of a cell line from a spontaneous human insulinoma (66). This cell line, designated CM, while expressing some islet antigens is difficult to grow and has lost much differentiated function, including insulin expression. Interestingly, human pancreatic cancers frequently have rare cells that express islet hormones (67,68) perhaps reflecting the origin of all pancreatic epithelial lineages from a common ductal precursor (69).

The first report of an attempt to develop a β-cell line was in 1935, when Murray and Bradley tried to culture human insulinoma cells (70). Despite the fact that human cells were the first target to develop β-cell lines, it has been difficult to establish functional human pancreatic endocrine cell lines (66,71-73).

Spontaneously and carcinogen-induced immortalized endocrine cell lines

A disadvantage of spontaneously or carcinogen-induced immortalized cell lines is the difficulty in determining the genetic events that lead to transformation and/or immortalization. Oncogene expression in many cell types leads to loss of some degree of differentiated function. This has been true for pancreatic endocrine cell lines. Creating cell lines that retain a high degree of differentiated function requires an understanding of the mechanisms by which this loss of differentiated function occurs. Such an understanding can be gained only if the nature of the genetic events that have contributed to cell line formation are understood.

Given the current limitations of our ability to maintain and expand primary islet cells in culture, and the lack of a fully differentiated spontaneous insulinoma cell line, a logical approach is to introduce growth-promoting genes (oncogenes) into β-cells. The advantage of this approach is that it provides a greater degree of control over the starting primary cell from which the cell line is to be derived.

Many different cell lines have been generated by transfer of dominant oncogenes into primary cells (reviewed in reference 74). Such cell lines have been constructed from a variety of different tissues, including brain, liver, bone marrow and pancreas. Because establishment of a cell line is a complex process, requiring multiple genetic alterations, many studies have used simultaneous or sequential introduction of two oncogenes into mammalian cells to achieve transformation or cell line formation (75,76). From these studies, it is clear that certain pairs of oncogenes act synergistically in transforming mammalian cells (77-79). For example, synergy between SV40 T antigen and activated H-ras has been observed (80).

SV40 induced human endocrine cell lines

There are significant differences between the biology of the human pancreas and that of other species. Rodents, for instance, have two copies of the insulin gene as opposed to the single human insulin gene and the duplicated rodent insulin gene exhibits a pattern of regulation that differs in some ways from the ancestral rodent insulin and human insulin genes (81). The response to growth factors such as HGF/SF also differs between species. While HGF/SF has been shown to be a potent mitogen for human β-cells and their precursors (20,45,47), it seems to be relatively inactive on rodent β-cells (82). Because of these biological differences and because of potential advantages of human β-cell lines for cell transplantation therapies, there has been considerable interest in developing human pancreatic β-cell lines.

Soldevila et al. reported a cell line derived from adult human islets that were transfected with an SV40 early region-expressing plasmid with a mutation in the early region promoter that eliminates SV40 T antigen-mediated transcriptional repression (71). Expression of multiple pancreatic hormones was found in early passages, but this rapidly disappeared. Since no selection for transfected cells, e.g., with a dominant selectable marker, was used in this experiment, it is unclear whether the transitory hormone production came from cells expressing the SV40 genes or was derived from primary cells that remained in the culture during early passages.

Because SV40 large T antigen alone is less efficient at transforming human than rodent cells, simultaneous transfer of multiple oncogenes has been used to develop cell lines from the epithelial cells of the human foetal pancreas as well as from adult islets (72,73). The oncogenes used in those studies were SV40 T antigen and H-ras^{val12}, because of the synergism that they exhibit in transforming human cells. These cell lines have some characteristics of endocrine cell precursors and mature endocrine cells, such as low levels of hormone expression, including insulin (72,73,83,84). However, the levels of hormones are low, and in the case of insulin, do not persist with increasing passage number. The reason for the accelerated loss of differentiated function in human pancreatic endocrine cell lines expressing SV40 T antigen plus H-ras^{val12} compared with rodent insulinomas expressing SV40 T antigen may be due to effects of H-ras^{val12} expression on differentiated function. Activated ras expression has been shown to inhibit cellular differentiation by a number of different mechanisms that in general converge to produce deleterious effects on both the ubiquitous and tissue-specific bHLH transcription factors (85,86). A major mechanism by which activated ras inhibits cellular differentiation is through its effects on c-jun. Expression of activated ras results in phosphorylation of c-jun with consequent c-jun activation (87). When activated ras was placed under the control of the insulin promoter in transgenic mice, islet cell destruction was observed in male mice (88,89). In rodent β-cell lines, c-jun acts to decrease insulin expression by inhibiting the ability of the ubiquitous E2A gene products to transactivate the insulin enhancer. H-ras^{val12} expression has also been shown to result in the downregulation of glucagon (90) and GLUT2 expression (91). Thus, there is increasingly strong evidence for an inverse relationship between differentiated function and activated ras expression.

A major difficulty with cell lines from many different cell types is the loss and/or alteration of differentiated function that occurs during their generation. In some cases, oncogene-expressing cell lines retain differentiated functions or the ability to differentiate *in vivo* (92). Unfortunately, in other cases, loss of differentiated function occurs, decreasing the usefulness of the cell line (87). The reason for these differences in cell lines is largely unknown (93,94).

Because they activate different growth promoting pathways in the cell, different oncogenes have widely varying effects on the differentiation state of the cell. For example, expression of the SV40 T antigen, activated ras, or myc oncogenes under the control of the rat elastase I promoter that directs expression to pancreatic acinar cells, results in different tumour types and kinetics of tumour formation (95). Expression of SV40 T antigen in β-cells under control of the insulin promoter results in insulinomas, while expression of activated ras results in β-cell death and diabetes (88,89). In cultured islet cells, the oncogenes src (96,97), myc (97) and ras (97,98) have been shown to stimulate DNA synthesis in β-cells to varying degrees (reviewed in reference 99).

Transformation has been shown to have significant effects on the expression of glucose transporters, with the general finding being downregulation of GLUT2 and upregulation of GLUT1 and GLUT3 (91,100). Many β-cell lines have been found to lose gap junctions, an important feature of normal islets. Expression of connexin 43 in the abnormal cell lines resulted in increased insulin gene expression and insulin content (101). As discussed in more detail below, insulin gene expression may also be downregulated by SV40 T antigen, acting through the transcriptional co-activator p300 (102,103).

In addition to the direct effects of oncogene expression on differentiated β-cell function, a significant problem with rodent and human β-cell lines is that they undergo loss of differentiated characteristics with increasing passage numbers (66,83,84,104,105). This has been a major drawback of cell lines that have been reported to exhibit glucose-responsive-insulin production (48,53,106). In human pancreatic endocrine cell lines, we have observed a progressive loss of insulin expression, even in the presence of nicotinamide, a potent inducer of pancreatic epithelial cell differentiation (83,84).

Growing cells on tissue culture plastic results in selection for growth on that substrate, rather than in the complex milieu that is normally present in the pancreatic islet that has been shown to contribute to the maintenance of proper function in β-cells (30,101,107) and other tissues (108). The most striking example of this phenomenon are cell lines that do not exhibit differentiated functions such as insulin expression and secretion *in vitro*, but do so following grafting *in vivo* (55,109).

Tumour formation with grafted cell lines

A potential problem with grafting partially or fully transformed and/or immortalized cell lines *in vivo* is the risk of tumour formation. Ordinarily, xenografted and allografted tumours are promptly rejected by the immune system. However, allogeneic tumours have been reported to grow in immunocompetent humans in rare cases (113). Protection from immunological rejection is important for transplantation results. Avoiding an immune response can take the form of physically isolating the cells from the immune system by encapsulation (3,4,11-13,15,16) inducing tolerance to the grafted cells (114-118) or modifying the grafted cells so that they are not recognized by the immune system (118-124). In all likelihood, multiple approaches will be required to avoid rejection, but these same approaches, with the exception of physical encapsulation, will make it more likely that a transformed cell line that is grafted will be able to form a tumour.

There are a number of approaches to eliminating the risk of tumour formation. One is to downregulate or eliminate the oncogenes that are used to create the cell line before transplantation. Cell lines that are created by transgenic techniques, or by *in vitro* oncogene transfer can be designed to be amenable to this approach by the use of inducible promoters (72,84,125,126) or by the Cre-loxP recombinase system that can mediate complete deletion of the introduced oncogenes (127,128). The cre recombinase from bacteriophage P1 catalyzes site specific recombination between two 34 bp loxP sequences. When the loxP elements are present in the same orientation, this recombination event results in excision from the genome and deletion of the sequences between the loxP elements (127). This reaction has been shown to work well in mammalian cells for conditional expression of a number of gene products, including SV40 T antigen (129). In particular, it is finding increasing application in transgenic mice for the tissue specific elimination of particular gene products (127).

An additional protection from uncontrolled tumour growth of transplanted cell lines can be accomplished by the use of so-called "suicide genes" that render the cell susceptible to selective elimination by drug treatment (130,131). The best known of these genes is the herpes virus thymidine kinase (TK) gene that makes cells expressing it susceptible to killing with ganciclovir. This method has been used to eliminate grafted Ltk^- cells expressing the human proinsulin gene (132). However, in this study, a problem was encountered with instability of TK expression leading to escape of some ganciclovir-treated cells and consequent tumour formation still remains a problem. Some degree of instability of TK expression may be acceptable because of the so-called "bystander effect", whereby cells neighboring those expressing TK are also killed by ganciclovir. This effect seems to be dependent on the presence of gap junctions between the TK-expressing and non-expressing cells (133,134).

GENE TRANSFER METHODS FOR PRIMARY β-CELLS

The goal of somatic cell therapy is treat human disease using a nucleic acid-based medicine. Effective gene therapy, permanent or transient, is dependent on the capacity to deliver nucleic acids into human cells. In addition, the development of cell lines by *in vitro* approaches, as opposed to making transgenic animals, requires the ability to transfer genes into primary β-cells. Of the different methods to introduce foreign DNA material into cells, (71,97,135,136,142-148), we will focus here, because of their high efficiency rates, on gene transfer with viral vectors.

Adeno-Associated vectors (AAV)

In a recent review, Jindal et al. (149) described the potential use of AAV for gene therapy as well as the general concepts for the construction of these vectors. Adeno-associated viruses are single-stranded DNA-containing human parvoviruses. Advantages of using these viruses as vectors include the fact that most humans have been exposed to the wild-type virus without causing any pathology while producing a stable infection in human cells following site-specific integration into the genome (149). Another advantage is that the virus has not been associated with malignant disease in humans. AAV replication requires co-infection with other viruses, either adenoviruses, herpes virus or vaccinia viruses. Disadvantages to the use of AAV include their small size which limits the size of DNA sequences that can be packaged, the inability to generate large quantities of high-titer vector stocks, and contamination with wild-type adenovirus that, although common, does not appear to be a serious problem for their use. As is the case with most vectors, AAV has been used more *in vitro* than *in vivo*. *In vivo*, the intravenous injection of these vectors in mice localized preferentially to liver (150). The same investigators have studied the efficacy of AAV vectors in rat hematopoietic stem cells transduced with the insulin gene to obtain transient alleviation of streptocotocin (STC) STZ diabetes.

Adenovirus

Adenovirus vectors have been used to transfer genes into pig (151) and rodent pancreatic islet cells *in vivo* (152) and *in vitro* (153). Adenoviruses have the attractive property of being able to infect non-dividing cells, but maintaining long-term gene expression from these vectors is a problem because they do not integrate into the genome (154) and stimulate a potent immune response against viral gene products (155). Adenoviruses require two distinct cell surface molecules to enter the cell. The first, required for initial binding by the adenovirus fiber protein, is as yet unknown. The second is binding by the adenovirus penton base protein to an a_v integrin, resulting in viral internalization (156). Injection of adenoviral vectors into the tail vein *in vivo* results in infection of a high percentage of islet cells (152). However, adenoviral vectors seem to be less efficient at infecting rodent islet cells *in vitro*. The difference could be the highly developed islet vasculature that delivers virus to each islet cell very efficiently (157). A variation on the use of adenoviruses to transfer genes into cells is inactivated adenovirus that is coupled covalently to polylysine, a polycation. Plasmid DNA binds non-covalently to the polylysine and this adenovirus/polylysine/DNA conjugate can then be used to transfer genes into cells (158,159). This method has been used to transfer plasmid DNA into human islets with up to 70% of dispersed human islet cells exhibiting staining for β-galactosidase. (145). However, due to endogenous β-galactosidase activity that can be present in human pancreatic endocrine cells, this number may be an overestimate (38). A drawback of all of the above techniques is that they do not result in integration of the transferred DNA into the host genome. Thus, they will only allow for transient gene expression in most cases. For gene therapy applications where prolonged gene expression is desirable, methods that result in stable integration of transferred DNA into the host genome are likely to be better.

Retroviral Vectors

Retroviral vectors are extremely efficient at infecting a wide variety of cell types, including primary cells from many tissues (160). They have the desirable property of integrating into the host genome, allowing for long-term, stable gene expression. The major drawback of the commonly used murine retroviral vectors is that mitotically active cells are required for the retroviral preintegration complex to enter the nucleus and integrate into the genome (161). Both rodent (162) and human (72,83) pancreatic endocrine cells have been infected with retroviral vectors. Slow transfection efficiency may be related to the low mitotic rate of these cells *in vitro*. Induction of mitosis in human β-cells and their precursors (20,45,47) has increased the efficiency with which retroviral vectors infect pancreatic endocrine cells. Lentiviral vectors such as the human immunodeficiency virus (HIV) are a new generation of retroviral vectors, that can infect both dividing and non-dividing cells, including pancreatic β-cells (163,164). Plasmid expression systems have been used to generate HIV-derived retroviral vectors (165) that have been made replication-defective. Besides initial *in vitro* applications, lentiviruses have successfully delivered genes *in vivo* into terminally differentiated neurons (165,166).

TRANSFER OF GENES TO HUMAN β-CELLS USING VIRAL VECTORS

We have recently studied the factors that influence the infection efficiency of human foetal and adult pancreatic endocrine cells with adenovirus (Ad-GFP), murine retrovirus (MLV-GFP) and lentivirus (Lenti-GFP) vectors all expressing the green fluorescent protein (GFP). Both adenoviral and lentiviral vectors are capable of transferring genes efficiently into insulin-expressing cells. MLV vectors, while inefficient at transferring genes directly into insulin-expressing cells, infect a substantial percentage of cells from both the foetal and adult pancreas (Table 2). Gene transfer to adult islets and foetal ICCs in suspension culture is attractive because it minimizes the extent to which the cells are manipulated, potentially increasing their viability. Infection of foetal ICCs and adult islets by retroviral vectors in suspension is poor, less than 3% of the cells being infected. Ad-GFP is the only viral vector that efficiently infected human islets in suspension, but infection of adult islet cells was only 50%. Adenoviral vectors infect rodent islets cells only in the periphery of the islets (167). β-cells are more abundant in the center of adult islets, therefore, very few β-cells are transduced by adenoviral vector infection of whole islets in suspension (167). It is likely that the geometry of the islet does not allow cells in the inner core of the islet/ICC to be exposed to viral particles. In line with this notion is the finding that human islets in suspension are more efficiently infected by Ad-GFP than foetal ICCs, although the infectivity in monolayer culture was similar.

In contrast to Ad-GFP, infection with MLV-GFP and Lenti-GFP is markedly increased by dispersion of the cells and HGF/SF treatment. Growth factors, including HGF/SF, have been shown to enhance the efficiency of infection of MLV and ecotropic retroviral vectors (168,169). This is considered to be because of effects of the growth factors on the mitotic rate of the target cells.

Both MLV-GFP and Lenti-GFP preferentially infected cells at the periphery of non-dispersed monolayer cultures, whereas transduction of dispersed cells is homogenous. Binding and internalization of virus to cells in single-cell suspension is efficient, but binding/internalization of viral particles is restricted to cells on the periphery of the monolayer cultures. It is conceivable that absence of virus binding/internalization explains the preferential transduction of dispersed cells and of cells in the periphery of the monolayer culture. Although the receptor for VSV-G protein is thought to be a ubiquitously present phospholipid, we have demonstrated previously that the binding of VSV-G pseudotyped retrovirus to human hematopoietic cells can be increased by soluble growth factors (169). Since both MLV and lentivirus vectors are pseudotyped with the VSV-G envelope protein, restriction of VSV-G binding/internalization may explain the pattern of infection observed for both viruses.

The rapid loss of transgene expression after Ad-GFP infection, in contrast to the increase in expression after MLV- and Lenti-GFP infection, demonstrated the importance of using integrating viral vectors in settings where both β-cell growth and prolonged transgene expression are required. With Ad-GFP adult β-cells are infected considerably more efficiently than foetal β-cells. Glucagon positive cells are hardly infected at all in either the foetal or adult pancreas. The explanation for this preferential infection is likely to be differences in the expression of adenovirus receptors on the cell surface of different cells. The difference in the efficiency of infection of adult α- and β-cells within the same tissue preparation indicates that the ability of different viral vectors to infect cells should be determined separately for each cell type. Thus, efficient gene transfer to human endocrine pancreatic cells with different viral vectors is feasible, but it depends on culture conditions and the cell type to be infected.

TRANSFER OF GENES OTHER THAN CLASSIC ONCOGENES

Expression of telomerase in cell lines

All normal cells have a finite capacity for cell division. After a limited lifespan they exit the cell cycle but remain viable in a non-dividing state called replicative senescence. The limiting factor for further cell division is directly related to insufficient telomerase activity and a measurable content of telomeric DNA that decreases as the cell undergoes further cell divisions. Replicative senescence can be bypassed by at least three mechanisms: 1) the activation of telomerase, 2) the activation of oncogenes, and 3) the loss of tumour suppressor function such as RB/p53.

If telomerase were all that is needed for immortalization, it would be practical to consider the expression of the gene in β-cells to prolong cell growth in culture. Expression of the catalytic component human telomerase reverse transcriptase (hTERT) has been accomplished in human fibroblasts and retinal pigment epithelial cells with continuous cell growth for longer than a year (170). However, the addition of hTERT in other cell types is, by itself, capable of inducing immortalization. In keratinocytes and mammary epithelial cells, immortalization requires not only telomerase activity but also inactivation of the Rb/p16 pathway by E7 or downregulation of p16 expression (171). A positive aspect of the immortalized hTERT-expressing fibroblast line is that it maintains a normal karyotype and does not exhibit the characteristic transformed properties of reduced serum requirements, anchorage-independent growth and tumour formation in immune-deficient mice (170). In a more recent example of the heterogeneous response to telomerase introduction to a human cell line, Halvorsen et al. showed that in the pancreatic cell lines TRM-6 and Blox5 it is possible not only to escape replicative senescence, but also a proliferative block *in vitro*, by the induction of telomerase activity alone via retroviral gene transfer (172).

Engineering glucose-responsive insulin secretion

Although it has been possible to develop insulinoma cell lines that express insulin, none of these cell lines exhibit physiologic secretion of insulin in response to glucose. Thus, attempts have been made to introduce the known components of the cellular apparatus involved in this function into both insulinoma cells lines as well as non-pancreatic cell lines. Despite significant progress in delineating the components of the glucose-sensing apparatus, our understanding of it remains incomplete (173-178). Therefore, it has not been possible to completely reconstitute physiologic glucose-responsive insulin secretion in any cell by transferring the genes that are thought to be involved in glucose-responsive insulin secretion.

Table 2a. Infectivity of adult islets and foetal ICCs with adenovirus, MLV and lentiviral vectors Virus (%GFP positive cells)

Tissue	Culture condition	Adenovirus	MLV	Lentivirus
Adult islets	Suspension	53.4 ± 15.5	< 1	2.6 ± 1.2
	Non-dispersed monolayer	90.7 ± 1.1	6.5 ± 0.4	17.2 ± 1.0
	Dispersed monolayer + HGF	ND‡	7.8 ± 0.8	28.1 ± 5.2
	Dispersed monolayer	ND	12.0 ± 0.15 *	39.2 ± 5.9 *
	Dispersed monolayer + HGF	ND	26.1 ± 4.2 *†	65.4 ± 7.2 *†
Foetal ICCs	Suspension	32.2 ± 12.7	< 1	< 1
	Non-dispersed monolayer	97.7 ± 0.5	1.9 ± 1.1	24.5 ± 3.3
	Non-dispersed monolayer + HGF	ND	3.45 ± 0.7	39.0 ± 4.6 !
	Dispersed monolayer	ND	15.2 ± 6.3 *	68.9 ± 10.1 *
	Dispersed monolayer + HGF	ND	33.1 ± 7.2 *†	84.9 ± 4.5 *

**Significant differences between dispersed and non-dispersed cultures; †Significant differences between HGF versus no-HGF treatment. Lenti-GFP infection was significantly higher than MLV-GFP under all conditions (P values <0.05 for non-dispersed cells and <0.01 for dispersed cells. In suspension, adenovirus and retroviruses infection was performed at an MOI of 10^6 CFU/islet and 10^4 CFU/islet, respectively. In monolayer culture, cells were infected at MOI of 20-50. ‡ND- not done. Infection of cultured pancreatic cells with Ad-GFP was very high and in preliminary experiments was not affected by HGF/SF; therefore the effect of cell dispersion on infection efficiency was not studied further. Reprinted with permission from Diabetes, 1999;48: 746.*

Table 2b. Infectivity of adult and foetal endocrine cells in monolayer culture

	% GFP positive β-cells*	% GFP positive α-cells
Adult islets		
Adenovirus	74.3 ± 5.4	1.8 ± 1.7
MLV	0	NA*
Lentivirus	25.7 ± 7.6	NA
Foetal ICCs		
Adenovirus	20.0 ± 6.7	NA
MLV	NA	NA
Lentivirus	NA	NA

**Only cells with bright red staining for insulin were considered positive; NA-not applicable (The number of positive cells was too low for meaningful quantification). Islet preparation from two independent donors, age 18 and 48 year-old were used for the analysis of infection of adult islets. Three foetal pancreases were used for the infection analysis of foetal ICCs. Reprinted with permission from Diabetes, 1999;48:746.*

GLUCOSE RESPONSIVE INSULIN SECRETION IN NON-β-CELLS

COS cells

In 1983, Rutter and co-workers used an SV40 virus vector to express the insulin gene in the CV-1 and COS cell lines that are permissive for SV40 virus replication (179,180). Although considerable amounts of insulin can be produced by this approach, the insulin is secreted in the form of proinsulin and there is no change in insulin secretion in response to changes in the glucose concentration. Since then, this approach has been applied to a wide range of cells in an attempt to find a cell line that would support insulin processing and glucose responsiveness without the need for extensive genetic modification of the cell (48). A disadvantage of cells other than β-cells is that even if it proves to be possible to engineer glucose-responsive insulin secretion into a non β-cell, this may not result in completely normal physiologic function following grafting into a diabetic patient. β-cells secrete hormones other than insulin such as neuropeptide Y and amylin (181) and the role of these substances in maintaining metabolic homeostasis is not completely understood. However, a potential advantage of using cells other than β-cells for cell transplantation therapies is that the autoimmune response to β-cells that exists in individuals with type 1 diabetes may not act against non-β-cells. Thus, transplanted cells would be a simple allograft, much easier to deal with immunologically than cells subject to an additional autoimmune attack. This principle has been demonstrated in transgenic NOD mice expressing the insulin gene in the pituitary under the control of the proopiomelanocortin promoter (182). Overall, despite considerable progress, the complex nature of the machinery involved in β-cell function has thus far precluded the development of a fully functional cell line by transferring or modifying components of the glucose-sensing apparatus.

Fibroblasts

Because of the ease with which they can be obtained, grown in culture, and grafted *in vivo*, fibroblasts have been a popular target for gene transfer studies (183-194). Both fibroblasts (195,196) and fibroblast cell lines (197-200) have been used as a cell type for insulin gene transfer and expression. The major problem with the use of fibroblasts for β-cell replacement strategies is that they do not possess any of the known elements of the glucose-sensing apparatus or regulated secretory pathway, such that insulin secretion is constitutive rather than glucose-responsive.

Most cell types, including fibroblasts, do not express the proinsulin processing enzymes necessary for conversion of proinsulin to insulin. Thus, only proinsulin is secreted by fibroblasts expressing the insulin gene. Although proinsulin does have some degree of insulin receptor binding, this is not adequate to produce normoglycaemia in diabetics. Therefore, animals that have been grafted with insulin-secreting fibroblasts do not achieve prolonged normoglycaemia. This problem can be dealt with by introduction of the prohormone convertase (PC)2 and PC3 endoproteases into the target cells (201-203) or by use of a modified proinsulin molecule that can be processed by the widely expressed endoprotease furin (204). The lack of any components of the complex apparatus involved in glucose responsive insulin secretion has prompted efforts to find cell types that more closely resemble β-cells.

Neuroendocrine cells

Because of the many similarities between β-cells and cells of the neuroendocrine system (205,206) including evidence for insulin gene expression in some neurons

(207), neuroendocrine cells have been proposed as candidates for engineering of glucose-responsive insulin secretion. Like β-cells, they are professional secretory cells that contain both the constitutive and regulated secretory pathways. Many neuroendocrine cell lines express the insulin processing enzymes PC2 and PC3, and thus have the ability to correctly process proinsulin to insulin without further genetic manipulation. Drawbacks of using neuroendocrine cell lines for β-cell replacement strategies include the fact that they already secrete other hormones and lack glucose-sensing.

AtT-20 cells are a mouse anterior pituitary cell line derived by alternate passage of LAF1 mouse pituitary tumour cells as tumours in animals and in cell culture (208,209). Consistent with its pituitary origin, AtT-20 cells produce and secrete considerable amounts of ACTH. Interestingly, AtT-20 cells have been found to express glucokinase (210), which raised the possibility that they might exhibit glucose-responsive secretion. AtT-20 cells also express high levels of PC3 and low levels of PC2 (211,212) suggesting that they might correctly process proinsulin to insulin. Genetically modified AtT-20 cells that secrete insulin (AtT-20ins) have been generated by transfection of the proinsulin gene (213-216). These cells store and secrete correctly processed insulin, but do not exhibit glucose-responsiveness (210,212,216). Although AtT-20 cells express glucokinase, they do not express GLUT2. Following transfer of the GLUT2 gene into AtT-20ins cells, glucose-responsive insulin secretion was observed, but with a maximal release at a subphysiologic glucose concentration of 10 mM (214). Unfortunately, because of the high ACTH production, grafting of AtT20ins cells into diabetic animals resulted in Cushing's syndrome (217).

The pro-opiomelanocortin promoter directs insulin gene expression in transgenic NOD mice to the anterior pituitary. The insulin is stored and secreted via secretory vesicles. Anterior pituitary tissue from these mice can be transplanted and partially reverse hyperglycaemia in non-transgenic NOD mice (218).

Hepatocytes

The liver is the major site of insulin action. Hepatocytes are the only primary cells other than pancreatic endocrine and pituitary cells that express glucokinase (219,220). Further, they are highly adapted for secretion of a variety of proteins. Hepatocytes and hepatoma cell lines have been targets for gene therapy for diabetic states. The first report of insulin expression in a liver cell was from Halban and colleagues (221). They transfected rat FAO hepatoma cells with either the human and rat II proinsulin genes and found constitutive secretion of proinsulin with a small amount of conversion to insulin (221). The human proinsulin gene has been introduced into the human hepatoma cell line HEPG2, to create the cell line HEPG2ins (222). The transfected cells stored proinsulin and insulin in secretory granules with a different morphology from β-cell insulin granules. HEPG2ins cells constitutively secreted both proinsulin and insulin, with eight-fold more proinsulin being secreted. Insulin, but not proinsulin secretion was stimulated by the secretagogues 8-Br cAMP or theophylline, but not glucose (222).

Kolodka et al. have examined primary hepatocytes as a target for insulin gene expression (223). In this study, the rat insulin 1 gene was cloned into a retrovirus and expressed from the Mouse Maloney Leukemia Virus Long Terminal Repeat promoter. This retrovirus was then injected into the portal vein of rats that had been subjected to partial hepatectomy in order to induce mitotic activity in hepatocytes.

Two weeks later, injected rats were treated with streptozocin to induce diabetes. Rats injected with the insulin vector had no difference in plasma glucose levels compared to control rats in the fed state, but seemed to be less prone to ketoacidosis. Moreover, proinsulin expressed in hepatocytes was not processed efficiently to mature insulin, as determined by low C-peptide: insulin ratios. Insulin secretion was not regulated by glucose levels as the animals became hypoglycaemic when fasted.

Muscle

Muscle is an attractive target for gene therapy because it is easily accessible and has been shown to secrete proteins produced by transgenes into the circulation (224-226). Myoblasts can also take up and express plasmid DNA that is directly injected *in vivo* (227). Bartlett et al. injected into the hamstring muscle of normal and streptozotocin (STZ) diabetic rats a vector in which the human insulin gene was driven by the CMV early promoter (228). Because of high levels of residual proinsulin in the STZ rats, it is difficult to determine whether the insulin gene was expressed and no data were presented on whether muscle can process and store insulin.

Glucose responsive insulin secretion in β-cells

Because of difficulties achieving normal glucose-sensing and coupling to insulin secretion in non-β-cells, genetic modification of primary β-cells and β-cell lines has been explored for β-cell replacement strategies. Most of the information comes from studies with β-cell lines, since it has been difficult to genetically modify and expand primary pancreatic endocrine cells in culture.

Madsen and colleagues introduced the human insulin gene under the control of the human insulin promoter into MSL-G2 cells, a variant of the New England Deaconess Hospital (NEDH) rat insulinoma that expresses high levels of glucagon and cholecystokinin, but very low levels of insulin *in vitro*, and switches to high levels of insulin expression upon passage *in vivo* (109). The human insulin gene was regulated in a manner similar to that of the endogenous mouse insulin II gene, but that the regulation of the mouse insulin I gene differed by virtue of longer duration of expression in a different subset of cells (229). Newgard and colleagues have genetically modified RIN 1046-38 cells that are also a derivative of the NEDH insulinoma, to try to improve its properties for β-cell replacement (230,231). In these cells they expressed the human insulin, glucokinase, and GLUT2 genes under the control of the cytomegalovirus (CMV) early promoter (230). The engineered cell lines exhibited high, stable, levels of human insulin expression and stored and processed insulin through the regulated pathway. Although the engineered cells had some alterations in the pattern of glucose-responsiveness, maximal insulin secretion still occurred at submillimolar glucose concentration. Transplantation of the engineered cells into nude rats resulted in hypoglycaemia and tumour formation.

Immunomodulation of grafted cells

Strategies for immune protection can be divided into physical and genetic approaches. Physical approaches encompass any strategy that physically isolates the grafted cells from the immune system. Genetic approaches encompass strategies to engineer the cell line so that it is not attacked by the immune system. It is likely that a combination of these approaches will be required to produce the goal of insulin independence without systemic immunosuppression.

Approaches to using gene therapy for reducing graft rejection can be divided into active and passive. Active approaches include engineering cells for local production of immunosuppressive molecules that actively downregulate immune responses to the grafted cells. Passive approaches include altering the cells so that they are not recognized by the immune system as foreign or in the case of autoimmunity, as β-cells. A third approach that does not involve altering the insulin-secreting cells is to directly manipulate the immune system to induce tolerance to the graft (reviewed in 235,236). To date, manipulating the immune cells directly is the best studied approach to prolong graft survival. For example, transfer of the gene for the transporter associated with antigen processing (TAP) into B lymphocytes from patients with type I diabetes increases the level of functional HLA class I molecules (139). This study was based on previous work suggesting that there is an antigen processing/antigen presentation defect involving TAP in NOD mice and patients with type 1 diabetes (237-239). However, this finding is controversial, as NOD mice did not exhibit an MHC-linked antigen processing defect. Interestingly, TAP expression can be induced in islets and has been found to be overexpressed in the islets of patients with IDDM (240).

More recently, using an HIV-based lentiviral vector, Galichan et al. (241) transduced interleukin 4 into mouse islets and prevented insulitis and graft destruction by the local production of the cytokine in the transduced cells.

Inducing tolerance to antigens involved in the autoimmune anti-β-cell response may be important for long-term graft survival (2). Infusion of donor bone marrow is a promising approach for induction of tolerance to islet grafts (116), but it is unclear whether this could be used in conjunction with β-cell replacement strategies since bone marrow syngeneic with the grafted cells would not be available. Other approaches such as *in vitro* culture and using antibodies to eliminate "passenger lymphocytes" have also shown some promise in prolonging graft survival (see references 122 and 239 for reviews). Tolerance induction using gene transfer technology has been shown to be possible in principle in a transgenic mouse model in which the β-cells express the lymphocytic choriomeningitis virus (LCMV) glycoprotein. Transfer of the LCMV glycoprotein into host bone marrow cells tolerized the host to the LCMV glycoprotein, preventing experimentally induced diabetes (242). Of more direct clinical relevance are studies of parenterally (243) or orally (244,245) administered insulin or other β-cell autoantigens in which tolerance is induced by the oral antigen. Although these studies have been directed at attempts to induce tolerance to β-cells in pre-diabetic individuals prone to autoimmune diabetes, they may also be relevant to the induction of tolerance to grafted β-cell replacements in diabetic patients.

REFERENCES

1. Hering B, Ricordi C. Islet transplantation for patient with type 1 diabetes. Graft 1999;2:12-27.
2. Tyden G, Reinholt FP, Sundkvist G, Bolinder J. Recurrence of autoimmune diabetes mellitus in recipients of cadaveric pancreatic grafts. New Engl J Med 1996;335(12):860-864.
3. Otsu I, Dunleavy K, Mullon CJP, Solomon BA, Monaco AP. Treatment of diabetes by xenogeneic islets without immunosuppression: use of vascularized bioartificial pancreas. Diabetes 1996;45:342-347.
4. Sun Y, Ma X, Zhou D, Vacek I, Sun AM. Normalization of diabetes in spontaneously diabetic cynomologus monkeys by xenografts of microencapsulated porcine islets without immunosuppression. J Clin Invest 1996;98(6):1417-1422.
5. Groth CG, Korsgren O, Tibell A, et al. Transplantation of porcine foetal pancreas to diabetic patients. Lancet 1994;344:1402-1404.
6. Xenotransplantation and xenogeneic infections. N Engl J Med 1999;333:1498-1501.

7. Patience C, Takeuchi Y, and Weiss RA. Infection of human cells by an endogenous retrovirus of pigs. Nature Med 1997;3:282-286.
8. Steinhuber S, Brack M, Hunsmann G, Schwelberger H, Dierich MP, Vogetseder W. Distribution of human endogenous retrovirus HERV-K genomes in humans and different primates. Hum Genet 1995;96:188-192.
9. Kazazian HHJ, Scott AF. "Copy and paste" transposable elements in the human genome. J Clin Invest 1993;91:1859-1860.
10. Larsen JL, Stratta RJ. Pancreas transplantation: a treatment option for insulin-dependent diabetes mellitus. Diabetes/Metab 1997;Rev 13(4):209-246.
11. Lacy PE, Hegre OD, Gerasimidi-Vazeou A, Genitle FT, Dionne KE. Maintenance of normoglycaemia in diabetic mice by subcutaneous xenografts of encapsulated islets. Science 1991;254:1782-1784.
12. Lim F, Sun AM. Microencapsulated islets a bioartificial endocrine pancreas. Science 1980;210:908-910.
13. Sullivan JS, Maki T, Borland KM, et al. Biohybrid artificial pancreas: long-term implantation studies in diabetic, pancreatectomized dogs. Science 1991;252:718-721.
14. Zhou D, Sun YL, Vacek I, Ma P, Sun AM. Normalization of diabetes in cynomologus monkeys by xenotransplantation of microencapsulated porcine islets. Transplant Proc 1994;26:1091-1994.
15. Scharp DW, Swanson CJ, Olack BJ, et al. Protection of encapsulated human islets implanted without immunosuppression in patients with type I or type II diabetes and in nondiabetic control subjects. Diabetes 1994;43:1167-1170.
16. Tziampazis E, Sambanis A. Tissue engineering of a bioartificial pancreas: modeling the cell environment and device function. Biotechnol Prog 1995;11:115-126.
17. Lanza RP, Sullivan SJ, Chick WL. Islet transplantation with immunoisolation. Diabetes 1992;41:1503-1510.
18. Gu D, Sarvetnik N. Epithelial cell proliferation and islet neogenesis in IFN-γ transgenic mice. Development 1993;118:33-46.
19. Vinik A, Pittenger G, Rafaeloff R, Rosenberg L. Factors controlling pancreatic islet neogenesis. Tumour Biol 1993;14:184-200.
20. Otonkoski T, Beattie GM, Lopez AD, Hayek A. Use of hepatocyte growth factor/scatter to increase transplantable human foetal islet cell mass. Transplantation Proceedings 1994;26:3334.
21. Miettinen PJ, Otonkoski T, Voutilainen R. Insulin-like growth factor-II and transforming growth factor-a in the developing human foetal pancreatic islets. J Endocr 1993;138:127-136.
22. Oberg C, Waltenberger J, Claesson-Welsh L, Welsh M. Expression of protein tyrosine kinases in islet cells: possible role of the Flk-1 receptor for beta-cell maturation from duct cells. Growth Factors 1994;10:115-126.
23. Brelje TC, Parsons JA, Sorenson RL. Regulation of islet beta-cell proliferation by prolactin in rat islet. Diabetes 1994;43:263-273.
24. Neilsen JH, Billestrup N, Moldrup A, et al. Growth of the endocrine pancreas: the role of somatolactogenic hormones and receptors. Biochem Soc Trans 1993;21:146-149.
25. Watanabe T, Yonemura Y, Yonekura H, et al. Pancreatic beta-cell replication and amelioration of surgical diabetes by reg protein. Proc Natl Acad Sci USA 1994;91:3589-3592.
26. Rafaeloff R, Pittenger GL, Barlow SW, et al. Cloning and sequencing of the pancreatic islet neogenesis associated protein (INGAP) gene and its expression in islet neogenesis in hamsters. J Clin Invest 1997;99(9):2100-2109.
27. Baeza N, Moriscot C, Figarella C, Guy-Crotte O, Vialettes B. Reg protein: a potential beta-cell specific growth factor? Diabetes/Metab 1996;22:229-234.
28. Shing Y, Christofori G, Hanahan D, et al. Betacellulin: a mitogen from pancreatic β cell tumors. Science 1993;259:1604-1608.
29. Mashima H, Ohnisi H, Wakabayashi K, et al. Betacellulin and Activin A coordinately convert amylase-secreting pancreatic AR42J cells into insulin secreting cells. J Clin Invest 1996;97:1647-1654.
30. Otonkoski T, Cirulli V, Beattie GM, et al. A role for hepatocyte growth factor/scatter factor in foetal mesenchyme-induced pancreatic β-cell growth. Endocrinology 1996;137(7):3131-3139.
31. Michael J.Shamblott, Joyce Axelman, Shunping Wang, et al. Derivation of pluripotent stem cells from cultured human primordial germ cells. Proc Natl Acad Sci USA 1998;95:13726-13731.
32. James A.Thompson, Joseph Itskovitz-Eldor, Sander S.Shapiro, et al. Embryonic stem cell lines derived from human blastocysts. Science 1998;6:1145-1147.
33. Gospodarowicz D. Preparation of extracellular matrices produced by cultured bovine corneal endothelial cells and PF-HR-9 endodermal cells: their use in cell culture. In: Barnes DW, Sirbasku DA, Sato GH, eds. Cell Culture methods for molecular and cell biology. 256th ed. New York, NY: Alan R Liss Inc, 1984:275-295.
34. Adamson ED. The effect of collagen on cell division, cellular differentiation and embryonic development. Collagen in Health and Disease 1982;218-243.
35. Bissell MJ, Barcellos-Hoff H. The influence of extracellular matrix on gene expression: is structure the message? J Cell Science Suppl 1987;8:327-343.

36. Beattie GM, Lappi DA, Baird A, Hayek A. Functional impact of attachment and purification in the short term culture of human pancreatic islets. J Clin Endocr Metab 1991;73:93-98.
37. Beattie GM, Rubin JS, Mally MI, Otonkoski T, Hayek A. Regulation of proliferation and differentiation of human foetal pancreatic islet cells by extracellular matrix, hepatocyte growth factor and cell-cell contact. Diabetes 1996;45:1223-1228.
38. Beattie GM, Levine F, Mally M, et al. Acid β-Galactosidase: A developmentally regulated marker of endocrine cell precursors in the human foetal pancreas. J Clin Endocrinol Metab 1994;78:1232-1240.
39. Langhofer M, Hopkinson SB, Jones JCR. The matrix secreted by 804G cells contains laminin-related components that participate in hemidesmosome assembly in vitro. J Cell Sci 1993;105:753-764.
40. Matsuit C, Wang CK, Nelson CF, Bauer EA, Hoeffer WK. The Assembly of Laminin-5 Subunits*
41. Ryle C, Breitkreutz D, Stark H, et al. Density-dependent modulation of synthesis of keratins 1 + 10 in the human keratinocyte line HaCat and in ras-transfected tumorigenic clones. Differentiation 1989;40:42-54.
42. Akaogi K, Okabe Y, Funahashi K, et al. Cell adhesion activity of a 30-kDa major secreted protein from human bladder carcinoma cells. Biochem Biophys Res Comm 1994;198(3):1046-1053.
43. Bourdrel L, Lin CH, Lauren SL, et al. Recombinant human transforming growth factor-beta 1: expression by Chinese hamster ovary cells, isolation, and characterization. Prot Expr & Pur 1993;4(2):130-140.
44. Bellusci S, Moens G, Thiery JP, Jouanneau J. A scatter factor-like factor is produced by a metastatic variant of a rat bladder carcinoma cell line. J Cell Sci 1994;107:1277-1287.
45. Hayek A, Beattie GM, Cirulli V, Lopez AD, Ricordi C, Rubin JS. Growth factor/matrix-induced proliferation of human adult β-cells. Diabetes 1995;44:1458-1460.
46. Eriksson PS, Perfilieve E, Bjork-Ericksson T, et al. Neurogenesis in the adult hippocampus. Nat Med 1998;4:1313-1317.
47. Beattie GM, Cirulli V, Lopez AD, Hayek A. Ex vivo expansion of human pancreatic endocrine cells. J Clin Endocrinol Metab 1997;82:1852-1856.
48. Newgard CB. Engineering and gene therapy strategies for insulin replacement in diabetes. Diabetes 1994;43:341-350.
49. Poitout V, Olsen LK, Robertson RP. Insulin-secreting cell lines: classification, characteristics and potential applications. Diabetes Metab 1996;22:72-14.
50. Efrat S. Genetic engineering of beta-cells for cell therapy of diabetes: cell growth function, and immunogenicity. Diabetes 1996;Rev 4:224-234.
51. Tiedge M, Lenzen S. Gene Therapy of diabetes mellitus: aims, methods and future prospects. Exp Clin Endocrinol Diabetes 1995;103:46-55.
52. Zhang Y, Warren-Perry M, Sakura H, et al. No evidence for mutations in a putative beta-cell ATP-sensitive K+ channel subunit in. Diabetes/Metab 1997;Rev 13(4):209-246.
53. Knaack D, Fiore DM, Surana M, et al. Clonal insulinoma cell line that stably maintains correct glucose responsiveness. Diabetes 1994; 43:1413-1417.
54. Levine F. Gene therapy for diabetes: strategies for β-cell modification and replacement. Diabetes 1997;13(4):209-246.
55. Rae PA, Yip CC, Schimmer BP. Isolation of cloned Syrian hamster insulinoma cell lines with limited capacity for insulin production. J Physiol Pharmacol 1979;57:819-824.
56. Chick WL, Warren S, Chute RN, Like AA, Lauris V, Kitchen KC. A transplantable insulinoma in the rat. Proc Natl Acad Sci USA 1977;74:628-632.
57. Santerre RF, Cook RA, Crisel RMD, et al. Insulin synthesis in a clonal cell line of simian virus 40-transformed hamster pancreatic β cells. Proc Natl Acad Sci USA 1981;78(7):-32768-4343.
58. Hanahan D. Heritable formation of pancreatic β-cell tumours in transgenic mice expressing recombinant insulin/simian virus 40 oncogenes. Nature 1985;315:115-122.
59. Radvanyl F, Christgau S, Baekkeskov S, Jolicoeur C, Hanahan D. Pancreatic β cells cultured from individual preneoplastic foci in a multistage tumorigenesis pathway: a potentially general technique for isolating physiologically representative cell lines. Mol Cell Biol 1993;13(7):4223-4232.
60. Drucker DJ. Molecular pathophysiology of glucagon-SV40 T antigen transgenic mice. Am J Physiol 1994; 267:E629-E635.
61. Christofori G, Naik P, Hanahan D. A Second signal supplied by insulin-like growth factor II in oncogene-induced tumorigenesis. Nature 1994; 369:414-418.
62. Yamaguchi N, Yamamura Y, Kunihiko K, Ohtsuji E, Imanish J, Ashihara T. Characterization of new human pancreatic cancer cell lines which propagate in a protein-free chemically defined medium. Cancer Res 1990;50:7008-7014.
63. Morgan RT, Woods LK, Moore GE, Quinn LA, McGavran L, Gordon SG. Human cell line(COLO 357) of metastatic pancreatic adenocarcinoma. Intl J Cancer 1980;25:591-598.
64. Vila MR, Lloreta J, Schussler MH, Berrozpe G, Welt S, Real FX. New pancreas cancer cell lines that represent distinct stages of ductal differentiation. Lab Invest 1995;72:395-404.
65. Lundqvist M, Oberg K. In vitro culture of neuroendocrine tumors of the pancreas and gut. Acta Oncol 1989;28:335-339.

66. Gueli N, Toto A, Palmieri G, Carmenini G, Delpino A, Ferrini U. In vitro growth of a cell line originated from a human insulinoma. JECCR 1987;6:281-285.
67. Pour PM, Permert J, Mogaki M, Fujii H, Kazakoff K. Endocrine aspects of exocrine cancer of the pancreas. Am J Clin Path 1993;100:223-230.
68. Permert J, Mogaki M, Andren-Sanberg A, Kazakoff K, Pour PM. Pancreatic mixed ductal-islet tumors. Intl J Pancreatol 1992;11:23-29.
69. Slack JMW. Developmental biology of the pancreas. Development 1995;121:1569-1580.
70. Murray MR, Bradley CR. Two islet cell adenomas of the human pancreases cultivated in vitro. Am J Cancer 1935;25:98.
71. Soldevila G, Buscema M, Marini V, et al. Transfection with SV40 gene of human pancreatic endocrine cells. J Autoimmun 1991;4:381-396.
72. Wang S, Beattie GM, Mally MI, et al. Isolation and characterization of a cell line from the epithelial cells of the human foetal pancreas. Cell Transplantation 1997;6(1):59-67.
73. Wang S, Beattie GM, Hayek A, Levine F. Development of a VSV-G protein pseudotyped retroviral vector system expressing dominant oncogenes from a lacO-modified inducible LTR promoter. Gene 1996;182:145-150.
74. Chou JY. Differentiated mammalian cell lines immortalized by temperature-sensitive tumor viruses. Mol Endocrinol 1989; 3:1511-1514.
75. Chang SE. In vitro transformation of human cells. Biochem Biophys Acta 1986;823:161-194.
76. Bradbury JM, Sykes H, Edwards PAW. Induction of mouse mammary tumours in a transplantation system by sequential introduction of the myc and ras oncogenes. Intl J Cancer 1995;48:908-915.
77. Ragozzino MM, Kuo A, DeGreori J, Kohl N, Ruley HE. Mechanism of oncogene cooperation: activation and inactivation of a growth antagonist. Environ Health Perspect 1991;93:97-103.
78. Oft M, Peli J, Rudaz C, Schwarz H, Geug H, Reichmann E. TGF-beta and Ha-Ras collaborate in modulating the phenotype plasticity and invasiveness of epithelial tumor cells. Genes Dev 1996;10:2462-2477.
79. van Leeuwen F, Nusse R. Oncogene activation and oncogene cooperation in MMTV induced mouse mammary cancer. Sem Cancer Biol 1995;6:127-133.
80. Adams JM, Cory S. Transgenic models of tumor development. Science 1991;254:1161-1167.
81. Lind K, Blume N, Michelsen BK, Bucchini D, Madsen OD. Differential expression of non allelic insulin genes in rodent islet tumour cells. J Mol Endocrinol 1993;11:305-318.
82. Sanvito F, Herrera P-L, Huarte J, et al. TGF-β1 influences the relative development of the exocrine and endocrine pancreas in vitro. Development 1994;120:3451-3462.
83. Wang S, Beattie GM, Mally MI, Lopez AD, Hayek A. Analysis of a human foetal pancreatic islet cell line. Transplantation Proceedings 1997;29:2219.
84. Levine F, Wang S, Beattie GM, et al. Development of a cell line from the human foetal pancreas. Transplantation Proceedings 1995;27(6 PT 3):3410.
85. Alema S, Tato F. Oncogenes and muscle differentiation: multiple mechanisms of interference. Semi Cancer 1994;5:147-156.
86. Kong Y, Johnson SE, Taparowsky EJ, and Koniezny SF. Ras p21val inhibits myogenesis with out altering the DNA binding or transcriptional activities of myogenic basic helix-loop-helix factors. Mol Cell Biol 1995;15:5202-5213.
87. Jehn B, Costello E, Marti A, Keon N, Deane R. Over-expression of myc, ras, src, and fos inhibits mouse mammary epithelial cell differentiation. Mol Cell Biol 1992;12:3890-3902.
88. Efrat S, Fleischer N, Hanahan D. Diabetes induced in male transgenic mice by expression of human H-ras oncoprotein in pancreatic beta cell. Mol Cell Biol 1990;10:1779-1783.
89. Efrat S. Sexual dimorphism of pancreatic beta cell degeneration in transgenic mice expressing an insulin-ras hybrid gene. Endocrinology 1991;128:897-901.
90. Robinson GLWG, Henderson E, Massari ME, Murre C, Stein R. c-Jun inhibits insulin control element-mediated transcription by affecting the transactivation potential of the E2A gene products. Mol Cell Biol 1995;15:1398-1404.
91. Tal M, Wu Y-J, Leiser M, et al. [Val12]HRAS downregulates GLUT2 in beta cells of transgenic mice without affecting glucose homeostasis. Proc Natl Acad Sci USA 1992;89:5744-5748.
92. Snyder EY, Deitcher DL, Walsh C, Arnold-Aldea S, Hartweig EA, Cepko CL. Multipotent neural cell lines can engraft and participate in development of mouse cerebellum. Cell 1992;68:33-51.
93. Hue E, Kin JB, Sarraf P, Spiegelman BM. Inhibition of adipogenesis through MAP kinase-mediated phosphorylation of PPARgamma. Science 1996;274:2100-2103.
94. Reichmann E. Oncogenes and epithelial cell transformation. Sim Cancer Biol 1994;5:157-165.
95. Sandgren EP, Quaife CJ, Paulovich AG, Palmiter RD, Brinster RL. Pancreatic tumor pathogenesis reflects the causative genetic lesion. Proc Natl Acad Sci USA 1991;88:93-97.
96. Welsh M, Andersson A. Transplantation of transfected pancreatic islets: stimulation of beta cell DNA synthesis by the src oncogene. Transplantation 1994;57:297-299.
97. Welsh M, Welsh N, Nilsson T, et al. Stimulation of pancreatic islet beta-cell replication by oncogenes. Proc Natl Acad Sci USA 1988;85:116-120.

98. Berggren P-O, Hallberg A, Welsh N, Arkhammar P, Nilsson T, Welsh M. Transfection of insulin-producing cells with a transforming c-HA-ras oncogene stimulates phospholipase C activity. Biochem J 1989;259:701-707.
99. Welsh M, Mares J, Oberg C, Karlsson T. Genetic factors of importance for beta-cell proliferation. Diabetes/Metab 1993;Rev 9:25-36.
100. Seino Y, Yamamoto T, Inoue K, et al. Abnormal facilitative glucose transporter gene expression in human islet cell tumors. J Clin Endocrinol Metab 1993;76:75-78.
101. Vozzi C, Ullrich S, Charollais A, Philippe J, Orci L, Meda P. Adequate connexin-mediated coupling is required for proper insulin production. J Cell Biol 1995;131(6:1):1561-1572.
102. Stein RW, Corrigan M, Yaciuk P, Whelan J, Moran E. Analysis of E1A-mediated growth regulation functions: binding of the 300-Kilodalton cellular product correlates with E1A enhancer repression function and DNA synthesis-inducing activity. J Virol 1990;64:4421-4427.
103. Stein RW, Whelan J. Insulin gene enhancer activity is inhabited by adenovirus 5 Ela gene products. Mol Cell Biol 1989;9:4531-4534.
104. Clark SA, Burnham BL, Chick WL. Modulation of glucose-induced insulin secretion from a rat clonal beta-cell line. Endocrinology 1990;127:2779-2788.
105. Ferber S, Beltrandel Rio H, Johnson JH, et al. Glut-2 gene transfer into insulinoma cells confers both low and high affinity glucose-stimulated insulin release. J Biol Chem 1994;269(15):11523-11529.
106. Noda M, Komatsu M, Sharp GWG. The BHC-9 B-cell lines preserves the characteristics of progenitor mouse islets. Diabetes 1996; 45:1766-1773.
107. Pictet RL, Rutter WJ. The molecular basis of the mescenchymal-epithelial interactions in pancreatic development in Cell Interactions in Differentiation, Karkinen-Jaaskelainen M, Saxen L, and Weiss L, Eds. Academic Press, London 1977;339-350.
108. Adams JC, Watt FM. Regulation of development and differentiation by the extracellular matrix. Development 1993;117:1183-1198.
109. Madsen OD, Andersen LC, Michelsen B, et al. Tissue-specific expression of transfected human insulin genes in pluripotent clonal rat insulinoma lines induced during passage in vivo. Proc Natl Acad Sci USA 1988;85:6652-6656.
110. Lengauern C, Kinzler KW, Vogelstein B. Genetic instability in colorectal cancer. Nature 1999;386:623-627.
111. Lengauer C, Kinzler KW, Vogelstein B. DNA methylation and genetic instability in colorectal cancer cells. Proc Natl Acad Sci USA 1997;94:2445-2550.
112. Fukasawa K, Choi T, Kuriyama R, Rulong S, Vande Woude GF. Abnormal centrosome amplification in the absence of p53. Science 1996;271:1744-1747.
113. Gartner H-V, Seidl C, Luckenbach C, et al. Genetic analysis of a sarcoma accidentally transplanted from a patient to a surgeon. N Engl J Med 1996;335:1494-1496.
114. Naji A. Induction of tolerance by intrathymic inoculation of alloantigen. Current Opinion in Immunology 1996;8:704-709.
115. Levey MM, Ketchum RJ, Park DH, et al. Engraftment and function of intrathymic pancreatic islet autografts in dogs. Tranplant Proc 1995;27:607-608.
116. Ricordi C, Murase N, Rastellini C, Behboo R, Demetris AJ, Starzl TE. Indefinite survival of rat islet allografts following infusion of donor bone marrow without cytoablation. Cell Trans 1996;5:53-55.
117. Gill RG, Coulombe M, Lafferty KJ. Pancreatic islet allograft immunity and tolerance: the two-signal hypothesis revisited. Immunol Rev 1996;149:75-96.
118. Parish NM, Hutchings PR, O'Reilly L, et al. Tolerance induction as a therapeutic strategy for the control of autoimmune endocrine disease in mouse models. Immunol Rev 1995;144:269-300.
119. Efrat S, Fejer G, Brownlee M, Horwitz MS. Prolonged survival of pancreatic islet allografts mediated by adenovirus immunoregulatory transgenes. Proc Natl Acad Sci USA 1995;92:6947-6951.
120. Osorio RW, Ascher NL, Melzer JS, Stock PG. Beta-2 microgolobulin gene disruption prolongs murine islet allograft survival in NOD mice. Transplant Proc 1994;26:752.
121. Markmann JF, Desai NM, Bassiri H, Kim JI, Baker CF. Prolonged survival of class I deficient mouse islet allograft but not xenografts. Transplant Proc 1994;26:748.
122. Faustman D. Strategies for circumventing transplant rejection: modification of cells tissues and organs. Trends Biotechnol 1995;13:100-105.
123. Bellgrau D, Gold D, Selawry H, Moore J, Franzusoff A, Duke RC. A role for CD95 ligand in preventing graft rejection. Nature 1995;377:630-632.
124. Qin L, Chavin KD, Ding Y, et al. Retrovirus-mediated transfer of viral IL-10 gene prolongs murine cardiac allograft survival. J Immunol 1996;156:2316-2323.
125. Efrat S, Fusco-DeMane D, Lemberg H, Emran OA, Wang X. Conditional transformation of a pancreatic β-cell line derived from transgenic mice expressing a tetracycline-regulated oncogene. Proc Natl Acad Sci USA 1995;92:3576-3580.

126. Wang S, Beattie G, Hayek A, Levine F. Transformation of human primary fibroblasts by pseudotype retroviral vectors expressing multiple dominant oncogenes from an inducible promoter. Gene 1996;182:145-150.
127. Zou Y-R, Muller W, Gu H, Rajewsky K. Cre-loxP-mediated gene replacement: a mouse strain producing humanizes antibodies. Current Biol 1994;4:1099-1103.
128. Metzger D, Clifford J, Chiba H, Chambon P. Conditional site-specific recombination in mammalian cells using a ligand-dependent chimeric Cre recombinase. Proc Natl Acad Sci USA 1995;92:6991-6995.
129. Westerman KA, Leboulch. Reversible immortalization of mammalian cells mediated by retroviral transfer and site-specific recombination. Proc Natl Acad Sci USA 1996;93:8971-8976.
130. Connors TA. The choice of prodrugs for Gene direct enzyme prodrug therapy of cancer. Gene Ther 1995;2:702-709.
131. Moolten FL. Drug sensitivity ("suicide") gene for selective cancer chemotherapy. Cancer Gene Ther 1994;1:279-287.
132. Rosengard AM, Cary NR, Langford GA, Tucker AW, Wallwork J, White DJ. Tissue expression of human complement inhibitor, decay-accelerating factor, in transgenic pigs: a potential approach for preventing xenograft rejection. Transplantation 1995;59:1325-1333.
133. Elshami AA, Saavedra A, Zhang H, et al. Gap junction play a role in the "bystander effect" of the herpes simplex virus thymidine kinase/ganciclovir system in vitro. Gene Ther 1996;3:85-92.
134. Misnil M, Piccoli C, Tirabt G, Willecke K, Yamasaki H. Bystander killing of cancer cells by herpes simplex virus thymidine kinase gene is mediated by connexins. Proc Natl Acad Sci USA 1996;93:1831-1835.
135. Berggren PO, Hallberg A, Welsh N, Arkahammar P, Nilsson T, and Welsh M. Transfection of insulin-producing cells with a transforming c-Ha-ras oncogene stimulates phospholipase C activity. Biochem J 1989;259:701-707.
136. German MS, Moss LG, Rutter WJ. Regulation of insulin gene expression by glucose and calcium in transfected primary islet cultures. J Biol Chem 1990;265(36):22063-22066.
137. Basudev F, Jones PM, Howell SL. Protein phosphorylation in the regulation of insulin secretion: the use of site-directed inhibitory peptides in electrically permeabilised islet of Langerhans. Acta Diabetol 1995;32:32-37.
138. Mucke S, Polack A, Pawlita M, et al. Suitability of Epstein-Barr virus-based episomal vectors for expression of cytokine genes in human lymphoma cells. Gene Ther 1997;4:82-92.
139. Wang F, Li X, Annis B, Faustman DL. Tap-1 and Tap-2 gene therapy selectively restores conformationally dependent HLA Class I expression in type I diabetes cells. Hum Gene Ther 1995;6:1005-1017.
140. Sun TQ, Livanos E, Vos JM. Engineering a mini-herpes virus as a general strategy to transduce up to 180 Kb of functional self-replicating human mini-chromosomes. Gene Ther 1996;3:1081-1088.
141. Mungal SA, Steinberg BM, Taichman LB. Replication of plasmid-derived human papillomavirus type II DNA in cultured keratinocytes. J Virol 1992;66:3220-3224.
142. Welsh N, Hallberg A, Sandler S, Hellerstrom C. Use of liposomes to introduce substance into pancreatic islet cells. Diabetes 1988;37:1123-1128.
143. Oberg C, Welsh N. Nonspecific delivery of substances into pancreatic islet cells by Ph sensitive liposomes in vitro. Diabetes Metab 1990;16:48-54.
144. Welsh N, Oberg C, Hellerstom C, Welsh M. Liposome mediated transfection of pancreatic islet cells. Biomed Biochem Acta 1990;49:1157-1164.
145. Saldeen J, Curiel DT, Eizirik DL, et al. Efficient gene transfer to dispersed human pancreatic islet cells in vitro using adenovirus-polylsine/DNA complexes or polycationic liposomes. Diabetes 1996;45:1197-1203.
146. Gainer AL, Korbutt GS, Rajotte RV, Warnock GL, Elliott JF. Successful biolistic transformation of mouse pancreatic islets while preserving cellular function. Transplantation 1996; 61(11):1567-1571.
147. Guo Z, Chong ASF, Jandeska S, et al. Gene gun-mediated gene transfer and expression in rats islet. Transplant Proc 1997;29:2209-2210.
148. Bartlett RJ, Secore SJ, Bottino R, Fernandez L, Inverardi L, Ricordi C. Use of biolistic particle accelerator to induce genes into isolated islets of Langerhans. Transplant Proc 1997;29:2201-2202.
149. Jindal RM, Sidner RA, Bocham MR. et al. Adeno-associated virus vectors: potential for gene therapy. Graft 1998;1:147-153.
150. Ponnazhagan S, Mukherjee P, Yonder MC. Adeno-associated virus 2-mediated gene transfer in vivo: organ-tropism and expression of transduced sequences in mice. Gene 1997;190:203-210.
151. Mirenda V, Charreau B, Sigalla J, et al. Xenoreactivity on the pig islet to human combination: feasibility of adenovirus-mediated gene transfer in to pig islet. Transplant Proc 1996;28:808-810.
152. Becker TC, BeltrandelRio H, Noel RJ, Johnson JH, Newgard CB. Overexpression of hexokinase I in isolated islets of Langerhans via recombinant adenovirus: enhancement of glucose metabolism and insulin secretion at basal but not stimulatory glucose levels. J Biol Chem 1994;269:21234-21238.

153. Csete ME, Benhamou PY, Drazan KE, et al. Efficient gene transfer to pancreatic islet mediated by adenoviral vectors. Transplantation 1995;59:263-268.
154. Smith TAG, Mehaffey MG, Kayda DB, et al. Adenovirus mediated expression of therapeutic plasma levels of human factors IX in mice. Nature Genet 1993;5:397-402.
155. Yang Y, Su Q, Wilson JM. Role of viral antigens in destructive cellular immune responses to adenovirus vector-transduced cells in mouse lungs. J Virol 1996;70:7209-7212.
156. Wickham TJ, Mathias P, Cheresh DA, Nemerow GR. Integrin alphaVbeta3 and alphaVbeta5 promote adenovirus internalization but not virus attachment. Cell 1993;73:309-319.
157. Brunicardi FC, Stagner J, Bonner-Weir S, et al. Microcirculation of the islets of Langerhans. Diabetes 1996;45:385-392.
158. Curiel DT, Agarwal S, Wagnerm E, Cotten M. Adenovirus enhancement of transferrin-polylysine-mediated gene delivery. Proc Natl Acad Sci USA 1991;88:8850-8854.
159. Michael SI, Curiel DT. Strategies to achieve targeted gene delivery via the receptor-mediated endocytosis pathway. Gene Ther 1994;1:223-232.
160. McLachlin JR, Cornetta K, Eglitis MA, Anderson WF. Retroviral-mediated gene transfer. Prog in Nuc Acid Res and Mol Biol 1990;38:91-135.
161. Roe TY, Reynold TC, Yu G, Brown PO. Integration of murine leukemia virus DNA depends on mitosis. EMBO J 1993;12:2099-2108.
162. Yoshida T, Hanahan D. Murine pancreatic ductal adenocarcinoma produced by in vitro transduction of polyoma middle T oncogene into the islets of Langerhans. Am J Pathol 1994;145:671-684.
163. Naldini L, Blomer U, Gallay P, et al. In vivo gene delivery and stable transduction of nondividing cells by a lentiviral vector. Science 1996;272:263-267.
164. Akkina RK, Walton RM, Chen ML, Li Q-X, Planelles V, Chen ISY. High-efficiency gene transfer in to CD34+ cells with a human immunodeficiency virus type 1-based retroviral vector pseudotyped with vesicular stomatitis virus envelope glycoprotein. J Virol 1996;70:2581-2585.
165. Luigi Naldini, Ulrike Blomer, Philippe Gallay, et al. In Vivo Gene Delivery and Stable Transduction of Nondividing Cells by a Lentiviral Vector. Science 1996;272:263-267.
166. Romain Zufferey, Dea Nagy, Ron J. Mandel, Luigi Naldini, Didier Trono. Multiply attenuated lentiviral vector achieves efficient gene delivery in vivo. Nature Biotechnology 1997;15:871-826.
167. Sigalla J, David A, Anegon I, et al. Adenovirus-mediated gene transfer into isolated mouse adult pancreatic islet: normal beta-cell function despite induction of an antiadenovirus immune response. Human Gene Therapy 1997;8:1625-1634.
168. Bosch A, McCray PB, Chang SM, et al. Proliferation induced by keratinocyte growth factor enhances in vivo retroviral-mediated gene transfer to mouse hepatocytes. J Clin Invest 1996;98:2683-2687.
169. Ott M, Stockert RJ, Ma Q, Gagandeep S, Gupta S. Simultaneous upregulation of viral receptor expression and DNA synthesis is required for increasing efficiency of retroviral hepatic gene. J Biol Chem 1998;273:11954-11961.
170. Titia de Lange, Ronald A.DePinho. Unlimited Mileage from Telomerase. Science 1999;283:947-949.
171. Tohru Kiyono, Scott A, Foster, et al. Both Rb/p16 INK4 inactivation and telomerase activity are required to immortalize human epithelial cells. Nature 1998;396:84-88.
172. Tanya L.Halvorsen, Gil Liebowitz, Fred Levine. Telomerase activity is sufficient to allow transformed cells to escape from crisis. Mol Cell Biol 1999;19 No.3:1864-1870.
173. Newgard CB, McGarry JD. Metabolic coupling factors in pancreatic β-cell signal transduction. Annu Rev Biochem 1995;64:689-719.
174. Hutton JC. Insulin secretory granule biogenesis and the proinsulin-processing endopeptidase. Diabetologia 1994;37 (Suppl 2):S48-S56.
175. Steiner DF, Rouille Y, Gong Q, Martin S, Caroll R, Chan SJ. The role of prohormone convertase in insulin biosynthesis: evidence for inherited defects in their action in man and experimental animals. Diabetes Metab 1996;22:94-104.
176. MacDonald MJ. Elusive proximal signals of beta-cells for insulin secretion. Diabetes 1990;39:1461-1466.
177. Dunne MJ, Harding EA, Jaggar JH, Squires PE. Ion channels and the molecular control of insulin secretion. Biochem Soc Trans 1994;22:6-12.
178. Prenki M. New insights into pancreatic beta-cell metabolic signaling in insulin secretion. Eur J Endocrinol 1996;134:272-286.
179. Laub O, Rall L, Bell GI, Rutter WJ. Expression of the human insulin gene in an alternate mammalian cell and in cell extracts. J Biol Chem 1983;258:6037-6042.
180. Laub O, and Rutter WJ. Expression of the Human insulin gene and cDNA in a heterologous mammalian system. J Biol Chem 1983;258:6043-6050.
181. Smith DM, Bloom SR. Paracine/autocrine control of the islet and the amylin family. Biochem Soc Trans 1995;23:336-340.
182. Lipes MA, Cooper EM, Skelly R, et al. Insulin-secreting non islet cells are resistant to autoimmune destruction. Proc Natl Acad Sci USA 1996;93:8595-8600.

183. St. Louis D, Verma I. An alternative approach to somatic cell gene therapy. Proc Natl Acad Sci USA 1988;85:3150-3154.
184. Palmer TD, Rosman GJ, Osborne WRA, Miller DA. Genetically modified skin fibroblasts persist long after transplantation but gradually inactivate introduced genes. Proc Natl Acad Sci USA 1991; 88:1330-1334.
185. Hsueh JL. Clinical protocol of human gene transfer for hemophilia B original covering memo. Hum Gene Ther 1992;3:543-552.
186. Liu Hong-W, Ofosu FA, Chang PL. Expression of human factor IX by microencapsulated recombinant fibroblast. Hum Gene Ther 1993;4:292-301.
187. Osborne WRA, and Miller AD. Design of vectors for efficient expression of human purine nucleoside phosphorylase in skin fibroblasts from enzyme-deficient humans. Proc Natl Acad Sci USA 1988;85:6851-6855.
188. Hoeben RC, van der Jagt RCM, Schoute F, et al. Expression of functional factor VIII in primary skin fibroblasts after retrovirus-mediated gene transfer. J Biol Chem 1990;265:7318-7323.
189. Moullier P, Bohl D, Heard J-M, Danos O. Correction of lysosomal storage in the liver and spleen of MPS VII mice by implantation of genetically modified skin fibroblasts. Nature Genet 1993;4:154-159.
190. Heartlein MW, Roman VA, Jiang J-L, et al. Long-term production and delivery of human growth hormone in vivo. Proc Natl Acad Sci USA 1994;91:10967-10971.
191. Veelken H, Jesuiter H, Mackensen A, et al. Primary fibroblasts from human adults as target cells for ex vivo transfection and gene therapy. Hum Gene Ther 1994;5:1203-1210.
192. Krueger GG, Morgan JR, Jorgensen CM, et al. Genetically modified skin to treat disease: potential and limitations. J Invest Dermatol 1994;103:76S-84S.
193. Naughton BA, Dai y, Sibanda B, et al. Long-term expression of a retrovirally introduced beta galactosidase gene in rodent cells implanted in vivo using biodegradable polymer meshes. Som Cell Mol Genet 1992;18:451-462.
194. Frueger GG, Liimatta AP, Jorgensen CM, Morgan JR. Prolongation of genetically modified human fibroblasts in culture in an extracellular nylon matrix enhances survival in vivo. J Invest Dermatol 1996;106:806.
195. Taniguchi H, Nakauchi H, Iwata H, Amemiya H, Fukao K. Treatment of diabetic mice with encapsulated fibroblasts producing human proinsulin. Transplant Proc 1992;24:2977-2978.
196. Simpson AM, Iland F, Clarke RA, Burn Al, Tuch BE. Transformation of pituitary and fibroblast cell lines using human insulin c-DNA and a dexamethasone-inducible promoter. Transplant Proc 1993;25:2915-2916.
197. Kawakami Y, Yamaoka T, Hirochika R, Yamashita K, Itakura M, Nakauchi H. Somatic gene therapy for diabetes with an immunological safety system for complete removal of transplanted cells. Diabetes 1992;41:956-961.
198. Yoskimoto K, Muakami R, Moritani M, et al. Loss of ganciclovir sensitivity by exclusion of Thymidine kinase gene from transplanted proinsulin-producing fibroblasts as a gene therapy model. Gene Ther 1996;3:230-234.
199. Selden RF, Skoskiewicz MJ, Russell PS, Goodman HM. Regulation of insulin-gene expression. N Engl J Medicine 1987;317:1067-1076.
200. Kasten-Jolly J, Aubrey MT, Conti DJ, Rosano TG, Ross IS, Freed BM. Reversal of hyperglycaemia in diabetic NOD mice by human proinsulin gene therapy. Transplant Proc 1997;29:2216-2218.
201. Smeekens SP, Montag AG, Thomas G, Albiges-Rizo C, et al. Proinsulin processing by the subtilisin-related proprotein convertases furin, PC2, and PC3. Proc Natl Acad Sci USA 1992;89:8822-8826.
202. Vollenweider F, Kaufmann J, Irminger J-C, Halban PA. Processing of proinsulin by furin, PC2 and PC3 in (co)transfected COS (monkey Kidney) cells. Diabetes 1995;44:1075-1080.
203. Kaumann JE, Irminger J-C, Mungall J, Halban PA. Proinsulin conversion in GH3 cells after coexpression of human proinsulin with the endoproteases PC2 and/orPC3. Diabetes 1997;46:978-982.
204. Groskreutz DJ, Slikowski MX, Gorman MX. Genetically engineered proinsulin constitutively processed and secreted as mature, active insulin. J Bio Chem 1994;269:6241-6245.
205. Alpert S, Hanahan D, Tietelman G. Hybrid insulin gene reveal a developmental lineage for pancreatic endocrine cells and imply a relationship with neurons. Cell 1988;53:295-308.
206. Teitelman G, Lee JK. Cell lineage analysis of pancreatic islet cell development: glucagon and insulin cells arise from catecholaminergic precursors present in the pancreatic duct. Dev Biol 1987;121:454-466.
207. Devaskar SU, Giddings SJ, Rajakumar PA, Carnaghi LR, Menon RK, Zahm DS. Insulin gene expression and insulin synthesis in mammalian neuronal cells. J Biol Chem 1994;269:8445-8454.
208. Furth J, Gadsen EL, Upton AC. ACTH secreting transplantable pituitary tumors. Proc Soc Exp Biol Med 1953;84:243-254.

209. Moore H-P, Walker MD, Lee F, Kelly RB. Expression a human proinsulin cDNA in a mouse ACTH-secreting cell: intracellular storage, proteolytic processing, and secretion on simulation. Cell 1983;35:531-538.
210. Hughes SD, Quaade C, Milburn JL, Cassidy LC, Newgard CB. Expression of normal and novel glucokinase mRNA in anterior pituitary and islet cells. J Biol Chem 1991;266:4521-4530.
211. Smeekens SP, Avruch AS, LaMendola J, Chan SJ, Steiner DF. Identification of a cDNA encoding a second putative prohormone convertase related to PC2 in AtT20 cells and islet of Langerhans. Proc Natl Acad Sci USA 1991;88:340-344.
212. Vindrola O, Lindberg I. Biosynthesis of the prohormone convertase mPC1 in AtT-20 cells. Mol Endocrinol 1992;6:1088-1094.
213. Stewart C, Taylor NA, Docherty K, Bailey CJ. Insulin delivery by somatic cell gene therapy. J Mol Endocrinol 1993;11:335-341.
214. Hughes SDF, Johnson JH, Quaade C, Newgard CB. Engineering of glucose-simulated insulin secretion and biosynthesis in non-islet cells. Proc Natl Acad Sci USA 1992; 89:688-692.
215. Irminger JC, Vollenweider FM, Neerman-Arbez M. Human proinsulin conversion in the regulated and the constitutive pathway of transfected AtT20 cells. J Biol Chem 1994;269:1756-1762.
216. Kaufmann JE, Irminger JC, Halban PA. Sequence requirement for proinsulin processing at the B-chain/C-peptide junction. Biochem J 1995;310:869-874.
217. Beltran del Rio H, Schnedl WJ, Ferber S, et al. Pancreatic Islet Transplantation 1994;Vol 1:169-178.
218. Lipes MA, Cavalli AM, Rhodes CJ, Skelly R, Cooper EM. Engineering insulin secretion in non-islet cells for beta-cell replacement in IDDM. Diabetes 1996;45 (Suppl 2):23A.
219. Liang Y, Jetton T, Zimmerman E, Najafi H, Matschinsky FM, Magnuson MA. Effects of alternate RNA splicing on glucokinase isoform activates in the pancreatic islet, liver and pituitary. J Biol Chem 1991;266:6999-7007.
220. Magnuson MA. Tissue-specific regulation of glucokinase gene expression. J Cell Biochem 1992; 48:115-121.
221. Vollenweider F, Irminger J-C, Gross DJ, Villa-Komaroff L, Halban PA. Processing of proinsulin by transfected hepatoma (FAO) cells. J Biol Chem 1992;267:14629-14636.
222. Simpson AM, Tuch BE, Swan MA, Tu J, Marshell GM. Functional expression of the human insulin gene in a human hepatoma cell line (HEP G2). Gene Ther 1995;2:223-231.
223. Kolodka TM, Finegold M, Moss L, Woo SLC. Gene therapy for diabetes mellitus in rats by hepatic expression of insulin. Proc Natl Acad Sci USA 1995;92:3293-3297.
224. Dhawan J, Pan LC, Pavlath GK, Travis MA, Lanctot AM, Blau HM. System delivery of human growth hormone by injection of genetically engineered myoblasts. Science 1991;254:1509-1512.
225. Barr E, and Leiden JM. System delivery of recombinant protein by genetically modified myoblasts. Science 1991;254:1507-1509.
226. Roman M, Axelrod JH, Dai Y, Naviaux RK, Friedmann T, and Verma IM. Circulating human or canine factor IX from retrovirally transduced primary myoblasts and established myoblast cell line grafted into murine skeletal muscle. Som Cell Mol Genet 1992;18:247-258.
227. Wolff JA, Malone RW, Williams P, et al. Direct gene transfer into mouse muscle in vivo. Science 1990;247:1465-1468.
228. Bartlett RJ, Secore SJ, Denis M, et al. Toward the biologic release of human insulin from skeletal muscle. Transplant Proc 1997;29:2199-2200.
229. Blume N, Petersen JS, Andersen LC, et al. Immature transformed rat islet beta-cells differentially express C-peptides from genes coding for I and II as well as a transfected human insulin gene. Mol Endocrinol 1992;6:299-307.
230. Clark SA, Quaade C, Constandy H, et al. Novel insulinoma cell lines produced by iterative engineering of GLUT, glucokinase, and human insulin expression. Diabetes 1997;46:958-967.
231. Hohmeier HE, Beltran del Rio H, Clark SA, Henkel-Rieger R, Normington F, Newgard CB. Regulation of insulin secretion from novel engineered insulinoma cell lines. Diabetes 1997;46:968-977.

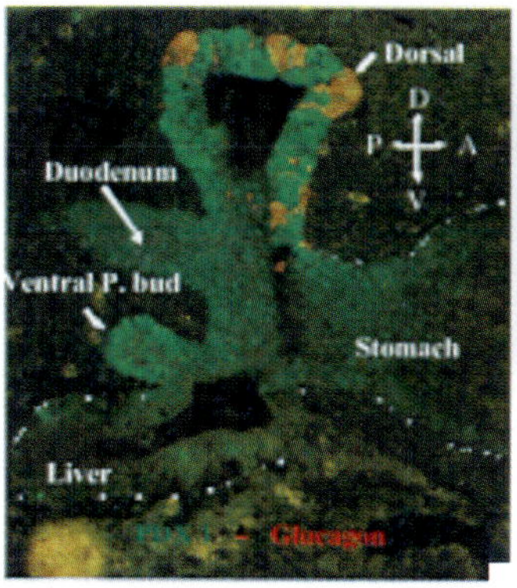

Madsen : Figure 3, page 9

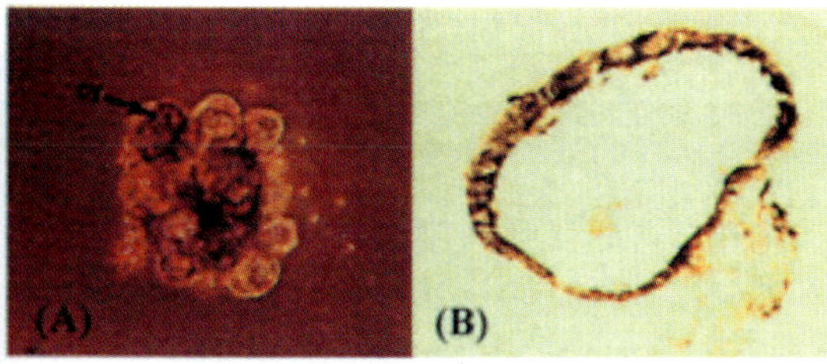

Maldonado : Figure 2, page 181

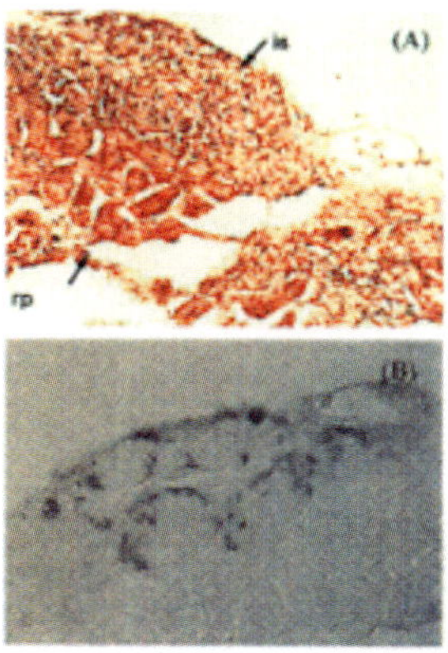

Maldonado : Figure 3, page 181

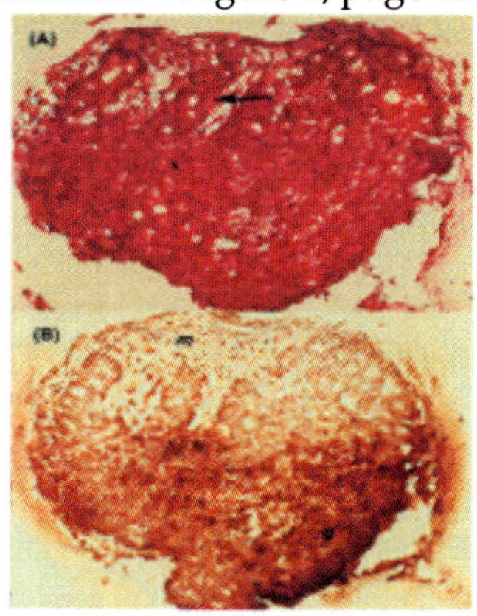

Maldonado : Figure 4, page 182

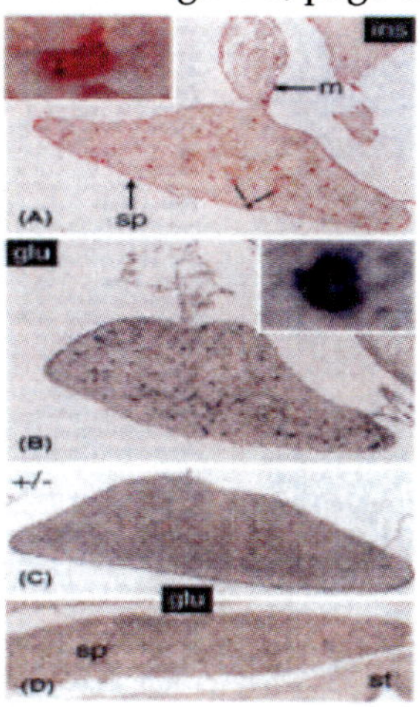

Maldonado : Figure 6, page 184

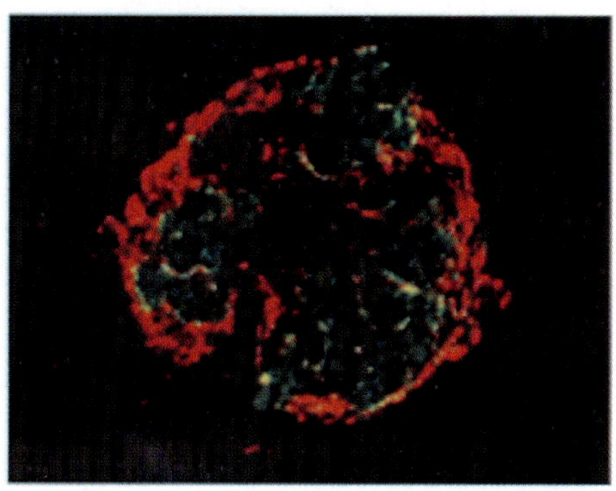

Maldonado : Figure 8, page 186

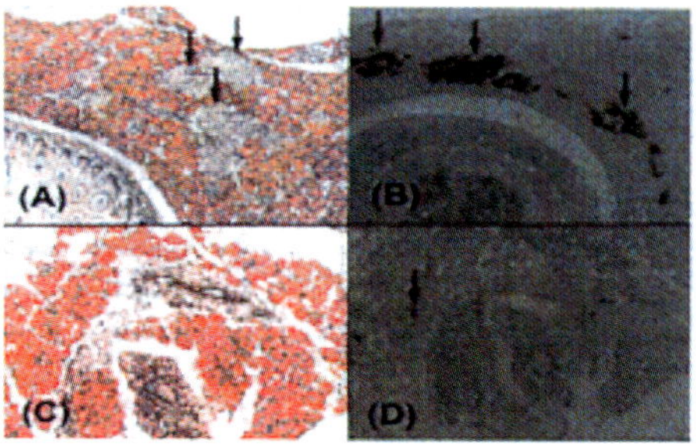

Maldonado : Figure 9, page 188

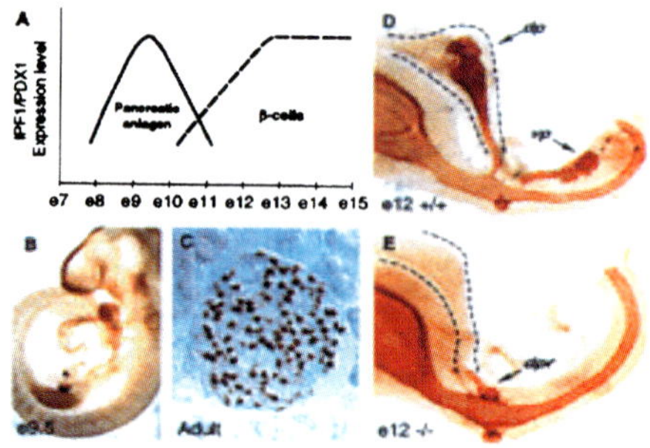

Ahlgren : Figure 2, page 201

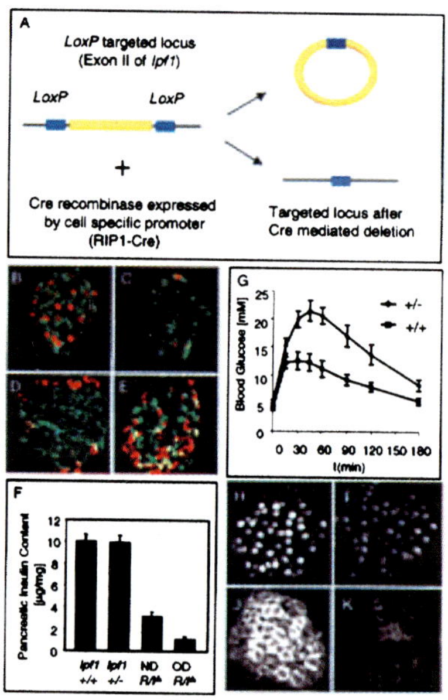

Ahlgren : Figure 3, page 202

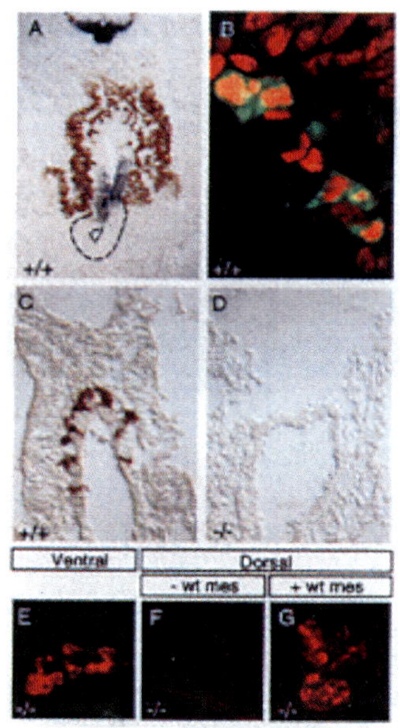

Ahlgren : Figure 4, page 206

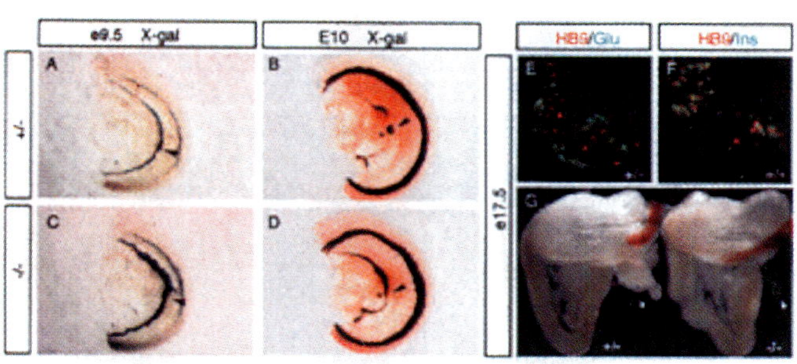

Ahlgren : Figure 5, page 207

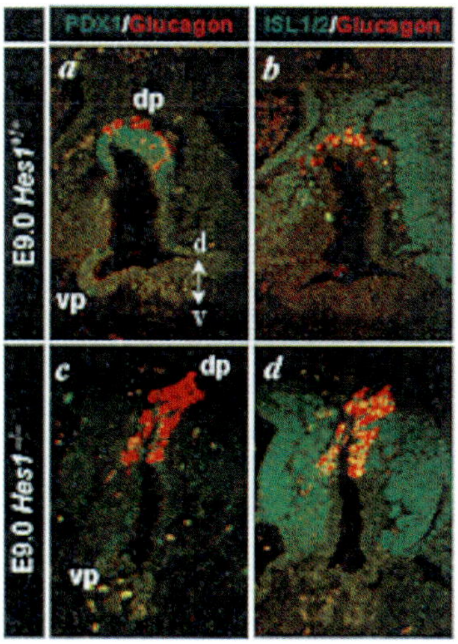

J ensen : Figure 1, page 219

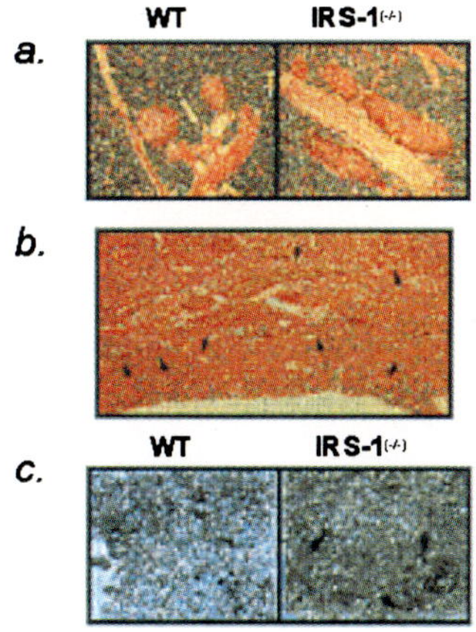

Kulkarni : Figure 2, page 303

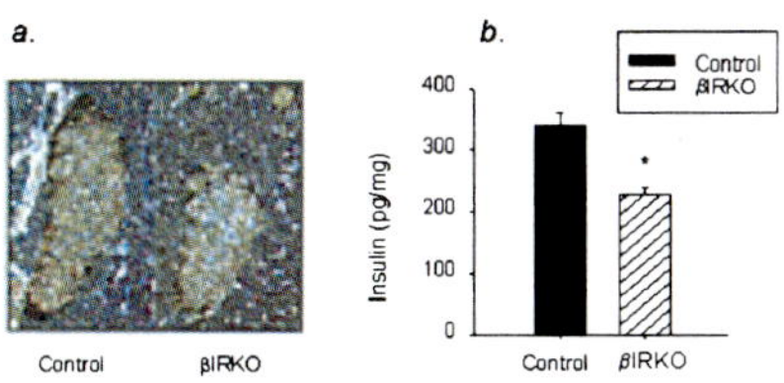

Kulkarni : Figure 8, Page 311

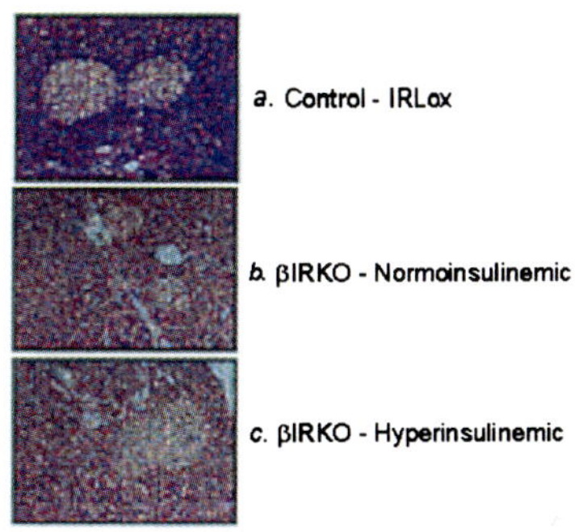

Kulkarni : Figure 9, page 312

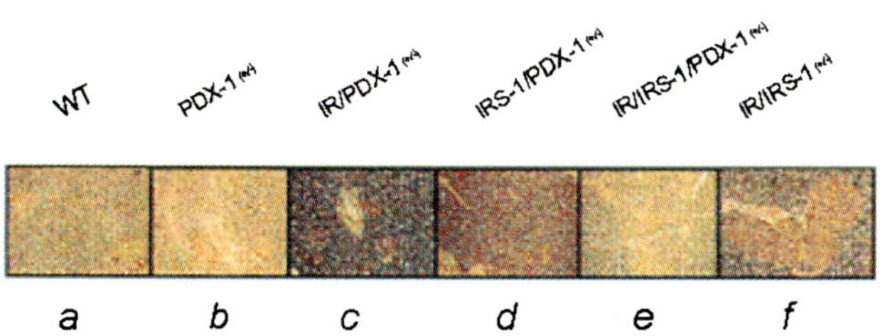

Kulkarni : Figure 11, page 316

A

B

C

D

J

K

L

M

N

O

Z